Schizophrenia Is a Misdiagnosis

C. Raymond Lake

Schizophrenia Is a Misdiagnosis

Implications for the DSM-5 and the ICD-11

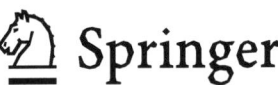

C. Raymond Lake, M.D., Ph.D.
Professor Emeritus
Department Psychiatry and Behavioral Sciences
University of Kansas, School of Medicine
Kansas City, KS 66160-7341, USA
craylake@hotmail.com

ISBN 978-1-4614-1869-6   e-ISBN 978-1-4614-1870-2
DOI 10.1007/978-1-4614-1870-2
Springer New York Dordrecht Heidelberg London

Library of Congress Control Number: 2011941582

© Springer Science+Business Media, LLC 2012
All rights reserved. This work may not be translated or copied in whole or in part without the written permission of the publisher (Springer Science+Business Media, LLC, 233 Spring Street, New York, NY 10013, USA), except for brief excerpts in connection with reviews or scholarly analysis. Use in connection with any form of information storage and retrieval, electronic adaptation, computer software, or by similar or dissimilar methodology now known or hereafter developed is forbidden.
The use in this publication of trade names, trademarks, service marks, and similar terms, even if they are not identified as such, is not to be taken as an expression of opinion as to whether or not they are subject to proprietary rights.
While the advice and information in this book are believed to be true and accurate at the date of going to press, neither the authors nor the editors nor the publisher can accept any legal responsibility for any errors or omissions that may be made. The publisher makes no warranty, express or implied, with respect to the material contained herein.

Printed on acid-free paper

Springer is part of Springer Science+Business Media (www.springer.com)

Preface

The mental health professions, the media and the public have accepted the diagnosis of schizophrenia as bona fide for over a century. Some have estimated that there are as many as two million patients with the diagnosis of schizophrenia. This book was written for diagnosing psychiatrists, mental health professionals and physicians, as well as patients diagnosed with schizophrenia and their families. It aims to provide information that will change their diagnosis and ensure their optimal treatment.

I began my research career in biological psychiatry at the NIMH, Bethesda, MD and published empirical papers on patients diagnosed with schizophrenia (Lake et al. 1980). At that time, there was little doubt in academic circles, nor did I doubt, that these patients who exhibited a certain constellation of psychotic symptoms should receive the diagnosis of schizophrenia. Subsequently, however, with increased clinical experience and familiarity with the comparative literature, I began to question the validity of the diagnosis of schizophrenia. Symptoms of mood disturbances were observed in psychotic patients diagnosed with schizophrenia, and I noted that some patients with "schizophrenia" improved with mood-stabilizing medications. This led me to the idea that many patients, initially diagnosed with schizophrenia, actually suffered from a psychotic mood disorder. A review of the descriptive historical and recent comparative scientific literature from patients diagnosed with bipolar disorder and with schizophrenia revealed, somewhat to my surprise, that others shared my opinion. Several recently published articles conclude there is only one disorder, a psychotic mood disorder, that accounts for the functional psychoses (Lake 2008a, b; Lake 2010a, b).

In this book, I have examined research data from a wide array of scientific disciplines as well as historical sources. The result of this investigation is my belief that at least two million patients have been misdiagnosed with schizophrenia. The question is not whether these patients suffer from a psychotic disorder; the vast majority do. The question is: Which psychotic disorder afflicts them? A correct diagnosis is mandatory for effective treatment. Without the correct diagnosis, patients receive substandard care and their prescribing physicians may be subject to malpractice claims. The purpose of this work is to improve the mental and emotional health of psychotic patients by discussing diagnostic strategies and appropriate treatments.

The book reviews the changing diagnostic concepts of schizophrenia and bipolar disorder within an historical perspective in order to clarify how the current conflict over diagnostic explanations for psychosis has arisen. The idea that two disorders, schizophrenia and bipolar, known as the Kraepelinian dichotomy, account for the functional psychoses has been a cornerstone of psychiatry for over 100 years, but this has recently been questioned because of substantial similarities and overlap between what for so long has been presumed to be two different disorders. One implication of the overlapping data is the question of whether to eliminate the diagnosis of schizophrenia from the psychiatric nomenclature.

Manic-depressive insanity or bipolar disorder has been consistently described in the literature for over 2,000 years. Its diagnostic criteria are disease-specific, validating bipolar disorder as a bona fide disease. Physicians through the centuries made clear that manic-depressive insanity included psychosis, chronicity of course and cycling episodes of mania and depression. It is only recently that some cases of bipolar disorder have been documented to involve deterioration through a chronic, non-cycling, persistently psychotic, treatment-resistant state. Well before the recognition of the possibility of such a chronic, non-cycling deterioration in bipolar patients, in the middle of the nineteenth century, several psychiatrists introduced a separate disease to account for such a condition of psychosis and chronicity. Critical to the establishment and maintenance of schizophrenia as a valid diagnosis has been the erroneous acceptance of two major conclusions: (1) schizophrenia is defined by chronicity and psychosis, i.e., hallucinations, delusions, disorganization and/or catatonia; (2) schizophrenia is separate from, more severe and more important than manic-depressive insanity, i.e., the Kraepelinian dichotomy. The most severe cases of manic-depressive insanity were, in retrospect, carved out and given a new name, schizophrenia. This new but redundant disease was then widely embraced, especially in the United States.

At least three famous psychiatrists initiated and promoted the concept of schizophrenia: Emil Kraepelin (1856–1926), Eugene Bleuler (1857–1939) and Kurt Schneider (1887–1967). All were prolific writers and lecturers and, as much or more than others, have influenced academic psychiatrists, mental health professionals, physicians, the press and the public with regard to schizophrenia. Because of the influence of their writings, each has been given a chapter in this book in which their most renowned publications have been extensively quoted in order to demonstrate how symptoms today considered diagnostic of a psychotic bipolar disorder were interpreted by them as diagnostic of schizophrenia. Thus, the early twentieth century concepts of schizophrenia that formed the foundation for current concepts of schizophrenia were flawed as they are explained by another disease, a psychotic mood disorder.

In 1933, Jacob Kasanin (1897–1946) published a now famous paper that introduced the diagnosis of schizoaffective disorder and that directly questioned the dogma that psychosis mandated a diagnosis of schizophrenia. He indirectly questioned the validity of the Kraepelinian dichotomy and schizophrenia itself. By the 1970s, several groups of psychiatrists provided support for Kasanin's position by reporting the presence of hallucinations, delusions, disorganization and catatonia in classic bipolar patients, thus discounting the specificity of the diagnostic criteria of schizophrenia. Specific diagnostic criteria are mandatory for a creditable psychiatric disease. Since the 1980s, basic and preclinical data began to steadily accumulate from laboratories around the world showing similarities and overlap between thousands of patients diagnosed with schizophrenia versus psychotic bipolar disorder. Persuasive data pointing to only one disease especially derive from the overlap recorded by comparative studies of molecular genetic and cognitive decline studies from these patients. There are also considerable data reported to be unique to either schizophrenia or bipolar disorder but if these were truly two separate diseases, there could not be such overlap. Such differences may be explained by differences between psychotic and non-psychotic mood-disordered patients. The psychotic mood-disordered patients can be misdiagnosed with schizophrenia. Currently there is a movement to return to the pre-1850s concept that severe, chronic and psychotic mood disorders can account for all of the criteria considered diagnostic of schizophrenia.

Four chapters in this book track the changing conceptualizations of the diagnosis of functionally psychotic patients from 100 BCE to the present. The impact of these conclusions, combined with the overlap and similarities in the diagnostic criteria in all of the editions of the DSM, is striking and leads to the question of how these two disorders can continue to be considered as separate entities.

The last three chapters in this book address respectively the extensive negative outcomes that can be a product of a diagnosis of schizophrenia, an explanation of how schizophrenia has survived as a clinical entity and finally what to do if you or a friend has a diagnosis of schizophrenia. The risk of murder, filicide and/or suicide is increased by a misdiagnosis of schizophrenia in psychotic bipolar or unipolar patients. Patients, families, friends, their psychiatrists and other mental health professionals are especially at an increased risk for violence.

The continuing acceptance of schizophrenia as a valid diagnosis is explained by a series of events discussed herein. These include the absence of any physical tests to rule in or out schizophrenia and a massive volume of research data published on schizophrenia. Patients and families are encouraged to use this book and to research the Internet for symptoms of a psychotic mood disorder, to question the diagnosis of schizophrenia and to seek a psychiatrist and treatment that emphasizes the first-line mood-stabilizing medications while minimizing the use of the antipsychotic drugs.

The DSM-5 proposes to eliminate the subtypes of schizophrenia. This revision, while welcome, does not go far enough. The elimination of the concept of the Kraepelinian dichotomy and the diagnoses of schizophrenia and schizoaffective disorder is necessary to achieve the proper standard of care for functionally psychotic patients. Ultimately such a change will hinge upon serious attention to the issues raised in this book by academic psychiatry. Such a discipline-altering change is warranted despite its radical nature.

Acknowledgments

The author thanks Anita Swisher; Sheryle Gallant, Ph.D., J.D.; Martha Breckenridge, Ph.D.; and Heather English, each of whom offered assistance and support that helped make the completion of this work possible. Especially critical were the efforts of Ms. Swisher.

About the Author

C. Ray Lake, M.D., Ph.D., is Professor Emeritus of Psychiatry at The University of Kansas, School of Medicine, Kansas City, KS.

Dr. Lake graduated from Tulane University, New Orleans, LA, in 1965. He received an MS in Insect Physiology, also from Tulane, in 1966. He graduated from Duke University, School of Medicine and Duke Graduate School (Department of Physiology and Pharmacology), Durham, NC, in 1971 and 1972. He studied at Oxford University and at St. Bartholomew's Hospital, London. His residency in Psychiatry was completed at Duke and at the National Institute of Mental Health (NIMH) Bethesda, MD. He remained at the NIMH, Laboratory of Clinical Sciences as a research associate and staff psychiatrist until 1979 when he moved across the pike to take a professorship of psychiatry and pharmacology at the new Uniformed Services University of the Health Sciences (USUHS), School of Medicine. He secured two RO1s continuing his research on the regulation of the sympathetic nervous system in health and in patients with neuropsychiatric and/or cardiovascular disorders.

In 1993, he accepted the chairmanship of Psychiatry at the University of Kansas, School of Medicine for 3 years after which he continued on the full-time faculty until his recent partial retirement. As Professor Emeritus, he continues to publish, teach students and residents about mood disorders, and follow his long-term patients. He has over 250 publications and has achieved life-fellowship status in the American Psychiatric Association and the American College of Neuropsychopharmacology. His current interests are the misdiagnosis of schizophrenia and a more effective strategy for teaching medical students about Psychiatry.

His wife has a Ph.D. in Psychology and was a member of the Clinical Psychology faculty at the University of Kansas for 10 years. She recently received her J.D. from Georgetown Law Center in Washington, DC. They have three wonderful children. Dr. Lake is competitive in tennis.

Contents

1 **Overview** 1
   1.1 Introduction 1
   1.2 The Impact of the Misdiagnosis of Schizophrenia 12
   1.3 Chapter Summaries 12
   1.4 Conclusions 19

2 **The Basic Data** 21
   2.1 Introduction 21
   2.2 Dementia, Insanity, and Psychosis 21
   2.3 The Types of Psychoses: Primary or Functional
       Versus Secondary or Organic 23
   2.4 Manic-Depressive Insanity and Bipolar Disorder 24
   2.5 Dementia Praecox and Schizophrenia 26
   2.6 The Controversy of the Kraepelinian Dichotomy
       Undermines the Diagnosis of Schizophrenia 30
   2.7 Conclusions 31

3 **A History of the Diagnoses of Psychotic Patients
Before 1950** 33
   3.1 Introduction 33
   3.2 A History of Manic Depressive Insanity or Bipolar
       Disorder Is Long and Consistent 38
   3.3 Early "Unitary" Hypotheses for the Psychoses
       (i.e., One Disorder Accounts for Bipolar Disorder
       and Schizophrenia) 41
   3.4 Dementia and Dementia Praecox (Schizophrenia) 48
   3.5 Dementia Praecox or Schizophrenia: Defined a Dichotomy
       with Manic-Depressive Insanity or Bipolar Disorder 49
   3.6 Kraepelin, Bleuler, Kasanin, and Schneider 53
   3.7 Conclusions 54

4 Psychiatric Disease and Diagnoses: The Scientific Basis for Establishing Validity ... 55
- 4.1 Introduction ... 55
- 4.2 Diagnostic Symptoms Must Be Unique and Consistent over Time ... 56
- 4.3 Patients with Such Unique Symptoms Must Have Other Consistent Findings ... 58
- 4.4 Conclusions ... 60

5 Emil Kraepelin (1856–1926) Established the Kraepelinian Dichotomy and Schizophrenia but Then Reneged ... 63
- 5.1 Introduction: A Dichotomy Meant Dementia Praecox/Schizophrenia Is a Real Disease ... 63
- 5.2 Selected Quotes from *Dementia Praecox and Paraphrenia*, by E. Kraepelin 1919/2002 ... 70
- 5.3 Selected Quotes from *Manic-Depressive Insanity and Paranoia*, by E. Kraepelin 1921/1976 ... 85
- 5.4 Kraepelin's Reversal of the Dichotomy: Implications for a Single Disease ... 90
- 5.5 Conclusions ... 90

6 Eugen Bleuler (1857–1939) Named and Dedicated Himself to Schizophrenia ... 93
- 6.1 Introduction ... 93
- 6.2 Bleuler's Fundamental Symptoms of Schizophrenia (1911/1950); Not Pathognomonic, Capture Eccentrics and Normals, and Suggest a Bipolar Disorder ... 95
- 6.3 Selected Quotes from Bleuler's Textbook, *Dementia Praecox or the Group of the Schizophrenias* (1911/1950) ... 101
- 6.4 Bleuler's Accessory Symptoms: Hallucinations and Delusions Embraced as Diagnostic of Schizophrenia ... 110
- 6.5 Functional Psychosis Does Not Equal Schizophrenia ... 120
- 6.6 Conclusions ... 120

7 Jacob Kasanin (1897–1946) and Schizoaffective Disorder ... 123
- 7.1 Introduction ... 123
- 7.2 Schizoaffective Disorder Contradicts the Concepts of Kraepelin and Bleuler About Schizophrenia ... 124
- 7.3 Schizoaffective Disorder Merges Schizophrenia and Psychotic Mood Disorders ... 125
- 7.4 Examples of Psychotic Mood Symptoms from Kasanin's Cases ... 126
- 7.5 Schizoaffective Disorder Ignored for 30 Years But Then Flourished ... 127
- 7.6 Schizoaffective Disorder Is a Compromise Diagnosis ... 132
- 7.7 Flawed Diagnostic Criteria for Schizoaffective Disorder ... 132
- 7.8 Conclusions ... 135

8	**Kurt Schneider (1887–1967): First- and Second-Rank Symptoms, Not Pathognomonic of Schizophrenia, Explained by Psychotic Mood Disorders**	137
	8.1 Introduction	137
	8.2 Selected Quotes From Schneider's Textbook *Clinical Psychopathology* (1959); Bleuler's Concept Reinforced: Psychosis Means Schizophrenia	139
	8.3 Schneider's First- and Second-Rank Symptoms of Schizophrenia Reflect Obsolescence but Remain in the DSM and ICD	143
	8.4 Conclusions	149
9	**Concepts of Schizophrenia and Bipolar Disorder in the 1950s and 1960s**	151
	9.1 Introduction	151
	9.2 The Effectiveness of New "Antipsychotic/Antischizophrenia" Medications in the 1950s Increased the Acceptance of Schizophrenia as a Bona Fide Disease	153
	9.3 Electroconvulsive Therapy (ECT) Initially Used to Treat Schizophrenia	155
	9.4 The National Institute of Mental Health (NIMH) and the Pharmaceutical Industry Focused on Schizophrenia Rather Than Mood Disorders	156
	9.5 The Use of Lithium in Bipolar Patients Was Delayed in the USA	157
	9.6 Discrepancies in Diagnostic Comparisons Between the USA and the UK	157
	9.7 Overlap of Diagnostic Symptoms Between Schizophrenia and Psychotic Mood Disorders from the Diagnostic and Statistical Manual for Mental Disorders-I (DSM-I) and the DSM-II	159
	9.7.1 The DSM-I (APA, DSM 1952)	160
	9.7.2 The DSM-II (APA, DSM 1968)	164
	9.8 The Timing of Schneider's Book (1959) Supported Schizophrenia	166
	9.9 Conclusions	166
10	**Changing Concepts in the 1970s and 1980s: The Overlap of Symptoms and Course Between Schizophrenia and Psychotic Mood Disorders**	167
	10.1 Introduction	167
	10.2 Symptoms and Course of Schizophrenia Observed in Severe Bipolar Patients: The Early Reports	168
	10.3 Thomas S. Szasz	178
	10.4 Harrison G. Pope and Joseph F. Lipinski	179
	10.5 I.F. Brockington	179

	10.6	Martin Harrow, Linda Grossman, Marshall Silverstein, Jay Himmelhoch, and Herbert Meltzer	180
	10.7	Reports from the NIMH	180
	10.8	Richard P. Bentall	181
	10.9	An Introduction to the Continuum Concept	181
	10.10	Overlap and Similarities Between Schizophrenia and Mood Disorders from the DSM-III (APA, DSM 1980) and the DSM-III-R (APA, DSM 1987)	182
		10.10.1 The DSM-III (APA, DSM 1980)	182
		10.10.2 The DSM-III-R (APA, DSM 1987)	184
	10.11	Conclusions	184
11	**Changing Concepts in the 1990s, 2000s, and 2010s: More Overlap and Similarities**		**187**
	11.1	Introduction	187
	11.2	Additional Reviews of Clinical Overlap and Similarities	197
	11.3	Overlap and Similarities from Basic Science and Preclinical Studies Comparing Schizophrenia and Mood Disorders	197
		11.3.1 Brain Metabolic and Neurochemical Studies	200
		11.3.2 Brain Imagining Studies	200
		11.3.3 Epidemiological Studies	202
		11.3.4 Psychopharmacological Studies	204
		11.3.5 Family and Heritability Studies	208
		11.3.6 Molecular Genetic Studies	211
		11.3.7 Neurocognitive, Selective Attention, and Insight Studies	220
	11.4	Overlap and Similarities Between Schizophrenia and Mood Disorders in the DSM from the DSM-IV (APA, DSM 1994) Through the DSM-5 (APA, DSM Proposed 2013)	224
		11.4.1 The DSM-IV (APA, DSM 1994)	224
		11.4.2 The DSM-IV-TR (APA, DSM 2000)	226
		11.4.3 The DSM-5 (APA, DSM Proposed 2013)	227
	11.5	Psychotic Depression Accounts for Many Patients Diagnosed with Schizophrenia	228
	11.6	C.M. Swartz and E. Shorter (2007)	230
	11.7	The Development and Implications of the Continuum Concept	230
	11.8	Conclusions	236
12	**The Subtypes and the Positive and Negative Diagnostic Symptoms of Schizophrenia Are Explained by Psychotic Mood Disorders**		**241**
	12.1	Introduction: The Subtypes Are the Same as the Diagnostic Criteria	241
	12.2	Catatonic Subtype	245

	12.3	Disorganized Subtype	248
	12.4	Paranoid Subtype, i.e., Hallucinations and Delusions: Paranoia Hides the Grandiosity and Guilt of Psychotic Mood Disorders	248
	12.5	Case Summaries of Psychotic Mood Disorders Misdiagnosed as Schizophrenia, Paranoid Subtype	250
	12.6	Paranoid Schizophrenia Is a Psychotic Mood Disorder	260
	12.7	Undifferentiated Subtype	262
	12.8	The Positive and Negative Symptoms of Schizophrenia	262
		12.8.1 The Positive Symptoms	263
		12.8.2 The Negative Symptoms	264
	12.9	Conclusions	267
13	**Psychotic Mood Disorders Are Disorders of Thought and of Mood**		271
	13.1	Introduction	271
	13.2	Selective Attention: The Brain's Filter-Prioritizer Mechanism	272
	13.3	Defective Selective Attention Is Epitomized by Manic Distractibility	274
	13.4	Student Case Conference: Schizophrenia Explained by Mania	275
	13.5	Conclusions	279
14	**Medical and Other Psychiatric Conditions Potentially Misdiagnosed as Schizophrenia**		281
	14.1	Introduction	281
	14.2	Medical and Surgical Causes of Psychosis	282
		14.2.1 Autoimmune Disorders	282
		14.2.2 Chromosomal Abnormalities	282
		14.2.3 Chronic Traumatic Encephalopathy (History of Head Trauma)	284
		14.2.4 Dementias and Delirium	285
		14.2.5 Demyelinating Diseases	285
		14.2.6 Electrolyte and Fluid Imbalance	285
		14.2.7 Endocrinopathies	285
		14.2.8 Epilepsy	286
		14.2.9 Hydrocephalus	286
		14.2.10 Infections	286
		14.2.11 Metabolic Diseases	287
		14.2.12 Narcolepsy	287
		14.2.13 Neuropsychiatric Diseases	287
		14.2.14 Nutritional Deficiencies	288
		14.2.15 Space-Occupying Lesions and Structural Brain Abnormalities	288
		14.2.16 Stroke	288

	14.3	Substances That Can Cause Psychosis...	289
	14.4	Tardive Psychosis Possibly Caused by Antipsychotic/"Antischizophrenia" Medications and Misdiagnosed as Schizophrenia...	290
	14.5	Obsessive-Compulsive Disorder and "Hallucinations and/or Delusions" in Normals Can Be Misdiagnosed as Schizophrenia	292
	14.6	Conclusions..	295
15	**The Negative Impact of the Misdiagnosis of Schizophrenia upon Patients, Their Families, and Their Caretakers**		297
	15.1	Introduction..	297
	15.2	The Absence of Mood-Stabilizing Medications due to Misdiagnoses of Schizophrenia Allows Recurrent Mood Disorders to Worsen	299
	15.3	Higher Dosages of Antipsychotic/"Antischizophrenia" Medications Are Given to Patients Diagnosed with Schizophrenia and for Longer Periods of Time	301
	15.4	The Stigma of Schizophrenia..	308
	15.5	Risk for Violence, Suicide, Homicide, and Filicide Is Increased in Psychotic Mood Disorders Misdiagnosed with Schizophrenia...	310
	15.6	The Negative Impact of the Misdiagnosis of Major Depressive Disorder or Postpartum Depression in Patients Who Have Bipolar Disorder, Depressed......................................	348
	15.7	Conclusions..	351
16	**How Has Schizophrenia Survived?**		353
	16.1	Introduction..	353
	16.2	The Overemphasis on Hallucinations and Delusions by Academic Psychiatry...	356
	16.3	Media Examples of the Endorsement of Schizophrenia...............	358
	16.4	The Neuroses Became Obsolete in 1980 with the DSM-III: Why Not Schizophrenia?	364
	16.5	The DSM and the ICD Perpetuate Schizophrenia and the Dichotomy..	365
	16.6	The Pharmaceutical Profit Motive Promotes Schizophrenia..	365
	16.7	Conclusions..	367
17	**What to Do if You, a Family Member, or Friend Is Diagnosed with Schizophrenia or Suffers with Psychotic Symptoms**...		371
	17.1	Introduction..	371
	17.2	How Do You Tell If There Is a Severe Psychiatric Problem?	374

	17.3	Journal Daily Symptoms, Dates, History, and Family History	374
	17.4	Learn About the Disorders: Study Diagnostic Symptoms and Compare to Your Symptoms	376
	17.5	Preparation for Seeing a Doctor/Psychiatrist	378
	17.6	Treatment Plans for Major Mood Disorders	379
		17.6.1 Major Depressive Disorder	380
		17.6.2 Bipolar Disorders	384
		17.6.3 Psychotherapy	386
	17.7	Conclusions	387
18	**Vision for the Future: Conclusions and Solutions**		**389**
	18.1	Introduction	389
	18.2	The Failure to Recognize Depression and the Risk for Suicide in Nonpsychiatric Clinical Settings	390
	18.3	The Responsibility of Academic Psychiatry for Improving the Recognition of Mood Disorders in Nonpsychiatric Clinical Settings	392
	18.4	Simplify and Consolidate the Functional Psychoses for DSM-5 and/or DSM-6	393
	18.5	Potential Judicial Sources for Change to Psychiatric Diagnostics	395
	18.6	Conclusions	396
References			**397**
Index			**419**

List of Tables

Chapter 1
Table 1.1 Selected quotes from reviews and books in support of no dichotomy 3
Table 1.2 Kraepelin, Bleuler, Kasanin, and Schneider: what they are remembered for and what they actually said 14

Chapter 2
Table 2.1 DSM-IV-TR psychoses due to secondary/organic causes versus the primary/functional psychoses 23
Table 2.2 Types of mood disorders 25
Table 2.3 DSM-IV-TR diagnostic criteria for mania or bipolar disorder 25
Table 2.4 DSM-IV-TR specifiers and features for mood disorders 25
Table 2.5 DSM-IV-TR diagnostic criteria for schizophrenia 28
Table 2.6 Definition and symptom overlap of psychotic mood disorders and schizophrenia from current sources 29
Table 2.7 The Kraepelinian dichotomy; two disorders explain severe mental illness 30

Chapter 3
Table 3.1 Bipolar disorder has a long and consistent history 35
Table 3.2 Historical links of paranoia with mood disorders not schizophrenia 39
Table 3.3 A history of the unitary or one disease hypothesis for the functional psychoses 43
Table 3.4 DSM-IV-TR subtypes of schizophrenia defined 51
Table 3.5 Diagnoses of 236 consecutive admissions with functional psychoses (hallucinations and/or delusions) 54

Chapter 4
Table 4.1 Concordance of monozygotic (MZ) and dizygotic (DZ) twins in the mood disorders 58
Table 4.2 Genetic loci associated with psychotic and nonpsychotic bipolar disorders (and schizophrenia) 59

Table 4.3	Characteristics initially attributed to schizophrenia are accounted for by psychotic mood disorders	59

Chapter 5

Table 5.1	A selection of publications of E. Kraepelin translated to English	64
Table 5.2	Selected quotes of symptoms Kraepelin assigned to schizophrenia that are diagnostic of mania and depression (Kraepelin 1919)	66
Table 5.3	Overlap of signs and symptoms between schizophrenia and psychotic mood disorders from two of Kraepelin's books	71

Chapter 6

Table 6.1	Bleuler's "pathognomonic" fundamental and accessory symptoms for schizophrenia	94
Table 6.2	Selected quotes from *Dementia Praecox or the Group of Schizophrenias* (E. Bleuler 1911/1950) raise questions as to the validity of schizophrenia	96
Table 6.3	Bleuler's subtypes of schizophrenia	100
Table 6.4	Additional characteristics Bleuler and others associated with schizophrenia	101
Table 6.5	Selected quotes from *Dementia Praecox or the Group of Schizophrenias* attributed to schizophrenia but diagnostic of a psychotic mood disorder	107

Chapter 7

Table 7.1	DSM-IV-TR diagnostic criteria for schizoaffective disorder	125
Table 7.2	PubMed literature cites of schizoaffective disorder	128
Table 7.3	Selected quotes discounting the validity of schizoaffective disorder: schizoaffective disorder is a psychotic mood disorder; there is no schizoaffective disorder	130

Chapter 8

Table 8.1	K. Schneider's "pathognomonic" first- and second-rank symptoms of schizophrenia	138
Table 8.2	Schneider's dichotomy	139
Table 8.3	Relevant quotes from *Clinical Psychopathology* (K. Schneider 1959)	140

Chapter 9

Table 9.1	Events in the 1950s and 1960s that promoted schizophrenia and demoted bipolar disorders	152
Table 9.2	PubMed literature cites of schizophrenia/schizophrenic	156
Table 9.3	DSM-I (APA, DSM 1952) classifications of the primary/functional psychotic reactions	162

| Table 9.4 | DSM-II (APA, DSM 1968): The neuroses and the psychoses not attributed to physical conditions listed previously | 165 |

Chapter 10

| Table 10.1 | Selected quotes showing overlap and similarity of symptoms and course between schizophrenia and psychotic mood disorders from the 1970s and 1980s and before | 169 |
| Table 10.2 | Classical and "atypical" symptoms in 20 manic patients | 177 |

Chapter 11

Table 11.1	Summary of areas of overlap between schizophrenia and mood disorders	188
Table 11.2	Selected quotes from clinical studies showing overlap of signs and symptoms comparing schizophrenia and psychotic mood disorders from the 1990s and 2000s	189
Table 11.3	Selected brain metabolic and neurochemical studies comparing schizophrenia and psychotic mood disorders	198
Table 11.4	Selected brain imagining studies comparing schizophrenia and psychotic mood disorders	201
Table 11.5	Selected epidemiological studies comparing schizophrenia and psychotic mood disorders	203
Table 11.6	Selected psychopharmacological studies comparing schizophrenia and psychotic mood disorders	206
Table 11.7	Selected heritability and family studies comparing schizophrenia and psychotic mood disorders	209
Table 11.8	Selected molecular genetic studies comparing schizophrenia and psychotic mood disorders	214
Table 11.9	Selected cognitive function, selective attention, and insight studies comparing schizophrenia and psychotic mood disorders	221
Table 11.10	Overlap and similarities in the DSM-IV-TR (2000) diagnostic criteria between schizophrenia and psychotic mood disorders	225
Table 11.11	Proposed for DSM-5 (2013): the subtypes eliminated as subtypes but retained as diagnostic criteria	226
Table 11.12	Proposed for DSM-5: nine dimensions of "schizophrenia" are more applicable to psychotic mood disorders	228
Table 11.13	Selected quotes supporting the continuum theory of a single disease encompassing schizophrenia and mood disorders	231
Table 11.14	Differences between schizophrenia and psychotic mood disorders resolved by one disorder	237

Chapter 12

| Table 12.1 | Changes and lack thereof of the subtypes and the positive and negative diagnostic symptoms of schizophrenia from the DSM-IV-TR to the DSM-5 (proposed) | 242 |

Table 12.2	Redundant descriptions of catatonia from the DSM-IV-TR chapters on schizophrenia versus the mood disorders	246
Table 12.3	Selected quotes discounting the validity of catatonia as diagnostic or even characteristic of schizophrenia	247
Table 12.4	Case summaries of psychotic mood disorders misdiagnosed as schizophrenia	257
Table 12.5	Symptoms indicating a psychotic mood disorder not schizophrenia in functionally psychotic patients	260
Table 12.6	Sources of paranoid delusional threats that suggest grandiosity of mania	261
Table 12.7	Take home messages for the diagnosis of psychotic patients	262
Table 12.8	A history of the negative symptoms of schizophrenia from Bleuler's accessory symptoms to the DSM-5	265
Table 12.9	The subtypes of schizophrenia explained by mood disorders; are a prerequisite for schizophrenia's existence	267
Table 12.10	Suggested initial screening questions for psychotic or paranoid patients (or their significant others)	268

Chapter 13

Table 13.1	Symptoms of disordered thought and speech traditionally indicative of schizophrenia or mania	272
Table 13.2	Psychotic mood disorders are disorders of mood and disorders of thought	279

Chapter 14

Table 14.1	Medical disorders with potential psychotic presentations	283
Table 14.2	Substances that can cause psychoses	289
Table 14.3	Suggested medical work-up for the rule out of secondary/organic psychoses	295

Chapter 15

Table 15.1	Department of Justice National Crime Victimization Survey for 1993-1999; Annual rate for nonfatal violet crime	298
Table 15.2	First-line mood-stabilizing medications	299
Table 15.3	Adverse effects of the first-line mood-stabilizing medications	300
Table 15.4	Antipsychotic/antischizophrenia medications; typical vs atypical	302
Table 15.5	Adverse effects of antipsychotic/antischizophrenia medications	304
Table 15.6	Movement disorders caused by the antipsychotic/antischizophrenia medications	305

Table 15.7	Violence, homicide, and suicide committed by patients misdiagnosed with schizophrenia	312
Table 15.8	Epidemiology of psychotic murderers and their victims	334
Table 15.9	Risk for filicide is increased in psychotic bipolar disordered patients misdiagnosed with schizophrenia, major depressive disorder, or postpartum depression	340

Chapter 16

Table 16.1	Factors prolonging the recognition of schizophrenia as valid	354
Table 16.2	Core beliefs of E. Kraepelin, E. Bleuler, and K. Schneider promoted schizophrenia	357
Table 16.3	Media emphasis on schizophrenia	361

Chapter 17

Table 17.1	Outline of what to do if you or a significant other has a diagnosis of schizophrenia	372
Table 17.2	Differentiating a bipolar disorder in a depression from a major depressive disorder	378
Table 17.3	Differentiating a bipolar disorder from the diagnosis of schizophreniaa	378
Table 17.4	Second-generation antidepressive medications	381

Chapter 18

Table 18.1	Suggested changes for the DSM-5 and/or the DSM-6	394
Table 18.2	Proposed additions to the DSM specifiers for mood disorders	395

List of Figures

Chapter 3
Fig. 3.1 Changing diagnostic concepts of the psychoses from 19th century (a) to 1933 (b) to 1986 (c) to current (d)......... 42
Fig. 3.2 Hypothesized history of diagnoses for the functional psychoses 50

Chapter 4
Fig. 4.1 Relationship between mean cycle length and episode number in recurrent mood disorders.. 57

Chapter 7
Fig. 7.1 PubMed literature cites of schizoaffective disorder 129

Chapter 9
Fig. 9.1 PubMed literature cites of schizophrenia/schizophrenic 153

Chapter 11
Fig. 11.1 Bipolar responsivity to lithium and antipsychotics along two axes 204
Fig. 11.2 Estimated diagnoses of functionally psychotic patients over 2000 years.. 212
Fig. 11.3 Continuum/dimensional concept explained by mood disorders: the original versus the current concept 236

Chapter 12
Fig. 12.1 Estimated diagnostic weight given to the positive and the negative symptoms and chronic course for the diagnosis of schizophrenia over time................................ 244
Fig. 12.2 Paranoia hides guilt and grandiosity: Psychotic mood disorders cause paranoid delusions... 249
Fig. 12.3 PubMed cites of the negative symptoms of schizophrenia........... 266

Chapter 13
Fig. 13.1 Psychotic mood disorders are disorders of thought: euthymia 273
Fig. 13.2 Psychotic mood disorders are disorders of thought: mania 277
Fig. 13.3 Psychotic mood disorders are disorders of thought: depression... 278

Chapter 16
Fig. 16.1 Feedback loop enhancing the promotion of the concept of schizophrenia. 355
Fig. 16.2 Schizophrenia: a covered wagon 368

Chapter 17
Fig. 17.1 Get the diagnosis right 373
Fig. 17.2 Daily mood, energy level, and sleep flow sheet for recurrent mood-disordered patients 375
Fig. 17.3 Medication treatment plan for unipolar depression (major depressive disorder, MDD). 382
Fig. 17.4 Medication treatment plan for bipolar disorder, manic or depressed.. 385

Chapter 1
Overview

> It must be assumed that these diseases [schizophrenia and affective illnesses] are genetically related. ... that the psychoses represent a continuum of variation at a single genetic locus.
>
> (Crow 1990a)
>
> There is a whole concept of major psychiatric illness as a single disease process, suggesting that schizophrenia might be the chronic untreated form of psychotic depression and of psychotic mixed manic-depressive states.
>
> (Swartz and Shorter 2007, pp. 19)

1.1 Introduction

In 1976, Professor Tom Szasz, a noted psychiatrist, published a controversial, if not heretical, article in the *British Journal of Psychiatry* in which he said, "There is, in short, no such thing as schizophrenia." In 1976, the current author was a resident in psychiatry and was appalled at Szasz's ideas because the esteemed professors at Duke thoroughly embraced the validity of schizophrenia and so, at that time, did this author. The curriculum, governed by the teachings of Kraepelin, Bleuler, and Schneider, fully accepted the Kraepelinian dichotomy, that is, the idea that schizophrenia is a disease distinct from mood disorders. Schizophrenia was taught as the "disorder of thought," while the affective or mood disorders were "disorders of the emotions," and there was no overlap. Schizophrenia was to be diagnosed in the presence of primary or functional psychosis and/or chronic dysfunctionality regardless of the presence of mood symptoms. Considerably more diagnostic weight was placed on psychotic than mood symptoms. While initially a strong proponent of schizophrenia and the Kraepelinian dichotomy for some 15 years between medical school and a fellowship, as this author coauthored a paper based on results from patients diagnosed with schizophrenia, there are now doubts about the validity of the diagnoses of schizophrenia in the patients from the 1980 publication (Lake et al. 1980).

Through subsequent decades, this author's experiences with psychotic patients and an examination of an emerging comparative literature led to doubt about a clear zone of rarity between patients diagnosed with schizophrenia and those with psychotic mood disorders. This author has never doubted that there are functionally psychotic patients who have a brain disease that warrants treatment, in contrast to what Dr. Szasz may have believed, that is, that "schizophrenia" fell within the normal spectrum.

In about 2000, one of this author's students discussed the 1978 paper by Pope and Lipinski from the *Archives of General Psychiatry*, and this article led to the review of several other publications that also appeared to question the prevalence and indirectly the validity of the Kraepelinian dichotomy and of schizophrenia (Table 1.1). These ideas were based on the presence of psychosis and chronicity of course in cases of severe mood disorders. Observations of acutely psychotic, manic, and depressed patients coupled with long-term follow-up of classic bipolar patients have revealed that the diagnostic criteria for schizophrenia from the Diagnostic and Statistical Manual (DSM) and The International Statistical Classification of Diseases and Related Health Problems (ICD) are not disease specific and can be accounted for by psychotic mood disorders.

Table 1.1 presents selected quotes from over 40 reviews or editorials beginning in 1905 but primarily from the 1970s to the present, most that express doubt as to meaningful differences between patients diagnosed with schizophrenia and psychotic mood disorders. For example, in 1905, the German psychiatrist, Professor G. Specht, believed that all primary/functional psychoses were due to disturbances in mood. He wrote that mania commonly developed a chronic course with no return to premorbid function; 6 years later, Bleuler said the same but about schizophrenia, not mania. Specht said that chronic mania was associated with paranoid delusions, "… judgment derailment born directly from passion and rage," manic incoherence, and deterioration to dementia paranoides (Specht 1905). These are characteristics specifically attributed to schizophrenia by Kraepelin, Bleuler, and later Schneider, and these views held sway over those of Specht for much of the twentieth century. Beginning in the 1970s, some psychiatrists resurrected the ideas of Specht questioning clinical differences between patients diagnosed with schizophrenia versus psychotic mood disorders.

For example, Kendell and Gourlay in 1970 said that schizophrenia and the affective psychoses were essentially indistinguishable (Table 1.1, quote 40). Ollerenshaw (1973) said that "… the schizophrenic syndrome is a nonspecific clinical entity…." Pope and Lipinski (1978) voiced their concern about the "overdiagnosis of schizophrenia and underdiagnosis of bipolar disorder." They stated that there are no valid diagnostic symptoms for schizophrenia bringing into question, "… all research that uses them [the DSM diagnostic criteria for schizophrenia] as the primary method of diagnosis." Brockington et al. (1980b) acknowledged that schizophrenia and mania had "… a number of properties in common…." (Table 1.1, quote #35) Yet, in response to such data, there has been minimal change in the DSM since 1980 with regard to the diagnostic criteria of schizophrenia.

In contrast to the DSM diagnostic criteria for schizophrenia (2000), the diagnostic criteria for classic bipolar disorder are disease specific with recurring cycles of mania and depression. Accurate diagnoses of such patients are made with a high degree of confidence. Historically, descriptions of cycles of mania and depression in the same

1.1 Introduction

Table 1.1 Selected quotes from reviews and books in support of no dichotomy

Quote no.	Journal (year)	Author(s)	Field of study	Selected quotes of summary/conclusions	Results
1	*Schiz Bull* (2008a)	Lake	Review	"Comparative clinical and recent molecular genetic data find phenotypic and genotypic commonalities lending support to the idea that paranoid schizophrenia is the same disorder as psychotic bipolar. Mania explains paranoia when grandiose delusions that one's possession are so valuable that others will kill for them. Similarly, depression explains paranoia when delusional guilt convinces patients they deserve punishment."	Paranoid schizophrenia same as psychotic mood disorder
2	*Schiz Bull* (2008b)	Lake	Review	"The zone of rarity between schizophrenia and psychotic mood disorders is blurred because severe disorders of mood are also disorders of thought. This relationship calls into question the tenet that schizophrenia is a disease separate from psychotic mood disorders."	Schizophrenia is a psychotic mood disorder
3	*Psychotic Depress* (Cambridge University Press) (2007)	Swartz and Shorter	Book	"There is a whole concept of major psychiatric illness as a single disease process, suggesting that schizophrenia might be the chronic untreated form of psychotic depression and of psychotic mixed manic-depressive states" (pp. 19).	Schizophrenia is psychotic depression
4	*AJP* (2007)	Crow	Review (molecular genetics)	"Epigenetic variation associated with chromosomal rearrangements that occurred in the hominid lineage and that relates to the evolution of language could account for predisposition to SZ and SAD and BP and failure to detect such variation by standard linkage approaches."	Continuum; schizophrenia and psychotic mood disorder similar/overlap
5	*Manic-Depressive Illn* (2007)	Goodwin and Jamison	Book	"It can be seen in Table 2-7 that delusions were present in 12-66% of bipolar depressive episodes and in 44-96% of manic episodes."	Schizophrenia and psychotic mood disorder similar/overlap

(continued)

Table 1.1 (continued)

Quote no.	Journal (year)	Author(s)	Field of study	Selected quotes of summary/conclusions	Results
6	Curr Opin Psychiatry (2007b)	Lake and Hurwitz	Review	"The concept of schizoaffective disorder promoted the coalescence of schizophrenia and bipolar eroding the Kraepelinian Dichotomy. A wide array of comparative data showing similarities and overlap led to the prediction of an end to the Kraepelinian Dichotomy, inviting the conclusion that a single disease [mood disorders] explains all the functional psychoses."	Schizophrenia and psychotic mood disorder similar/same
7	Curr Psychiatry (2006a)	Lake and Hurwitz	Review	"Three disorders – schizophrenia, schizoaffective disorder and psychotic bipolar disorder – have been evoked to account for the variance in severity in psychotic patients, but psychotic bipolar disorder expresses the entire spectrum."	Schizophrenia and psychotic mood disorder similar/same
8	Psychiatry Res (2006b)	Lake and Hurwitz	Review	"We conclude that the data overall are compatible with the hypothesis that a single disease, a mood disorder, with a broad spectrum of severity, rather than three different disorders, accounts for the functional psychoses."	Schizophrenia and psychotic mood disorder similar
9	AJP (2006)	Fink and Taylor	Editorial	"Catatonia is more frequently associated with mania, melancholia, and psychotic depression than it is with schizophrenia."	Schizophrenia and psychotic mood disorder similar
10	Acta Psychiatr Scand (2006)	Maier	Editorial	"Taken together, there is growing evidence that a substantial proportion of etiological factors is shared between schizophrenia and bipolar disorder…. In summary, the historical starting point of the concept of schizoaffective disorders is not valid anymore…. The task forces for new versions of the DSM-and ICD-diagnostic systems and manuals… would be badly advised if they would just continue the historical and current concepts of schizoaffective disorders into the future."	Schizophrenia, schizoaffective disorder, and psychotic mood disorder similar/ overlap; schizoaffective disorder invalid

1.1 Introduction

11	*Curr Opin Psychiatry* (2006)	Maier et al.	Review	"... the validity of the diagnostic distinction between schizophrenia and bipolar disorder is increasingly challenged.... The diagnostic split between schizophrenia and bipolar disorder is unable to define distinct etiological and/or pathophysiological entities."	Schizophrenia and psychotic mood disorder similar/overlap
12	*BJP* (2005)	Craddock and Owen	Editorial (molecular genetics)	"The beginning of the end for the Kraepelinian dichotomy." [article title] "Now molecular genetic studies are beginning to challenge and will soon, we predict, overturn the traditional dichotomous view [that schizophrenia and bipolar are separate]."	Schizophrenia and psychotic mood disorder similar
13	*J Med Genet* (2005)	Craddock et al.	Review (molecular genetics)	"Increasing evidence suggests an overlap in genetic susceptibility across the traditional classification system that dichotomized psychotic disorders into schizophrenia or bipolar disorder, most notably with findings at DAOA(G72), DISC1, and NRG1.... we can expect that over the coming years molecular genetics will catalyze a re-appraisal of psychiatric nosology as well as providing a path to understanding the pathophysiology [of bipolar and schizophrenia]."	Schizophrenia and psychotic mood disorder similar
14	*Schiz Res* (2005)	Hafner et al.	Review	"The high frequency of depressive symptoms at the prepsychotic prodromal stage and their increase and decrease with the psychotic episode suggests that depression in SZ might be expression of an early, mild stage of the same neurobiological process that causes psychosis."	Ambivalent; Schizophrenia and psychotic mood disorder similar
15	*AJP* (2005)	Fawcett	Editorial	"... of the [eleven] chromosome loci found for the transmission of schizophrenia and bipolar disorder, eight have been found to overlap...."	Schizophrenia and psychotic mood disorder similar

(continued)

Table 1.1 (continued)

Quote no.	Journal (year)	Author(s)	Field of study	Selected quotes of summary/conclusions	Results
16	*Medscape Psychiatry Mental Health* (2004)	Korn	Review	"Schizophrenia and Bipolar Disorder: An Evolving Interface" [article title]; "... there is increasing evidence of connections between the two disorders;.... It is also becoming increasingly evident that there are many similarities.... in family studies, genetic analysis, common symptoms complexes, psychopharmacologic responses, as well as other areas."	Schizophrenia and psychotic mood disorder similar
17	*J Psychiatry Res* (2004)	Ketter et al.	Review	"Psychotic bipolar disorders have characteristics such as phenomenology, biology, therapeutic response and brain imaging findings suggesting both commonalities with and dissociations from schizophrenia.... Taken together, these characteristics are in some instances most consistent with a dimensional view, with psychotic bipolar disorders being intermediate between non-psychotic bipolar disorders and schizophrenia spectrum disorders. However, in other instances, a categorical approach appears useful."	Ambivalent; schizophrenia and psychotic mood disorder similar; continuum
18	*Schiz Res* (2004)	Murray et al.	Review (cognitive)	"Finally, following the onset of illness, common factors are likely to underlie the deterioration in brain structure in cognitive and social function, which can occur in both illnesses [SZ and BP]."	Ambivalent; schizophrenia and psychotic mood disorder overlap
19	*Psychiatr News* (2003)	Rosack	Editorial/review	"A common molecular pathway may lead to variations in dopamine dysfunction that manifests as either schizophrenia or bipolar disorder, tying the two disorders together as 'chemical cousins.'"	Schizophrenia and psychotic mood disorder similar

1.1 Introduction

20	*J Clin Psychiatry* (2003)	Moller	Review	"Bipolar Disorder and Schizophrenia: Distinct Illnesses or a Continuum" [article title]; "Family and twin studies suggest hereditary overlap between the two disorders.— Certain susceptibility markers appear to be located on the same chromosomes.… [the two] also demonstrate some similarities in neurotransmitter dysfunction.… A conceptual case can be made for a relationship between schizophrenia and bipolar disorder.… the Kraepelinian dichotomy between bipolar disorder and schizophrenia may be gradually succumbing to a theory of disease overlap and continuum."	Continuum; schizophrenia and psychotic mood disorder similar
21	*AJP* (2003)	Kendell and Jablensky	Review	"Diagnostic categories defined by their syndromes should be regarded as valid only if they have been shown to be discrete entities with natural boundaries that separate them from other disorders.… Unfortunately, once a diagnostic concept such as schizophrenia… has come into general use, it tends to become reified. That is, people too easily assume that it is an entity of some kind that can be evoked to explain the patient's symptoms and whose validity need not be questioned."	Schizophrenia and psychotic mood disorder similar/overlap
22	*Am J Med Genet* (2003a)	Berrettini	Review (molecular genetics)	"…there are five genomic regions for which evidence suggests shared genetic susceptibility of BPD and SZ.… Family and linkage studies are consistent with the concept that SZ and BPD share some genetic susceptibility. Multiple regions of the genome, including 18p11, 13q32, 22q11, 10p14, and 8p22, represent areas with potential BPD/SZ shared genetic susceptibility."	Schizophrenia and psychotic mood disorder similar

(continued)

Table 1.1 (continued)

Quote no.	Journal (year)	Author(s)	Field of study	Selected quotes of summary/conclusions	Results
23	*Psychiatr Times* (2002a)	Swartz	Review	"Apathetic major depression with catatonic features (catatonic depression), completely overlaps with schizophrenia and schizophreniform disorder (depending on duration).... The term schizophrenia pays homage to our professional predecessors.... Of course many organizations and individuals are invested in the name schizophrenia, e.g., clinicians, grantees, authors, the US Food and Drug Administration and pharmaceutical companies."	Schizoaffective disorder is a psychotic mood disorder
24	*Bipolar Disord* (2001)	Berrettini	Review (molecular genetics)	"Two of these regions [18p11 and 22q11] [implicated repeatedly in bipolar disorders] are also implicated in genome scans of schizophrenia, suggesting that these two distinct nosological categories may share some genetic susceptibility."	Schizophrenia and psychotic mood disorder similar
25	*Biol Psychiatry* (2000)	Berrettini	Review (epidemiology, family, and molecular genetics)	"Are Schizophrenic and Bipolar Disorders Related?... [article title]; "Schizophrenic and bipolar disorders are similar in several epidemiologic respects, including age at onset, lifetime risk, course of illness, worldwide distribution, risk for suicide, gender influence, and genetic susceptibility.... our nosology will require substantial revision during the next decade, to reflect this shared genetic susceptibility, as specific genes are identified."	Schizophrenia and psychotic mood disorder similar
26	*Psychiatr Ann* (1996)	Dieperink and Sands	Review/symptoms (psychotic features)	"Psychosis is prevalent in bipolar disorder.... When differentiating from schizophrenia and schizoaffective disorder, presenting signs and symptoms are usually not helpful...."	Continuum; schizophrenia and psychotic mood disorder similar

1.1 Introduction

27	*Compr Psychiatry* (1994)	Taylor and Amir	Review (clinical symptoms)	"Our findings do not fully support the present classification system, and suggest that its emphasis on hallucinations and delusions is overvalued…. our analyses repeatedly yielded a single discriminate function, indicating that… schizophrenics and affectives can be represented on a continuous distribution of clinical features representing a single underlying process."	Continuum; schizophrenia and psychotic mood disorder similar/ same
28	*Can J Psychiatry* (1994)	Lapierre	Review (symptoms and family history)	"… there is no compelling evidence to indicate a common pathophysiology for schizophrenia and bipolar disorder."	Schizophrenia and psychotic mood disorder different
29	*AJP* (1992)	Taylor	Review	"Future research should focus on factors that may reveal overlap between schizophrenia and affective disorder…"	Ambivalent; continuum; schizophrenia and psychotic mood disorder similar
30	*AGP* (1991)	Kendler	Review (symptoms, psychotic features)	"… Mood-incongruent psychotic affective illness is a distinct subtype of affective illness… diagnostic validators tend to support this the second (of four) viewpoints.…"	Schizophrenia and psychotic mood disorders similar
31	*BJP* (1990a)	Crow	Review (genetics)	"It must be assumed that these diseases [schizophrenia and affective illnesses] are genetically related. … that the psychoses represent a continuum of variation at a single genetic locus."	Continuum; schizophrenia and psychotic mood disorders similar
32	*Acta Psychiatr Scand* (1990b)	Crow	Review (molecular genetics)	"The recurrent psychoses… manic depressive illness and schizophrenia,… may be distributed along a continuum that extends from unipolar depressive illness through bipolar and schizoaffective psychosis to schizophrenia with increasing severities of defect state. It is proposed that this continuum rests on a genetic base……. such variation relates to changes at a single genetic locus."	Continuum; schizophrenia and psychotic mood disorders similar

(continued)

Table 1.1 (continued)

Quote no.	Journal (year)	Author(s)	Field of study	Selected quotes of summary/conclusions	Results
33	*Br J Clinic Psychol* (1988)	Bentall et al.	Clinical	"One possible reason for this lack of progress [in discovering the etiology of schizophrenia] is that schizophrenia is not a valid object of scientific enquiry. Data from published research [mainly carried out by distinguishing psychiatrists] are reviewed casting doubt on: (i) the reliability, (ii) the construct validity, (iii) the predictive validity, and (iv) the aetiological specificity of the schizophrenia diagnosis."	Schizophrenia invalid
34	*Hosp Community Psychiatry* (1983)	Pope	Clinical symptoms	"The presence of putative 'schizophrenic' symptoms is no longer held to be valuable in distinguishing between manic-depressive illness and schizophrenia."	Schizophrenia and psychotic mood disorder similar/overlap
35	*Psycho Med* (1980b)	Brockington et al.	Clinical symptoms	"They [schizophrenia and mania] have a number of properties in common, including heritability, response to neuroleptics and the tendency to post-psychotic depression. In the area of psychotic phenomena such as delusions, hallucinations and passivity phenomena, the overlap is almost complete."	Schizophrenia and psychotic mood disorder similar/overlap
36	*AGP* (1978)	Pope and Lipinski	Review (symptoms, family history, and treatment response)	"The over diagnosis of schizophrenia and under diagnosis of bipolar disorder is a particularly serious problem in contemporary America. There are no known pathognomonic symptoms for schizophrenia, nor even any cluster of symptoms,… to be valid in diagnosing schizophrenia. The non-specificity of 'schizophrenic' symptoms brings into question all research that uses them as the primary method of diagnosis."	Schizophrenia invalid
37	*AGP* (1974)	Abrams et al.	Review (symptoms, psychotic features)	"… many patients whose conditions are diagnosed as paranoid schizophrenia actually suffer from an affective illness.…"	Paranoid schizophrenia same as psychotic mood disorder

1.1 Introduction

38	*BJP* (1973)	Ollerenshaw	Review (symptoms)	"… the schizophrenic syndrome is a non-specific clinical entity which can be symptomatic … of manic-depressive psychosis … particularly the manic phase … as well as schizophrenia itself."	Schizophrenia and psychotic mood disorder similar
39	*AGP* (1972)	Fowler et al.	Review (symptoms, psychotic features)	"… family studies do not validate good prognosis schizophrenia as schizophrenia and suggests that most good prognosis cases are variants of affective disorder…. the presence or absence of an affective syndrome is of considerably more diagnostic importance than schizophrenic symptoms."	Schizophrenia and psychotic mood disorder similar
40	*BJP* (1970b)	Kendell and Gourlay	Review (symptoms, psychotic features)	"… the results of this further analysis do not lend support to the view that schizophrenic and affective psychoses are distinct entities…. as most of American psychiatrists do, by glossing over the affective symptoms and regarding the illness as a form of schizophrenia…."	Schizophrenia and psychotic mood disorder similar
41	*Themes and Variations in European Psychiatry* (1920/1974)	Kraepelin	Book	"It is becoming increasingly clear that we cannot distinguish satisfactorily between these two illnesses [dementia praecox/schizophrenia and manic-depressive insanity/bipolar] and this brings home the suspicion that our formulation of the problem may be incorrect."	Dementia praecox and manic-depressive insanity similar
42	*Zbl Nervenheilk* (1905)	Specht	Clinical symptoms	He "argued that all psychoses derive from an abnormal affect." (Doran et al. 1986) Specht associated mania with both chronicity and paranoia. He wrote that chronic mania was "not at all a rare occurrence." He believed that once chronic mania took hold, there was no return to normal and that with advancing age, the condition worsened.	Dementia praecox and manic-depressive insanity similar

individuals have been quite consistent and frequent for over 2,000 years (Chap. 3; Table 3.1). Upon reviewing the ancient literature through the twentieth century, Goodwin and Jamison (1990, 2007) make clear that psychosis and chronicity are consistent with a bipolar disorder diagnosis. Many physicians from different countries through the centuries recorded observations that such bipolar patients could be psychotic and sustain a downhill, cognitively impaired course leading to "dementia." "Dementia" implies an absence of continued cycling, chronic cognitive decline, and permanent dysfunctionality, a course and prognosis that, in the mid-to-late 1800s, Morel and then Kraepelin, Bleuler, and others reassigned to a new disease.

In the mid-nineteenth century, despite knowledge at that time and earlier that classic bipolar patients could become psychotic and develop a chronically impaired course, dementia praecox or schizophrenia was named to account for young psychotic patients who incurred "severe intellectual deterioration." Because such patients were relatively young and suffered cognitive decline superficially akin to dementia of old age, the disease was first called dementia praecox (Morel 1851). Dementia praecox or schizophrenia was not an entity in and of itself but was made up of subtypes (Bleuler 1911; Kraepelin 1919; APA, DSM-II 1968 through APA, DSM-IV-TR 2000).

1.2 The Impact of the Misdiagnosis of Schizophrenia

The overriding goal of this book is to improve the lives of patients with primary/functional psychoses. The key to improvement is effective treatment, and the key to correct treatment is an accurate diagnosis. The clinical literature asserts that psychotic patients are frequently misdiagnosed as suffering from schizophrenia when they really suffer from a psychotic mood disorder or a subtle secondary/organic disease presenting with a psychosis. Such patients, their families, and their caretakers suffer significant disadvantages from the misdiagnosis of schizophrenia. Psychotic mood-disordered patients misdiagnosed with schizophrenia receive substandard care regarding their medications, thus allowing their mood conditions to worsen. Other adverse effects are substantial and are detailed in Chap. 15. These include stigma, hopelessness, and an increased risk for suicide due to a lack of recognition and treatment for depression. There is liability for medical malpractice for the mental health professionals who make the majority of the diagnoses of schizophrenia.

The impact to the taxpayers of the cost of schizophrenia specifically is significant. According to Wu et al. (2005), "… the overall U.S. 2002 cost of schizophrenia was estimated to be $62.7 billion, with $22.7 billion direct health care cost ($7.0 billion outpatient, $5.0 billion drugs, $2.8 billion inpatient, $8.0 billion long-term care)."

1.3 Chapter Summaries

An understanding of basic terms such as insanity, psychosis, dementia, dementia praecox, schizophrenia, manic-depressive insanity, bipolar disorder, and the Kraepelinian dichotomy is important before their discussions. Chapter 2 gives these

1.3 Chapter Summaries

definitions and also discusses the dependence of schizophrenia on the Kraepelinian dichotomy.

Chapter 3 details the history of the diagnoses of psychotic patients from BCE until 1950. The idea that one disease caused psychosis was common until between 1850 and 1900 when two diseases, dementia praecox and manic-depressive insanity, were cited to explain the functional psychoses. The discovery of the infectious cause of general paresis of the insane supported the acceptance of schizophrenia as a bona fide disease.

Since no psychiatric disorder has a recognizable pathophysiology, Chap. 4 reviews the criteria for establishing the scientific validity of a psychiatric disorder.

Four psychiatrists from the nineteenth and twentieth centuries have had such a major impact upon the diagnoses of psychotic patients, primarily dementia praecox/schizophrenia, that each is given a chapter. Extensive direct quotations of their descriptions of some of their patients from their most respected books are reproduced, allowing an understanding of how they reached their ideas and beliefs. Three of these, Kraepelin, Bleuler, and Schneider, could be called "Psychiatry's Grand Masters of the Psychotic Disorders." A review of their original publications shows that signs and symptoms that today are considered indicative of a psychotic mood disorder were often thought diagnostic of schizophrenia by these early authors. The contribution of Kasanin (1933) was bold for its rejection of established Bleulerian tradition.

Often the theories and ideas that these highly influential Psychiatrists became famous for are in conflict with some of what they wrote at other times (Table 1.2). For example, world psychiatry and especially academic psychiatry promoted the Kraepelinian dichotomy, but ignored the publication of Kraepelin's later reversal of his opinion that schizophrenia and manic-depressive insanity were so different (Table 1.1, quote #41).

Chapter 5 focuses on the writings of Emil Kraepelin (1856–1926) and his contributions to modern psychiatry. Quotations of Kraepelin's descriptions of some of his patients are given from two of his most famous books: "Manic-Depressive Insanity and Paranoia" (1921/1976) and "Dementia Praecox and Paraphrenia" (1919/2002). Kraepelin was a prolific writer, and the volumes of his work that consisted of multiple editions were published over decades from the late nineteenth century well into the twentieth century. Mid career, Kraepelin believed dementia praecox or schizophrenia was distinct from manic-depressive insanity or bipolar disorder based on course and prognosis. His "Kraepelinian dichotomy" became a cornerstone of psychiatry. The validity of schizophrenia as a bona fide disease has been sustained by the acceptance of the Kraepelinian dichotomy. Ignored until relatively recently was Kraepelin's later reversal in 1920, from his initial opinion to his belief that there was considerable overlap between schizophrenia and bipolar disorder (Table 1.1, quote #41).

Chapter 6 reviews the contributions and influence of Eugene Bleuler (1857–1939). Bleuler's famous textbook titled *Dementia Praecox or the Group of Schizophrenias* (1911) may have had more influence upon academic psychiatry, especially in the USA, than any other single work with the exception of the DSM's which have been heavily influenced by Bleuler's ideas. Extensive quotations from his case descriptions are given. Many academic departments of psychiatry through the 1970s required the study of his textbook. Bleuler changed the name dementia

Table 1.2 Kraepelin, Bleuler, Kasanin, and Schneider: what they are remembered for and what they actually said

Author DOB/DOD	Reference	Remembered/famous for	Actually said (pp.)	Comments
Kraepelin (1856–1926)	Themes and Variations in European Psychiatry (1920/1974)	(1) Kraepelinian dichotomy, (2) SZ defined by psychosis and chronicity, and (3) three SZ subtypes: catatonia, disorganized, and paranoid.	"It is becoming increasingly clear that we cannot distinguish satisfactorily between these two illnesses [dementia praecox/schizophrenia and manic-depressive insanity/bipolar] and this brings home the suspicion that our formulation of the problem may be incorrect."	Kraepelin rejected his initial dichotomy theory, admitting that SZ and BD are similar, but this reversal was ignored for almost a century.
Bleuler (1857–1939)	Dementia Praecox or the Group of Schizophrenias (1911)	(1) SZ defined by hallucinations and delusions, (2) psychosis nor chronicity necessary for SZ, (3) four SZ subtypes: catatonia, disorganized, paranoid, and added simple (later dropped), and (4) "no restituto ad integrum."	"Manic and depressive moods may occur in all psychoses: flight of ideas, inhibition and ... hallucinations and delusions, are partial phenomena of the most varied diseases. Their presence is often helpful in making the diagnosis of a psychosis, but not in diagnosing the presence of schizophrenia.... As far as the true schizophrenic symptoms have been described up to the present." they are distortions and exaggerations of normal processes" (pp. 294).	Academic psychiatry by means of the DSM has erroneously considered functional hallucinations, delusions, paranoia, disorganization, and catatonia as disease specific and diagnostic for SZ.
Kasanin (1897–1946)	AJP (1933)	Schizoaffective disorder.	Published a paper titled, "The Acute Schizoaffective Psychoses." Concluded that psychotic patients with symptoms of mood disturbances, a brief psychotic course with full remission and productivity did not have SZ. Unwilling to diagnose them with psychotic mood disorders, he used schizoaffective psychoses (AJP 13, pp. 97–126).	Broke with Bleuler's dogma and enabled the exploration of similarities and overlap between patients diagnosed with SZ and psychotic mood disorders.
Schneider (1878–1967)	Clin Psychopathol (1959)	The first-rank symptoms (FRS) are pathognomonic of SZ, irrespective of course.	Schneider divided the functional psychoses into cyclothymia and schizophrenia, suggesting that there could be no psychotic mood disorder (pp 88). Schneider's second-rank symptoms include "... perplexity, depressed and elated moods, experiences of flattened feeling and so on. If only symptoms of this order are present, diagnosis will have to depend wholly on the coherence of the total clinical picture.... Symptoms of first-rank importance do not always have to be present for a diagnosis [of schizophrenia] to be made;... we are often forced to base our diagnosis on the symptoms of second-rank importance..." (pp. 134–135).	Schneider was mistaken as his FRS are not disease specific but readily explained by psychotic mood disorders that he apparently did not recognize. His second-rank symptoms of SZ appear to include mood-disordered subjects and subjects on the eccentric side of the normal spectrum, certainly not warranting the diagnosis of SZ.

1.3 Chapter Summaries

praecox to schizophrenia and essentially dedicated his life to diagnosing and writing about schizophrenia (Fig. 3.2). Not explicitly clear in Bleuler's definition of schizophrenia is the fact that his diagnosis of schizophrenia was not limited to psychotic patients or to those who had a deteriorating course. Rather, his diagnostic criteria were so broad as to encompass subjects with eccentric, idiosyncratic, or "odd" behavior who did not develop psychotic or cognitive deterioration. Undoubtedly, as a result of this overbroad conceptualization, there were patients who were misdiagnosed and treated for schizophrenia whose eccentricities may have fallen within a range of "normal limits" as suggested by Szasz, Bentall, van Os, and others (Szasz 1976; Bentall et al. 1988; Bentall 1990, 2004, 2006; Verdoux and van Os 2002). Thankfully most, although not all, of Bleuler's very broad "fundamental symptoms" have been dropped from diagnostic consideration with the publication of the DSM-III (APA, DSM 1980) but only after seven decades of use. Remnants of his fundamental symptoms have been retained in the "negative symptoms" still considered by many as diagnostic of schizophrenia (APA, DSM 2000). Bleuler's most damaging influence has been the wide acceptance of his beliefs that nonorganic/functional psychosis, hallucinations, delusions, catatonia, and disorganization of thought and behavior, although not necessary, mandated the diagnosis of schizophrenia regardless of the presence or even predominance of mood symptoms. It was Bleuler's influence that led psychiatry in general for generations to fully endorse the view that a primary/functional psychosis was equated with schizophrenia; there could be no mood disorder diagnosis if the patient had hallucinations, delusions, catatonia, or disorganization. Catatonia, disorganization, and paranoid (hallucinations and delusions) became and continue as the essential subtypes as well as the core diagnostic symptoms of schizophrenia. He supported the Kraepelinian dichotomy and minimized the role of mood disorders.

The influence of Jacob Kasanin (1897–1946) is discussed in Chap. 7. Just as Kraepelin's reversal (1920) was largely ignored, so was Kasanin's publication in 1933 that recognized that Bleuler was wrong in his belief that psychosis dictated the diagnosis of schizophrenia. Kasanin described case studies of nine psychotic patients with symptoms of depression and/or mania and remissions to functionality. Kasanin did not diagnose these patients with schizophrenia or with a psychotic mood disorder. Today, his patients likely would have received the diagnosis of a psychotic mood disorder. Rather, he compromised with the creation of a new diagnosis, acute schizoaffective psychosis, that became schizoaffective disorder. This diagnosis linked schizophrenia and bipolar disorder, initiating a merger that would take some 80 years to close. Although this author believes the diagnosis of schizoaffective disorder has been a disservice to patients, Kasanin's break with Bleuler enabled doubt about the validity of schizophrenia as different from psychotic mood disorders. For this brave step, Kasanin deserves considerable credit. The reasons that these two diagnoses, schizophrenia and schizoaffective disorder, are detrimental to patients is discussed in Chaps. 7 and 15.

Chapter 8 addresses the work of Kurt Schneider (1887–1967) and his widely embraced teachings memorialized in his textbook titled *Clinical Psychopathology* (1959) in which he promoted his first- and second-rank symptoms as diagnostic of schizophrenia (Table 8.1). Schneider reinforced the beliefs of Bleuler that psychoses, especially auditory hallucinations, were pathognomonic of schizophrenia. It is troubling that some of his first-rank symptoms, when present, still mandate a diagnosis of schizophrenia according to our current DSM, despite having been described in psychotic mood-disordered patients. His second-rank symptoms of schizophrenia are revealing of his broad concept of schizophrenia. Belief in the Kraepelinian dichotomy was bolstered by Schneider by default since he, as Bleuler, minimized the role of mood disorders and emphasized schizophrenia as a separate disease.

Several critical occurrences in the 1950s and 1960s that solidified the belief that schizophrenia was defined by psychosis and chronicity and indeed was a valid disease are highlighted in Chap. 9 (Table 9.1). The first DSM was published in 1952 and codified schizophrenia as a valid disease. Chlorpromazine (Thorazine) and ECT were discovered effective in psychotic patients who were diagnosed with schizophrenia. The devastation attributed to the disease called schizophrenia stimulated publicity and major efforts by pharmaceutical, private, and federal government funding sources and psychopharmacologists to understand and cure it. The use of lithium in bipolar disorder was inhibited due to its reputation as dangerous. Physicians tended to diagnose the disorder for which there was treatment, that is, schizophrenia. The consistency of the diagnostic descriptions and criteria of schizophrenia and major mood disorders are traced through seven DSM editions.

The decades of the 1970s and 1980s are marked by a growing doubt by some psychiatrists about the disease specificity of the DSM diagnostic criteria of schizophrenia. Chapter 10 reviews this literature, primarily from the UK and the USA, that reflected recognition of the clinical overlap between the diseases called schizophrenia and severe bipolar disorders (Table 10.1). Comparative clinical data questioned the concept that psychosis and chronicity were unique to schizophrenia because these same symptoms and chronicity were documented in psychotic bipolar and unipolar disorders. The idea that chronic, psychotic mood disorders do occur was still a minority view, and the authors of such publications must have struggled for acceptance (Tables 1.1 and 10.1). For example, psychotic bipolar patients were reported to suffer bizarre, mood-incongruent hallucinations and paranoid delusions, gross disorganization, catatonia, the "negative symptoms" (during depression), cognitive impairment, and chronic, deteriorating, treatment-resistant courses (Kendell and Gourlay 1970a, b; Lipkin et al. 1970; Fowler et al. 1972; Carlson and Goodwin 1973; Carpenter et al. 1973; Ollerenshaw 1973; Abrams et al. 1974; Taylor et al. 1974; Guze et al. 1975; Procci 1976; Szasz 1976; Tsuang et al. 1976; Abrams and Taylor 1976a, b; Pope and Lipinski 1978; Brockington and Leff 1979; Brockington et al. 1979, 1980a, b; Harrow et al. 1982; Pope 1983; Grossman et al. 1986; Bentall et al. 1988; Goodwin 1989; Post 1992; Taylor and Amir 1994; Borkowska and Rybakowski 2001; Swartz 2002a, b; Fink and Taylor 2006; Lake and Hurwitz 2006a, b; Lake 2008a, b; Demily et al. 2009). Such bipolar patients can become persistently dysfunctional, complicating accurate diagnosis because psychotic symptoms can obscure mood symptoms that may not be aggressively pursued in psychotic presentations (Carlson and Goodwin 1973; Post 1992). Although the

1.3 Chapter Summaries

diagnosis of schizophrenia over bipolar in psychotic patients has been challenged and its validity questioned (Pope and Lipinski 1978), such doubt has been stymied by the broad acceptance of schizophrenia (Kendell and Jablensky 2003) (Table 1.1, quote #21). Based on the lessons of Bleuler and Schneider, mood symptoms were either ignored or dismissed in the presence of psychotic symptoms and psychotic patients usually continued to receive the diagnosis of schizophrenia through the 1970s, 1980s, and well into the 1990s.

From the 1990s through the present, there has been a shift in the frequency of the three diagnoses of primary/functionally psychotic patients away from schizophrenia, first to schizoaffective disorder and then to psychotic mood disorders, with the frequency of schizoaffective diagnoses decreasing through the late 2000s (Figs. 3.1 and 3.2). By 2001, at one major academic department of psychiatry, a psychotic mood disorder was the diagnosis in over 75% of admissions with a primary/functional psychosis; schizophrenia accounted for about 12% and schizoaffective disorder about 10% (Pini et al. 2001). In this author's judgment, these data are not at all representative of diagnostic ratios among mental health professionals in general. As indicated in Fig. 3.2, these percentages represent points on changing curves, with the percentage of schizophrenia and schizoaffective disorder approaching zero over the coming decade.

The importance of the comparative literature from the 1990s, 2000s, and 2010s (Chap. 11), with regard to the validity of the Kraepelinian dichotomy, derives from an accumulating body of evidence from myriad basic science, preclinical, and additional clinical comparative works demonstrating surprising overlap and similarities between patients diagnosed with schizophrenia and psychotic bipolar disorder. Such data come from neurochemical, neuroimaging, neuropsychological (insight, sensory gating, cognitive impairment), neurodevelopmental, psychopharmacological, epidemiological, and genetic disciplines (Tables 11.2, 11.3, 11.4, 11.5, 11.6, 11.7, 11.8, and 11.9). Molecular genetic studies show several susceptibility loci common to both disorders. These data caused further skepticism about differences between the two. Acknowledging blurred zones of rarity between bipolar disorder, schizoaffective disorder, and schizophrenia, Professor Tim Crow and others have proposed the "continuum theory" stating that the propensity for psychosis is heritable, irrespective of diagnosis. The continuum theory is consistent with the one-disease hypothesis since the full spectrum of severity and chronicity can be explained by psychotic bipolar disorders.

Schizophrenia and bipolar disorder were thought to "breed true" for decades, indicating two different diseases. However, the recent data suggest that psychosis "breeds true," irrespective of diagnosis, that is, that psychotic bipolar disorder and nonpsychotic "classic" bipolar disorder tend to "breed true." This understanding can resolve the conflict with the older family studies when the psychotic bipolar patients are assumed to have been misdiagnosed with schizophrenia. It is the psychosis that is heritable.

In 2009, data from a large Swedish heritability study now reveal that there is considerable overlap of the two diagnoses (schizophrenia and bipolar disorder) in the same families, suggesting one disease and some overlap of heritability of psychotic and nonpsychotic mood-disordered patients (Lichtenstein et al. 2009).

Chapter 12 reveals how the current core subtypes of schizophrenia (paranoid, catatonic, and disorganized) as well as the "negative symptoms" (alogia, avolition, flat affect) are accounted for by psychotic mood disorders. The subtypes, the positive and the negative symptoms of schizophrenia are synonymous with the DSM diagnostic criteria for schizophrenia. The absence of meaningful change of the subtypes, negative symptoms, and diagnostic criteria for schizophrenia for decades if not a century, despite the growing recognition of overlap with psychotic mood disorders, shows the lasting impact of Kraepelin, Bleuler, and Schneider. An exception "to only minimal change" in the diagnostic criteria for schizophrenia was the elimination of most of Bleuler's extremely broad fundamental symptoms with the publication of the DSM-III in 1980 (APA, DSM 1980). Since 1980, changes to the DSM diagnostic criteria for schizophrenia have been trivial.

These subtypes of schizophrenia that have defined schizophrenia for a century (there could be no schizophrenia without its subtypes) may be eliminated from the DSM-5, due to be published in 2013. Presumably, this is because of some doubts as to their validity. Eliminating the subtypes does not solve the problem of overlap of diagnostic symptoms of schizophrenia with psychotic mood disorders because the positive symptoms of the diagnostic criteria of schizophrenia are synonymous to the subtypes. The same diagnostic criteria will be retained to diagnose schizophrenia (Tables 2.5, 11.10, and 11.11). If the subtypes are to be dropped, what about the identical criterion A diagnostic criteria?

Chapter 13 documents that psychotic mood disorders are disorders of thought as well as of mood, making schizophrenia redundant.

In Chap. 14, a number of secondary or organic disorders that can present with psychotic symptoms are discussed because such disorders can be misdiagnosed as a psychotic mood disorder or schizophrenia. Examples are legal and illegal drugs as well as many medical and surgical disorders. Some of these, such as a previous use of phencyclidine (PCP) and the concept of tardive psychosis, account for some cases of misdiagnoses of schizophrenia. An underlying secondary/organic defect likely explains a small percentage of psychotic patients without a mood disturbance and diagnosed with schizophrenia.

The negative impact of a misdiagnosis of schizophrenia on patients, relatives, caretakers, and society in general is large (Chap. 15).

Many in the mental health field, physicians and scientists as well as the public and the media are certainly skeptical of any question as to the validity of schizophrenia. Chapter 16 explores explanations for the continued acceptance of schizophrenia. Schizophrenia remains the most widely known and feared mental health disease worldwide. This is documented by the hundreds of millions of dollars, if not more, devoted to research and drug development for schizophrenia by government and the pharmaceutical industries. Hundreds of thousands of patients are diagnosed and/or treated for schizophrenia or schizoaffective disorder. There are hundreds, if not thousands, of articles and books published, lectures, talks, seminars given, and conferences held that focus on schizophrenia. There are at least three international psychiatric journals with schizophrenia in the journal name. The public and the media, on a daily basis, misuse "schizophrenic" to mean ambivalent behavior typically referencing political "flip-flopping." Schizophrenia is often the diagnosis presumed in the media in high-profile murder cases perpetrated under bizarre circumstances such as the John Hinckley and Andrea Yates cases, the West Virginia and Tucson shooters, and the case of "Willie," as reported on Anderson Cooper 360 degrees. Schizophrenia is often the featured psychiatric condition of psychotic characters in movies and television.

Chapter 17 suggests some strategies for patients and families when there is a diagnosis of schizophrenia. Chapter 18 offers ideas for shifting the concepts of the Kraepelinian dichotomy, schizophrenia, and schizoaffective disorder from diagnostic to historical relevance and focusing more time helping medical students learn to recognize depression and a risk for suicide.

1.4 Conclusions

The primary driving force behind this work has been the motivation to provide the best psychiatric care for patients who suffer from psychotic episodes; a misdiagnosis of schizophrenia is an extremely heavy burden. The strategy has been to document, collate, and interpret data suggesting similarities from a variety of scientific disciplines to justify approaching the elimination of the diagnosis of schizophrenia from the nomenclature, hopefully for the benefit of patients, their families, the physicians who treat them, the mental health professions, and the public in general. This author is now convinced that patients diagnosed with schizophrenia are misdiagnosed and that the vast majority suffer from a psychotic mood disorder and the rest, with an absence of mood symptoms, from subtle, unrecognized, organic etiologies. However, readers must judge for themselves whether there are two diseases, that is, the Kraepelinian dichotomy, a continuum or only a single disease. The author has not conducted research with comparative studies but has reviewed the research literature by others relevant to this subject. The accurate diagnosis and treatment of psychotic bipolar or unipolar mood disorders, even if severe and chronic, offers hope of correct medications, functional improvement, and a decrease in the chances of adverse medication side effects from the long-term administration of antipsychotic/antischizophrenia medications.

Advances in molecular genetic linkage and association studies, identifying contributions of allele variants to phenotypic outcome, will eventually link DNA sequence polymorphisms to specific diagnostic behaviors and resolve this question. Yet, the data currently available, especially overlap from comparative clinical, molecular genetic, and cognitive decline studies, warrant extending the hypothesis that there is no dichotomy and that schizophrenia is the same disease as a psychotic mood disorder. If schizophrenia and psychotic mood disorders are in fact different, then one would not expect to find the similarities and overlap reviewed from a broad literature and presented in this book.

"A touch of schizophrenia (psychosis) is schizophrenia" must evolve to "A touch of a mood disturbance in psychotic patients is a psychotic mood disorder" (Figs. 3.1

and 3.2). "The beginning of the end of the Kraepelinian dichotomy" has already been predicted by Craddock and Owen (2005). No dichotomy, a continuum, and overlap suggest a single disorder. This would be a mood disorder, not schizophrenia, because bipolar disorder is scientifically grounded with very specific and unique diagnostic symptoms; schizophrenia has no such grounding because its diagnostic criteria are disease nonspecific and explained by psychotic mood disorders (Chap. 4).

In general, mood disorders and risk for suicide are not effectively treated because they are inadequately recognized; psychotic mania and depression are too often misdiagnosed as schizophrenia (Lake 2008c, d; Lake and Baumer 2010). Substantial time and money now invested in schizophrenia might be more productively redirected to research on the causes, recognition, treatment, and prevention of severe mood disorders and suicide as well as the development of new mood-stabilizing medications. Such a change can be fostered by increased academic focus on mood disorders.

The validity of two basic psychiatric concepts is questioned in this discussion: (1) the equation of functional psychosis with a single disease, schizophrenia and (2) the persistent idea that schizophrenia and bipolar are different diseases (Chap. 4). The concept put forward in this work, if accurate, will have a discipline-altering impact.

Chapter 2
The Basic Data

> *Psychosis is prevalent in bipolar disorder.... When differentiating from schizophrenia and schizoaffective disorder, presenting signs and symptoms are usually not helpful....*
>
> (Dieperink and Sands 1996)
>
> *... the validity of the diagnostic distinction between schizophrenia and bipolar disorder is increasingly challenged.... The diagnostic split between schizophrenia and bipolar disorder is unable to define distinct etiological and/or pathophysiological entities.*
>
> (Maier et al. 2006)

2.1 Introduction

Definitions and explanations of the terms and diseases referred to in this book are derived from various sources including the American Psychiatric Association's (APA) current DSM and the American Psychiatric Glossary as well as Wikipedia and other sources. Examples include the definitions of the functional or primary versus the organic or secondary psychoses, insanity, dementia, dementia praecox, schizophrenia, manic-depressive insanity, bipolar disorder, major depressive disorder, and the Kraepelinian dichotomy.

2.2 Dementia, Insanity, and Psychosis

Clarification of such terms is relevant because dementia praecox/schizophrenia and manic-depressive insanity/bipolar disorder were considered by some in the nineteenth century as overlapping psychoses that both could lead to dementia (Morel 1851; Berrios & Beer 1994; Angst 2002; Conrad 1958). According to Wikipedia (2011),

Dementia (taken from Latin, originally meaning "madness", from *de-*"without" + *ment*, the root of *mens* "mind") is a serious loss of cognitive ability in a previously unimpaired person, beyond what might be expected from normal aging. … Although dementia is far more common in the geriatric population, it may occur in any stage of adulthood. Dementia is a non-specific illness syndrome (set of signs and symptoms) in which affected areas of cognition may be memory, attention, language, and problem solving. It is normally required to be present for at least 6 months to be diagnosed;… In all types of general cognitive dysfunction, higher mental functions are affected first in the process. Especially in the later stages of the condition, affected persons may be disoriented in time (not knowing what day of the week, day of the month, or even what year it is), in place (not knowing where they are), and in person (not knowing who they are or others around them). Dementia, …, is usually due to causes that are progressive and incurable.

(Wikipedia 2011)

According to the APA's Psychiatric Glossary (2003), dementia is

A cognitive disorder characterized by deficits in memory, aphasia, apraxia, agnosia, and deficits in executive functioning.

The concept of dementia as it is known today evolved during the twentieth century. Prior to the early 1900s, dementia was broadly defined as mental dysfunctionality. The terms madness, dementia, insanity, and psychosis might have been used interchangeably before and even into the early years of the twentieth century. Dementia praecox or dementia of the young (a precursor to what was later labeled as schizophrenia) was initially confused with dementia of old age. The distinctions between secondary/organic and primary/functional psychoses were not recognized before the twentieth century (see below).

Psychosis is the modern term for insanity. According to the American Psychiatric Glossary, eighth edition (2003), "psychosis" is defined by,

A severe mental disorder characterized by gross impairment in reality testing, typically manifested by delusions, hallucinations, disorganized speech, or disorganized or catatonic behavior.

Note that this definition of a primary or functional psychosis is identical to the DSM core diagnostic symptoms of schizophrenia (Chap. 2; Table 2.5), and for almost a century, primary/functional psychosis was erroneously equated with schizophrenia due in large measure to the substantial influence of Eugene Bleuler (1911) and Kurt Schneider (1959) on academic psychiatry in the USA. Their ideas are described in detail in Chaps. 6 and 8, respectively. The misconception of schizophrenia as isomorphic with primary/functional psychosis has gradually waned in acceptance as psychosis has been recognized as common to severe mood disordered patients.

A state of psychosis is

… often characterized by aggressive behavior, inappropriate mood, diminished impulse control, … and delusions and hallucinations.

Aggressive behavior and diminished impulse control are characteristics of psychotic mania and inconsistent with avolition attributed to schizophrenia and major depression. The psychotic behaviors of several murderers over the past decades have been consistent with manic episodes but have been called schizophrenia (Chap. 15). The APA also characterizes psychosis as "a major mental disorder of organic or

Table 2.1 DSM-IV-TR psychoses due to secondary/organic causes versus the primary/functional psychoses

- Psychoses due to organic or secondary causes
  - Multiple drugs (illegal, over-the-counter, and prescription)
  - Toxins
  - Medical/surgical disorders
- Functional or primary psychoses
  - Psychotic mood disorders (Bipolar or Unipolar)
  - Schizophrenia
  - Schizoaffective disorders
  - Delusional disorders
  - Psychoses, not otherwise specified (NOS)

emotional/functional origin" (Shahrokh and Hales 2003). The disorder must be sufficiently severe as to grossly interfere with the individual's capacity to meet the ordinary demands of life. While there are only five primary/functional disorders in the DSM currently said to have the potential to involve psychosis (Table 2.1), there are dozens of pharmacological, medical, and surgical (secondary/organic) causes of altered brain function and psychosis (Chap. 14; Tables 14.1, 14.2, and 14.3).

2.3 The Types of Psychoses: Primary or Functional Versus Secondary or Organic

The psychoses can be artificially divided into two major subtypes: (1) primary or functional and (2) secondary or organic (Table 2.1). This work will focus primarily on the functional psychoses because it is this subtype that includes schizophrenia and psychotic mood disorders. A primary/functional psychosis is one for which no causal pathophysiology has been reliably identified, but since all valid diseases must at some level be represented by pathophysiology, there must be a neurochemical abnormality in brain function in the valid "primary/functional psychoses." Thus, the primary/functional psychoses that can be scientifically grounded as valid, distinct diseases are actually in a fundamental sense also secondary/organic. A secondary/organic basis for dementia praecox/schizophrenia was postulated by Kraepelin and Bleuler around 1900 and even earlier for manic-depressive insanity/bipolar disorder. However, to date, no clinically reliable pathophysiology has been discovered for any psychiatric disorder despite massive efforts.

A discussion of secondary/organic causes of psychosis is presented in Chap. 14. Many of the secondary/organic psychoses are a consequence of medical/surgical disorders or drug/medication effects that can present predominately with psychotic symptoms. The typical clinical symptoms of each medical/surgical disorder can be so subtle initially, or the causative drug cleared from the body, that they are missed and the psychosis mistakenly labeled as functional. The possibly misdiagnoses include bipolar disorder, major depression, schizoaffective disorder, and schizophrenia (Chap. 14; Tables 14.1, 14.2, and 14.3). There are substantial negative consequences of such misdiagnoses (Chap. 15). For example, a patient with a brain tumor can develop psychotic and/or mood symptoms first before neurological signs are obvious, and if the diagnosis of a functional psychosis is made, there is no early treatment of the tumor.

The DSM is the most widely accepted authority on classifications and definitions of mental disorders. The most recent edition, the DSM-IV-Text Revision (DSM-IV-TR), lists five diagnoses with potential for "functional psychosis": (1) mood disorders, (2) schizophrenia, (3) schizoaffective disorder, (4) delusional disorders, and (5) psychotic disorders not otherwise specified (Table 2.1) (APA, DSM 2000). The latter two diagnoses have been included relatively recently in contrast to the first three disorders that date to the first century, the nineteenth century, and 1933, respectively (Chap. 3). The delusional disorders are a relatively rare group of disorders, characterized by a focused rather than generalized dysfunctionality (APA, DSM 2000). These patients display various nonbizarre delusions of paranoia, such as having an imaginary illness, of being loved by another at a distance, of the replacement of a significant other, etc. The relevance of the delusional disorders to the present work is that they may account for a small percent of patients misdiagnosed with schizophrenia, especially paranoid schizophrenia. The erotomanic type of delusional disorder involves the delusion that another person, typically of a higher social and economic status, is in love with the individual. Such grandiosity also fulfills one of the criteria for mania and thus indicates a consideration of a diagnosis of bipolar disorder. However, to qualify for a diagnosis of bipolar disorder, the other DSM diagnostic criteria must be present (Tables 2.3 and 2.4).

Labeling an individual with the category of psychotic disorder, not otherwise specified, suggests diagnostic uncertainty as to the cause of the psychosis, whether primary/functional or secondary/organic, and if considered primary, which one. This label is sometimes used in forensic psychiatry with the goal of avoiding a specific diagnosis; it is not recommended and should not be used as a permanent diagnosis but may be appropriate for a brief period while a more definitive diagnosis is sought.

2.4 Manic-Depressive Insanity and Bipolar Disorder

Manic-depressive insanity was the early name for bipolar disorder, and the two are synonymous. That "insanity" was used for bipolar patients for centuries suggests that such patients are capable of exhibiting psychosis. The mood disorders, also previously called affective disorders, are common and have been subdivided into bipolar and unipolar (Table 2.2). Bipolar is defined by the occurrence of one or more manic and/or hypomanic episodes with or without depression, while unipolar patients suffer only episodes of depression, that is, they never experience a manic or hypomanic episode (Table 2.3). When only hypomanic episodes occur and not full blown mania, bipolar-II is the diagnosis, while bipolar-I requires a full manic episode. The depressions that can occur in both bipolar-I and bipolar-II disorders, as well as in recurrent unipolar or major depressive disorder, are indistinguishable with regard to severity, signs, symptoms, psychosis, and risk for suicide. Further, moderate to severely depressed patients, whether bipolar or unipolar, typically

Table 2.2 Types of mood disorders

- Bipolar disorders
  Bipolar-I[a,b]
  Bipolar-II[b]
  Bipolar-III[c]
  Cyclothymia[d]
- Unipolar depression (major depressive disorder)[b]
  Single Episode
  Recurrent
  Dysthymia[e]

[a]Manic episodes can be associated with psychosis, i.e., hallucinations, delusions, disorganization, catatonia, paranoia
[b]Depressive episodes can be associated with psychosis, i.e., hallucinations, delusions, disorganization, catatonia, paranoia
[c]Manic and/or hypomanic episodes occur only after use of antidepressant medications
[d]Cycles of mild hypomania and mild depression lasing several days to a week or two, occurring continually for two years or more
[e]Persistent mild depression, i.e., the glass half empty person with symptoms lasting two years or more; often also associated with the occurrence of major depressive episodes

Table 2.3 DSM-IV-TR diagnostic criteria for mania or bipolar disorder (Modified for brevity)

A. Distinct period for at least *1 week* (or inpatient hospitalization necessary) of abnormal and persistently elevated, expansive, or irritable mood
B. In the period, three symptoms (four if mood is only irritable) persist to a significant degree:
   1. Distractibility
   2. Insomnia with increased energy
   3. Grandiosity/increased self-esteem
   4. Flight of ideas
   5. Increased activities: including phoning, spending, travel, investing, gambling, sex; excessive involvement in pleasurable activities with high potential for negative outcome
   6. Speech: pressed to *incoherent*[a]
   7. Thoughts: racing, *loose, tangential*[a]
C. Symptoms cause *marked impairment in functioning*[a] (job, social, family) or *hospitalization*[a] *warranted* because of severity of symptoms
D. Symptoms not due to substance or general medical condition

Note: See Table 2.4 for specifiers that overlap with schizophrenia
[a]Signs and symptoms associated or confused with schizophrenia

Table 2.4 DSM-IV-TR specifiers and features for mood disorders

A. Presenting state: for BP: manic, depressed, mixed; for UP: single episode or recurrent
B. Severity: mild, moderate, severe without, *severe with psychotic features*,[a] partial, full remission
C. Course/onset: *chronic (symptoms over 2 years)*,[a] seasonal affective disorders, *rapid cycling*[a] (at least four episodes/year), postpartum onset (within 4 weeks), with or *without full interepisode recovery*[a]
D. Features: *catatonic*,[a] melancholic, *atypical*[a]

Abbreviations: *BP* bipolar, *UP* unipolar
[a]Signs and symptoms associated or confused with schizophrenia

experience the "negative symptoms" that are considered diagnostic of schizophrenia (Table 2.5) (Chap. 12).

Although psychotic mood disorders are called "primary or functional," which means that no consistent pathophysiology has been identified, data from patients with bipolar disorder, such as that from genetic studies, show differences between patients diagnosed with bipolar disorder and a nonaffected population; the limitation is that the specific brain pathophysiology remains elusive. Heritability and molecular genetic evidence substantiating bipolar as a bona fide disease is discussed in Chaps. 3, 4, and 11.

Another definition is found in Wikipedia (2011):

> Bipolar Disorder and Manic-Depressive Disorder [or originally manic-depressive insanity], which is also referred to as Bipolar Affective Disorder or Manic Depression, is a psychiatric diagnosis that describes a category of mood disorders defined by the presence of one or more episodes of abnormally elevated energy level, cognition, and mood with or without one or more depressive episodes. The elevated moods are clinically referred to as mania or, if milder, hypomania. Individuals who experience manic episodes also commonly experience depressive episodes, or symptoms, or mixed episodes in which features of both mania and depression are present at the same time. These episodes are usually separated by periods of "normal" mood; but, in some individuals, depression and mania may rapidly alternate, which is known as rapid cycling. Extreme manic episodes can sometimes lead to such psychotic symptoms as delusions and hallucinations. The disorder has been subdivided into Bipolar I, Bipolar II, cyclothymia, and other types, based on the nature and severity of mood episodes experienced; the range is often described as the bipolar spectrum....

Bipolar-III is designated for patients with episodes of mania or hypomania that occur only after use of an antidepressant.

> Data from the United States on lifetime prevalence varies; but it indicates a rate of around 1% for Bipolar-I, 0.5%–1% for Bipolar-II or cyclothymia,... The onset of full symptoms generally occurs in late adolescence or young adulthood. Diagnosis is based on the person's self-reported experiences, as well as observed behavior. Episodes of abnormality are associated with distress and disruption and an elevated risk of suicide, especially during depressive episodes. In some cases, it can be a devastating long-lasting disorder. In others, it has also been associated with creativity, goal striving, and positive achievements. There is significant evidence to suggest that many people with creative talents have also suffered from some form of Bipolar Disorder. ... People with Bipolar Disorder exhibiting psychotic symptoms can sometimes be misdiagnosed as having Schizophrenia, another serious mental illness.

(Wikipedia 2011)

As a general reference, this Wikipedia description of the signs and symptoms of the bipolar disorders is accurate and reasonably comprehensive.

2.5 Dementia Praecox and Schizophrenia

Emil Kraepelin (1856–1926) in his 1919 textbook defined dementia praecox as

> ... a series of clinical states which have as their common characteristic a peculiar destruction of the internal connections of the psychic personality with the most marked damage of the emotional life and of volition.

(Kraepelin 1919)

2.5 Dementia Praecox and Schizophrenia

Kraepelin wrote that a chronic, downhill course of intellectual or cognitive deterioration was the defining common feature to all of the subtypes and thus to dementia praecox overall. The references to "… damage of the emotional life and volition …" are striking in this definition of dementia praecox by Kraepelin, a disease supposedly separate from mood disorders, when these characteristics are so closely associated with mood. Avolition, universal in severe depression, has survived for a century as a diagnostic "negative symptom" of schizophrenia in the DSM-IV-TR (APA, DSM 2000).

Eugene Bleuler (1857–1939) renamed dementia praecox, schizophrenia and defined schizophrenia as

> … a group of psychoses whose course is at times chronic, at times marked by intermittent attacks and which can stop or retrograde at any stage, but does not permit a full "restituto ad integrum."

(Bleuler 1911/1950)

Thus, Bleuler said, once one has a diagnosis of schizophrenia, they can never get back to their prediagnosis functional baseline. This concept added substantial stigma and hopelessness to a diagnosis of schizophrenia. Thus, dementia praecox and schizophrenia were synonymous, and with time, the former label fell into disuse. Not reflected in these early and influential definitions was the prevalence of mood symptoms in many of the psychotic patients who Kraepelin and Bleuler depended on to develop their concepts of dementia praecox and schizophrenia. Mood symptoms were actually interpreted as symptoms of schizophrenia in psychotic patients (Chaps. 3, 5, and 6).

According to Wikipedia, schizophrenia is derived from the Greek roots "*schizein*," meaning "to split" and "*phren*," the "mind." Despite its etymology, schizophrenia is not associated with multiple personality disorder, "split personality," or dissociative identity disorder. It

> … is a psychiatric diagnosis that describes a mental disorder characterized by abnormalities in the perception or expression of reality. It most commonly manifests as auditory hallucinations, paranoid or bizarre delusions, catatonia or disorganized speech and thinking in the context of significant social or occupational dysfunction. Social problems, such as long-term unemployment, poverty and homelessness, are common and life expectancy is decreased; the average life expectancy of people with the disorder is 10–12 years less than those without, owing to increased physical health problems and a high suicide rate.

(Brown et al. 2000)

The high suicide rate quoted in patients diagnosed with schizophrenia may be explained by the high suicide rate in misdiagnosed and mismedicated patients actually suffering from psychotic depression (Swartz and Shorter 2007). "… Significant social or occupational dysfunction…. Social problems, such as long-term unemployment, poverty, and homelessness,…" are common to severe or psychotic mood disorders (APA, DSM 2000).

According to the APA Guidelines, schizophrenia is a

> … chronic and debilitating mental illness in which patients often have a diminished capacity for learning, working, self-care, interpersonal relationships, and maintaining general living skills.

According to the current APA Psychiatric Glossary, eighth edition (2003), schizophrenia is defined as

Table 2.5 DSM-IV-TR diagnostic criteria for schizophrenia (modified)[a]

A. Characteristic symptoms: patient must have two symptoms during a 1-month (active) phase (except as noted below):
   1. Delusions[b]
   2. Hallucinations[b]
   3. Disorganized speech (frequent derailment, incoherence)[b]
   4. Grossly disorganized[b] or catatonic[b] behavior
   5. Negative symptoms (affective flattening, alogia, and avolition)[b]

Note: Only one symptom is required if delusions are bizarre or hallucinations are a voice commenting on one's behavior/thoughts, or if two or more voices are conversing with each other[b,c]

B. Social/occupational dysfunction: work, interpersonal relations, or self-care have markedly deteriorated[b]
C. Duration: continuous signs for 6 months with 1-month active phase symptoms and may include prodromal or residual symptoms[b]
D. Exclude schizoaffective and mood disorders with psychotic features[d]
E. Exclude substance and general medical condition[b]
F. Exclude preexisting pervasive developmental disorder[b]
  • Subtypes: paranoid, disorganized, catatonic, undifferentiated, residual

[a]Abbreviated format without change in meaning or substance
[b]These symptoms/criteria are disease nonspecific and occur frequently in mood disorders, severe with psychotic features
[c]These qualifications that allow a diagnosis of schizophrenia with only one of the characteristic symptoms in Sect. A are from K. Schneider's first-rank symptoms (Chap. 8)
[d]This criterion is often underemphasized or ignored; a diagnosis of schizophrenia is made before reaching criterion D due to the presence of psychotic features

> A group of psychotic disorders characterized by both positive and negative symptoms associated with disturbance in one or more major areas of functioning, such as work, academic development or achievement, interpersonal relations, and self-care.

The positive and negative symptoms of schizophrenia are discussed in detail in Chap. 12. The "positive" of positive symptoms suggests an increased chance for improvement with antipsychotic/antischizophrenia medications compared to the negative symptoms. Positive symptoms include delusions, which may be bizarre in nature; hallucinations, especially auditory; catatonia; disorganized speech; and disorganized behavior. Negative symptoms include flat or inappropriate affect, avolition, alogia and anhedonia, and associate with a poor prognosis (Shahrokh and Hales 2003):

> Duration is variable: the International Classification of Diseases, Tenth Edition (ICD-10) requires that continuous signs of the disturbance persist for at least one month; the DSM-IV-TR requires a minimum of six months.
>
> (Shahrokh and Hales 2003)

Perhaps surprisingly, schizophrenia is defined and understood today much as it was over a century ago with some narrowing of the diagnostic criteria from Bleuler's very broad concept that occurred in 1980 with the publication of the DSM-III (Table 2.5) (APA, DSM 2000).

Table 2.6 Definition and symptom overlap of psychotic mood disorders and schizophrenia from current sources

Source	Schizophrenia	Bipolar disorder
DSM-IV-TR (APA, DSM 2000)	(A) Characteristic symptoms: (1) delusions, (2) hallucinations, (3) disorganized speech (e.g., frequent derailment or incoherence), (4) grossly disorganized or catatonic behavior, (5) negative symptoms, that is, affective flattening, alogia, or avolition. (B) Social/occupational dysfunction. (C) Duration: continuous signs for at least six months.	According to the DSM-IV-TR, episodes of mania and depression can display, "Mood-incongruent psychotic features: delusions or hallucinations … persecutory delusions … thought insertion, thought broadcasting, and delusions of control or being controlled." Episodes can be "… continuous for at least the past two years." Major depressive and manic episodes can display "catatonic features" that are identical to the definition of catatonia in the chapter on schizophrenia in the DSM-IV-TR. The three "negative symptoms of schizophrenia" are readily accounted for by moderate to severe unipolar or bipolar depression. Note: Thus, according to the current DSM, psychotic mania or depression can explain all of the supposedly disease-specific diagnostic criteria for schizophrenia including symptom severity, chronicity, and catatonia.
ICD-10 (2007)	"… characterized … by fundamental and characteristic distortions of thinking and perception, and affect that are inappropriate or blunted. The most important psychopathological phenomenon includes thought echo; thought insertion or withdrawal; thought broadcasting; delusional perception and delusions of control, influence or passivity; hallucinatory voices commenting or discussing the patient in the third person…"	"… delusions … or hallucinations are present … flight of ideas are so extreme that the subject is incomprehensible or inaccessible to ordinary communication. [also] Mania with: mood congruent [or] mood incongruent psychotic symptoms … manic stupor. … [For] Severe depressive episode with psychotic symptoms… hallucinations, delusions, psychomotor retardation, or stupor so severe that ordinary social activities are impossible;… danger to life from suicide, dehydration or starvation." Note: Psychotic mood disorders explain any, and all of the "… fundamental and characteristic distortions of 'thinking and perception…'" held in the ICD-10 (2007) as specific for schizophrenia.
Wikipedia (2011)	"F20.4: Post schizophrenia depression… with an increased risk of suicide…" "… most commonly manifests as auditory hallucinations, paranoid or bizarre delusions, or disorganized speech and thinking, and it is accompanied by significant social or occupational dysfunction… [such as] social withdrawal; sloppiness of dress and hygiene, and loss of motivation and judgment… social isolation commonly occurs,… the person may be largely mute, remain motionless… Negative symptoms are deficits of normal emotional responses…. They commonly include flat or blunted affect and emotion, poverty of speech (alogia), inability to experience pleasure (anhedonia), lack of desire to form relationships (asociality), and lack of motivation (avolition)…. [Disorganization] may range from loss of train of thought, to sentences only loosely connected in meaning, to incoherence known as word salad… The onset … occurs in young adulthood with a global lifetime prevalence of about 0.3 to 0.7%…. People with schizophrenia are likely to have additional (comorbid) conditions, including major depression… the lifetime occurrence of substance abuse is almost 50%…. suicide rate is about 5%."	Postschizophrenic depression is likely psychotic depression, not schizophrenia. "… psychotic symptoms as delusions and hallucinations…;" "… onset … in late adolescence or young adulthood…;" "lifetime prevalence … of around 1% for Bipolar-I …;" "…episode … associated with distress and disruption [of life] and an increased rate of suicide…;" "… can be misdiagnosed as schizophrenia…" Note: Psychotic mood disorders can suffer each and every sign and symptom given under schizophrenia. The negative symptoms (of schizophrenia) are common to moderate to severe depression, both bipolar and unipolar, specifically flat or blunted affect and emotion, alogia, anhedonia, asociality, avolition.

The "group" of schizophrenias refers to the subtypes canonized by Kraepelin, Bleuler, and academic psychiatry. These early concepts of Kraepelin and Bleuler directly influenced the definitions in textbooks and in all DSM editions. Also of note, the current DSM diagnostic signs and symptoms for schizophrenia, that were once considered disease specific, are now recognized in the same DSM to occur in severe mood disorders as well (compare Tables 2.3, 2.4, 2.5, and 2.6).

2.6 The Controversy of the Kraepelinian Dichotomy Undermines the Diagnosis of Schizophrenia

From 100 CE to about 1850, some psychotic patients were consistently described with behaviors meeting criteria for manic-depressive insanity; dementia praecox/schizophrenia had yet to be named. Throughout the eighteenth and nineteenth centuries, several prominent psychiatrists believed that only one disease explained all the psychoses (Sect. 3.3). The concept of the Kraepelinian dichotomy emerged in the last half of the nineteenth century with the idea that manic-depressive insanity could not encompass young, functionally psychotic patients with a chronic course.

A dichotomy, credited to Kraepelin (1856–1926), was entertained by others including Kahlbaum (1828–1899) and Griesinger (1817–1868). Kahlbaum was,

> Initially taken by the idea that all insanities were stages of one disease, [but] he progressed on to offer a classification which included many.

(Berrios and Beer 1994)

Angst (2002) notes that Kahlbaum's classification system was not successful because it was too complex. Griesinger's later publications indicate that he believed that there were two groups of insanities: the affective ones and then the primary disturbances of perception and will. This idea seems a precursor of the Kraepelinian dichotomy. A new disease, dementia praecox or schizophrenia was named, and "the dichotomy" was born (Table 2.7). The Kraepelinian dichotomy was simple and widely embraced and has been a cornerstone of the mental health professions for over a century. Its acceptance guaranteed the acceptance of schizophrenia as a bona fide disease.

Modern skepticism as to the validity of the Kraepelinian dichotomy was actually initiated by Kraepelin himself in 1920 when he said:

> It is becoming increasingly clear that we cannot distinguish satisfactorily between these two illnesses [dementia praecox/schizophrenia and manic-depressive insanity/bipolar] and this brings home the suspicion that our formulation of the problem may be incorrect.

(Kraepelin 1920)

Table 2.7 The Kraepelinian dichotomy; two disorders explain severe mental illness

- Dementia praecox or schizophrenia
- Manic depressive insanity or bipolar disorder

The 1933 introduction of schizoaffective disorder (Kasanin 1933) recognized the diagnostic relevance of mood symptoms in psychotic patients, linked schizophrenia (psychosis) and mood disorders, and eroded the concept of the Kraepelinian dichotomy and the dogma that psychosis was schizophrenia (Procci 1976; Brockington and Leff 1979; Brockington et al. 1979; Pope et al. 1980; Lake and Hurwitz 2006a, b). The concept of schizoaffective disorder facilitated a narrowing of zones of rarity between schizophrenia and psychotic mood disorders, but further closure did not progress for another 50 years (Figs. 3.1 and 3.2) (Schwartz et al. 2000; Swartz 2002a, b; Averill et al. 2004; Maier 2006; Vollmer-Larsen et al. 2006; Lake and Hurwitz 2007a, b). Pope and Lipinski (1978) raised the idea that many psychotic patients were misdiagnosed with schizophrenia and actually suffered from bipolar disorder. More recently, persuasive overlap and similarities across a wide spectrum of clinical and basic science fields have led to the idea that the disease we have called schizophrenia, since the time of Bleuler (1911), may actually be a severe, psychotic mood disorder. Craddock and Owen (2005) have recently predicted "The Beginning of the End of the Kraepelinian Dichotomy" (article title) in the *British Journal of Psychiatry*.

2.7 Conclusions

Before the early 1900s, there was not a clear distinction between primary and secondary psychoses as many of the surgical, medical, and drug causes of secondary psychoses were unknown. Before the twentieth century, dementia was considered the end stage for many diseases including schizophrenia and manic-depressive insanity suggesting overlap in course and symptom severity.

From the inception of schizophrenia in the 1850s through the present DSM, the definitions of bipolar disorder and schizophrenia contain striking clinical similarities and overlap. It is surprising to this author that there has not been earlier doubt about the Kraepelinian dichotomy and the validity of schizophrenia as separate from psychotic bipolar disorders (Table 2.6). The Kraepelinian dichotomy has been questioned if not discounted; having been a cornerstone of psychiatry for over a century, it now seems best represented by a tombstone.

Chapter 3
A History of the Diagnoses of Psychotic Patients Before 1950

> *In my opinion melancholia is without any doubt the beginning and even part of the disorder called mania. ... The patient who previously was gay, euphoric, and hyperactive suddenly has a tendency to melancholy; he becomes, at the end of the [manic] attack, languid, sad, ... he complains ... about his future, he feels ashamed. When the depressive phase is over, such patients go back to being gay, they laugh, they joke, they sing, they show off in public with crowned heads as if they were returning victorious from the games; sometimes they laugh and dance all day and all night. In serious forms of mania, called furor, the patient 'sometimes kills and slaughters the servants;' ...in less severe forms, he often exalts himself: without being cultivated he says he is a philosopher ... others yet are suspicious and they feel that they are being persecuted ...*
>
> (Aretaeus of Cappadocia ca150 CE, from Goodwin and Jamison, 1990)

> *Specht (1905) argued that all psychoses derive from an abnormal affect. Specht associated mania with both chronicity and paranoia. He wrote that chronic mania was not at all a rare occurrence. He believed that once chronic mania took hold, there was no return to normal, and that with advancing age, the condition worsened.*
>
> (Specht 1905)

3.1 Introduction

Drawings in Sanskrit on cave walls suggest psychotic behaviors may date to 4,000 years ago. Some have said such writings represent schizophrenia (Doran et al. 1986). This attribution highlights the "catch 22" of the acceptance of schizophrenia as a valid disease. The assumption that the cave wall writings described schizophrenia depends entirely on the understanding that psychosis means schizophrenia. However, despite the linkage of psychosis with schizophrenia for the past 100 years, psychosis does not define schizophrenia or any other disease. Schizophrenia was initiated in the mid-nineteenth century as dementia praecox and regrettably, until recently, was thought to be defined by primary or functional psychosis and a chronic course.

Manic-depressive insanity or bipolar disorder has a long and consistent history of unique diagnostic criteria spanning 2,000 years (Tables 2.3, 2.4, and 3.1). Descriptions of psychotic bipolar patients in the ancient literature have been tabulated by Goodwin and Jamison (1990) (Table 3.1). The early literature frequently referred to the mixing of manic and depressive symptoms with psychosis and chronicity, dysfunctionality and a progression to a final stage of "dementia" (Table 3.1). From at least 100 BCE, the literature contained repeated and consistent descriptions of patients who suffered from cycling episodes now recognizable as depression and mania and eventually known as manic-depressive insanity. Despite the above, in the mid-1800s, a new disease was named for the most psychotic and chronic patients having an early age of onset of their disease (Bruijnzeel and Tandon 2011). This new disease, dementia praecox or schizophrenia, was considered different from manic-depressive insanity or bipolar disorder. With the acceptance of dementia praecox or schizophrenia, the Kraepelinian dichotomy was initiated; acceptance of a dichotomy assumes and promotes the validity of schizophrenia. The influence of Kraepelin, Bleuler, and later Schneider caused a shift in concepts among psychiatrists, away from a focus on the classic symptoms of manic-depressive insanity/bipolar disorder as disease defining and encompassing psychosis and chronicity. Chronicity and psychosis began to define dementia praecox or schizophrenia. Psychosis began to be diagnostically overvalued as disease defining compared to mood symptoms that began to be considered as secondary or ancillary. Bleuler especially discounted the diagnostic relevance of mood symptoms teaching that all of the symptoms of manic-depressive insanity/bipolar disorder could occur in schizophrenia, but that none of the symptoms of schizophrenia (which came to mean psychotic symptoms) could occur in manic-depressive insanity/bipolar disorder or the diagnosis would be schizophrenia (Chap. 6). Bleuler essentially eliminated the possibility of psychotic mood disorders; some 50 years later, Schneider reinforced Bleuler's emphasis on psychosis, especially auditory hallucinations, as defining schizophrenia. Schneider divided major mental illness into cyclothymia and schizophrenia, concurring with Bleuler that there could be no psychotic disorder of mood. From the late 1800s through the present time, a majority of mental health workers around the world have considered schizophrenia to be different from bipolar disorder and that "the dichotomy" or two diseases account for major mental illness. The concept of a dichotomy overwhelmed opinions of a single disease to explain functional psychoses. Those continuing to support a "unitary hypothesis" became a minority from around 1900 until the late twentieth century (Chaps. 4, 10, and 11).

Controversy about a dichotomy actually began with "Kraepelin's reversal" in the early 1900s and Specht's belief that all psychoses derived from an abnormal affect (1905). Further doubt regarding a dichotomy included Kasanin's introduction of schizoaffective disorder (1933) that suggested a link between patients diagnosed with schizophrenia and those diagnosed with manic-depressive insanity or bipolar disorder (Chaps. 5 and 7). None of these authors' statements appeared to have any substantial impact until very recently on the acceptance of schizophrenia as a disease different from bipolar, that is, the dichotomy.

3.1 Introduction

Table 3.1 Bipolar disorder has a long and consistent history (adapted from Goodwin and Jamison, 1990, pgs 57–60, 70–73)

Quote no.	Approx. date	Author	Quote
1	ca. 400 BCE	Hippocrates (and his followers)	Described "melancholia as a condition associated with an aversion to food, despondency, sleeplessness, irritability, restlessness and … when prolonged … means melancholia." Health was explained as "equilibrium of the four humors of blood, yellow bile, black bile, phlegm and illness as a disturbance of the equilibrium." Melancholia means black bile and was thought to be caused by an excess of black bile; mania, by an excess of yellow bile.
2	ca. 400 BCE	Aristotle	Believed that the heart was the dysfunctional organ in melancholia and that gifted people were particularly susceptible such as Plato and Socrates.
3	ca 100 BCE	Themison	Considered "melancholy a form of the disease of mania."
4	ca 100 CE	Soranus of Ephesus	Thought that mania involved an impairment of reason with delusions: fluctuating states of anger and merriment, although sometimes of sadness and futility and sometimes "an overpowering fear of things which are quite harmless; continual wakefulness, the veins are distended, cheeks flushed, and body hard and abnormally strong;" and a tendency for there to be "attacks alternating with periods of remission." Melancholia involved being "downcast and prone to anger and…. practically never cheerful and relaxed"; "signs ……as follows: mental anguish and distress, dejection, silence, animosity toward members of the household, sometimes a desire to live and at other times a longing for death, suspicion… that a plot is being hatched against him, weeping without reason, meaningless muttering, and again, occasional joviality; and various somatic symptoms, many of them gastrointestinal."
5	ca 150 CE	Galen of Pergmon	Firmly established that "melancholia was a chronic and recurrent condition."
6	ca 150 CE	Aretaeus of Cappadocia	"In my opinion melancholia is without any doubt the beginning and even part of the disorder called mania. The melancholic cases tend towards depression and …..if, however, respite from this condition… occurs, gaiety and hilarity in the majority of cases follows, and this finally ends in mania. Summer and autumn are the periods of the year most favorable for the production of this disorder, but it may occur in spring." "The patient who previously was gay, euphoric, and hyperactive suddenly has a tendency to melancholy; he becomes, at the end of the attack, languid, sad, taciturn, he complains… about his future, he feels ashamed. When the depressive phase is over, such patients go back to being gay, they laugh, they joke, they sing, they show off in public with crowned heads as if they were returning victorious from the games; sometimes they laugh and dance all day and all night." In serious forms of mania, called furor, the patient "sometimes kills and slaughters the servants; in less severe forms, he often exalts himself: without being cultivated he says he is a philosopher…and the incompetent [say they are] good artisans…others yet are suspicious and they feel that they are being persecuted, for which reasons they are irascible."
7	ca 575	Alexander of Trallus	"Those affected with such a condition are not suffering from melancholia only, for they tend to become maniacal periodically and in a cycle. Mania is nothing else but melancholia in a more intense form."
8	ca 1000	Avicenna	"Undoubtedly the material which is the effective producer of mania is of the same nature as that which produces melancholia."
9	ca 1300	Jon. Gaddesden	"Mania and melancholia are different forms of the same thing."

(continued)

Table 3.1 (continued)

Quote no.	Approx. date	Author	Quote
10	ca 1500	Joan Manardus	"[Melancholia] manifestly differs from what is properly called mania; there is no doubt, however, that at some time or other, authorities agree that it replaces melancholia."
11	ca 1549	Jason Pratensis	"Most physicians associate mania and melancholia (truly dreadful diseases) as one disorder, because they consider that they both have the same origin and cause, and differ only in degree and manifestation. Others consider them to be quite distinct."
12	ca 1600	Felix Platter	"Perturbation of the spirit of the brain when mixed with and kindled by other matter can produce melancholia, or if more ardent, mania."
13	ca 1672	Thomas Willis	"[Manics and melancholics] are so much akin, that these Distempers often change, and pass from one into the other; for the Melancholick disposition growing worse, brings on Fury; and Fury or Madness [mania] growing less hot, oftentimes ends in a Melancholick disposition. These two, like smoke and flame, mutually receive and give place to one another."
14	ca 1735	Herman Boerhaave	"If Melancholy increases so far, that from the great Motion of the Liquid of the Brain, the Patient be thrown into a wild Fury, it is called Madness [mania]. Which differs only in Degree from the sorrowful kind of Melancholy, is its Offspring, produced from the same Causes, and cured almost by the same Remedies."
15	ca 1744	Robert James	"There is an absolute Necessity for reducing Melancholy and Madness [mania] to one Species of Disorder, and consequently of considering them in one joint View....We find that melancholic Patients..... easily fall into Madness, which, when removed, the Melancholy again discovers itself, though the Madness [mania] afterwards returns at certain Periods."
16	ca 1751	Richard Mead	"Medical writers distinguish two kinds of Madness, and describe them both as a constant disorder of the mind without any considerable fever; but with this difference, that the one is attended with audaciousness and fury, the other with sadness and fear; and that they call mania, this melancholy. But these generally differ in degree only. For melancholy very frequently changes, sooner or later, into maniacal madness; and, when the fury is abated, the sadness generally returns heavier than before."
17	ca 1845	Jean-Etienne-Dominique Esquirol	"Several distinguished masters, Alexander de Tralles, and Boerhaave himself, were of the opinion, that melancholy... was only the first degree of mania. This is in some cases true. There are in fact, some persons who, before becoming maniacs, are sad, morose, uneasy, diffident and suspicious."
18	ca 1854	Jules Baillarger	"There exists a special type of insanity characterized by two regular periods, the one of depression and the other of excitement....This type of insanity presents itself in the form of isolated attacks; or, it recurs in an intermittent manner; or, the attacks might follow one another without interruption." He called it "la folie a double forme, emphasizing that the manic and depressive episodes were not two different attacks but rather two different stages of the same attack."

3.1 Introduction

19	ca 1854	J.P. Falret	"There is a certain category of patient who continually exhibits a nearly regular succession of mania and melancholia. This seemed sufficiently important to us to serve as a basis for a specific mental disorder, which we call circular insanity because these patients repeatedly undergo the same circle of sickness, incessantly and unavoidably, interrupted only by rather brief respites of reason." Described a circular disorder (la folie circulaire), which for the first time expressly defined an illness in which "this succession of mania and melancholia manifests itself with continuity and in a manner almost regular."
20	ca 1867	W. Griesinger	"Provided rich clinical descriptions of melancholia and mania, although he described primarily chronic states with poor prognosis. As Aretaeus had centuries before, Griesinger conceived of mania as an end-stage of a gradually worsening melancholia and both as different stages of a single, unitary disease."
21	ca 1881	E. Mendel	"Was the first to define hypomania as that form of mania which typically shows itself only in the mild stages abortively, so to speak."
22	ca 1882	K. Kahlbaum	"Described circular disorders (cyclothymia), which were characterized by episodes of both depression and excitement but which did not end in dementia, as chronic mania or melancholia could."
23	ca 1899	Emil Kraepelin	"Used the term manic-depressive to encompass the circular psychoses and simple manias, and expressed doubt that melancholia and the circular psychoses were really separate illnesses."
24	ca 1905	G. Specht	He wrote a paper titled, "Chronic Mania and Paranoia" in which he said that "all psychoses derived from an abnormal affect." (Doran et al. 1986) Specht associated mania with both chronicity and paranoia. He wrote that chronic mania was "not at all a rare occurance."
25	ca 1911	Eugene Bleuler	"Although he departed from Kraepelin by conceptualizing the relationship between manic-depressive (affective) illness and dementia praecox (schizophrenia) as a continuum without a sharp line of demarcation, he so minimized mood disorders, subservient to schizophrenia, that schizophrenia comprised the vast majority of his continuum. Any hint of psychosis demanded the diagnosis of schizophrenia regardless of a predominance of mood symptoms.
26	ca 1913	Emil Kraepelin	"Virtually all of melancholia was subsumed under manic-depressive illness." "Kraepelin placed special emphasis on the features of the illness that most clearly differentiated it from dementia praecox: the periodic or episodic course, the more benign prognosis, and a family history of manic-depressive illness" [Note: He essentially reversed himself in 1920 saying that differences between schizophrenia and bipolar were obscure].
27	ca 1979	K. Leonhard	"It was the work of Angst and Perris that helped spread my theory that unipolar and bipolar diseases...have different clinical pictures. The bipolar form displays a considerably more colorful appearance; it varies not only between the two poles, but in each phase offers different pictures. The unipolar forms...return, in a periodic course, with the same symptomatology."

Adapted from Goodwin and Jamison (1990)

3.2 A History of Manic Depressive Insanity or Bipolar Disorder Is Long and Consistent

Goodwin and Jamison (1990, pp. 56–60) summarized a chronological history of manic-depressive insanity/bipolar disorder. This history is long and consistent and confirms that bipolar disorder has been established as a specific disorder (Table 3.1, 3.2, 3.3; Chap. 4). As Goodwin and Jamison (1990, p. 56) said,

> Medical conceptions of mania and depression are as old as secular medicine itself. From ancient times to the present, an extraordinary consistency characterizes descriptions of these conditions. Few maladies in medical history have been represented with such unvarying language. …the essential features are recognizable in the medical literature through the centuries. ….

An accurate concept of depression, called melancholia, dates to at least 400 BCE when Hippocrates described a condition associated with "an aversion to food, despondency, sleeplessness, irritability, restlessness, …." An excess of black bile was thought to be the cause of depression, while too much yellow bile or a mixture of yellow and black bile was associated with mania, suggesting the potential for an association of mania and depression. As shown in Table 3.1, the relationship of depression and mania (at least according to current understanding) was consistently and accurately described BCE. Mania and melancholy were directly linked as early as 100 BCE by Themison (Goodwin and Jamison 1990, p. 57). Soranus of Ephesus, in 100 Current Era (CE), apparently believed that melancholia and mania were two distinct diseases but with common prodromal symptoms requiring the same treatments (Goodwin and Jamison 1990, p. 57).

Several ancient descriptions connect mania with paranoia as well as with depression (Table 3.2). Soranus described symptoms of mania to include paranoia, that is, having a "… suspicion … that a plot is being hatched against him, …" and wrote that manic patients "… sometimes have an overpowering fear of things …." Soranus accurately described the signs and symptoms of both mania and depression that are consistent with current observations and DSM diagnostic criteria (Tables 2.3 and 2.4).

By 150 CE, Aretaeus of Cappadocia also believed depression was,

> "… part of the disorder called mania" since he observed that, "Some patients after being melancholic have fits of mania … so that mania is like a variety of being melancholy." He described mania as "… furor, excitement and cheerfulness." This "… serious form of mania" was called "furor." He suggested that "… mania was an end-stage of melancholia, …." Aretaeus accurately described the cycling of such patients between depression and mania saying that, "… the patient who previously was gay, euphoric, and hyperactive suddenly has a tendency to melancholy; he becomes, at the end of the [manic] attack, languid, sad, taciturn, he complains that he is worried about his future, he feels ashamed. When the depressive phase is over, such patients go back to being gay, they laugh, they joke, they sing, … sometimes they laugh and dance all day and all night. … sometimes [the patient] kills and slaughters the servants."

He even observed that spring and autumn were the most common seasons for these disorders suggestive of seasonal affective disorder. Like Soranus, Aretaeus associated "… a paranoid psychosis" with mania. According to Goodwin and Jamison (1990, p. 57), "Aretaeus included syndromes (as mania) that today would

3.2 A History of Manic Depressive Insanity or Bipolar Disorder Is Long and Consistent

Table 3.2 Historical links of paranoia with mood disorders not schizophrenia

Date	Name	Quote
ca 400 BCE	Hippocrates	"Described melancholia as a condition associated with … fear or depression that when prolonged means melancholia."
ca 100 CE	Soranus of Ephesus	Thought that mania sometimes involved "an overpowering fear of things which are quite harmless. … sometimes …. suspicion that a plot is being hatched against him…."
ca 150 CE	Aretaeus of Cappadocia	"… others [manics] yet are suspicious and they feel that they are being persecuted…."
1799	Sims, James	Sims convincingly linked severe depression (melancholia) with paranoid delusions (Swartz and Shorter 2007, pp. 24–25).
1905	Specht, G	"Chronic Mania and Paranoia" (article title) Specht associated mania with both chronicity and paranoia and believed these combinations were common.
1921	Kraepelin, E	Kraepelin wrote a book titled, "Manic-Depressive Insanity and Paranoia." (1921) Described "paranoid depression" as a disorder with a high rate of suicide, marked depression, auditory hallucinations, paranoia, and agitation.
1967	Beck, A.T	He found that 46% of severely depressed patients suffered delusions of having sinned or committed terrible crimes. They then suffered paranoid delusions that torture and execution were imminent (Swartz and Shorter 2007, p. 137).
1974	Abrams et al.	They published a paper titled, "Manic-Depressive Illness and Paranoid schizophrenia," in which they implied that about 95% of their sample of patients diagnosed with paranoid schizophrenia actually suffered from mania because classic bipolar patients were observed to suffer paranoid delusions.
1976	Hamilton, M	"Several British investigators … argue that delusions in a depressed individual usually arise from guilt and a depressed mood. Persecutory thoughts, in this context, are a derivative of these guilt feelings and a mood disorder, and not primary in themselves. For example, the patient may say 'I have committed terrible crimes and I'm going to be punished,' or even, 'the police are pursuing me and will hang me for my crimes.' Initially, these thoughts appear persecutory in nature, but they really stem from the delusion of guilt and the basic mood disorder" (Doran et al. 1986).
2008	Lake, CR	He attributes paranoia to either psychotic manic grandiosity or psychotic depressive guilt resulting in delusional persecutory fears for one's life, thus discounting the validity of paranoid schizophrenia.

be classified as schizophrenia, ..." Aretaeus was likely accurate when he classified the severe, paranoid, psychotic patients as manic, that today by DSM criteria might be diagnosed with schizophrenia rather than severe psychotic bipolar disorder because of the predominance of psychotic symptoms. Aretaeus has been called "The clinician of mania, ..."

Alexander of Trallus in about 575 CE said, "... mania is nothing else but melancholia in a more intense form." Gaddesden (1300) said, "... mania and melancholia are different forms of the same thing." In 1549, Pratensis said, "Most physicians associate mania and melancholia .... as one disorder, ..." In 1600, Platter used the term "kindled" to describe an onset of melancholia or mania. Willis in 1672 said that, "These two [manics and melancholics], like smoke and flame, mutually receive and give place to one another." In 1744, James said that, "There is an absolute necessity for reducing melancholy and madness [mania] to one species of disorder, ..." By 1845, Baillarger accurately characterized what we now know as classic bipolar cycling when he said:

> There exists a special type of insanity characterized by two regular periods, the one of depression and the other of excitement ... calling it "la folie a double forme," emphasizing that the manic and depressive episodes were not two different attacks but rather two different stages of the same attack.

In that same year, Falret

> ... described a circular disorder [la folie circulairle], which expressly defines an illness in which this succession of mania and melancholia manifests itself with continuity and in a manner almost regular.

It is curious that one of Falret's assistants, Benedict Morel, initiated the separate disease, dementia praecox, in the mid-1800s for the most severe psychotic patients. In 1867, Griesinger recognized that such patients [manic-depressive] could progress to chronic states with poor prognoses. Kraepelin in 1899 used the term "manic-depressive insanity," and he initially differentiated it from dementia praecox by "... the periodic or episodic course, a more benign prognosis and a family history of Manic-Depressive Illness." Later in his career, Kraepelin apparently reversed his belief that there are clear differences between dementia praecox/schizophrenia and manic-depressive insanity/bipolar disorder (Table 1.1, quote #41). In 1979, Leonhard differentiated unipolar from bipolar mood disorders (Tables 2.2, 3.1, quote #27).

An important point to be taken from the history of bipolar disorder is the linkage of psychotic paranoia with mania and depression that has spanned some 2,000 years, long before a new diagnosis of paranoid schizophrenia was used for paranoid patients (Table 3.2). Such an association between paranoia and a mood disorder is found in the writings of Hippocrates and his followers in about 400 BCE, from the writings of Soranus of Ephesus (ca 100 CE), Aretaeus of Cappadocia (ca 150 CE), Specht (1905), Kraepelin (1921), Abrams et al. (1974), and Lake (2008a, b, c) (Table 3.2). Kraepelin considered at least two subtypes of paranoia, one he associated with mood in which the paranoid delusion was relatively specific, organized, and stable and the other, which he listed as the paranoid subtype of dementia praecox or schizophrenia, had generalized suspiciousness that rapidly changed from one source to another in a disorganized way. This distinction has subsequently been discounted as psychotic mood-disordered patients have been observed to display generalized paranoia that can rapidly change from one source to another in a disorganized way.

The early association between paranoid psychosis and mood disorders was lost by the subsequent association of paranoia with schizophrenia due to the substantial influences of Kraepelin (1919), Bleuler (1911), and later Schneider (1959). Since the early twentieth century, paranoia associated with psychosis has uniformly been diagnosed as paranoid schizophrenia, by far the most common subtype of schizophrenia (Chap. 12). From the 1970s through the present, other authors have again attempted to link paranoid psychosis to psychotic mood disorders, not schizophrenia, but without changes to the DSM's use of paranoid delusions as a specific diagnostic criterion for schizophrenia (Kendell and Gourlay 1970a, b; Abrams et al. 1974; Pope and Lipinski 1978; Brockington et al. 1980 a, b; Taylor and Amir 1994; Dieperink and Sands 1996; Lake 2008a, b, c). Undermining the validity of schizophrenia in general is the increasing belief that the diagnosis of paranoid schizophrenia can be accounted for by either psychotic mania or psychotic depression (Chaps. 11 and 12) (Figs. 3.1, 3.2, 12.2).

A second point to be noted from the history of bipolar disorder that reflects negatively upon the concept of schizophrenia is the early and consistent recognition of a relationship of severity of symptoms, chronicity of course, and poor prognosis associated with psychotic mood disorders, all criteria that became accepted as diagnostic of schizophrenia around 1900. For example, in 1867, Griesinger noted that patients with manic-depressive insanity "… could progress to a chronic state with a poor prognosis." Specht (1905) said that chronic mania, leading to cognitive deterioration, was common. That manic patients could become psychotic was made clear even earlier in the writings of Aretaeus (ca 150 CE) when he referred to the "serious form of mania" as "furor" when his manic patient "… kills and slaughters the servants."

A third point to be taken from this 2,000-year history of bipolar disorder is the consistency of the descriptions of patients who suffered cycles of mania and depression. Such a consistency and uniqueness of signs and symptoms over such an extensive period of time described in detail by a wide variety of physicians from around the world, strongly supports the scientific validity of bipolar illness as a bona fide disease (Chap. 4). There is no other condition with such characteristics, and in its classic form, there is wide separation from healthy nonbipolars and any other group of psychiatric patients. As seen below, this has not been the case for the disease named schizophrenia.

3.3 Early "Unitary" Hypotheses for the Psychoses (i.e., One Disorder Accounts for Bipolar Disorder and Schizophrenia)

The validity of schizophrenia depends in large part upon schizophrenia and bipolar disorder being different diseases, that is, the Kraepelinian dichotomy. That the two are explained by one disease is not a new concept (Table 3.3). At least four authors or groups of authors reviewed aspects of the history of the idea that severe mental

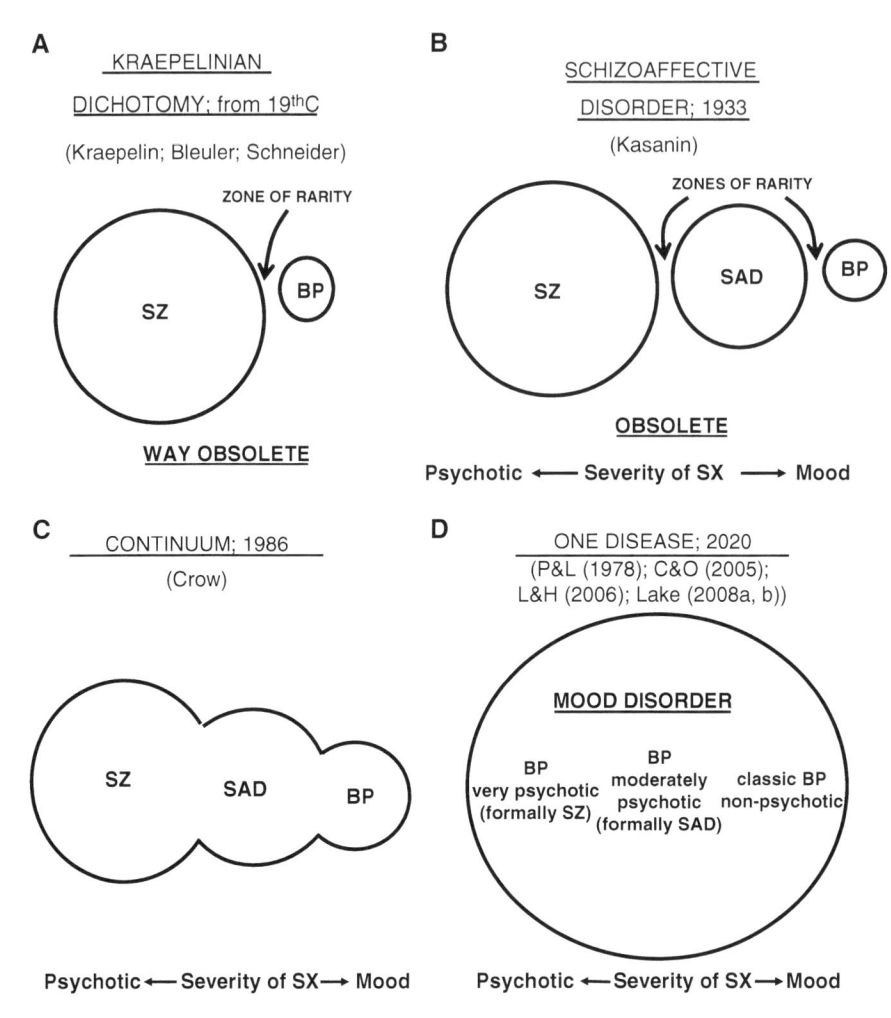

Fig. 3.1 Changing diagnostic concepts of the psychoses from 19th century (**a**) to 1933 (**b**) to 1986 (**c**) to current (**d**)

Before the 1850s, there was no dichotomy. The dichotomy began when Kraepelin and Bleuler established the new disease called schizophrenia. As shown by the circle sizes, schizophrenia became the dominate diagnosis over bipolar disorder for functionally psychotic patients. This occurred rapidly between 1850 and the early 1900s and continued well into the 1980s.

Although Kasanin in 1933 initiated yet a third diagnosis for psychotic patients, schizoaffective disorder, this diagnosis did not become popular until the late 1960s through the 1980s and 1990s. As shown in Fig. 3.2, schizoaffective disorder became very popular as a diagnosis for psychotic patients with mood abnormalities. Initially, clear zones of rarity were described between schizophrenia, schizoaffective disorder, and bipolar disorder.

A continuum or dimensional concept developed during the 1980s and continues to be popular. Crow has been a major proponent of this theory which joins all three diagnoses together.

Extending the continuum concept, some have proposed that a single disorder, a psychotic mood disorder explains all of the functional psychoses. It is suggested that this one disease, a psychotic mood disorder, will eliminate the need for the diagnoses of schizophrenia and schizoaffective disorder. *Abbreviations*: *SZ* schizophrenia, *BP* bipolar disorder, *SAD* schizoaffective disorder, *SX* symptoms, *P & L* Pope and Lipinski, *C & O* Craddock and Owen, *L & H* Lake and Hurwitz

3.3 Early "Unitary" Hypotheses for the Psychoses... 43

Table 3.3 A history of the unitary or one disease hypothesis for the functional psychoses

Approx Year of Quote/Source	Author of quote (life span)	Description of beliefs
1700s/Berrios and Beer (1994)	Cullen (1710–1790)	"… these varieties [of different diagnoses of psychoses] appear to me to be often combined together and to be often changed into one another in the same person.…"
1813–1818/Berrios and Beer (1994)	Pinel (1745–1826)	"… the common sources of mental alienation are related to sadness and loss.…"
1805/Berrios and Beer (1994)	Reil (1759–1813)	Believed that insanity had an organic basis caused by irritation of the brain; variations in intensity of the "irritability" caused mania, rage, insanity, melancholia, idiocy and dementia.
1830/Berrios and Beer (1994)	Jacobi (1775–1858)	Considered "… mental symptoms as nonspecific, changeable in time and space, and as providing a poor basis for classification … in my view, there are no mental illnesses which are independent.…"
1799	Sims (1741–1799)	Convincingly linked severe depression (melancholia) with paranoid delusions.
1833/Angst (2002)	Guislain (1797–1860)	Proposed a unitarian causal model of all psychiatry. He wrote, "… all the phenomenology of the mental diseases, all their forms of presentation may be found combined … or they change into each other with some symptoms disappearing and others reappearing … melancholia [major depression] could be transformed into… mania, paraphrenia, epilepsy, delirium and dementia."
1837/Angst (2002)	Zeller (1804–1877)	Credited by Angst (2002) as the founder of the "unitary psychosis" idea. He believed that all psychotic syndromes were only different stages of one pathological process. He said that, "… in the course of one case all the main forms of mental disorder [psychotic symptoms] may occur.… All four types of madness [melancholia, mania, paranoia and finally dementia] were but stages of the same pathological process."
1851/Angst (2002)	Morel (1809–1873)	Introduced a classification based on etiology and popularized the influence of heredity, known as the "degeneration theory" that appeared to be a longitudinal form of "unitary psychosis." "Thus, melancholia or mania may lead to dementia and eventually idiocy" (Berrios and Beer 1994).
1859/Angst (2002)	Neumann (1814–1884)	Wrote that "… every classification of mental illness is artifical … there is only one form of mental illness, that is insanity [psychosis], which does not have different forms but different stages."
1845/Angst (2002)	Griesinger (1817–1868)	"… considered melancholy [major depression] to be the fundamental disorder leading in due course to disturbances of thought and of will [mania, partial madness, confusion] and then dementia" (His later publications indicated two groups of insanities) (Berrios and Beer 1994).
1863–1874–1878/Angst (2002)	Kahlbaum (1828–1899)	"Initially taken by the idea that all insanities were stages of one disease, [but] he progressed on to offer a classification which included many" (Berrios and Beer 1994).
1866/Berrios and Beer (1994)	Sankey (1800s)	Said that there were, "… no different species of insanity.… which commences with a stage of depression and passes through those of delusion and excitement to mental torpor and decay."

(continued)

Table 3.3 (continued)

Approx Year of Quote/Source	Author of quote (life span)	Description of beliefs
1888/Angst (2002)	Clouston (1840–1915)	Described a disease that he called "adolescent insanity" or "secondary dementia of adolescence" that encompassed both dementia praecox and manic-depressive insanity.
1899/Angst (2002)	Kraepelin (1856–1926)	"It is becoming increasingly clear that we cannot distinguish satisfactorily between these two illnesses [dementia praecox/schizophrenia and manic-depressive insanity/bipolar] and this brings home the suspicion that our formulation of the problem may be incorrect."
1905	Specht	Believed that the functional psychoses were caused by mood disorders so that dementia praecox/schizophrenia was the same condition as manic-depressive insanity.
1909/Angst (2002)	Bunke (1877–1950)	Bipolar frequently does not recover; 15% chronicity.
1919/Angst (2002)	Kretschmer (1888–1964)	Disputed two separate disorders (p. 9); believed that dementia praecox and manic-depressive insanity were not really independent: "… they are not separate, but flow into each other." According to Angst (2002), "Kretschmeyer (1919a, b) disputed the whole notion of the existence of two separate disorders and described circular insanity and schizophrenia as disorders of the same stratum…."
1924/Angst (2002)	Kehrer and Kretschmer	Intermediate/mixed psychosis.
1926–1939/Angst (2002)	Gaupp (1870–1953)	Mixtures of symptoms of both (schizophrenia and manic-depressive insanity) common.
1946–1954/Berrios and Beer (1994)	Llopis (1906–1964)	Suggested that all syndromes were "quantitative gradations of a single fundamental disorder."
1958/Berrios and Beer (1994)	Conrad (1905–1961)	Believed patients with mania or depression could develop delusions and "deterioration of personality."
1963/Angst (2002)	Ey (1900–1977)	"Supported the existance of a 'monopsychose' with all clinical types resulting from variations in the same mechanisim…."
1965/Angst (2002)	Rennert	Universal origin of psychosis; believed that a common disease process operated in all psychoses. "… There is only one psychosis…."
1969/Angst (2002)	Janzarik	Unitary psychosis.
1983/Angst (2002)	Angst et al. (1926–)	Believed that there are no schizophrenia symptoms cluster without symptoms of mania and/or depression, thus mood symptoms are common to all functional psychoses.
2007	Swartz and Shorter	"There is a whole concept of major psychiatric illness as a single disease process, suggesting that schizophrenia might be the chronic untreated form of psychotic depression and of psychotic mixed manic-depressive states. It is indeed possible that there exists no separate entity of schizophrenia, and that the chronic psychotic state we call schizophrenia is initially the same disease as psychotic depression."

illness derives from a single disorder: Maier (1992), Berrios and Beer (1994), Angst (2002), Maier et al. (2006), and Swartz and Shorter (2007). Jules Angst (2002) reviewed the "Historical Aspects of the Dichotomy between Manic-Depressive Disorders and schizophrenia," and Berrios and Beer (1994) published "The Notion of Unitary Psychosis: a Conceptual History."

The term "… unitary psychosis … is the name for a collection of views which have in common the assertion that there is only one psychosis." (Berrios and Beer 1994). Berrios and Beer (1994) made an important point that "… early unitarians … have changed their minds or have contradicted themselves." Kraepelin is a good example since he initially implied only one psychotic process but then cemented the dichotomy of dementia praecox and manic-depressive insanity and finally appeared to return to his original unitary belief. His unitary ideas were ignored, and the Kraepelinian dichotomy became the basis of the concept of the primary psychoses for a century.

A discussion of a unitary hypothesis for the psychoses is complicated by advancements in medical science that occurred around the turn of the nineteenth century when many more secondary/organic causes of psychosis were elucidated, finally leaving only psychiatric disorders as functional. Before the middle of the nineteenth century, there was not an appreciation of primary versus secondary psychoses, so all were grouped together with a few exceptions. For example, alcoholism and epilepsy were recognized as organic disorders that could cause psychosis, but most of the causes of secondary psychoses, such as infections, toxins, endocrine, head trauma, space-occupying CNS lesions, stroke, and other medical and surgical disorders, were unknown as causes of psychosis. General paresis of the insane that accounted for a substantial percent of the psychotic or demented population and manic-depressive insanity were not initially differentiated as organic and functional, respectively, until the discovery of *T. pallidum*. From the early 1900s, the Kraepelinian dichotomy versus a unitary hypothesis has referred to the functional psychoses only, that is, psychotic mood disorders, schizophrenia, and later, schizoaffective disorder that has been associated with schizophrenia rather than the mood disorders (APA, DSM 2000).

Early "unitarians" based their belief that there is only one form of psychosis on observations that diagnoses were longitudinally unstable, often changing from one disease to another, and that boundaries between the psychoses were unreliable. Cullen (1710–1790) classified mental disorders based on anatomical, functional, symptomatic, and outcome features, but at one point in his life, he criticized classifications and supported a unitarian view. He said that

> … these varieties [of different diagnoses] appear to me to be often combined together, and to be often changed into one another, in the same person; in whom we must therefore suppose a general cause of the disease.

(Berrios and Beer 1994)

Swartz and Shorter (2007, pp. 24–25), however, credit Cullen with moving away from the "unitary insanity" view by beginning to enumerate separate psychiatric diseases. Pinel (1745–1826) used terms such as mania, melancholia, and dementia, but he apparently believed "… that the common sources of mental alienation related to sadness and loss…." Berrios and Beer (1994) also included Kant (1724–1804) and Battie (1704–1776) as unitarians. However, Kant referred to three categories that he called "confusion, delusion, and mania." Today, mania or bipolar disorder is associated with confusion, delusions, and cognitive deterioration.

Shorter (2005) noted that German psychiatry endorsed a single disorder then called "einheitspsychose" to explain psychosis in the early nineteenth century (Swartz and Shorter 2007, p. 19). Berrios and Beer (1994) thoroughly discussed "German-speaking [unitarian] psychiatrists prior to Kraepelin." For example, Reil (1759–1813) believed that insanity had an organic basis and that mental illness was caused by irritation of the brain. He wrote that variations in "brain irritability" caused mania, rage, insanity, melancholia, idiocy, and dementia. Jacobi (1775–1858) considered "… mental symptoms … as nonspecific, changeable in time and space, and as providing a poor basis for classification …" He said that,

> … in my view, there are no mental illnesses which are independent … all are caused by an organic disturbance and should be seen as organic illnesses ….

Guislain (1797–1860), a Belgian psychiatrist, in 1852 wrote that,

> … all the phenomenology of the mental diseases, all their forms of presentation may be found combined … or they change into each other with some symptoms disappearing and others reappearing. …. Given the right irritants, melancholia could be transformed into other brain diseases such as mania, paraphernia, epilepsy, delirium and dementia.

Although Guislain's unitarian causal theory may have led to the concept of "unitary psychosis," Angst (2002) credits Zeller (1837), who translated Guislain, as the founder of the "unitary psychosis theory," encompassing all psychotic syndromes that he believed were different stages of one pathological process. Zeller (1804–1877) claimed that,

> "… the insanities were but stages of a common disease, '… in the course of one case all the main forms of mental disorder may occur.'" He believed that, "All four types of madness [melancholia, mania, paranoia and finally dementia] were but stages in the same pathological process."

Neumann (1814–1884) and Griesinger (1817–1868), an assistant of Zeller, also supported the "unitary psychosis" idea. Neumann wrote that,

> … every classification of mental illness is artificial. We should throw it all overboard … there is only one form of mental illness, that is insanity, which does not have different forms but different stages.

Griesinger, who was an early leader of German psychiatry and who was professor of psychiatry in Zurich and then in Berlin, linked severe depression (melancholia) with a poor prognosis, a gradual onset and a chronic duration (Swartz and Shorter 2007, p. 26).

> In the early days of psychiatric diagnosis, melancholy and mania were thought of as way stations on a long road that led from wellness to dementia [dementia praecox/schizophrenia]: First the patient would develop melancholy, then progress to mania, then to dementia.
>
> (Swartz and Shorter 2007, p. 24)

Berrios and Beer (1994) also noted that Griesinger

> … considered melancholy to be the fundamental disorder leading in due course to disturbances of thought and of will (mania, partial madness, confusion) and then dementia.

Specht (1905) concurred and included dementia praecox as deriving from a core disturbance of mood.

Berrios and Beer (1994) discussed the French-speaking psychiatrists who proposed a single disease to explain mental illness, at least in some of their writings. "Pinel set the pattern for psychiatric classifications." Morel (1809–1873) introduced a classification based on etiology. He popularized the influence of heredity that after 1857 was known as the "degeneration theory" (Berrios and Beer 1994).

> Degeneration theory seemed to entail a longitudinal form of unitary psychosis, i.e., the same "invariant" was passed on from generation to generation, although on each occasion it caused a "different" clinical picture. ... Thus, melancholia or mania may lead to dementia and eventually idiocy.

However, in 1851, Morel introduced dementia praecox as different from manic-depressive insanity and was one of the first to begin the concept of a dichotomy of two primary/functional diseases, dementia praecox and manic-depressive insanity.

In 1799, London physician James Sims convincingly linked severe depression (melancholia) with paranoid delusions (Angst 2002). As British "unitarians," Berrios and Beer (1994) also counted Monro and Sankey who published in 1857 and 1866, respectively. Sankey said that there were

> ... no different species of insanity, ... which commences with a stage of depression and passes through those of delusion and excitement to mental torpor and decay.

Kraepelin (1856–1926) initially appeared to endorse the unitarian hypothesis when he said that mental disorders "... merged into one another" but by 1899 had reversed himself in concluding that there were two separate disorders to explain insanity: dementia praecox and manic-depressive insanity. Kraepelin reversed himself again in his famous 1920 paper on

> The manifestation of madness [when] he abandoned his belief in pathognomonic symptoms: [when he said] "It is incorrect to attribute signs to specific disease processes ... symptoms are not limited to a distinct disease process but occur in the same form in response to different morbid insults."

Kraepelin appeared to question a distinction between dementia praecox and manic-depressive insanity when he said:

> We shall have to get used to the fact that our much used clinical check-list does not permit us to differentiate reliably between Manic-Depressive Illness and Dementia Praecox.
>
> (Berrios and Beer 1994)

Berrios and Beer (1994) listed the following psychiatrists as twentieth-century unitarians: Bonheoffer, Hoche, Kretschmer, Specht, Conrad, Llopis, Ey, Menninger, Rennert, Janzarik, Kendell, and Crow.

Kretschmer (1888–1964),

> ... believed that Dementia Praecox and Manic-Depressive Insanity were not really independent: ... "they are not separate, but flow into each other."

Conrad (1905–1961) believed patients with mania or depression could develop delusions and a "deterioration of personality." Llopis (1906–1964) "... suggested that all syndromes were 'quantitative gradations of a single fundamental disorder.'"

Ey (1900–1977) "... supported the existence of a 'monopsychose' with all clinical types resulting from variations in the same mechanism ...." Rennert

> ... supported the view that a common disease process operated in all psychoses, and that personality factors accounted for the differences [in presenting symptomatology] ... There was only one psychosis but it appeared as if there were many for [because] symptoms had different distribution[s] in the population.

Swartz and Shorter (2007) supported the concept of "unitary psychosis," meaning that there is only one underlying brain disease that produces the symptoms of psychotic depression and schizophrenia when they said:

> There is a whole concept of major psychiatric illness as a single disease process, suggesting that schizophrenia might be the chronic untreated form of psychotic depression and of psychotic mixed manic-depressive states. It is indeed possible that there exists no separate entity of "schizophrenia," and that the chronic psychotic state we call schizophrenia is initially the same disease as psychotic depression. Perhaps the mild form is affective disorder, the severe acute form is psychotic depression and the extreme persistent form is schizophrenia.
>
> (Swartz and Shorter 2007, pp. 19, 24)

Others have recently expressed their beliefs that psychosis and paranoia are characteristics of severe depression and mania and have asserted that psychotic mood disorders explain schizophrenia (Kendell and Gourlay 1970b; Abrams et al. 1974; Pope and Lipinski 1978; Brockington et al. 1980a, b; Lake and Hurwitz 2006a, b; 2007a, b).

3.4 Dementia and Dementia Praecox (Schizophrenia)

An important time in the history of the psychoses and psychiatry was the mid-seventeenth century when madhouses or insane asylums began to be built (Szasz 1976). In retrospect, most of the psychotic patients institutionalized suffered from secondary/organic conditions that were not recognized as organic. One of the most common of which was general paresis of the insane or neurosyphilis.

Although the causes of some organic psychoses began to be discovered in the 1800s, Guislain (1833), "... considered the cause of all psychiatric disturbances to be the consequences of psychic pain ... ultimately resulting in dementia." "Dementia" was thought to be the end result of most cases of psychosis or insanity including patients that were diagnosed with manic-depressive insanity (bipolar disorder), general paresis of the insane, alcoholism, epilepsy, and dementia of old age (Angst 2002) (Table 3.3). Dementia praecox (schizophrenia) was named "dementia" of the young because of the severity of symptoms (psychosis) and chronicity of course, similar to the other "dementias" of that time.

The history and timing of the elucidation of the etiology of general paresis of the insane is critical to the naming of dementia praecox and the acceptance of schizophrenia. From the eighteenth century, Esquirol had recorded his observations of psychosis complicated by paralysis which was called general paresis of the insane.

Before 1800, the dominant disease model was still that of "humoral pathology," an imbalance in the four body fluids or humors, that is, blood, phlegm, yellow bile, and black bile. In the mid-1700s, an Italian anatomist said that disease was due to the dysfunction of an organ and not humoral dysregulation. The publications of Bayle in 1822 clarified the pathophysiology of general paresis of the insane, later shown to be caused by an infection with the treponema and called syphilis. In 1858, Virchow established the cellular model of disease. For over a century, psychiatrists who treated paresis in institutions did not understand it as an organic disease. Prior to the mid-1800s, psychiatrists thought paresis was caused by masturbation, alcohol, tobacco, or genetics. Like manic-depressive insanity, general paresis of the insane could have been considered a functional psychosis until the microscope allowed the identification of the infectious cause.

Also around this same time that an infection was proved to be causative of a psychosis, a group of relatively young patients without an infection, alcoholism, or epilepsy were recognized to suffer dysfunctionality, psychosis, and some cognitive impairment, superficially similar in some ways to dementia of old age. The similarity was the dysfunctionality, and the new disease was initially called dementia praecox (Morel 1851). Dementia praecox/schizophrenia was initially thought of as a form of "dementia." With the recognition over some 50 years, that dementia praecox did not have the same degree of cognitive dysfunction as dementia of old age, the name was changed to schizophrenia (Bleuler 1911).

The connections of the psychotic behaviors of patients with general paresis of the insane to syphilis and to myriad *Treponema pallida* in those patients' brains gave psychiatry a pathophysiological model to apply to other unexplained primary/functional psychoses. This paresis model also promoted the confidence of eventually finding an organic etiology for dementia praecox/schizophrenia described around the same time and lent support to its validity (Szasz 1976).

The recognition that one pathological organism (the *Treponema*) and thus one disease explained a wide array of symptoms previously thought to be caused by several different diseases, substantiated the concept of Ockham's razor in clinical medicine, that is, that if one disease can explain a wide spectrum of symptoms, rather than two or more diseases, there is likely only one disease. This concept can be applied to the psychotic disorders with severe mood disorders explaining the signs and symptoms of the "primary/functional" psychoses.

3.5 Dementia Praecox or Schizophrenia: Defined a Dichotomy with Manic-Depressive Insanity or Bipolar Disorder

Despite the long and consistent descriptions of manic-depressive insanity as encompassing psychosis and chronicity (Table 3.1; Sect. 3.2), the modern concept of schizophrenia as a distinct and separate disease from manic-depressive insanity or bipolar disorder, as noted above, was generated in the mid-nineteenth century. As indicated but not directly shown in Fig. 3.2, manic-depressive insanity would have

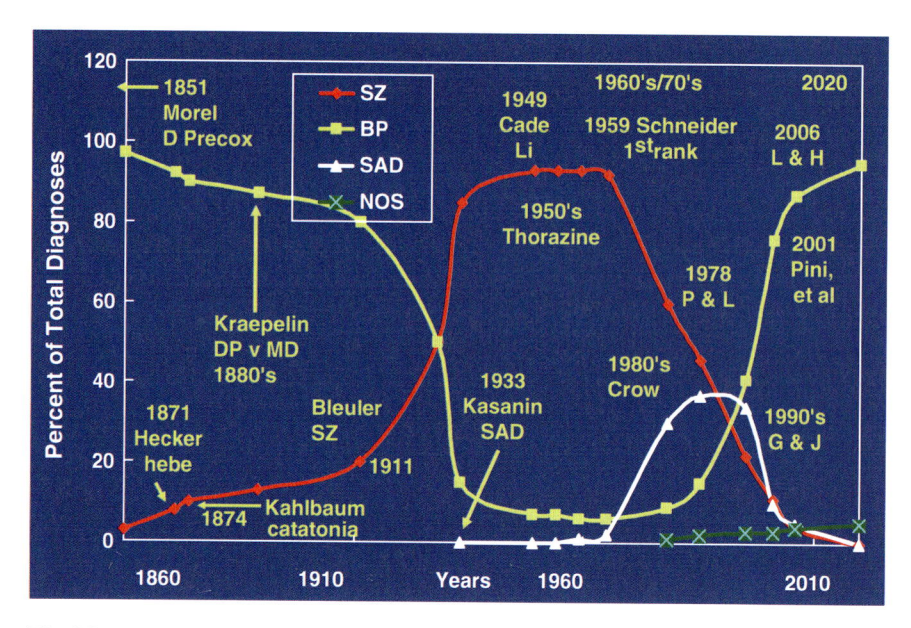

Fig. 3.2 Hypothesized history of diagnoses for the functional psychoses

Abbreviations: *SZ* schizophrenia, *BP* bipolar disorder, *SAD*, schizoaffective disorder, *NOS* psychosis not otherwise specified, *DP* dementia praecox, *MD* manic depressive insanity, *hebe* hebephrenia, *cat* catatonia, *Kraep* Kraepelin, *P & L* Pope and Lipinski, *G & J* Goodwin and Jamison, *L & H* Lake and Hurwitz, *Li* Lithium, *1st rank* Schneider's first-rank symptoms of SZ (*References*: Estimated percentages are based on the following references: Kramer (1961), Kramer et al. (1969), Cooper et al. (1972), Edwards (1972), Stoll et al. (1993), and Pini et al. (2001)).

accounted for essentially 100% of functionally psychotic patients prior to the 1850s. Morel (1851) may have been one of the first to use the diagnosis of dementia praecox in an attempt to separate these "dementias" of youth that occurred in adolescence or early adulthood from the more classic senile dementias, alcoholic dementia, epilepsy, general paresis of the insane, and classic manic-depressive insanity. Morel based his new diagnosis on his observations of some of his relatively young patients with severe personality and intellectual deterioration. In 1871, E. Hecker initiated the subtype of dementia praecox he called hebephrenia (now called disorganized schizophrenia that remains in the DSM as both a subtype of schizophrenia and a core DSM diagnostic criterion) (Fig. 3.2; Table 3.4). His patients had symptoms similar to those described by Morel but had a very early onset (in puberty) of a particularly severe, psychotic deterioration that often included inappropriate affect and regressed behaviors characterized by giggling, silliness, sexual exhibitionism, and coprophagia. In retrospect, such descriptions may have been consistent with acute mania. In 1879, Karl Kahlbaum, a prolific psychiatric author in the nineteenth century, described catatonia that was also considered a subtype of dementia praecox or schizophrenia (Angst 2002). These patients were described as having "tension insanity" and usually exhibited a peculiar posturing of the limbs called "waxy flexibility."

Table 3.4 DSM-IV-TR subtypes of schizophrenia defined

295.30 Paranoid type

A type of schizophrenia in which the following criteria are met:
- A. Preoccupation with one or more delusions or frequent auditory hallucinations
- B. None of the following is prominent: disorganized speech, disorganized or catatonic behavior, or flat or inappropriate affect

295.10 Disorganized type

A type of schizophrenia in which the following criteria are met:
- A. All of the following are prominent:
  1. Disorganized speech
  2. Disorganized behavior
  3. Flat or inappropriate affect
- B. The criteria are not met for catatonic type

295.20 Catatonic type

A type of schizophrenia in which the clinical picture is dominated by at least two of the following:
1. Motoric immobility as evidenced by catalepsy (including waxy flexibility) or stupor
2. Excessive motor activity (that is apparently purposeless and not influenced by external stimuli)
3. Extreme negativism (an apparently motiveless resistance to all instructions or maintenance of a rigid posture against attempts to be moved) or mutism
4. Peculiarities of voluntary movement as evidenced by posturing (voluntary assumption of inappropriate or bizarre postures), stereotyped movements, prominent mannerisms, or prominent grimacing
5. Echolalia or echopraxia

295.90 Undifferentiated type

A type of schizophrenia in which symptoms that meet criterion A are present, but the criteria are not met for the paranoid, disorganized, or catatonic type

295.60 Residual type

A type of schizophrenia in which the following criteria are met:
- A. Absence of prominent delusions, hallucinations, disorganized speech, and grossly disorganized or catatonic behavior
- B. There is continuing evidence of the disturbance as indicated by the presence of negative symptoms or two or more symptoms listed in criterion A for schizophrenia, present in an attenuated form (e.g., odd beliefs, unusual perceptual experiences)

Dates	Events
1850s	Morel names dementia praecox (DP)
1871	Hecker describes a subtype, hebephrenia (hebe) (renamed disorganized SZ)
1874	Kahlbaum specifies catatonia (cat) as another subtype
1880s	Kraepelin differentiates dementia praecox (DP) from manic depressive insanity (MD); names paranoid as a subtype; the Kraepelinian dichotomy is initiated
1911	Bleuler names schizophrenia (SZ) in place of DP; says very broad symptoms are pathognomonic; includes subtypes
1933	Kasanin initiates schizoaffective disorder (SAD) linking SZ to bipolar (BP)
1949	Cade discovers efficacy of lithium (Li) in mania; not used extensively in USA until 1980s

(continued)

Dates	Events
1950s	Thorazine discovered effective and used extensively for SZ (psychoses); government and pharmaceuticals research focus on SZ
1959	Schneider publishes his first- and second-rank symptoms (auditory hallucinations and delusions) pathognomonic for SZ; his ideas are widely accepted
1960s/1970s	SAD increases in popularity for patients with psychoses and mood symptoms
1978	Pope and Lipinski publish their review concluding that patients with SZ often are unrecognized psychotic BP
1980s	SAD continues its popularity at the expense of SZ; BP begins to increase following Pope and Lipinski's article
1990s	Goodwin and Jamison publish the "bible" of BP disorder; Crow suggests a common genetic defect for psychoses
2001	Pini, et al. publish the diagnostic percentages of psychotic patients
2006	Lake and Hurwitz suggest SZ and SAD are psychotic BP
2020	Projected percentages of the diagnoses for psychotic psychiatric patients

Although Kahlbaum also believed at some point that melancholia was often a malignant psychotic disease that progressed to dementia (or schizophrenia), contradicting the dichotomy idea, he was one of the first to formally introduce a dichotomy based on symptoms, course, and outcome, differentiating two groups of primary/functional psychotic disorders. He called these two conditions (1) "vecordia" that he said was "a limited disturbance with a continuous but remitting course" and (2) "vesania" that he said was "a complete disturbance of the mind" which was progressive leading to dementia. "Vesania typica" led to the diagnoses of dementia praecox or schizophrenia that he said progressed to dementia. While the "milder" group of disorders called "vecordia" encompassed what we now call dysthymia and depression, the more severe group of disorders encompassed by "vesania" also included "melancholia, mania, progressive paralysis, stroke, and dementia." These descriptions emphasize the confusion at that time between dementia praecox or schizophrenia, manic-depressive insanity or bipolar disorder, paresis, and dementia. Angst (2002) states that, "From today's perspective, these two groups appear as a clear description of Mood Disorders and Schizoaffective Disorders." There seems to have been considerable overlap of mania and depression in both of Kahlbaum's groups with the differentiating characteristic being the course and severity of dysfunctionality in outcome.

His writings influenced Emil Kraepelin to emphasize chronicity and a poor prognosis in grouping hebephrenia and catatonia with the addition of the paranoid subtype under the diagnosis of dementia praecox or schizophrenia some 30 years later (Swartz and Shorter 2007, p. 27). The establishment of dementia praecox initiated the dichotomy (Table 2.7). Dementia praecox or schizophrenia was conceived as a group of subtypes, and a patient could not suffer from schizophrenia without being subtyped.

As shown in Fig. 3.2, the percent of psychotic patients diagnosed with manic-depressive insanity began to decrease sharply between the late 1800s and the 1960s. Making up for the decrease in psychotic patients diagnosed with manic-depressive insanity was the diagnosis of schizophrenia which increased rapidly with the publication of Bleuler's textbook in 1911. Neither the naming of schizoaffective disorder in 1933 nor the discovery of the effectiveness of lithium in bipolar patients in Australia affected the percentages of the diagnoses of psychotic patients. The effectiveness of the phenothiazines in the 1950s kept the percentage of psychotic patients diagnosed with schizophrenia high as did the publication and popularity of Schneider's 1959 book. It was only after the 1960s that schizoaffective disorder and bipolar disorder began to increase their percentages of the diagnoses of functionally psychotic patients at the cost of schizophrenia (Fig. 3.2).

3.6 Kraepelin, Bleuler, Kasanin, and Schneider

These four authors have influenced our current concepts of the diagnoses of functionally psychotic patients. Kraepelin, Bleuler, and Schneider published widely; Kraepelin may have published as many as seven textbooks, several with revisions. Bleuler and Schneider each published a book that was very influential. In contrast, Kasanin wrote one major paper titled, "The Acute Schizoaffective Psychosis" published in the American Journal of Psychiatry in 1933. Although the theme of his paper appeared to contradict Bleuler's dogma that psychotic symptoms meant a diagnosis of schizophrenia, he was largely ignored until about 1965. The number of PubMed citations to his diagnosis of schizoaffective disorder in their titles rose from 0 in 1963 to 289 in 1965, increasing steadily to 1,840 cites in 2008 before falling to 1,478 in 2010 (Table 7.2).

Kraepelin, Bleuler, and later Schneider promoted the concept that functional psychosis (especially Bleuler and Schneider) and chronicity (especially Kraepelin and Bleuler) warranted the diagnosis of schizophrenia, not a mood disorder based on the presence of a chronic deteriorating course (Kraepelin) or of hallucinations and/or delusions (Bleuler and Schneider). All three emphasized to a varying degree a dichotomy, that is two main diseases, schizophrenia versus bipolar disorder to account for the major psychiatric conditions. Bleuler's textbook (1911) may have had the most influence on the acceptance of schizophrenia as the diagnosis in not only all functionally psychotic patients but also in subjects with odd and eccentric behavior until 1980 and the DSM-III. Bleuler and later Schneider minimized mood disorders and emphasized schizophrenia in diagnosing functionally psychotic patients. Schneider published his book in 1959 and essentially reinforced Bleuler's notion that functional psychosis meant schizophrenia. Schneider deemphasized chronicity of course in contrast to Kraepelin and emphasized his first-rank symptoms that described various auditory hallucinations as pathognomonic of schizophrenia (Table 8.1). The timing of Schneider's book almost 50 years after Bleuler's enhanced Bleuler's influence, further promoting the acceptance of schizophrenia. More details of each of these authors' writings, Kraepelin, Bleuler, Kasanin, and Schneider, are given in Chaps. 5, 6, 7, and 8, respectively.

3.7 Conclusions

The idea that only one disease explained all severe psychiatric disorders was popular through the nineteenth century, but after about 1910, only a minority of psychiatrists endorsed the "unitary hypothesis" until recently. Despite knowledge that patients with manic-depressive insanity could exhibit psychosis and a chronic downhill course to "dementia," beginning in the mid- to late 1800s, poor prognosis and functional psychosis began to be considered as pathognomonic of a new disease first called dementia praecox and then schizophrenia. This dichotomy between schizophrenia and bipolar disorder has been broadly embraced by mental health professionals around the world, and this concept extended for over a century and is still very popular. Although psychosis and chronicity in the mood disorders are documented and widely accepted as common, the misconcept that schizophrenia is defined by psychosis continues as exemplified by its diagnostic criteria given in the current DSM (Table 2.5), the ICD, and the draft of the next DSM edition, the DSM-5. Psychotic symptoms, hallucinations, delusions, catatonia, disorganization of thought and behavior, the "negative symptoms," and chronicity are disease nonspecific and are explained by several diseases most notably, the severe mood disorders over 75% of the time (Table 3.5) (Pini et al. 2001). That psychosis and chronicity mean schizophrenia has been a costly error.

Table 3.5 Diagnoses of 236 consecutive admissions with functional psychoses (hallucinations and/or delusions) (adapted from Pini et al. 2001)

A. *All functionally psychotic patients (n = 236) (%; n)*				
Mood disorders		Schizophrenia		Schizoaffective D/O
77.5%; 183		12.3%; 29		10.2%; 24
B. *Only mood D/O patients (n = 183) (%; n)*				
Bipolar (83.6%; 153)				Unipolar 16.4%; 30
Manic	Mixed	Depressed	Unknown	
36.6%; 67	25.1%; 46	20.2%; 37	1.6%; 3	

Chapter 4
Psychiatric Disease and Diagnoses: The Scientific Basis for Establishing Validity

> *Medical conceptions of mania and depression [the mood disorders] are as old as secular medicine itself. From ancient times to the present, an extraordinary consistency characterizes descriptions of these conditions. Few maladies in medical history have been represented with such unvarying language. ... the essential features [of bipolar disorders] are recognizable in the medical literature through the centuries. ...*
>
> (Goodwin and Jamison 1990, p. 56)

> *Diagnostic categories defined by their syndromes should be regarded as valid only if they have been shown to be discrete entities with natural boundaries that separate them from other disorders.... Unfortunately, once a diagnostic concept such as schizophrenia... has come into general use, it tends to become reified. That is, people too easily assume that it is an entity of some kind that can be evoked to explain the patient's symptoms and whose validity need not be questioned.*
>
> (Kendell and Jablensky 2003)

4.1 Introduction

There are no pathophysiological tests that are diagnostic for any psychiatric disorder including bipolar disorder. Psychiatric diseases have been established based on individual psychiatrists' subjective observations and opinions, sometimes from more than several hundred years ago. It should not be surprising that a disease described in the nineteenth century could be found flawed when its diagnostic symptoms, initially conceived as disease specific, turn out to be nonspecific and accounted for by another disease. An early example was the multiple "established" medical and psychiatric diseases that were utilized to explain varied symptom complexes of syphilis, such as general paresis of the insane. Another changing variable has been the diagnostic weight given to certain symptoms (Table 13.1). From the mid-nineteenth century, psychosis and chronicity trumped mood symptoms, resulting in the diagnoses of schizophrenia, not bipolar disorder in psychotic manic and depressed patients. This is changing as psychosis and chronicity have been recognized as common to psychotic mood disorders. Psychosis, including hallucinations, delusions and disorganization, and chronicity are nondisease specific and inappropriate to use as diagnostic of schizophrenia or any other disease. Mood symptoms have gained in diagnostic importance over the last two decades but are sometimes not pursued in psychotic patients because of the misconception that psychosis means schizophrenia. Diagnostic symptoms of mania and depression have proved to be disease specific and consistent for over 2,000 years in contrast to the psychotic symptoms that are still considered to be the defining criteria for schizophrenia in the DSM-IV-TR (Table 2.5) (APA, DSM 2000).

Given the above, strict criteria are necessary to scientifically support the existence of any psychiatric disease (Feighner et al. 1972; Winokur 1973; Welner et al. 1977a, b, 1979; Procci 1976). These include: (1) symptoms that are clearly unique to one disease only, (2) consistent epidemiology, (3) consistent response to medications (some that relieve and others that exacerbate symptoms), (4) generally consistent course and outcome, (5) an increased heritability in first-degree relatives including monozygotic twins, (6) the identification of specific genetic susceptibility loci, (7) consistent signs and symptoms over time in patients diagnosed with a particular disorder, and (8) a high consistency of the same diagnosis by evaluating psychiatrists (Cohen's kappa).

4.2 Diagnostic Symptoms Must Be Unique and Consistent over Time

First and most critical, the signs and symptoms of classic bipolar disorder are so striking (in contrast to the nonbipolar population) with repeating cycles of mania and depression in the same individuals, that classic patients are reliably identified. Such cycling has been recognized for over 2,000 years when mania and melancholia were described in the same individuals in accurate detail (Table 3.1) (Evans 2000; Goodwin and Jamison 1990, 2007). Homogeneous groups of bipolar patients have been rigorously diagnosed, gathered on research units at the NIMH and elsewhere, and studied for months to decades (Carlson and Goodwin 1973; Goodwin and Jamison 2007; Post 1992). Consistent and disease-specific diagnostic symptoms have been confirmed that reliably identify typical bipolar patients for whom organic and substance use causes have been eliminated (Tables 2.3, 2.4, 14.1, 14.2, and 14.3). Confusion about a misdiagnosis of bipolar patients derives in part from a wide variability in severity of symptoms, course, and outcome. The cycle length in bipolar disorder can vary from hours to decades. Severity of symptoms also demonstrates a very wide spectrum from mild cyclothymia to the overwhelming predominance of mood incongruent, bizarre psychosis (Tables 2.2, 2.3, and 2.4). Despite this variability in course, outcome, and severity, there is a consistent, general pattern of course with the cycle length decreasing with each episode (Fig. 4.1). The core diagnostic criteria are consistently present enough, even across the wide spectrum of

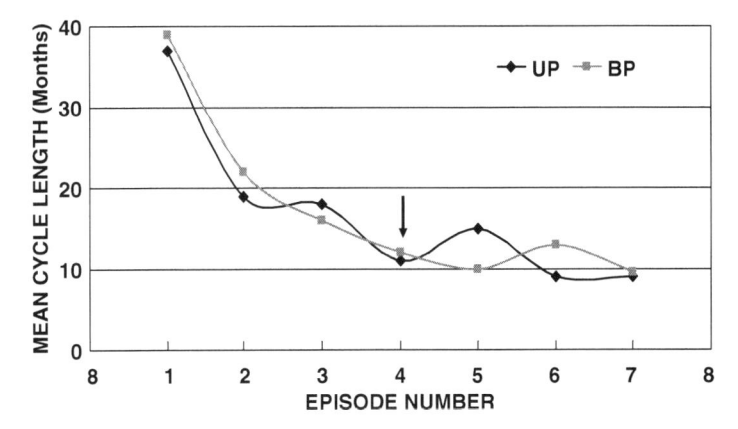

Fig. 4.1 Relationship between mean cycle length and episode number in recurrent mood disorders (adapted from Goodwin and Jamison, 1990, pg 135)

For both unipolar and bipolar mood disorders with each episode, of either mania or depression, the next episode of either comes faster. By the fourth episode as denoted by the *arrow*, patients suffer, on average, an episode of mania or depression every 12 months. Given that the average major depressive episode lasts about 6 months and a manic episode, about 3 months, one's life is disrupted in a major way with an episode every 12 months (*Abbreviations*: *UP* unipolar or major depressive disorder, *BP* bipolar disorder)

course and severity, to enable accurate mood disorder diagnoses (Tables 2.3 and 2.4) (Goodwin and Jamison 2007). Course and outcome vary from acute episodes with remissions to treatment resistance, perpetual chronicity without remissions and global deterioration (Post 1992, 2010). These chronic, persistently psychotic patients are difficult diagnostically without knowledge of a past or family history of cycles of mania and depression. Patients whose courses were cycling before can deteriorate to a noncycling, subtly psychotic, dysthymic, and irritable state without typical symptoms of mania or major depression; they can appear flat and emotionless except for anger. Such patients fit descriptions of "terminal dementia" or "burned out" schizophrenia and can easily be misdiagnosed.

The DSM diagnostic criteria reliably indentify bipolar disorder patients although there are certainly false positives when the criteria are not strictly applied or are not determined to be present during the same time period. False negatives typically occur at both ends of the severity spectrum. Mild symptoms may cause only minimal life problems, lead to substantial productivity, and be denied even when such individuals do get into trouble. In the most severe cases with florid psychoses, the mood symptoms in classic bipolar patients may be temporarily overwhelmed and obscured by patients' emersion in and focus on their own psychotic distortions that often involve fear for their lives (Carlson and Goodwin 1973; Goodwin 1989; Post 1992, 2010). Patient focus on their psychotic symptoms can be quite misleading in the time-limited, initial diagnostic interview, leading to misdiagnoses of schizophrenia and/or schizoaffective disorder (Lake 2008c, d; Lake and Baumer 2010). Bipolar symptoms may only be revealed with a diagnostic interview that focuses on eliciting manic and depressive symptoms from a patient's significant other(s) if the psychotic patient is unable to provide such.

4.3 Patients with Such Unique Symptoms Must Have Other Consistent Findings

The epidemiology of bipolar disorder has been recently reviewed by Berrettini (2000) and is quite consistent. This epidemiology for bipolar does not differ from that described for the diseases called "schizophrenia" and "schizoaffective disorder." For example, clinical, heritability and epidemiological findings historically thought unique to schizophrenia, but consistent with bipolar, include severity of symptoms, chronicity of course, prognosis, age of onset, lifetime risk, worldwide distribution, risk for suicide, gender influence and genetic susceptibility.

There are pharmacological consistencies. Lithium and other mood stabilizers usually reduce cycling in bipolar disorders while all classes of antidepressants switch bipolar-depressed patients to mania about 10% of the time. Stimulant drugs including caffeine, pseudoephedrine and methylphenidate (Ritalin) can trigger mania in stable bipolar disordered patients. The most compelling scientific evidence that establishes bipolar disorder as a specific biological disease derives from a consistent monozygotic concordance for bipolar approaching 70% (Bertelsen et al. 1977; McGuffin et al. 2003) and the localization of several bipolar susceptibility loci (Tables 4.1 and 4.2) (Detera-Wadleigh et al. 1999; Berrettini 2001; Craddock and Owen 2005; Craddock et al. 2005; Green et al. 2005).

Two other criteria support the validity of bipolar disorders: (1) the stability of the diagnosis over time and (2) a high interrater reliability (Cohen's kappa). In general, for classic bipolar disorder, once a manic or hypomanic episode has been documented, cycles of depression and mania or hypomania continue to occur with an increase in frequency with each subsequent episode (Fig. 4.1). Complicating this factor is a large variability across bipolar patients regarding length of cycles and time spent euthymic.

The interrater reliabilities for diagnosing bipolar disorder and major depressive disorder are high, 0.71 and 0.82, respectively (Brockington and Leff 1979; Brockington et al. 1979, 1980b; Maj et al. 2000). In contrast, the Cohen's kappa for schizoaffective disorder is only 0.22 and 0.19, based on Maj's and Brockington's calculations, respectively.

These data are in contrast to the absence of scientific data supporting schizophrenia or schizoaffective disorder as separate or distinct bona fide disorders. Not only is there no pathophysiology identifying schizophrenia (or bipolar disorder), there are no unique symptoms, course, outcome, or epidemiology for schizophrenia (compare Tables 2.3 and 2.4 with 2.5 and 4.3).

Table 4.1 Concordance of monozygotic (MZ) and dizygotic (DZ) twins in the mood disorders (adapted from Faraone et al. 1987)

	#Studies	#MZ pairs	%MZ concordance	#DZ pairs	%DZ concordance
Unipolar Proband	4	50	42	53	13
Bipolar Proband	8	117	69	263	23

4.3 Patients with Such Unique Symptoms Must Have Other Consistent Findings 59

Table 4.2 Genetic loci associated with psychotic and nonpsychotic bipolar disorders (and schizophrenia)

Association findings at gene/locus	Chromosomal location[a]
DAOA (G72/G30) (D-amino acid oxidase activator)[b]	13q33
DTNBP1 (dysbindin)[b]	6p22
DISC 1, 2 (disrupted in schizophrenia)[a,b]	1q42
NRG1 (neuregulin 1)[b]	8p12
COMT (catechol-O-methyl transferase), its deletion is associated with VCFS (velocardiofacial syndrome)[b]	22q11[c]
BDNF(brain-derived neurotrophic factor)[b]	11p13
AY070435 (slynar)[d]	12q24
	4p16[e]
	12q24[e]
	18q22[e]
	18p11[e]
PFK (phosphofructokinase)[e]	21q21[e]
	2p11-q14[e]
	13q21–33[e]

[a]Variation at these genes appear to confirm risk to schizophrenia and bipolar disorder
[b]Craddock et al. (2005)
[c]Berrettini (2001)
[d]Kalsi et al. (2006)
[e]Goes et al. (2007)

Table 4.3 Characteristics initially attributed to schizophrenia are accounted for by psychotic mood disorders

Criterion	Traditional dogma	Current concepts
Course	SZ – chronic vs BP – acute	BP can be chronic
Symptoms	SZ – psychoses vs BP – mild	BP can be psychotic
Epidemiological	SZ unique	BP similar to SZ
Heritability	SZ and BP "breed true"	Psychotic BP and non-psychotic BP "breed true"; Psychotic BP and SZ "cross breed"
Basic science/ preclinical data	SZ unique vs controls	Considerable overlap between SZ and BP
Genetic loci and linkage	SZ unique: DISC-1 and DAOA/G72	Considerable overlap between SZ and BP; unique loci are unique to psychotic vs non-psychotic BP
Pharmacological responsivity	Typicals in SZ; Li in BP	Typicals for psychotic Sx and Li for mood Sx
Cognitive deficits	SZ unique	BP can develop persistent cognitive deficits (even when euthymic)
Depression	"Post-SZ depression;" suicide in SZ, "negative Sx" of SZ	All explained by psychotic BP or UP depression

Abbreviations: *SZ* schizophrenia, *BP* bipolar, *UP* unipolar, *Li* lithium, *Sx* symptoms

If schizophrenia and bipolar disorder are separate diseases, then the symptoms, course, outcome, epidemiology, family heritability, genetics, pharmacological responsivity, and cognitive defects should not overlap. However overlap and similarities are substantial as summarized in the previous and subsequent chapters (Tables 1.1, 10.1, and 11.2).

4.4 Conclusions

The concepts of schizophrenia and psychotic bipolar disorder have developed separately. Before the mid-nineteenth century, manic-depressive insanity accounted for essentially all of the actual functional psychoses. Manic-depressive insanity has been described since about 200 BCE (Table 3.1); dementia praecox or schizophrenia was conceived about 1850 (Fig. 3.2) and split the most severe cases of manic-depressive insanity, those with an early age of onset, psychosis, and chronicity into a new disease. Dementia praecox/schizophrenia soon obscured manic-depressive insanity as the diagnosis for functionally psychotic patients with a chronic course and early onset. Psychosis, hallucinations, delusions, and a chronic course somehow became diagnostic of schizophrenia despite the long history of psychosis and chronicity in manic-depressive insanity. This concept that equated schizophrenia with psychosis continued in all the editions of the DSM beginning in 1952, including the DSM-5 (APA, DSM 2013), and in all textbooks in spite of psychotic features being simultaneously described in manic and depressed patients in the chapters on mood disorders (Tables 2.3, 2.4, 9.3, and 11.10). By the 1970s authors attacked the concept of schizophrenia from two sides of the severity spectrum: (1) overlaps with normal eccentric behavior (Szasz 1976; Bentall et al. 1988; Verdoux and van Os 2002) and (2) overlap and similarities with psychotic mood disorders (Kendell and Gourlay 1970a, b; Pope and Lipinski 1978). In 1980 and the publication of the DSM-III, the mild end of the severity spectrum of schizophrenia was addressed with the elimination of Bleuler's subtype of simple schizophrenia and at least some of his fundamental symptoms of schizophrenia. This narrowed the concept of schizophrenia to psychotic patients and strengthened support for the validity of schizophrenia.

Despite dozens of reports of hallucinations, delusions, catatonia, disorganization, and chronicity of course in mood disorders beginning in the 1970s and continuing through the present, the current and future DSM diagnostic criteria for schizophrenia continue to include these symptoms as diagnostic of schizophrenia. Schizophrenia continues to be taught in medical, psychology, nursing, and social work schools and in psychiatry residency training programs. The validity of schizophrenia has been accepted by all mental health and medical professions, scientists, mental health patients, the public, and the media.

4.4 Conclusions

A decline in function to perpetual dysfunctionality, a chronic course, and an early onset of severe mental illness are quite consistent with psychotic mood disorders yet these characteristics are offered as diagnostic signs of schizophrenia. Schizophrenia continues to be diagnosed in most patients with chronic psychotic courses with subtle disturbances of mood depending upon the bias of the training of the diagnostician.

If overlap and similarities suggest a single disease, not a dichotomy, why choose bipolar disorder rather than schizophrenia? The diagnostic criteria for bipolar disorder are disease specific with such a wide spectrum of unique behaviors, cycling from depression to mania and back, that identification of such patients has been consistent and reliable through 2,000 years. When one disease can account for the symptoms of two or more diseases, Ockham's razor suggests that there is only one disease, in this case, a psychotic mood disorder.

Chapter 5
Emil Kraepelin (1856–1926) Established the Kraepelinian Dichotomy and Schizophrenia but Then Reneged

> *It is becoming increasingly clear that we cannot distinguish satisfactorily between these two illnesses [dementia praecox/ schizophrenia and manic-depressive insanity/bipolar] and this brings home the suspicion that our formulation of the problem [the Kraepelinian dichotomy] may be incorrect.*
>
> (Kraepelin 1920/1974)
>
> *"The beginning of the end for the Kraepelinian dichotomy" [article title]. "Now molecular genetic studies are beginning to challenge and will soon, we predict, overturn the traditional dichotomous view [that schizophrenia and bipolar are separate]."*
>
> (Craddock and Owen 2005)
>
> *But such was the power of a simple binary classification [the Kraepelinian dichotomy] that a century of clinicians, textbook writers, and examiners adopted the system with uncritical enthusiasm and regardless of the reservations of its progenitor.*
>
> (Crow 2010)

5.1 Introduction: A Dichotomy Meant Dementia Praecox/Schizophrenia Is a Real Disease

Emil Kraepelin, a German psychiatrist, was a prolific writer. He began his training at the University of Leipzig. He became a professor of psychiatry, first in 1882 at the University of Tartu (then Dorpot) in what is today Estonia, then in Heidelberg in the 1890s, and later in Munich. At his first post, Kraepelin also became the director of an 80-bed university hospital where he observed and recorded in detail many patients' behaviors, symptoms, family histories, and courses because he "… wanted to create a nosology that would provide a basis for successful prognosis, therapy and prevention" (Roelcke 1997). In 1908, he was elected to the Royal Swedish Academy of Sciences.

Table 5.1 A selection of publications of E. Kraepelin translated to English

Volume 1
Lectures on Clinical Psychiatry, (1904; 3rd edition 1913)
Volume 2
Clinical Psychiatry: A Text-Book for Students and Physicians (1883). Abstracted and adapted from the seventh German edition of Kraepelin's *"Lehrbuch der Psychiatrie"* by A. Ross Diefendorf (1907)
Volume 3
General Paresis (1913)
Volume 4
Dementia Praecox and Paraphrenia (1919)
Volume 5
Manic-Depressive Insanity and Paranoia (1921)

He focused primarily on the clinical courses of his patients in order to separate two diseases, dementia praecox or schizophrenia and manic-depressive insanity or bipolar disorder, thus breaking with the prevalent concept before the mid- to late 1800s that manic-depressive insanity explained the functional severe mental illnesses. He communicated his ideas with several textbooks, many with subsequent editions (Table 5.1). For example, his *Clinical Psychiatry: A Textbook for Students and Physicians* that was first published in 1883 and translated to English in 1907 had several editions. He published a book on schizophrenia in 1919 and one on manic-depressive insanity in 1921. Both of these texts are excerpted herein because they convey a striking overlap of symptoms of these two disorders that became accepted as mutually exclusive. The Kraepelinian dichotomy has become a cornerstone of the mental health professions everywhere (Table 2.7). He has been referred to as "… the founder of contemporary scientific Psychiatry" (Wikipedia 2011).

Morel and Kahlbaum may have laid the groundwork for Kraepelin's dichotomy by the mid-1800s as they apparently named and separated dementia praecox from manic-depressive insanity. In 1871, Hecker described hebephrenia as a subtype of dementia praecox (Kraepelin 1919, p. 4), and 8 years later, Kahlbaum added catatonia as a second subtype. In 1893, Kraepelin incorporated the subtypes of hebephrenia and catatonia with his own subtype, "dementia paranoia," that became the most common subtype of schizophrenia, paranoid schizophrenia. According to Angst (2002), "In comparison with Kahlbaum [Kahlbaum's classification system], Kraepelin's terminology was simpler and his comprehensive text much easier to read and understand." From the sixth edition of his textbook, his text on dementia praecox (1919), and his text on manic-depressive insanity (1921), Kraepelin, not Morel, Hecker, or Kahlbaum, gained credit for the dichotomy (Angst 2002).

Kraepelin believed that there were "certain fundamental disturbances" that were common to all three subtypes so that an overriding diagnosis of dementia praecox was warranted. Kraepelin characterized his dementia praecox as had his predecessors, as having an onset in one's youth of a marked deterioration in intellect, personality, emotional life, volition, and social withdrawal. For example, he discussed, "The disintegration of the psychic personality …" with disruption of emotions and of volition which he said, "… dominate the morbid state" in dementia praecox.

It should be noted that disturbances of the emotions and of volition are accepted characteristics of mood disorders, but, as this chapter and Chaps. 6 and 8 will demonstrate, such characteristics were thought to be indicative of dementia praecox or schizophrenia by Kraepelin and others rather than diagnostic of a major depressive disorder or bipolar disorder.

Kraepelin initially differentiated these two disorders based on what he considered differences in longitudinal course, prognosis, and the pattern and severity of current symptoms. According to Kraepelin, the most distinguishing feature of dementia praecox was based on his misconception that only dementia praecox could have a chronic, nonremitting, downhill, psychotic course. Over the past three decades, such symptoms as cognitive decline and chronicity of course have been documented in patients with psychotic mood disorders, especially major depressive disorder, chronic and severe with psychotic features. However, dementia praecox was considered to separate from manic-depressive insanity as the more severe of the two disorders and became predominant as the diagnosis among severely ill mental health patients (Figs. 3.1 and 3.2).

Even as early as 1919, Kraepelin admitted that his "… assertion that this [dementia praecox] is a distinct disease has met with repeated and decided opposition…" (Kraepelin 1919, p. 3). For example, in 1888, Sir Thomas Clouston described a disease that he called "adolescent insanity" or "secondary dementia of adolescence" that encompassed both dementia praecox and manic-depressive insanity. Specht (1905) also believed that the functional psychoses were caused by mood disorders implying that dementia praecox or schizophrenia was redundant to manic-depressive insanity. Kraepelin (1920) later reversed himself on the dichotomy.

Despite his reversal of his dichotomy, unitary ideas were overshadowed by the embracement of Kraepelin's dichotomy by Bleuler, Schneider, the 1978 publication of the Research Diagnostic Criteria (Sptizer et al. 1978), and academic psychiatry. Again, his reversal to question his own dichotomy had little if any influence upon any edition of the DSM or ICD including the draft proposal of the DSM-5 scheduled for publication in 2013. This acceptance of the dichotomy carries the understanding that schizophrenia is bona fide and different from psychotic mood disorders.

As noted below, many of Kraepelin's manic-depressive patients apparently experienced psychotic episodes and chronicity (Kraepelin 1921; Swartz and Shorter 2007, p. 32), but these observations were largely ignored, as were similar prior recordings from several other physicians from as early as 100 BCE (Table 3.1). Even more striking from his 1919 book *Dementia Praecox and Paraphrenia*, reviewed below, is how often Kraepelin cited symptoms, today considered diagnostic of psychotic mania or depression, as diagnostic of dementia praecox, not manic-depressive insanity (Table 5.2) (Kraepelin 1919). After reviewing Kraepelin's two books, *Dementia Praecox and Paraphrenia* (1919) and *Manic-Depressive Insanity and Paranoia* (1921), it is understandable why he reneged on his initial idea that these were separate disorders. The overlap in signs, symptoms, and behaviors is extensive as demonstrated in the case vignettes quoted below from these two books.

Table 5.2 Selected quotes of symptoms Kraepelin assigned to schizophrenia that are diagnostic of mania and depression (Kraepelin 1919)

Quote no.	Page no.	Selected quote	Current author's comment
1	6–7	Kraepelin refers to a defect in attention in schizophrenia: "… a certain unsteadiness of attention … an irresistible attraction of the attention to casual external impressions. The patients involuntarily introduce into their speech words that they have heard, react to each movement of their neighbors, or imitate them."	This defect in attention that Kraepelin assigns to schizophrenia is the same as the distractibility that is diagnostic of mania (see Chaps. 12 and 13).
2	9	Kraepelin assigns auditory hallucinations usually "unpleasant and disturbing" to schizophrenia. He quoted a patient to say, "The voices rushed in on me at all times as burning lions…. The patient is everywhere made a fool of and teased, mocked, grossly abused and threatened. … he hears voices, 'Rascal, vagrant, miserable scoundrel, … good-for-nothing, rogue, thieving murderer … swine, filthy swine, town whore, convict.…'"	"The voices rushed in on me at all times …" is consistent with racing thoughts and flight of ideas diagnostic of mania. The unpleasant and degrading voices are consistent with the auditory hallucinations characteristic of the delusions of sin and punishment of psychotic depression either bipolar or unipolar.
3	10	Kraepelin also assigns auditory hallucinations of "… good wishes, praise …" to schizophrenia: "He hears that he is a King's son, an officer's son, that he is very musical; he has a splendid life …. The voice calls out: 'King, King!, St. Joseph!, I am God … you have already the divine bride.'"	Such auditory hallucinations are grandiose and consistent with psychotic mania.
4	25	Kraepelin assigned poor judgment to schizophrenia. He said that, "… the faculty of judgment in the patient [with schizophrenia] suffers without exception severe injury. … the most nonsensical ideas can be uttered by them and the most incomprehensible actions carried out. … they not infrequently commit the grossest blunders."	Poor judgment is a core symptom of moderate to severe mania.
5	26–27	Kraepelin associated delusions involving ideas of sin and of persecution with schizophrenia. "The patient has by a sinful life destroyed his health of body and mind, he is a wicked fellow, the greatest sinner, … has denied God, scorned the Holy Ghost. …. The devil dwells in him, will fetch him, God has forsaken him, he is eternally lost, is going to hell … he is considered a spy, he is under police control, he is watched by detectives …. People spy on him; … persecute him, poison the atmosphere with poisonous powder, the beer with prussic acid, …. He must die, will be shot, beheaded, poisoned by the state …."	As discussed in Chaps. 12 and 13, delusional ideas of sin and persecution are consistent with psychotic depression.

5.1 Introduction: A Dichotomy Meant Dementia Praecox/Schizophrenia... 67

6	29	Kraepelin believed that exalted ideas were common to schizophrenia. "The patient is 'something better,' born to a higher place, the 'glory of Israel', an inventor, a great singer, ... He is noble, of royal blood, an officer of the dragoons, heir to the throne of Bulgaria; Wilhelm Rex, a Kaiser's son, the greatest man in Germany, ... is the chosen one, the prophet, influenced by the Holy Ghost, guardian angel, second Messiah, Savior of the world, the God, ... more than the Holy Ghost, the Almighty."	Such grandiosity is consistent with psychotic mania.
7	30–31	Kraepelin believed that delusional "sexual ideas [held] a conspicuously large place in the clinical picture of dementia praecox ..." "The patient has committed sin with his step-daughter, with his sister, ... Women feel that they have lost their virtue, that their honor has been tarnished; their father, their clergyman has abused them, their master, the Kaiser comes at night to them. Gentlemen are sent to them for sexual intercourse, someone lies on them every night. They are raped in anesthesia, 'spiritually abused,' are pregnant by a cup of coffee, by a shadow, by the devil."	Hypersexuality is consistent with moderate to severe mania. The ideas of sin and abuse are consistent with psychotic depression.
8	32–33	Kraepelin associated "emotional dullness" with schizophrenia. "Hopes and wishes, cares and anxieties are silent; the patient accepts without emotion dismissal from his post, being brought to the institution, sinking to the life of a vagrant, the management of his own affairs being taken away from him, ... feels ... no satisfaction; he lives one day at a time in a state of apathy."	Such loss of emotion, lack of satisfaction, apathy and a deterioration in life status are consistent with severe depression.
9	34	Kraepelin associates "... the disappearance of delicacy of feeling" to schizophrenia. "The patients have no longer any regard for their surroundings; they do not suit their behaviour to the situation in which they are, they conduct themselves in a free and easy way, laugh on serious occasions, are rude and impertinent towards their superiors, challenge to duels, loose their deportment and personal dignity; they go about in untidy and dirty clothes, unwashed, unkempt, ... speak familiarly to strangers, decorate themselves with gay ribbons. The feeling of disgust and of shame is also lost .... The want of a feeling of shame expresses itself in regardless uncovering of their persons, in making sexual experiences public, in obscene talk in improper advances and in shameless masturbation. ... they make little balls of feces, collect their evacuation in handkerchiefs or cigar boxes, smear themselves with urine, ..."	Such behavior can be consistent with psychotic depression and mania. Coprophilia has been associated with psychotic mood disorders (Chap. 12).

(continued)

Table 5.2 (continued)

Quote no.	Page no.	Selected quote	Current author's comment
10	35	Kraepelin wrote that "… sudden oscillations of emotional equilibrium of extraordinary violence …" were characteristic of schizophrenia. "In particular, sudden outbursts of rage with or without external occasion are not infrequent and can lead to most serious deeds of violence. The patients destroy objects, smash windows,… . A patient stabbed a girl's arm, another killed his master, a third killed a companion by whom he felt himself influenced. On the other hand the patents may suddenly fall into the most unrestrained merriment with uncontrolled laughter, seldomer into states of intense anguish. All these emotions are distinguished by the suddenness of their onset and disappearance and the often quite sudden change of mood."	This description is common to irritable mania and rapid cycling of mood that signifies a disorder of mood rather than any other disorder.
11	37	Kraepelin associated a "… weakening of volitional impulses" to schizophrenia. "The patients have lost every independent inclination for work and action; they sit about idol, trouble themselves about nothing, do not go to their work, neglect their most pressing obligations, although they are perhaps still capable of employing themselves in a reasonable way… they have 'no more joy in work,' but can lie in bed unoccupied for days and weeks…".	Such behavior is characteristic of severe depression, either bipolar or unipolar.
12	49–50	Kraepelin assigned autism to schizophrenia (as did Bleuler), "It is a common experience that the patients with dementia praecox are more or less inaccessible, that they shut themselves off from the outer world. … they do not look up when spoken too, perhaps turn away their head, or turn their back …. The hand offered in greeting is refused. …. Many patients close their eyes, cover their faces with their hands, cover themselves up, draw the bedcover over their head, and convulsively hold it fast;… one notices very distinctly… the resistance which they oppose to any searching into their inner life. Frequently the patients have already shut themselves off from their family and their surroundings … [they] do not appear any more at the common meals, avoid all friendly intercourse, bolt themselves in, take lonely walks. … there is developed the picture of negativistic stupor, the rigid, impenetrable shutting up of themselves from all outer influences."	Such behavior is consistent with major depression, either bipolar or unipolar, that is severe with psychotic features.

| 13 | 56–69 | Kraepelin believed that incoherence of the train of thought was indicative of schizophrenia. "The most different ideas follow one another with most bewildering want of connection even when the patients are quite quiet. ... similarity in sound ... is a certain link in the disconnected utterances of the patients. They rhythm, ... they play senselessly with words and sounds. ... derailments in linguist expression form a specially important domain in the speech disorders of dementia praecox. Vocal speech itself can be changed in the most varied way by side and cross impulses. Patients in speaking, ... often pass suddenly from low whispering to loud screaming. The flow of speech is frequently hurried and rapid ... it was already a case of new unintelligible words ... there may be produced also quite senseless collections of syllables, here and there still having a sound reminiscent of real words. ... the tendency to silly plays on words and neologisms can get the upper hand in our patients to such an extent, that they fall into a wholly incomprehensible gibberish; they usually then give it out as a foreign language ...." | Such incoherence, derailments in linguistic expression, neologisms, etc. are explained by the distractibility of mania accounted for by a defect in the manic brain of selective attention (see Chap. 13). |

5.2 Selected Quotes from *Dementia Praecox and Paraphrenia*, by E. Kraepelin 1919/2002

There are 13 chapters and 331 pages in Kraepelin's book titled *Dementia Praecox and Paraphrenia*, published in 1919. Two hundred eighty-one pages are dedicated to Kraepelin's discussion of dementia praecox, 46 to paraphrenia. In Chap. 2 titled "Psychotic Symptoms," Kraepelin recorded what his patients said, their behaviors, and their activities that he initially believed were diagnostic of dementia praecox or schizophrenia and separated them from manic-depressive insanity or bipolar disorder. Several are reproduced here to demonstrate the overlap of psychotic symptoms with mood symptoms that were considered diagnostic of dementia praecox, not manic-depressive insanity.

Kraepelin referred throughout his book to several core symptoms which he believed were common to all of his subtypes and diagnostic of dementia praecox. These included defects in attention, emotions, volition, train of thought, judgment, personality, hallucinations, delusions, ideas of sin, ideas of persecution, exalted ideas, sexual ideas, ideas of influence and reference, automatic obedience, incoherence, and derailments in linguistic expressions. However, in his next book published 2 years later on manic-depressive insanity (1921), he attributes many of these same signs and symptoms to manic-depressive insanity or bipolar disorder (Table 5.3). For example, under the subheading of "Hallucinations," Kraepelin noted that "… hallucinations of hearing" or "the hearing of voices … are almost never wanting … [in dementia praecox]."

Kraepelin observed that the voices of patients with schizophrenia are:

> … as a rule, unpleasant and disturbing (consistent with symptoms of depression in this author's view).

Kraepelin noted that his patients told him that,

> … someone calls out [to them]: rascal, vagrant, miserable scoundrel … good-for-nothing … anarchist, rogue, thieving murderer, filthy fellow, filthy blockhead, filthy beast, filthy swine, town whore, criminal …. The patient is said to have assaulted a child, seduced a girl … had sexual intercourse with his children …. He is threatened with having his ears cut off, his feet chopped off … with being beheaded; there is a command from the Government to stab him … he must be arrested …. Just come along, and you'll be killed.

As suggested here and throughout Kraepelin's writings, the above quotes are most consistent with psychotic depression with delusions of sin and guilt. Also consistent with depression are the delusions of persecution for the delusional criminal acts, sins, or worthlessness (Table 3.2). This often leads to presenting symptoms of paranoia and the misdiagnosis of paranoid schizophrenia (Lake 2008b).

Kraepelin then states that,

> … there are also frequently "good voices, good wishes, praise" ….
> He hears that he is a King's son, an officer's son, that he is very musical; he has a splendid life; … The voice calls out: "King, King!, Saint Joseph!, I am God;" a dove says at night: "You have already the divine bride."

These quotes exemplify grandiosity that is the hallmark of mania.
Kraepelin thought that,

5.2 Selected Quotes from *Dementia Praecox and Paraphrenia*, by E. Kraepelin...

Table 5.3 Overlap of signs and symptoms between schizophrenia and psychotic mood disorders from two of Kraepelin's books

From *Dementia Praecox and Paraphrenia* (Kraepelin 1919)	From *Manic-Depressive Insanity and Paranoia* (Kraepelin 1921)
Auditory hallucinations (p. 7), either unpleasant (p. 9) or grandiose (p. 10)	Auditory hallucinations, negative, unpleasant, disturbing, or grandiose (p. 21)
Delusions, paranoid (p. 26), persecutory (pp. 26–28), sinfulness (pp. 27, 109, 112), grandiosity (pp. 29–30), hypochondriacal/incurable disease (p. 26), poison (p. 48)	Delusions, paranoid, persecutory (pp. 20, 84, 89–97), grandiosity. Sinfulness (p. 20), evilness (pp. 20–21), incurable illness (p. 19), poison, "Profound confusion and perplexity, also well developed delusions."
Distractibility (pp. 20, 23)	Distractibility (p. 20)
Pressure of activity/persistence of impulse to movement (p. 59), loquacious (p. 97), verbose (p. 98), "many preach..." (p. 115) "Manic pressure of activity, ... often in great excitement ... the flight of ideas ... and the inhibition of will ... [attributed by Kraepelin to his subtype of dementia praecox he called "catatonic raving mania"]" (p. 262)	Pressure of activity, speech (pp. 26–31) [mania is mania, not schizophrenia]
Hypersexuality (pp. 16, 30), sexual excitement (improper talk, violent masturbation) (p. 115)	Hypersexuality (p. 22)
Rage, violence (p. 35), obscene speech (p. 98)	Irritability, rage, fury, violence (pp. 24, 64) [common to psychotic mania]
Poor judgment (pp. 25–26), spending money (p. 97), senseless journeys (p. 98), land in prison (p. 98)	Poor judgment (pp. 26, 27) [common to moderate to severe mania]
Waxy flexibility (pp. 39–41)	Waxy flexibility (pp. 36–37)
Echolalia, echopraxia (p. 39)	Echolalia, echopraxia (p. 36)
Rhyming (pp. 19, 61–62), [clanging and punning currently associated with schizophrenia]	Rhyming, clanging (32–100% of manic patients clang), punning (pp. 31–34, 72)
Mutism (p. 98), apathy (p. 33), indifference (p. 33), avolition (pp. 37, 106–107), negativism (pp. 47–52)	Mutism, indifference, apathy, avolition (pp. 34, 38, 63, 87)
[Blocking associated with schizophrenia]	Blocking [see Chap. 13 in current book]
Ideas of influence/reference (pp. 12–14, 28–29, 31–32)	Ideas of influence/reference (p. 63)
Chronicity of course "... more or less complete remissions ... of a few days or weeks, but also to years and even decades ..." (p. 181)	Chronicity of course (pp. 3, 73, 161); "... in exceptional cases of Manic-Depressive Insanity [there was progression] to a chronic course without further cycling: and with a permanent peculiar psychotic weakness." (p. 3) "... a periodic and circular insanity .... The Duration of manic excitement is also subject to great fluctuations. While occasionally attacks run their course within a few weeks or even a few days, the great majority extend over many months. Attacks of two or three years' duration are very frequent; isolated cases may last considerably longer, for ten years and more." (p. 73)

(continued)

Table 5.3 (continued)

From *Dementia Praecox and Paraphrenia* (Kraepelin 1919)	From *Manic-Depressive Insanity and Paranoia* (Kraepelin 1921)
Depersonalization [associated with schizophrenia]	Depersonalization "… their own body feels as it not belonging to them…" (p. 75)
Age of onset: teens to early adulthood	Age of onset for bipolar disorder: before 20th year (p. 197)
Neologisms (pp. 67–70)	Neologisms [see Chap. 13 in current book]
[Coprophilia, smearing associated with schizophrenia, not bipolar disorder]	Coprophilia (pp. 65, 71)
"Despondent, no joy in life, despair, they weep and lament, would like to die, frequently make attempts at suicide." (p. 106)	[Depression]

> … it is quite specially peculiar to dementia praecox that the patients' own "thoughts appear to them to be spoken aloud."

However, if thoughts that are reported as heard spoken aloud are rational or eccentric, even mentally healthy subjects may be misdiagnosed as having schizophrenia based on saying they "hear voices" when actually they mistake the "voices" for their thoughts. E. Bleuler and K. Schneider were also overinclusive in interpreting schizophrenia based on reports of "hearing voices" even though Schneider warned against misinterpretations by patients of hearing actual voices (Chap. 8).

Kraepelin's next subheading in his text on dementia praecox is "Influence on Thought." He gave as an example that,

> … the patient sometimes "knows the thoughts of other people," is "connected by telephone with M Kinley," can "speak with the Kaiser, tones constantly with God, is in constant communication with the Holy Ghost." [Another] … patient heard the unborn Virgin Mary speak in his belly; another carried God's voice in his heart.

These examples are consistent with the grandiosity of mania rather than a separate disease.

Under the subheading "Sexual Sensations," Kraepelin said that these "… play a considerable role in our [schizophrenic] patients' experiences." As examples, Kraepelin said that,

> At night lustful deeds are committed, …; lustful men approach her.

Hypersexuality has also been identified as a characteristic of mania more so or rather than schizophrenia.

Kraepelin emphasized that orientation and memory were minimally, if disordered at all.

However, "train of thought" and associations "… sooner or later suffer considerably." Kraepelin referred to Bleuler in noting that,

> "… the patients [with schizophrenia] lose in a most striking way the faculty of logical ordering of their trains of thought." Kraepelin discussed these patients', "… irrational associations, omissions; … tendency to indirect associations, tendency to rhyme, … to play with words, …. In certain circumstances the incoherence may go on to complete loss of connection and to confusion. … On the whole, however, we have before us a completely unintelligible and aimless series of words and fragments of thoughts."

The symptom of distractibility causes disorganization of thought and each of the abnormalities of speech noted above and is now considered central to mania (Chap. 13) (Lake 2008a, b).

The next subtopic is "Judgment" where Kraepelin said that the judgment of patients with dementia praecox

> ... suffers without exception severe injury. ... they not infrequently commit the grossest blunders. ... In this respect they resemble dreamers in whom likewise the ability to sift the ideas which come into the mind, to arrange them and to correct them according to the standards gained by former experiences and general ideas is abolished.

These ideas of a defect in sensory gating have been recently discussed in the literature in relationship to psychotic mania, not schizophrenia (Lake 2008a). Poor judgment is an accepted symptom of moderate to severe mania and is given as a diagnostic criterion of mania in the DSM (Table 2.3).

The next heading involves "Delusions, either transitory or permanent, [that] are developed with extraordinary frequency ... created by dementia praecox." Under the heading of "Delusions," Kraepelin listed the subheadings of "Ideas of Sin" immediately followed by "Ideas of Persecution." He said that,

> "These delusions are frequently accompanied by ideas of sin." Such as, "The patient has by a sinful life destroyed his health ..., he is a wicked fellow, the greatest sinner, ... has denied God, scorned the Holy Ghost, ... the devil dwells in him, will fetch him, feels as if the devil wished to take hold of him ... is watched by detectives, ... is to be driven to death." Kraepelin emphasized that, "In connection with these ideas of sin, ideas of persecution are invariably developed in the shaping of which hallucinations of hearing generally play an important part." Kraepelin gave examples that such patients believed that they, "... must die, will be shot, beheaded, poisoned by the State, petroleum is poured over him and set on fire, he comes into the iron maiden, into a vault with toads and broken glass."

This relationship of delusions of sin coupled with ideas of persecution is compatible with psychotic depression as detailed by Swartz and Shorter (2007) as well as Beck (1967, 1972) and Lake (2008a, b). Because the delusional threat to one's life obscures the delusions of sin, the typical chief complaint involves paranoia and fear of punishment or death, and a misdiagnosis of paranoid schizophrenia can be made (Chap. 12).

Kraepelin next addressed "Exalted Ideas":

> In a large number of cases [of dementia praecox] ... are added to the ideas of persecution, sometimes from the beginning, more frequently first in the further course when they often come quite into the foreground of the clinical picture. ... The patient is ... born to a higher place, the "Glory of Israel," an inventor, a great singer, ... He is noble, of royal blood, an officer of the Dragoons, heir to the throne of Bulgaria; Wilhelm Rex, the Kaiser's son, the greatest man in Germany, more than King or Kaiser. ... Or he is the chosen one, the prophet, influenced by the Holy Ghost, guardian angel, second Messiah, Savior of the world, God, ... more than the Holy Ghost, the Almighty. ...conquered death, turned the axis of the earth, can make weather, can walk on the waves. ... will get a great inheritance. ... Female patients are countesses, princesses, queens; they possess the whole world, have the dignity of the Mother of God, get gold-embroidered clothes, children from the Grand Duke and from the Kaiser, will marry the surgeon-major or a prince, their uncle has left [them] millions.

Kraepelin did not address how such grandiosity is diagnostic of mania or how such manic grandiosity can lead to paranoid delusions (Lake 2008a, b).

Kraepelin associated "Sexual Ideas," his next subheading, with dementia praecox rather than mania. He said that sexual ideas have

> "A conspicuously large space in the clinical picture of dementia praecox, ..." Kraepelin linked, the "Ideas of Sin" with sexual ideas. For example, "The patient has committed sin with his step-daughter, with his sister, has had intercourse with cows so that hybrids have been produced; he has committed a crime against decency, has ruined himself by sexual excess, ... is a sadist."

Under his subheading of "Emotion," Kraepelin discussed

> "Very striking and profound damage occurs as a rule in the emotional life of our patients." He emphasized "emotional dullness" in which, "Hopes and wishes, cares and anxieties are silent; ... sinking to the life of a vagrant, the management of his own affairs being taken from him; ... he feels no satisfaction; ... he lives ... in a state of apathy. ... Loss of empathy is shown in indifference."

To these symptoms of depression, which Kraepelin attributed to dementia praecox, he also linked symptoms and behavior consistent with mania. Kraepelin said that,

> One of the most characteristic features of the disease [dementia praecox] is a frequent, sudden outburst of laughter, ... sudden outbursts of rage with or without external occasion and not infrequent and can lead to most serious deeds of violence. The patients destroy objects, smash windows, force open doors, deal out boxes on the ear. A patient stabbed a girl's arm, another killed his master, a third killed a companion by whom he felt himself influenced. On the other hand the patients may suddenly fall into the most unrestrained merriment with uncontrollable laughter, seldomer into states of intense anguish. All these emotions are distinguished by the suddenness of their onset and disappearance and the often quite sudden change of mood. (p. 35)

Rather than any new disease, these descriptions are consistent with cycles of mania and depression (Tables 3.1 and 3.2).

The next two headings by Kraepelin are "Volition" and "Automatic Obedience." Kraepelin commented on the

> ... weakening of volitional impulses. Patients have lost every independent inclination for work and action; they sit about idol ... neglect their most pressing obligations, ... have no more joy in work, but can lie in bed unoccupied for days and weeks ....

Today, such symptoms are recognized as common to depression rather than any other disease.

Kraepelin next addressed "Catatonic Excitement" which now is likely considered manic excitement. Kraepelin said that,

> The patients hop, jump, turn summersaults, scream, grunt, see-saw, drum, screech, go through the movements of ringing, of playing the violin, usually with the expenditure of all of their energy, but without any recognizable aim.

Kraepelin attributed another subheading, "Negativism," to dementia praecox, but the behaviors described are compatible with psychotic depression (Swartz and Shorter 2007).

Under "Incoherence of the train of thought, ...," Kraepelin noted that it

> ... is usually distinctly noticeable in the conversation of the patients.

Incoherence has been associated with the defect in manic processing of incoming stimuli (Chap. 13).

5.2 Selected Quotes from *Dementia Praecox and Paraphrenia*, by E. Kraepelin...

Kraepelin uses examples of patients' writing and drawings to demonstrate incoherence. However, these examples demonstrate an excess of detail, although incomprehensible, that speak to mania. Kraepelin described his patients' behavior as a

> ... persistence of impulse to movement, ... senseless, childish drawings which a patient produced in large numbers daily; there are wonderful combinations of strokes and flourishes with hints of stereotypy. ... there were endless variations of the same recurring fundamental form.
>
> (Kraepelin 1919, pp. 58–61)

Also compatible with manic distractibility, Kraepelin noted that,

> ... the purely outward connection of ideas by the similarity of sound that appears here clearly the persistence in the direction of the thought which is once come into view (mountain, huntsman, cliffs, birdsman, Desuvius and so on).

Kraepelin next discussed "Derailments in Linguistic Expression" and "Neologisms":

> "... disorders in connected speech ...," the use of "... new unintelligible words, ... composed of sensible component parts ..." and "...senseless collections of syllables, here and there still having a sound reminiscent of real words ... ."

The speech of these patients was attributed by Kraepelin to dementia praecox but is consistent with mania. The manic thought processes of distractibility and disorganization may be accounted for by a breakdown of sensory gating mechanisms and would appear to explain these phenomena misattributed to schizophrenia (Chap. 13) (Lake 2008a).

In a brief Chapter III, titled "General Psychic Clinical Picture," Kraepelin organized conclusions drawn from Chapters I and II based on his observations of about "1,000 cases" (Kraepelin 1919, p. 74). He divided dementia praecox into

> "... two principal groups, ... On the one hand we observe a weakening of those emotional activities which permanently form the mainsprings of volition. ... The second group ... consists in the loss of the inner unity of the activities of intellect, emotion and volition in themselves and among one another." Kraepelin further detailed that: "This annihilation presents itself to us in the disorders of association described by Bleuler, in incoherence of the train of thought, in the sharp change of moods as well as in desultoriness and derailments in practical work. ... The patients laugh and weep without recognizable cause, without any relation to their circumstances and their experiences, smile while they narrate the tail of their attempts at suicide; they are very much pleased that they 'chatter so foolishly,' ... on the most insignificant occasions they fall into violent terror or outbursts of rage, and then immediately break out into a neighing laugh." This phenomena has been referred to as an "ataxia of the feelings." (p. 35)

These two divisions initially attributed by Kraepelin to cases of dementia praecox are accounted for by psychotic depression and rapidly cycling or mixed bipolar disorder.

Chapter IV, "Bodily Symptoms," is summarized to demonstrate an absence of a clear understanding of a distinction between organic and functional psychoses early in the twentieth century when Kraepelin and Bleuler published their observations and conclusions. Attributed to schizophrenia were abnormalities of:

> "... behavior of the pupils, tendon reflexes and seizures," encompassing "attacks of vertigo, thinking fits or epileptiform convulsions, ... aphasia, vasomotor disorders, [abnormalities

in] blood-pressure, secretion of saliva, temperature, sleep and food." Kraepelin said that behavior of the pupils was "… of great significance" in dementia praecox and that "… in conditions of excitement, conspicuously wide, …" He said that, "The tendon reflexes are often more or less considerably increased …."

Sympathetic tone is increased in mania. Other physical signs Kraepelin thought were associated with dementia praecox are unrelated to functional psychoses and indicative of organicity. A bona fide seizure disorder may well have explained a small but significant percent of Kraepelin's psychotic patients diagnosed with dementia praecox. Kraepelin described aphasia as: "… disappearing again after a few hours." Kraepelin believed that vasomotor disorders in dementia praecox were:

… very widely spread in our patients. … blood-pressure was as a rule lowered; … the secretion of saliva was frequently increased usually only temporarily, much seldomer permanently; … temperature was usually low. …

Kraepelin was accurate in his description of the disturbance of sleep and in the "taking of food" that he said fluctuated

"… from complete refusal to the greatest voracity. The body-weight usually falls at first often a considerable degree, even to extreme emaciation, …" Kraepelin went on to say that: "Later on the contrary, we may see the weight not infrequently rise quickly in the most extraordinary way …"

Such changes in appetite resulting in weight changes are most likely due to mood cycles in psychotic patients rather than schizophrenia.

Chapter V, "Clinical Forms," is the longest chapter numbering 92 pages. Kraepelin dictated three subtypes of dementia praecox: hebephrenic, catatonic, and paranoid. He stated that this classification was based on:

"… about 500 cases in Heidelberg which had been investigated by myself, …" Kraepelin said that, "Recovered cases were not taken into account because of the uncertainty of their significance … but only such cases as have led to profound dementia or to distinctly marked and permanent phenomena of decreased function."

This exclusion of patients who had "recovered" possibly eliminated milder cases of bipolar disorder. Further complicating the study subjects was the difficulty in differentiating functional from organic psychoses such as that secondary to alcohol dependence, epilepsy, general paresis of the insane, as well as other organic disorders which may not have been appreciated at that time.

Under the subheading of "Silly Dementia" or hebephrenia (now called disorganized schizophrenia), Kraepelin referenced Hecker who described this group of patients as initially having "… an introductory stage of melancholy, [but then] a stage of mania develops and rapidly makes room for a quite peculiar weak-minded condition." Thus, the subtype of schizophrenia called hebephrenia, even in the nineteenth century, appeared to encompass the cycles between depression and mania, diagnostic of bipolar disorder rather than schizophrenia. Hecker and Kraepelin also recognized the potential for a later onset of a chronic, persistently dysfunctional course that they misattributed to dementia praecox rather than a chronic, psychotic mood disorder. Kraepelin further discussed the delusions of this subgroup noting that during:

> ... passing states of depression ... The patients are dispirited and dejected, they think they are syphilitic, ... they have a feeling of oppression in their brain, ... the disease is in all their limbs. ... [they] are damned, have committed sins, are said to have killed someone; they wish to make confession, read the Bible zealously, search out clergymen. ... People are ... persecuting [him] ... giving him poison in his food, assaulting him at night ... He must be slaughtered, ... broken on the wheel. Thoughts of suicide often rise to the surface; a patient thought he would have liked to kill his child in order that it might not be so unhappy as himself.

This description is consistent with psychotic depression. A psychotically depressed parent killing children to spare them "from this hell on earth" is a tragedy that continues to occur with some frequency (Sects. 15.5 and 15.6).

Kraepelin's next subheading under his subtype of dementia praecox called "hebephrenia" is "Exalted Ideas." His descriptions of such patients are diagnostic of mania and bipolar disorder rather than any other disease such as schizophrenia. For example, he described the exalted ideas of patients he diagnosed with hebephrenic schizophrenia:

> "A patient hopes to become 'a general with 250 marks yearly income;' a female patient ... declares that she was the Empress Augusta. ... They cannot any longer manage money; they make aimless purchases, give away and squander their property; ... A poor patient fooled away an inheritance of 5,000 marks within two years; ... Many patients fall into drinking habits and in this way come down in the world with remarkable rapidity. ... they wear conspicuous clothing, tie cigar ribbons in their button-hole, stick paper in their ears ... a lawyer bound flowers onto his stick and umbrella, hung a garland round his neck, stuck brooches and pictures on himself, ... The patients ... play the harmonica at night, ... burn their own hair and beard and those of other people with their cigar, cut up their linen and clothing; they destroy the furniture and throw it about; ... make senseless journeys, often without money and without a ticket, want to get into the Castle, to go to America; a patient wandered for days in the forest without food. They are very changeable in their behavior, at times ... irritable, flaring up easily, at one moment loquacious and verbose, at another taciturn and mute. ... Their mode of speech is ... sometimes noisy or purposely obscene. The substance of their conversation is often confused and unintelligible. ... they easily become vagrants, beg, commit small thefts and land in this way in prison ..." Kraepelin said that, "Nearly a quarter of my male patients met this fate [of incarceration]."

The descriptions above are diagnostic of mania, and Kraepelin's high rate of incarceration is compatible with figures today for patients with bipolar disorder.

Kraepelin discussed other clinical forms of his dementia praecox that he called "simple depressive dementia," "delusional depressive dementia," "circular dementia," "agitated dementia," "periodic dementia," "catatonia," and the "paranoid dementias." His descriptions of these clinical forms were redundant with the descriptions just given. For example, under the headings "Hallucinations" and "Delusions," Kraepelin stated that,

> The voices torment them all day long, reproach them that they have lived an immoral life, that they have committed a moral offense ... that they are wanted by the police ... should have a sound thrashing ... be executed, slaughtered ....
>
> Very frequently there are also ideas of sin .... He is a wicked fellow, ... has told lies and committed theft, ... has killed his children, has said something about the Kaiser ... everyone has died on his account. He is the last Judas, is rejected, is damned for time and eternity, is the Anti-Christ, cannot be saved, is to vow allegiance to Satan; his children are in hell ... he must die for the sins of the world.

> Not less various are the ideas of persecution that are developed. ... They are watched, starred at, spied on ... chloroformed, hunted like a wild animal in flight. ... the policemen are coming to drag them to court ... there are serpents in their bed ... hellish spirits are threatening. ... The patient is murdered, executed, burned ... dissected alive, trampled by a horse.
>
> In a number of cases exalted ideas are present also, mostly for the first time in a more advanced period. The patient will be rich, ... get a situation on the railroad of the Grand Duke, ... possesses needs to make people omniscient, has the "imperial attack," .... An inheritance of 1,000,000 is being kept back for him; ... his father is a Count, Prince of Leiningen, the Grand Duke, the Emperor Fredrick; he himself is a millionaire, Prince of Hesse, possesses a third part of the world; ... is the Vicar of Christ, the son of Almighty God, ... lives eternally; the spirit goes forth from him; .... Women are the bride of a gentleman in a white suit, ... they are countesses, angels, mother of the world, the bride of Christ, their sons are princes ....
>
> Mood is at first anxious and depressed. The patients mourn, ... they break out into convulsions of weeping, ... Very frequently ideas of suicide come to the surface; the patients beg that ... they should be killed ... they should be beheaded .... Many patients also make attempts at suicide .... Not at all infrequently exalted moods are interpolated in the periods of anguish, giggling, grinning and laughing, especially in the further course of the malady; also states of irritated excitement, outbursts of obscene abuse, and sudden dangerous assaults on the surroundings often occur. ... Sexual excitement is expressed by undressing, ... improper talk, violent masturbation, ...

These hallucinations and delusions are mood congruent with mania and/or depression suggesting the diagnosis of a psychotic mood disorder rather than any other psychotic disorder.

Kraepelin described the course of his "circular dementia [praecox]" as follows:

> The course of the disease, which in general progresses from depression to excitement to a terminal state, was interrupted in 53% of the cases by periods of considerable improvement, in nearly 14% even several times. These remissions lasted in the half of the patients concerned up to three years, in the other half up to ten years. In 70% of the cases the improvement was interpolated after the preliminary depression; several times periods of depression preceded, separating by more lucid intervals. After the improvement, the disease then generally continued with a state of excitement leading to dementia; less frequently a state of depression was again interpolated and the first excitement followed. ... Seizures occurred in one-fifth of the patients.

This description is typical of cycles of bipolar disorder. Apparently, 20% of patients that Kraepelin diagnosed with dementia praecox actually suffered from a seizure disorder that could have accounted for all of the symptoms used to diagnose dementia praecox.

Later in this same chapter, Kraepelin continued with a description of the course of his patients that he diagnosed with dementia praecox. At that time, a course of "progressive dementia" was incorrectly thought to rule out bipolar disorder. Kraepelin said,

> The recurrence of the disease occurs usually with fresh states of excitement, somewhat seldomer in the form of progressive dementia, now and then also perhaps with a state of depression to which excitement may again follow, terminating in dementia. When there are repeated remissions of the disease, the states of excitement may return more frequently.

The "progressive dementia" described by Kraepelin and attributed by him to dementia praecox is compatible with a chronic psychotic mood disorder characterized by the onset of a chronic, persistent, treatment-resistant, psychotic dysfunctionality that can replace a classic, cycling course of either bipolar or unipolar disorder. Such a change in course can be marked by avolition, social withdrawal, poverty of thought, emotional dullness, and depression.

5.2 Selected Quotes from *Dementia Praecox and Paraphrenia*, by E. Kraepelin...

Kraepelin said that, "The outbreak of the disease occurred in two thirds of my cases before the 20th year, sometimes at 14 years of age," consistent with today's estimated average age of onset of bipolar disorder and an increasing recognition of bipolar disorder in children and adolescents.

Under the subtype of dementia praecox Kraepelin called "periodic dementia," he described,

> ... intervals often [of a] very few weeks, sometimes only once a year, [in which] confused states of excitement appear which run a rapid course. In the female sex they are frequently connected with the menstrual periods .... After, at most, slight indications of the commencing attack, [it can] cause less laughter, ... wandering about, ... there is developed from one day to another, often in the middle of the night, the picture of maniacal excitement. Sometimes it is limited to heightened irritability, change of mood ... incessant chatter; but gradually the excitement becomes worse, going on even to raving mania of the most severe type, often with delusions and hallucinations. The body weight invariably decreases rapidly, sometimes as much as five to eight pounds in 24 hours. ... The excitement often lasts only a few days or weeks, more rarely it continues for months and then is interrupted by only a few quiet days. Usually the intervals are somewhat longer, a few weeks or months. In course of time the duration of the attacks may be extended. ... In a small number of cases there may finally be developed a quite regular alternation lasting for decades between short periods of the most severe excitement and of quietness. ... But it invariably comes to the development of marked psychic decline which sometimes has more the features of a simple weak-mindedness with poverty of thought, lack of judgment, emotional dullness and weakness of volition, sometimes is accompanied by incoherence and affectation.

Kraepelin then stated that:

> "Formally I regarded these forms as belonging to manic-depressive insanity." However he concluded that: "... the states of excitement themselves, with their monotony, impulsive character, and poverty of thought, resemble much more those of dementia praecox than those of mania. Again the circumstance might be pointed out, that periodic states of excitement are also otherwise very frequent in dementia praecox."

Kraepelin began to have more questions about his idea of clear differences between dementia praecox or schizophrenia and manic-depressive insanity or bipolar disorder. His final opinion was that there are no clear differences between patients diagnosed with schizophrenia versus psychotic bipolar disorder or major depressive disorders. Today, the description above is certainly considered typical if not diagnostic of bipolar disorder even with the worsening and increased frequency of attacks with recurring episodes (Fig. 4.1).

Under the subtype of "catatonia," Kraepelin refers to Kahlbaum and states that:

> The really characteristic pictures of the state are rather the "mania" of Kahlbaum, which today we more correctly name [dementia praecox] catatonic excitement and stupor. I think, therefore, that I may group together as catatonic forms of dementia praecox those cases in which the conjunction of peculiar excitement with catatonic stupor dominates the clinical picture. ... In 47% of the cases a state of depression forms the introduction; ... The patients become reserved, shy, introverted, absent-minded, distracted, indifferent, irritable, taciturn; they stand about, carry on unintelligible conversations, pray, go often to church, get up at night, eat and sleep badly. ... They have evil thoughts, feel themselves lost and abandoned, proscribed. They feel uneasy, as if someone were persecuting them; their life is no longer of any value; everything has turned out badly; no one can help them. ... they are to be taken to the convict prison, condemned to death, slaughtered, buckled onto the railway; ... people are coming to fetch them; their daughter is being murdered; their children are going to the scaffold. ...

Their food is poisoned, ... poison is being blown on them; ... The patient is more wicked than Judas ... has nailed the Savior to the Cross, murdered his children, ... the devil is hiding in him; he wishes to do penance. ... they ... do not want to be killed. ... Here and there ideas of exaltation appear beside those of depression. The patient is ... King of Hungry, a great athlete, will go to Vienna and there become Kaiser, inherits money from his fiancée, gets 60,000 marks from God ... is the Emperor/angel ... wants milk from angels. Female patients are "Queen on the Rhine," "Heaven's child," become engaged to the Kaiser, wish to marry Jesus, an officer, have a secret love affair, are pregnant, possess castles, 10 millions. ... After the introductory depression there usually next follows a state of stupor especially in men, and then excitement; more rarely it is the other way. ... The patients become restless, sleepless, run about, ... their actions are impulsive and aimless, and they fall more or less rapidly into severe excitement; sometimes raving mania may break out quite suddenly, ... Mood is usually exalted. The patients laugh, try to be witty, make jokes, tease other patients, boast, carry on unrestrained conversations; here and there religious ecstasy is observed. But very frequently the patients are also irritated, angry, threatening; they break out into wild abuse, fly into a passion on the slightest occasion, make dangerous attacks without consideration. ... Many patients laugh and weep confusedly, and sing merry couplets amid tears. Very frequently there is extreme sexual excitement, which is made known by ... shameless utterances, movements of coitus, regardless exposure and masturbation. A female patient tore her chemises down the front; others grasp at the genitals of the physicians; ... During the menses the states of excitement usually grow worse. ... The irritable mood leads to sudden deeds of violence, megalomania, to the squandering and giving away of their goods ... the exalted mood [can lead] to wonderful decorations. ... In more severe excitement the activities of the patients are resolved into a disordered series of unconnected and unrelated impulses. They dart through the room with arms stretched out in front of them, slide on the polished floor, run violently up and down or round about in small circles. ... Others lie down on their belly and carry out swimming movements, glide, roll about on the floor, frisk about, hop, stamp with their feet ...

Compatible with current data showing that "catatonia" is most frequently associated with a psychotic mood disorder, Kraepelin's descriptions of his catatonic dementia praecox patients are suggestive if not pathognomonic of a classic psychotic bipolar disorder.

Under Kraepelin's subheading "The Paranoid Dementias," he described,

...the essential morbid symptoms of which are delusions and hallucinations; we call them paranoid forms.

Kraepelin discussed these patients' delusions stating that:

Gradually there come "forebodings," "things come to light." ... The patient acquires the conviction that he has very powerful enemies and is threatened with frightful danger. People want to behead him, ... to crush, to burn him, to throw him to wild animals; sparrows, rats, dogs with goats' hoofs are called out against him. ... He is going to be brought before a secret military tribunal, is being treated as a political prisoner; ... There is poison in the beer, soap in the drinking water, morphia, hydrochloric acid, iodine in the food; ... Female patients hear "immoral stuff," sexual accusations; forest-whore, married man's whore, strolling whore; ... A patient heard that he was God. ... The patients feel themselves used sexually from behind; ... Women are ... violated at night, turned into whores ... The physician has given them desire in their bath; ... At night there are 17 or 18 gentlemen in their bed; the hospital is a brothel; ... The patient has supernatural gifts, has made important inventions, ... he possesses numerous patents, a factory, a hospital, a country, all kingdoms belong to him. He has money in the safe, has great riches, ... he has a claim to 32 millions, which have been deposited for him by Rothschild and the Shah of Persia; ... The ideas of persecution lead to violent outbursts of rage and dangerous attacks on these supposed

5.2 Selected Quotes from *Dementia Praecox and Paraphrenia*, by E. Kraepelin...

> enemies. A patient threatened a clergyman that he would shoot him; ... A female patient wished to cut her father's throat, another suffocated her friend, ... a fourth hit her husband on his head with an ax "in order to redeem him." ... The motives of these attacks are often very obscure. A patient felt himself suddenly forced to injure his sister with whom he was on good terms, went up to her on the road and stabbed her in the back. ... Ideas of poisoning may lead to refusal of food; ... a female patient for a considerable time only ate eggs; one patient only drank milk; another spat a great deal in order to get rid of the poison again. Many patients suddenly fling their food away, because it appears suspicious to them. Occasionally it comes also to attempts at suicide; a patient tried to remove his testicles by ligature; a female patient swallowed needles. ... Sexual excitement causes the patients to commit dissolute acts, to decide to be divorced, to make an attempt to approach any wholly unknown person whatever of the opposite sex, and to commit immoral acts on children.

The descriptions above that Kraepelin gave of his patients diagnosed with dementia praecox or schizophrenia would today warrant the diagnosis of bipolar disorder. Grandiosity, hyperactivity, hypersexuality, nihilistic ideation, expectations of punishment, weight loss, indifference, insomnia, and suicidality are symptoms of mood disorders. The presence of seizures in 20% of his patients diagnosed with dementia praecox raises a question as to an organic source of their psychotic behavior and their diagnoses. In Chap. 12 of the current work, similar case vignettes are given that explain how delusions of grandiosity and of guilt and sin in psychotic mood disorder patients lead to delusional paranoia.

Chapter VI is titled "Course and Remissions." Kraepelin stated that,

> The general course of dementia praecox is very variable. On the one hand there are cases which very slowly and insidiously bring about a change in the personality, ... On the other hand the malady may without noticeable prodromata suddenly break out, ... In the majority of cases ... a certain terminal state with unmistakable symptoms of weak-mindedness is usually reached at the latest in the course of about two to three years. ... The fact is of great significance that the course of the disease, as we have seen is frequently interrupted by more or less complete remissions of the morbid phenomena; the duration of these may amount to a few days or weeks, but also to years and even decades and then give way to a fresh exacerbation with terminal dementia. ... The beginning of the improvement takes place as a rule very gradually. The excited patients become quiet; the stuporous, more accessible and less restrained; delusions and hallucinations become less vivid; the need for occupation and for taking up again of former relationships becomes active. At the same time sleep, appetite, and body-weight usually improve considerably.

The above descriptions of course remissions and relapses are inconsistent with the attribution of academic psychiatry that Kraepelin differentiated dementia praecox from manic-depressive insanity based on a chronic, persistent, dysfunctional course. At least Kraepelin documented that he changed his mind; Bleuler did not and was convinced that chronicity of course and psychosis mandated the diagnosis of schizophrenia (Chap. 6). In 1933, Kasanin recognized that a cycling course with remissions was incompatible with Bleuler's concept of schizophrenia (Chap. 7).

In Chapter VII, titled "Issue-Terminal States," Kraepelin discussed recovery. His observations were that: "... about 8%" of patients he diagnosed with hebephrenic schizophrenia recovered, about 13% of those he diagnosed with catatonic schizophrenia recovered, and there was no recovery in the paranoid subtype of dementia praecox. No recovery in patients diagnosed with paranoid schizophrenia is inconsistent with current thought since this subtype may have the best prognosis for periods of recovery compared to the other subtypes of schizophrenia. Kraepelin quoted other authors of the day who reported a range of recovery from zero to one third. It should be noted that it is likely that some of the cases diagnosed as having dementia praecox or schizophrenia in the early 1900s included patients with unrecognized organic causes of their psychoses and a downhill course of cognitive and personality decline without symptoms of a mood disorder. Possible examples of such organic diseases are dementia, alcoholism, general paresis of the insane, toxins, space-occupying brain lesions, and seizure disorders (Chap. 14). Kraepelin described his patients who did not recover as suffering from a "weakness of judgment" that he described as an absence of insight or understanding of their cognitive defects and a diminished ability to function in work, family, and social roles. He said a

> "... lack of deep emotion, however, is the characteristic feature. The patients regard with indifference the events of life, live a day at a time without endeavor, without wishes, without hopes or fears." He said that the "... outward conduct of the patients is in general reasonable; only they often exhibit a stiff, constrained demeanor or a somewhat odd behavior, singular clothing, neglect of their person, small peculiarities in speech, gate and movement." Kraepelin used the term "cured with defect."

These descriptions can fit various forms of dementia as well as advanced cases of bipolar disorder observed by Carlson and Goodwin (1973), Goodwin (1989), Post (1992, 2010), Goodwin and Jamison (1990, 2007), Swartz and Shorter (2007), and Lake (2008a, b), when patients with initial classic, cycling bipolar deteriorate into a noncycling, dysfunctional, cognitively impaired, perpetually psychotically depressed, downhill course. Such a state in the early 1900s and before was referred to as a "terminal dementia."

Again suggestive of some confusion between organic and functional disease, Kraepelin used various terms for subtypes of dementia, such as "driveling, dull, silly, manneristic and negativistic," to characterize a potential end stage of his dementia praecox. Even here, Kraepelin described the mood of "silly dementia" as impulsive:

> ... invariably confident and cheerful, more rarely and only temporarily depressed and lachrymose. But for the most part the patients are easily excited and fall suddenly into lively agitation or into quickly passing outbursts of rage, sometimes with periodic return.

In Chapter IX titled "Frequency and Causes," Kraepelin stated that, "Dementia Praecox is without doubt one of the most frequent of all forms of insanity." Kraepelin estimated that between 10% and 80% of mental hospital admissions suffered from dementia praecox. Undoubtedly, at least in this author's opinion, around 1900, a significant percent of such patients diagnosed with dementia praecox or schizophrenia actually suffered from an unrecognized organic disorder or a chronic psychotic mood disorder.

Chapter XI is titled "Diagnosis." Kraepelin discussed distinguishing dementia praecox from imbecility, idiocy, alcoholism, epilepsy, "paralysis," infections, and cerebral syphilis. Kraepelin said that the differential diagnosis between schizophrenia and manic-depressive insanity was difficult.

> By far the most important point in diagnosis, but at the same time also the most difficult, is the distinguishing of dementia praecox from isolated attacks of Manic-Depressive Insanity. ... Opinions still differ widely as to whether here greater weight must be attributed to the catatonic or to the circular symptoms for the classification of the case.

5.2 Selected Quotes from *Dementia Praecox and Paraphrenia*, by E. Kraepelin...

This statement expresses one of the core issues of the current book, that is, the weight given in diagnostics to the psychotic symptoms and chronic unremitting course versus episodes of cycling symptoms accepted as diagnostic of mania and/or depression. Academic psychiatry, especially in the USA, heavily weighted the former and therefore the diagnosis of schizophrenia despite the presence of symptoms of mania and depression. The idea that "a touch of Schizophrenia [psychotic symptoms such as hallucinations and delusions] means Schizophrenia [despite mood symptoms]" dominated world psychiatry and especially that in the USA.

Kraepelin attributed "Manic pressure of activity, ... often in great excitement ...; the flight of ideas ... [and] the inhibition of will ..." to "catatonic raving mania," a subtype of his dementia praecox. Kraepelin referred to "intrapsychic ataxia," the lack of "inner-logical arrangement" of thoughts and ideas as diagnostic of dementia praecox, not mania. Kraepelin quoted Bornstein who attributed "clang associations" with mania. This is a curious attribution since clang associations subsequently became associated with schizophrenia and not mood disorders. Kraepelin said that in the "depressive forms [of dementia praecox], the early appearance of numerous hallucinations of hearing and of nonsensical delusions, in particular the idea of influence on will, makes dementia praecox probable, ... hallucinations of hearing are in Manic-Depressive Insanity much rarer ...."

Despite Kraepelin's emphasis on the necessity to observe the long-term course of a patient in order to make the correct diagnosis, he discussed his ability to make a diagnosis upon greeting the patient. Kraepelin said:

> Even the behavior at the approach and greeting of the physician permits certain conclusions [about diagnosis] to be made. The negativistic patient [with dementia praecox] does not look up, hides himself, perhaps turns away or stares straight in front of him, and does not portray by any movement of muscle that he is aware of anything. All the same he usually perceives better than the manic-depressive patient, who indeed also perhaps remains mute and motionless, but still in his glance, in the expression of his face, in slight attempts at movement, acceleration of the pulse, flushing, stoppage of respiration, lets it be seen that he has felt the impressions. ... For distinguishing the states of excitement of dementia praecox from manic seizures, it must first be noticed, that the faculty of perception and ordinary sense are usually more severely injured in mania than in the former. ... Not infrequently we meet in the excitement of dementia praecox a striking want of relation between pressure of speech and pressure of movement, ... The patients [with dementia praecox] may be in violent movement without at the same time saying a word, or they chatter incessantly without moving from the spot and even without lively gestures. ... the manic on the contrary seeks everywhere for the opportunity to occupy himself, runs about, busies himself with the other patients, follows the physician, carries on all sorts of mischievous tricks. In other words, in mania, perception, thought, orientation, are relatively more profoundly disordered than in the excitement of dementia praecox, while in the latter it is especially emotions, actions and speech expression which are injured in a peculiar way. Special difficulties in the differentiation, ... are presented by the mixed states of manic-depressive insanity. ... The content of the delusions offers in general few effective points for the differentiation of the two diseases here discussed. Delusions of sin, ideas of persecution, ... may in both [schizophrenia and bipolar] appear in very similar forms. ... The delusion of physical, especially sexual, influence points with great probability, the idea of influence on thoughts and will almost certainly, to dementia praecox. ... exalted ideas are connected with the delusion of influence on will and perhaps persistent vivid hallucinations of hearing ... the assumption of dementia praecox will be justified. ... Sudden and abrupt change of

the states, as also shortness and irregularity of attacks and intervals, especially with more frequent recovery, will arouse rather the suspicion of dementia praecox. … the persistence of those peculiarities [in action and behavior] … allows the conclusion to be made that dementia praecox is present, ….

Kraepelin did say that "On the other hand I have still doubts of all kinds."

Most of the symptoms given above that Kraepelin attributes to dementia praecox, such as "pressure of movement or speech, … excitement, … delusions of sin, … ideas of persecution, … sexual delusions, … sudden and abrupt changes of the states [depression and mania], … shortness and irregularity of attacks and intervals and more frequent recovery" are now considered indicative of a psychotic mood disorder. Also incongruent with attributions to Kraepelin is his statement that, "… the faculty of perception and ordinary sense are usually more severely injured in mania than in [dementia praecox] …."

In this chapter, Kraepelin gave a hint to his subsequent reversal of his dichotomy when he said,

As little as we can doubt that here we have to keep separate two morbid processes quite different in their character, and as simple as the delimitation is in the great majority of cases, just as insufficient do our distinguishing characteristics yet appear in those cases in which we have before us a mingling of morbid symptoms of both psychoses.

Chapter XII titled, "How to Combat It," also allows critical assessment of the state of clinical understanding and expertise at the time regarding these disorders. Treatments for dementia praecox discussed in this chapter include bilateral castration, immunization with

"… sensitized goat's serum" or "dead bouillon cultures," "partial excision of the thyroid gland." "Rest in bed, supervision, care for sleep and food, … prolonged baths, … moist warm packs and tube feeding" when necessary. Kraepelin emphasized that, "frequent weighing is here indispensible. Likewise the regular evacuation of the bowels has to be kept in mind, and because of the negativistic retention of urine, which sometimes occurs, of the bladder as well." Kraepelin recognized that, "Not all together infrequently one sees the psychotic condition of the patients essentially improve under the influence of a fever, even in terminal states which have already lasted a long time without change."

This last observation of improvement "under the influence of a fever" suggests an infective etiology for the psychosis and not schizophrenia or bipolar disorder.

In Chapter XIII titled, "Paraphrenia," Kraepelin essentially differentiates what is now called delusional disorder and paranoid personality disorder from patients diagnosed with paranoid schizophrenia. In differentiating paranoid schizophrenia, Kraepelin emphasized the "disintegration of the psychic personality [that] is in general accomplished in dementia praecox in such a way that in the first place the disorders of emotions and of volition dominate the morbid state." Kraepelin's association of "disorders of emotions and volition" to dementia praecox or schizophrenia speaks to the bias of diagnosing schizophrenia over mood disorders since "disorders of emotion and volition" are core to mood disorders. Further, Kraepelin believed that a high percentage of patients initially diagnosed with "paraphrenia" and who did not initially demonstrate global dysfunctionality eventually did deteriorate and warranted the diagnosis of dementia praecox.

According to Kraepelin, hyperactivity, grandiose or erotic delusions, depressed mood, despair, delusions of sinfulness, and social withdrawal should not lead to diagnoses of mania or depression in psychotic patients but rather to diagnoses of schizophrenia. Again, Kraepelin's descriptions of such patients are entirely compatible with diagnosis of mania or depression.

For example, Kraepelin recorded the behavior of patients he diagnosed with paraphrenia and paranoid schizophrenia as follows:

> After being ill for some years a woman directed a letter to the Emperor with the inquiry how she could be rid of her husband; later she praised her own brilliant talk, her voice clear as a bell, her fine tact, her high endowment. ... Very commonly the patients make claims to money. From some source or another large sums should come to them which are being kept back; they have been left an inheritance which has been suppressed. ... another [female patient] was convinced that an Arch Duke had settled some money on her for their marriage. ... In a further group of cases it is an affair of erotic relations with highly-placed persons. ... A Duke made known to a female patient by hypnotic waves that he wished intercourse with her. ... Another female patient wrote letters to a man, already married, with the address, "Peter the Great of Russia, Incognito" and then made complaints at the post office that the letters were not dispatched. ... In a small number of cases the exalted ideas acquire a somewhat religious content, ... The patient is sent by God, ... A female patient declared that she was a saint, ... could read the hearts of men, ... another was called the bride of Christ.

The symptoms of other patients or these same grandiose patients as noted above but at different stages are compatible with depression. For example,

> Mood is at first for the most part anxious, depressed, even despairing, but then becomes more and more suspicious, strained, hostile, threatening. Later, when the exalted ideas come more distinctly into the foreground, the patients become self-conscience, haughty, scornful. They withdraw themselves from those round them, avoid intercourse, ... go lonely ways, ... shut themselves up and become gloomy and taciturn ...

5.3 Selected Quotes from *Manic-Depressive Insanity and Paranoia*, by E. Kraepelin 1921/1976

The editor's preface by Dr. George M. Robertson, at the University of Edinburgh stated that, "Professor Kraepelin's account of Manic-Depressive Insanity, co-joined with that of dementia praecox, forms probably his greatest achievement in psychiatry."

In Chapter I titled "Definition," Kraepelin described a "periodic and circular insanity" that included mania and melancholia. He said he was convinced that this condition was

> "... a single morbid process ... that all the morbid forms brought together here as a clinical entity, not only pass over the one into the other without recognizable boundaries, but that they may even replace each other in one in the same case." Kraepelin accurately observed that: "... we see in the same patient not only mania and melancholia, but also states of the most profound confusion and perplexity, also well developed delusions ... There are indeed slight and severe attacks which may be of long or of short duration but they alternate irregularly in the same case."

"… the attacks of manic-depressive insanity … never lead to profound dementia, not even when they continue throughout life almost without interruption. Usually all morbid manifestations completely disappear; but where that is exceptionally not the case, only a rather slight, peculiar psychic weakness develops …" Kraepelin distinguished, "… all manic states with the essential morbid symptoms of flight of ideas, exalted mood, pressure of activity, and melancholia or depressive states with sad or anxious moodiness and also sluggishness of thought and action." He also described, "… mixed forms, in which the phenomena of mania and melancholia are combined with each other …."

Kraepelin later seemed to contradict himself about manic-depressive insanity, "… never lead[ing] to profound dementia," saying that, "… only in exceptional cases of Manic-Depressive Insanity was the course chronic without further cycling: and with a permanent peculiar psychotic weakness." He later acknowledged that, "Many patients remain permanently quiet, depressed, uninterested, stand about in corners…" (see below).

In Chapter II titled "Psychotic Symptoms," Kraepelin discussed all of the symptoms currently given as diagnostic in the ICD and the DSM. He discussed an

Extraordinary distractibility of attention … [as] an essential part in defective perception. The patients gradually loose the capacity for the choice and arrangement of impressions; each striking sense-stimulus obtrudes itself on them with a certain force, so that they usually attend to it at once. Accordingly, if their attention can for the most part be quickly attracted by the exhibition of objects or by the calling out of words, yet it digresses again with uncommon ease to any fresh stimulus.

Kraepelin continued later in this chapter in discussing,

The Train of Ideas of our patients … [when] in states of excitement they are not able to follow systematically a definite train of thought, but they continually jump from one series of ideas to a wholly different one and then let this one drop again immediately. Any question directed to them is at first perhaps answered quite correctly, but with that are associated a great many side remarks which have only a very loose connection, or soon none at all, with the original subject.

Here Kraepelin associates loose associations and thought blocking (no connections between thoughts) with mania, but the ideas of Bleuler influenced academic psychiatry to interpret these signs as indicative of schizophrenia, not bipolar disorder.

Kraepelin discussed as part of this manic syndrome a

… confusion with flight of ideas … [when] they complain that they cannot concentrate or gather their thoughts together. The thoughts come of themselves, obtrude themselves, impose upon the patients. "I can't grasp all the thoughts which obtrude themselves," said a patient. … "I am not master over my thoughts, … One thought chases the other; they just vanish like that," …

Kraepelin also discussed an "Inhibition of Thought" that he said:

… appears to form the exact opposite to flight of ideas. It is observed, … almost everywhere in depression …

5.3 Selected Quotes from *Manic-Depressive Insanity and Paranoia*, by E. Kraepelin...

Later in this chapter, in association with mania, Kraepelin detailed the symptoms today considered typical of mania: pressure of activity and pressure of speech. Kraepelin said that,

> By far the most striking disorders in manic-depressive insanity are found in the realm of volition and action. ... Every chance impulse seems to lead forthwith to action, while the normal individual usually suppresses innumerable volitional impulses immediately as they arise. ... The patients make all sorts of plans, wish to train as singers, to write a comedy; they send suggestions for reform to the police magistrate or to the railway managers; ... they start senseless businesses, buy houses, clothes, hats, give large orders, make debts; they wish to set up an observatory, they go to America ... they make plans of marriage, enter into doubtful acquaintanceships, kiss strange ladies on the streets, frequent public houses, commit all possible acts of debauchery. ... While they appear in company as jovial fellows, give large tips, ... they quarrel with their superiors, neglect their duty, give up their situations for trifling causes, leave the public houses without paying. ... in very severe excitement ... the patients ... roll about on the floor, hop, bellow, turn summersaults, beat rhythmically on the mattress, throw their legs about, ... behave convulsively, ... spit and bite about them.

This description of mania is strikingly similar to that given in Kraepelin's description of his patients diagnosed with dementia praecox (Sect. 5.2; Table 5.3).

Kraepelin continued to describe his manic patients in keeping with current concepts:

> Pressure of Speech, which is often very marked in the patients, ... as corresponding sounds and rhymes, usurp more and more the place of the substantive connection of ideas. ... the pure clang-associations, in which every trace of an inner-relation of ideas has vanished, ... rhymes, even though quite senseless, gain more and more the upper hand.

Kraepelin presented a graph, his Figure 7, on page 32 of his book, indicating that manic patients use "clang associations" about 6–50 times more frequently than normal (Kraepelin 1921). Despite this association of "clang associations" with mania, psychiatry subsequently attributed such to schizophrenia until recently (Lake 2008a, b). Kraepelin described pressure of speech and flight of ideas:

> He cannot be silent for long; he talks and screams in a loud voice, makes a noise, bellows, howls, whistles, is over-hasty in speech, strings together disconnected sentences, words, syllables, mixes up different languages, preaches with solemn intonation and passionate gestures, ... threats, ... and obscenity, or suddenly coming to an end in unrestrained laughter. ... talking in self-invented languages which consist partly of senseless syllables, partly of strangely clipped and mutilated words. Among these are interpolated quotations, silly puns, poetical expressions, vigorous abuse.

Of note is that Kraepelin associated clang associations, rhyming, punning, and delusional preaching with both schizophrenia and mania. Also in schizophrenia and in the depressed state of manic-depressive insanity, Kraepelin associated the signs and symptoms of waxy flexibility, mutism, and avolition (Table 2.5). These symptoms became associated with schizophrenia and not bipolar disorders.

Kraepelin's description of the disordered thought processes in mania from the early twentieth century comports with the idea of a defective sensory filter in mania as discussed in Chap. 13.

Although hallucinations and delusions became and remain diagnostic of schizophrenia, Kraepelin recognized and gave numerous examples of both auditory and visual hallucinations as well as delusions in patients whom he diagnosed with manic-depressive insanity. He described in detail that,

> Delusions are in manic-depressive insanity very frequent, especially in states of depression. ... Ideas of Sin are almost more frequent. He reflects on his past life, ... has committed many sins, ... has not taken good care of his children, has treated them badly, ... has neglected religion, has been dishonest about taxes, has masturbated, has committed adultery, ...

Kraepelin said that,

> Even these ideas may become more and more remote not only from reality, but also from possibility. The patient has committed perjury, offended a highly placed personage without knowing it, carried on incest, set his house on fire, killed his brothers and sisters. He has poisoned a Prince, is a five-fold murderer, is to blame for every misfortune, is a dammed soul, the refuse of humanity.

Kraepelin recognized that,

> Ideas of Persecution ... are frequently connected with the delusion of sin. The patient sees that he is surrounded by spies, is being followed by detectives, has fallen into the hands of the secret court of justice, ... is going into the convict prison, is to be slaughtered, executed, burned, nailed to the cross; all his teeth are being drawn out, his eyes dug out; he is inoculated with syphilis; he must ... die in a filthy manner. ... There are illusions in the newspapers; the sermon is aimed at him; his sins are publicly made known on large placards. Burglars, anarchists, force their way into his house; people are hidden in the cupboards. The patient notices that there is poison in the coffee, in the water for washing. ... There is a conspiracy against him. His relatives also become involved. ... Satan has power over him, he is hiding inside him ... hellfire is already burning under the bed.

These descriptions are similar, if not identical, to those found in his 1919 book about patients he diagnosed with dementia praecox.

Kraepelin next discussed

> Ideas of Greatness ... which not infrequently accompany the manic state, often bare more the stamp of half jocular swaggering and boastful exaggeration, ... [such as] the assertions of the patients that they are Messiah, the pearl of the world, the Christ child, the Bride of Christ, Queen of Heaven, Emperor of Russia, Almighty God, ... a great artist or author, a Baron, physician by birth, honorary doctor of all the sciences, a knight of high orders, illegitimate son of a Prince ... speaks seven languages ....

Under "Insight," Kraepelin said that,

> A clear understanding of the morbidity of the state is, as a rule, present only in the slightest states of depression; ....

This statement accurately implies that insight in mania and severe depression as well as in schizophrenia is lacking.

Kraepelin said that,

> Mood is mostly exalted in mania, ... The patients are pleased, over merry or quietly happy, visionary, more than satisfied, ... they feel well, ready for all possible sport ... they laugh, sing and jest. ... Sexual excitability is increased and leads to hasty engagements, marriages by the newspaper, improper love adventures, conspicuous behavior, fondness for dress, on the

other hand to jealousy and matrimonial discord. ... It easily acquires the stamp of foolishness and silliness ... the disposition of the manic may assume the form of angry irritation. ... The patients become arrogant and high flown; when they are contradicted, or on other trifling occasions, they fall into measureless fury, which is discharged in outburst in rank abuse and violence.

Kraepelin used such descriptions of patients he diagnosed with dementia praecox (Sect. 5.2).
Kraepelin accurately described

... mood in the states of depression [as] most frequently a sombre and gloomy hopelessness. ... The torment of the states of depression, which is nearly unbearable, according to the perpetually occurring statements by the patients, engenders almost in all, at least from time to time, weariness of life, only too frequently also a great desire to put an end to life at any price. ... The patients, therefore, often try to starve themselves, to hang themselves, to cut their arteries; ...

Kraepelin addressed "Pressure in Writing." Chapters IV, V, and VI focused on "Manic States," "Depressive States," and "Mixed States." In these chapters, Kraepelin again associated behaviors to mania or depression that subsequently became indicative if not diagnostic of schizophrenia (Table 5.3). Examples are ideas of influence (p. 63), use of clang associations and senseless rhyming (p. 72), marked depression lasting for months or even years (p. 72), depersonalization (p. 75), marked stupor (p. 79), deep apathy (p. 79), avolition (p. 87), and delusions and hallucinations (pp. 89–97).

In the next chapter, Chapter VII, titled "Fundamentals States," Kraepelin accurately described cyclothymia as

... characterized by frequent, more or less regular fluctuations of the psychic state to the manic or to the depressive side. It was found in only three to four percent of our patients, but without doubt in reality is much more frequent, ...

In Chapter IX titled "Prognosis," Kraepelin acknowledged the poor prognosis of bipolar patients stating that,

... with increase of attacks, in certain circumstances perhaps also with very severe single attacks extending over many years and in advanced age, there exists the greater or less danger of the development of the psychic decline. ... The states of weakness, which appear in such cases, invariably let the after effects of past attacks be recognized. Many patients remain permanently quiet, depressed, uninterested, stand about in corners with dejected or anxious appearance, ... They are inactive, irresolute, timid, have to be forced to do everything, resist energetically when much interfered with. Frequently also the residua of depressive delusions still persist; the patients call themselves the devil, ask for forgiveness, for a mild punishment, are afraid that they will be sent away, that they will have to remain there forever.

This description of "psychotic decline" in manic-depressive insanity here was attributed to "many patients" and is consistent with more recent observations of the potential for a chronic deterioration from classic bipolar cycles to a permanent, noncycling, psychotic, and treatment-resistant depressed state. Kraepelin has been remembered as having said such a course was diagnostic of schizophrenia and could rule out bipolar disorder.

In Chapter X titled "Causes," Kraepelin said that he demonstrated a

Hereditary taint in about 80% of cases in Heidelberg.

Kraepelin was mistaken when he apparently concluded that bipolar disorder is more common in females than males. He said that he found alcoholism in about 25% of his male bipolar patients and syphilis in about 8% of his male patients. Infectious diseases, hypothyroidism, and epilepsy were also discussed as contributors to bipolar disorders.

5.4 Kraepelin's Reversal of the Dichotomy: Implications for a Single Disease

As noted by Swartz and Shorter (2007, p. 34), toward the end of his life in 1921, Kraepelin "… admitted that it had been a mistake to erect a firewall between dementia praecox (Schizophrenia) and Manic-Depressive Insanity (Bipolar), that in fact the two largely overlapped" when he wrote, "It is becoming increasingly clear that we cannot distinguish satisfactorily between these two illnesses [dementia praecox/schizophrenia and manic-depressive insanity/bipolar] and this brings home the suspicion that our formulation of the problem may be incorrect" (Kraepelin 1920). This reversal was largely ignored for over 50 years obscured by Kraepelin's original "dichotomy" that the "two supposedly separate diseases of Schizophrenia and affective illness" are different. The Kraepelinian dichotomy has recently been challenged again (Craddock and Owen 2005, 2010a, b).

5.5 Conclusions

Considering the tremendous influence that Emil Kraepelin has had upon the mental health professions through academic psychiatry, he deserves his place as "… the founder of contemporary scientific psychiatry" (Wikipedia 2011). As noted in Sect. 3.3, several psychiatrists in the late 1800s and early 1900s changed their minds about whether a single disease entity or two diseases explained severe mental illness. Kraepelin was no exception. What is striking in considering Kraepelin's legacy is that he is remembered for his dichotomy despite later in his life writing that he questioned differences between schizophrenia and psychotic bipolar disorders. The influence of his contemporary, Eugene Bleuler, who did not change his mind about schizophrenia existing as a disease separate from bipolar disorders, reinforced acceptance of the dichotomy.

A major point deserves reemphasis: the acceptance of a dichotomy requires the acceptance of schizophrenia as a separate and bona fide disease. Data from the past two decades have led several psychopharmacologists to conclude that there is no Kraepelinian dichotomy. No dichotomy implies that schizophrenia and psychotic mood disorders are one and the same disorder with a continuum of severity.

5.5 Conclusions

The two major books reviewed in this chapter are titled *Dementia Praecox and Paraphrenia*, published in 1919, and *Manic-Depressive Insanity and Paranoia*, published in 1921/1976. These books contain Kraepelin's recordings of his patients' behaviors and speech followed by his interpretations as to the diagnostic meanings of the symptoms he observed. It is not surprising that Kraepelin, later in his career after writing these two books, decided that he could not differentiate schizophrenia from psychotic mood disorders. As demonstrated above in extensive selected quotes, especially from his 1919 book on dementia praecox, the signs, symptoms, and behaviors Kraepelin attributed to dementia praecox are suggestive, if not diagnostic, of psychotic mood disorders (Tables 5.2 and 5.3). Even more striking is that the psychotic signs, symptoms, and behaviors Kraepelin attributed to dementia praecox in his 1919 book are similar, if not identical, with the signs, symptoms, and behaviors Kraepelin recorded in his 1921 book as diagnostic of manic-depressive insanity.

Despite both of these textbooks being available for almost a century, such overlap and redundancy in signs and symptoms attributed to patients diagnosed with dementia praecox and with manic-depressive insanity have not been adequately addressed in the DSM, the ICD, psychiatry textbooks, or by Academic psychiatry. If such overlap had been recognized earlier in the modern history of the development of diagnoses for functionally psychotic patients, the Kraepelinian dichotomy and schizophrenia may have already been eliminated as redundant with psychotic mood disorders.

In Kraepelin's time, a misdiagnosis of schizophrenia versus bipolar disorder had much less impact regarding treatment. The treatments for insanity or psychosis were the same regardless of the diagnosis. It was not until the 1970s with the recognition and use of lithium for bipolar patients that the correct diagnosis became critical for adequate standard of care.

Chapter 6
Eugen Bleuler (1857–1939) Named and Dedicated Himself to Schizophrenia

> *As far as we know, the fundamental symptoms are characteristic of schizophrenia, while the accessory symptoms [hallucinations and delusions] may also appear in other types of illness [bipolar disorders]. ... A number of these patients [catatonic schizophrenics] are manifestly manic (with demonstrable flight of ideas); others are melancholic; ... or feel themselves persecuted. ... The masturbation insanity described by various authors must obviously be included in schizophrenia.*
>
> (Bleuler 1911, pp. 13, 214, 289)

> *The presence of putative "schizophrenic" symptoms is no longer held to be valuable in distinguishing between manic-depressive illness and schizophrenia.*
>
> (Pope 1983)

> *Bleuler and his many disciples, especially Academic Psychiatry in the U.S., called "any and all serious mental illness schizophrenia" as well as less severe mental illness.*
>
> (Swartz and Shorter 2007, p. 31)

6.1 Introduction

Bleuler was born near Zurich, Switzerland in 1857, a year after Kraepelin. He studied medicine first at the University of Zurich and then in Paris, London, and Munich before returning to Zurich for an internship at the Burgholzli, a large university hospital. In 1886, he took the directorship of a psychiatric clinic at Rheinau where he improved patient conditions. In 1989, he returned to the Burgholzli hospital in Zurich as the director. In 1911, while a professor of psychiatry in Zurich, he published his famous book titled *Dementia Praecox or the Group of Schizophrenias*, renaming dementia praecox to schizophrenia, because

> "[Dementia praecox] seems too awkward. It only designates the disease, not the diseased; moreover it is impossible to derive from it an adjective denoting the characteristics of this

Table 6.1 Bleuler's "pathognomonic" fundamental and accessory symptoms for schizophrenia

a. *Fundamental symptoms/Four A's of schizophrenia*[a]:
   1. Ambivalence[b] (can be normal or due to distractibility)[c]
   2. Affect, inappropriate[b,d] (can be due to anxiety and embarrassment)
   3. Associations, loose[b] (likely represents distractibility, racing thoughts, and flight of ideas associated with mania)[d,e]
   4. Autistic thinking (only means delusional, unable to distinguish fantasy from reality)[d,e]
b. *Accessory symptoms*[a,d,e]:
   1. Hallucinations
   2. Delusions

[a]None of these symptoms alone or in any combination, are disease specific; they occur frequently in severe mood disorders with psychotic features
[b]These signs and symptoms can overlap with normal behavior or be caused by multiple circumstances or causes other than a psychotic process
[c]Statements in parentheses added by author
[d]Retained in current and proposed DSMs as diagnostic of schizophrenia
[e]Common in severe mood disorders

illness, ..." Bleuler said, "Without such a new term, a thorough work on differential diagnosis would be hard to write and even harder to read." Bleuler then emphasized "… a far more important and practical reason why it seems so unavoidable to me to propose a new designation [schizophrenia instead of dementia praecox]: … The older form [dementia praecox] is a product of a time when not only the very concept of dementia, but also that of precocity, was applicable to all cases at hand. But it hardly fits our contemporary ideas of the scope of this disease-entity. Today we include patients whom we would neither call "demented" nor exclusively victims of deterioration early in life."

Thus, Bleuler broadened schizophrenia to include all ages with or without psychoses and with or without a deteriorating course. His addition of "simple" schizophrenia as a fourth subtype enabled assigning the diagnosis to older, eccentric but functional individuals. As judged by some of his statements quoted below, it is unclear if he recognized whether or not his patients with the diagnosis of schizophrenia suffered some of the same characteristics of the dementias of old age such as confusion, loss of memory, and disorientation. But, if he did recognize the differences, this was not the major motivation for Bleuler's change in the name of the disease. For example, Bleuler believed that in most patients with schizophrenia, the presence of psychotic symptoms typically led to deterioration or dementia. He admitted that, "There were always some cases, however, which exhibited these symptoms [psychoses], yet seem to recover." This is in contrast to another statement for which he became famous noted below.

He chose schizophrenia because of its Greek translation (schizein, "to split," and phren, "mind"). Bleuler's concept of splitting is obtuse and has been misinterpreted as a splitting of personality leading to myriad multiple personality diagnoses and confusion. Bleuler's splitting reflected his observations in some of his hospitalized patients of an apparent disconnect between their content of speech and thought, and their affect; that is, inappropriate affect which became one of Bleuler's four fundamental diagnostic symptoms that has still been retained for a diagnosis of schizophrenia (Table 6.1). He said

> In every case we are confronted with a more or less clear-cut splitting of the psychic functions.

"… the personality looses its unity; at different times different psychic complexes seem to represent the personality." He elaborated that, "… groups of ideas or drives are "split off" and seem either partly or completely impotent. Often ideas are only partially worked out, and fragments of ideas are connected in an illogical way to constitute a new idea. Concepts loose their completeness, …"

(Bleuler 1911/1950, pp. 8, 9)

Inappropriate affect came to encompass "flat affect" that today continues to be considered as especially indicative of schizophrenia as one of the three "negative symptoms" of schizophrenia. Bleuler may have also initiated two additional words that have been widely accepted by psychiatry and the public in general. "Autism" and "ambivalence" were thought by Bleuler to characterize two additional "fundamental symptoms" of his disease of schizophrenia. Autistic thinking means one is unable to distinguish their delusions from reality, and examples of ambivalence are given below.

Throughout Bleuler's book are statements by him that raise some concern as to the applicability of his concepts today and subsequently the validity of schizophrenia (Table 6.2). Despite this, Bleuler's ideas continue to have considerable influence upon the development of the next addition of the DSM, the DSM-5 due in 2013.

6.2 Bleuler's Fundamental Symptoms of Schizophrenia (1911/1950); Not Pathognomonic, Capture Eccentrics and Normals, and Suggest a Bipolar Disorder

Bleuler greatly expanded the diagnostic criteria for schizophrenia by establishing his quite subjective four fundamental symptoms as pathognomonic. These became known as Bleuler's four As of schizophrenia. Bleuler's "fundamental" diagnostic criteria were so broad that eccentric and even normals on a bad day could warrant the diagnosis of schizophrenia, a lifetime diagnosis (Tables 6.1 and 6.3). Since schizophrenia only existed through subtypes and all of the three existing subtypes required psychotic symptoms, Bleuler had to define a new subtype. To capture such patients, Bleuler added simple schizophrenia to Kraepelin's three subtypes of schizophrenia (Table 6.3). These patients "suffered" only his "fundamental symptoms" and did not necessarily have any psychotic symptoms. As stated by Swartz and Shorter (2007, p. 31), Bleuler's "fundamental symptoms" were much milder than psychosis, and he included for his diagnosis of schizophrenia a much milder prognosis than Kraepelin. Bleuler felt that patients with schizophrenia did not necessarily "go on to complete the deterioration" and also said that,

We designate a group of psychoses whose course is at times chronic, at times marked by intermittent attacks, and which can stop or retrograde at any stage, but does not permit a full *restituto ad integrum.*

(Bleuler 1911/1950, pp. 8, 9)

According to Swartz and Shorter (2007, p. 31),

Bleuler and his many disciples, especially Academic Psychiatry in the U.S., called "any and all serious mental illness Schizophrenia" as well as less severe mental illness.

Table 6.2 Selected quotes from *Dementia Praecox or the Group of Schizophrenias* (E. Bleuler 1911/1950) raise questions as to the validity of schizophrenia

Quote no.	Page no.	Selected quotes	Current author's comments
1	4	"Nevertheless we believe that an advance has been made which is even greater than the progress made by the discovery of the etiology of general paresis.... We feel that the dementia praecox problem involves much more deeply the entire complex of the systematics of all the psychoses than the problem of general paresis ever did in its day."	Bleuler may have been overconfident in considering his disease of schizophrenia to have been more important than the resolution of general paresis. He believed schizophrenia would subsume a spectrum of psychotic disorders as had syphilis.
2	4	"... catatonia [schizophrenia] passes through the stages of melancholia, mania, stupor, confusion, and finally dementia ...."	This statement demonstrates some confusion in differentiating these disorders as separate and suggests that schizophrenia/dementia praecox might be an end stage of a chronic, psychotic mood disorder.
3	9	"In every case [of schizophrenia] we are confronted with a more or less clear-cut splitting of the psychic functions."	Bleuler himself appeared "ambivalent" when he said, "… a more or less clear-cut splitting." His concept of splitting has been a source of confusion, and even in rereading his original text, his concept is obtuse.
4	13	"As far as we know, the fundamental symptoms are characteristic of schizophrenia, while the accessory symptoms [hallucinations and delusions] may also appear in other types of illness [bipolar disorders]."	The interpretation of Bleuler's concept of schizophrenia is inconsistent with this statement since functional psychosis became equated with schizophrenia. Academic psychiatry, textbooks of psychiatry, the DSM, and all other diagnostic manuals interpreted hallucinations and delusions as disease specific and diagnostic for schizophrenia despite Bleuler saying they occur in other illnesses.
5	39	"In manic phases of schizophrenia, flight of ideas, is added to the typically schizophrenic association disturbances. In depressive episodes [of schizophrenia], we find inhibition of thinking and disturbances of association brought about by abnormal affective reactions."	Flight of ideas and disturbances of association and inhibition of thinking are consistent with psychotic mania and psychotic depression, respectively, so that the use of a new diagnosis, schizophrenia, is redundant.
6	159	"The very appearance of a piece of writing often permits one to recognize the presence of schizophrenia.... Paranoids have the peculiar habit of leaving no margin and are inclined to fill the page completely. Conversely a catatonic uses an entire sheet to write:…."	A majority of the writing samples Bleuler gave as examples of schizophrenia indicated hyperactivity, grandiosity, and/or an erotic focus that are indicative of mania. Making a diagnosis based on the percent of a sheet of paper the patient uses dates Bleuler's diagnostic judgment.

6.2 Bleuler's Fundamental Symptoms of Schizophrenia (1911/1950)... 97

7	208	"The melancholic symptom triad of depressive affect, inhibition of thinking and of action is one of the most frequent acute disturbances in schizophrenia."	This "melancholic symptom triad" is most likely explained by psychotic depression and not any other psychotic disease.
8	210	"Ordinarily the schizophrenic manic is capricious rather than euphoric.... Outbursts of wild rage are even more common in these people [schizophrenics] than in the usual type of manic...."	Differentiating "capricious" versus "euphoric" or the frequency of "outbursts of wild rage" to make a differential diagnosis between schizophrenia and bipolar disorder is itself capricious and subjective. Psychotic mania explains both.
9	211	"In schizophrenia I have not as yet seen Manic-Depressive mixed states, ... but it is quite possible that they also exist."	Bleuler's statement is despite his discussion of "Manic Conditions" in schizophrenia when he elaborates both the classic symptoms of mania as well as cycling with melancholia that he attributes to schizophrenia, not bipolar disorder. On the previous page, Bleuler refers to "... transient shifts to tearful sadness [from manic rage]." Bleuler subsumes all symptoms of mood disorders under his overriding diagnosis of schizophrenia.
10	214	"A number of these patients [catatonic schizophrenics] are manifestly manic (with demonstrable flight of ideas); others are melancholic; still others are irritable, anxious, or feel themselves persecuted."	Instead of a new disease, schizophrenia, such descriptions of patients' manic and depressive symptomatology warrant diagnoses of psychotic mania or psychotic depression.
11	223–224	"Special attention has to be given to these confusional states [in schizophrenia] which are a direct consequence of the fragmentation of the associations. This type of incoherence represents an acute syndrome in almost all cases [of schizophrenia]. The patients speak completely disconnectedly, often in half-broken sentences. They are quite restless and constantly busy doing something, but their activities lack purpose and are not carried through to the end...."	Bleuler's descriptions of his psychotic patients' confusion, incoherence, and hyperactivity are again entirely compatible with manic distractibility, racing thoughts, flight of ideas, confusion, and incoherence (see Chap. 13 of the current book).
12	232	"The nature of the agitation [in catatonic schizophrenia] may alter many times, in an irregular way, betwixt manic and melancholic conditions, confusional and stuporous states."	It seems more likely that the symptoms of depression and mania define a psychotic bipolar disorder rather than any other disorder.
13	232	"But after each of them [psychotic episodes], the deterioration usually becomes more and more pronounced."	Bleuler's description is compatible with the deterioration observed after increasing episodes of mood disorders (Fig. 4.1 of the current book).

(continued)

Table 6.2 (continued)

Quote no.	Page no.	Selected quotes	Current author's comments
14	235	"Melancholic and manic excitements, twilight states, etc., can appear at anytime in the course of the disease [hebephrenic schizophrenia] just as well as at the beginning."	It seems more likely that the symptoms of depression and mania define a psychotic bipolar disorder rather than any other disorder.
15	254	Under subsection C, The "Termination of the Disease [schizophrenia]," subheading #1" "Death" Bleuler said, "The immediate causes [of death in schizophrenia] may be cerebral pressure due to cerebral edema or increased cerebral-spinal fluid; metabolic disturbances (including auto-intoxications) and cerebral paralysis as seen in catatonic or epileptiform attacks."	Such causes of death raise questions as to whether the psychotic symptoms utilized by Bleuler to diagnosis schizophrenia were actually due to organic disease negating the diagnosis of schizophrenia.
16	268	"Manic and melancholic symptoms are so common in our [schizophrenic] patients that we must assume that they are usually released by the disease process itself, and thus are part of the schizophrenia."	This statement epitomizes Bleuler's inaccurate belief that schizophrenia or psychosis trumps any mood disorder diagnosis.
17	282	"Chronic alcohol-paranoia has frequently been diagnosed by others; I, however, have not yet seen such a patient, who gave me even the slightest reason to see in him anything other than an ordinary schizophrenic who also drank…. schizophrenia, itself, also predisposes to delirium tremens…. I have also seen alcoholic hallucinosis develop on the basis of schizophrenia."	Thus, Bleuler tended to diagnosis patients who abused alcohol with schizophrenia.
18	288	"Obviously almost all of Wernicke's 'motility psychoses' are also schizophrenias …Of the chronic diseases, all those designated as dementing types….belong to our disease [schizophrenia]. …."	Thus, Bleuler tended to diagnosis psychotic demented patients with schizophrenia.
19	288	"A large number of women whom I considered schizophrenics passed for hysterically insane in other places …."	As seen here and in other entries from Bleuler's book, he seemed to diagnose schizophrenia readily in women.
20	289	"'Nervous' persons, too, whose conversations are often confused, who refuse nourishment and exhibit delusions of jealously, are, as far as our experience goes, neither neurasthenics nor narcoleptics, but [schizophrenic] catatonics."	Diagnosing "nervous persons" with schizophrenia speaks to Bleuler's broad application of his disease and raises questions about the wide acceptance of his clinical judgments.

6.2 Bleuler's Fundamental Symptoms of Schizophrenia (1911/1950)…

21	289	"Many, although not all, of the very severe form of compulsive conditions, of folie du doute …, and of impulsive behavior undoubtedly belong to schizophrenia … These clinical pictures termed pyromania, kleptomania, etc., are sometimes schizophrenics."	Diagnosing people with "compulsive and impulsive behaviors" with schizophrenia speaks to Bleuler's broad application of his disease.
22	289	"The masturbation insanity described by various authors must obviously be included in schizophrenia."	Diagnosing people who "masturbate even excessively" with schizophrenia speaks to Bleuler's broad application of his disease.
23	294	"Character abnormalities, indifference, lack of energy, unsociability, stubbornness, moodiness, … 'whimsical,' hypochondriacal complaints, etc., are not necessarily symptoms of an actual mental disease; they are, however, often the only perceptible signs of schizophrenia."	As demonstrated by this quote as well as the others in this table, Bleuler might diagnose a high percent of the healthy population with his disease, schizophrenia.
24	295	"It is of no pathological significance if someone draws stereotype 'doodles' on the paper in front of him during a boring lecture; but when the same 'doodles' are included in a serious letter, they may assure for themselves a diagnosis of schizophrenia."	One might wonder how many patients received the diagnosis of schizophrenia for "doodles" on a "serious letter."
25	304	"All the phenomena of manic-depressive psychosis may also appear in our disease [schizophrenia]; the only decisive factor is the presence or absence of schizophrenic symptoms. Therefore, neither a state of manic exaltation nor a melancholic depression, nor the alternation of both states has any significance for the diagnosis. Only after careful observation has revealed no schizophrenic features, may we conclude that we are dealing with a manic-depressive psychosis."	Thus, Bleuler denies the possibility of a psychotic mood disorder since psychotic symptoms such as hallucinations and delusions were considered diagnostic of schizophrenia regardless of prominent mood disturbances. It is this concept that is Bleuler's legacy as demonstrated by the current DSM, ICD, and textbooks of psychiatry.
26	332	"The appearance of unprovoked and unmotivated short outbursts of peevishness and agitation, be they regular or not, seem to have a bad prognostic significance [for that patient with schizophrenia]."	Diagnosing individuals with schizophrenia based on "unprovoked short outbursts of peevishness and agitation" speaks to Bleuler's broad application of his disease.
27	332	"Young individuals who chronically do not work, who are without drive and initiative, who show poor vasomotor control and who cannot be moved or interested by reproaches concerning their behavior - these youths must all be considered hopeless cases [of schizophrenia],…"	Diagnosing young people who "do not work and are without drive and initiative" with schizophrenia speaks to Bleuler's broad application of his disease.

Table 6.3 Bleuler's subtypes of schizophrenia (Bleuler 1911/1950, p. 10)

1. *Paranoid*. "Hallucinations or delusions continuously hold the forefront of the clinical picture."
2. *Catatonia*. "Catatonic symptoms dominate continuously, or for rather long periods of time."
3. *Hebephrenia*. "Accessory symptoms appear but do not dominate the picture continually."
4. *Simple schizophrenia*. "Throughout its whole course only the specific, basic symptoms can be found. ... This group is rarely found in hospitals but outside it is as common as any of the other forms. In private practice, we often see it, indeed, as frequently in the relatives who bring the patients as in the patients themselves. On the lower levels of society, the simple schizophrenics vegetate as day laborers, peddlers, even as servants. They are also vagabonds and hoboes as are other types of schizophrenics of mild grade. On the higher levels of society, the most common type is the wife (in a very unhappy role, we can say), who is unbearable, constantly scolding, nagging, always making demands but never recognizing duties. Her family never considers the possibility of illness, suffers for many years a veritable hell of annoyances, difficulties, unpleasantnesses from the 'mean' woman. They usually employ every possible means to conceal the true state of affairs in the home from the prying eyes of the outside world. The possibility of keeping the anomaly secret is facilitated by the fact that many of these patients still manage to conduct themselves in an entirely unobtrusive way." (Bleuler 1911/1950, p. 236)

His "four As" of schizophrenia, Bleuler's fundamental symptoms, were taught in medical schools and psychiatry residency training programs in the USA and around the world at least through the 1970s if not later (Table 6.1). Bleuler did not require psychosis (hallucinations and/or delusions), referred to as accessory symptoms, for a diagnosis of schizophrenia, but if present, felt that the diagnosis was a certainty, and this has been his legacy. Demonstrating the longevity of his remarkable impact, schizophrenia, as defined by his accessory symptoms and subtypes (except simple schizophrenia) and at least one of his fundamental criteria, remains today in the DSM-IV-TR (Table 2.5; compare Tables 3.4 and 6.3). The DSM-5 draft proposal continues to define schizophrenia with some nineteenth century concepts.

Of more lasting impact than his fundamental symptoms, Bleuler's accessory symptoms, hallucinations, and delusions, that is, psychosis, have been equated with schizophrenia and continue to be diagnostic in the DSM-IV-TR and the DSM-5 draft proposal. Bleuler discounted mood symptoms as secondary to the primary diagnosis of schizophrenia. According to interpretations of Bleuler's teachings, there could be no psychotic mood disorder since psychosis without an organic cause warranted the diagnosis of schizophrenia. Schneider in 1959 reemphasized this by substituting cyclothymia for manic-depressive insanity. Cyclothymia does not offer the possibility of psychosis (Chap. 8).

Bleuler and psychiatry in general continued to consider schizophrenia as a group of subtypes (until the DSM-5 draft); there was no schizophrenia without the subtypes (Table 3.4; Chap. 12). Further examples of the continuing influence from the nineteenth to early twentieth centuries in the current DSM-IV-TR and ICD-10 include the presence of most of the original subtypes (paranoid, catatonic, and disorganized (hebephrenic)); some of which (catatonia and disorganization) also comprise two of the core diagnostic criteria of schizophrenia coupled with Bleuler's accessory symptoms of hallucinations and delusions (compare Tables 2.5 and 3.4). Paranoid schizophrenia featured hallucinations and delusions. The subtypes,

6.3 Selected Quotes from Bleuler's Textbook, *Dementia Praecox*...

Table 6.4 Additional characteristics Bleuler and others associated with schizophrenia[a]

1. Loner, poor premorbid personality[b]
2. Onset of psychotic illness in late adolescence or early adulthood[c]
3. A disorder of thought; formal thought disorder[c]
4. Derailment, tangentiality, loose associations, disorganization, blocking, incoherence, word salad, clanging, echolalia, echopraxia, speaking in tongues[c]
5. Catatonia[c]
6. Coprophagia, coprophilia[c]
7. Downward drift in society and employment[b,c]
8. Multiple, brief jobs[b,c]
9. Street person[b,c]
10. Ideas of control or reference, paranoia[b,c]
11. Mood-incongruent hallucinations and/or delusions[c]
12. No "restituto ad integrum"[c]
13. Character anomalies[b,d]
14. Indifference[b,d]
15. Lack of energy[b,d]
16. Unsociability[b,d]
17. Stubbornness[b,d]
18. Moodiness[b,d]
19. "Whimsical"[b,d]
20. Hypochondriacal complaints[b,d]

[a]None of these symptoms alone or in any combination are disease specific
[b]These signs and symptoms can overlap with normal behavior or be caused by multiple circumstances or causes other than a psychotic process
[c]Common in severe mood disorders
[d]From Bleuler's textbook, p. 294

therefore, became synonymous with the diagnostic criteria. Misconcepts of Bleuler include his belief of the disease specificity of his fundamental and accessory symptoms, and of his subtypes, and the belief that being a "loner," having a course of a "downward drift" in society, coprophagia, early onset, odd or eccentric behavior, and "no restituto ad integrum," etc. were indicative of schizophrenia (Table 6.4).

6.3 Selected Quotes from Bleuler's Textbook, *Dementia Praecox or the Group of the Schizophrenias* (1911/1950)

Bleuler's book, published in 1911, was translated into English by Dr. Joseph Zinkin, M.D., in 1950. Gregory Zilboorg, who encouraged the translation of Bleuler's monograph said that, "… it was the classic work of 20th century Psychiatry." The book is 548 pages including indices. It is divided into 11 sections each with chapters and subheadings.

Curiously, in some parts of his book, Bleuler, the only author, used the pronouns "we" and "our" instead of "I" possibly suggesting consensus with his statements. Bleuler gave other hints of his confidence in the validity of his concepts.

For example, in his Preface, he essentially warned readers that they needed to pay close attention to what he wrote:

> Whoever does not take the trouble to follow the thought of the author closely, will soon come to understand a specific term in a sense other than the one intended by the author, and thus develop a wrong picture of the basic issue.

In his "General Introduction," he said,

> In the present state of our knowledge, therefore, the delineation of this disease-group [schizophrenia] is not only permissible, it is mandatory.

Bleuler continued:

> Furthermore, it has been established that all these forms of deterioration that begin without any prominently acute phase, but slowly and insidiously, have identical symptoms [to schizophrenia] and can at no time be differentiated from the so-called "secondary" types. Thus we must include in this disease [schizophrenia] all those types known under a wide variety of names, such as "primary deterioration," "deteriorating paranoia," etc. [He then said] Nevertheless we believe that an advance has been made which is even greater than the progress made by the discovery of the etiology of general paresis. The latter syndrome too was for a long time obscured by many other symptom-pictures. We feel that the dementia praecox problem involves much more deeply the entire complex of the systematics of all the psychoses than the problem of general paresis ever did in its day.

Bleuler was certainly optimistic if not narcissistic when he implied that his concept of schizophrenia would be more productive than the elucidation of general paresis. He implied that schizophrenia, like syphilis, included a wide spectrum of psychotic disorders.

He continued:

> The development of the concept of dementia praecox constitutes a considerable part of the whole development of theoretical psychiatry.
>
> (Bleuler 1911/1950, p. 4)

Bleuler concurred with Kahlbaum that, "... catatonia [schizophrenia] passes through the stages of melancholia, mania, stupor, confusion, and finally dementia ..." This statement suggests the interchangeability of schizophrenia with mania and depression and thus raises the question of there being only one disease process. Bleuler thought the one disease was schizophrenia.

Under the heading of "The Definition of the Disease," Bleuler stated his definition of schizophrenia as given above. He continued that,

> The disease is characterized by a specific type of alteration of thinking, feeling, and relation to the external world which appears no where else in this particular fashion. ...
>
> Thus, the process of association often works with mere fragments of ideas and concepts. This results in associations which normal individuals will regard as incorrect, bizarre, and utterly unpredictable. Often thinking stops in the middle of a thought; ... (blocking) ... Instead of continuing the thought, new ideas crop up which neither the patient nor the observer can bring into connection with the previous stream of thought.
>
> (Bleuler 1911/1950, p. 9)

6.3 Selected Quotes from Bleuler's Textbook, *Dementia Praecox*... 103

Yet, psychotic mood-disordered patients suffer the same alterations of thinking, feeling, and relating as described by Bleuler and attributed by him "specifically" to schizophrenia. Blocking, considered specific for schizophrenia, has been postulated to be explained by a defectively porous filter mechanism in the manic brain (Chap. 13).

In his book, Bleuler recorded word for word many of his patients' conversations and writings to demonstrate symptoms he considered suggestive or diagnostic of schizophrenia. In rereading Bleuler's book, what is most striking is that many of the symptoms and examples that he cited as specific for schizophrenia today seem more suggestive of psychotic mania or depression (Tables 6.2 and 6.5). For example, in Section I, "Symptomatology," Chapter 1 titled, "The Fundamental Symptoms," subheading "*Association*," he states that,

> ... we know of two disturbances peculiar to schizophrenia... pressure of thoughts, that is, a pathologically increased flow of ideas, and the particularly characteristic "blocking".
>
> (Bleuler 1911/1950, p. 14)

These "... disturbances of association," his first fundamental symptom, that Bleuler linked with schizophrenia are explained by manic distractibility and flight of ideas discussed in detail in Chap. 13. As an example of Bleuler's attribution of manic speech to schizophrenia, he gives the following quote below from "... a young schizophrenic who had first appeared as either paranoid or hebephrenic and then some years later became markedly catatonic...,"

> At the time of the new moon, Venus stands in Egypt's August-sky and illuminates with her rays the commercial ports of Suez, Cairo, and Alexandria. In this historically famous city of the Califs, there is a museum of Assyrian monuments from Macedonia. There flourish plantain and olives. Olive-oil is an Arabian liquor-sauce which the Afghans, Moors and Moslems use in ostrich-farming. The Indian plantain-tree is the whisky of the Parsees and Arabs. The Parsee or Caucasian possesses as much influence of his elephant as does the Moor over his dromedary. The camel is the sport of Jews and Arabs. Barley, rice, and sugar-cane called artichoke, grow remarkably well in India. The Brahmins live as castes in Beluchistan. The Circassians occupy Manchuria in China. China is the Eldorado of the Pawnees.
>
> (Bleuler 1911/1950, pp. 14–15)

See another case example in Chap. 13 with a different diagnostic interpretation of a similarly loosely associated and disorganized discussion. Another example of manic distractibility and flight of ideas that Bleuler attributes to "a hebephrenic [Schizophrenic] patient, ill for 15 years but still able to work and still full of ambitions," is the following answer given to him by his patient to his question of "Who was Epaminondas?": [author's clarification: Epaminondas (425–362 BC) was a famous Greek general from Thebes. He defeated the heavily favored Spartans and other armies using an ingenious military strategy.]

> Epaminondas was one of those who are especially powerful on land and on sea. He led mighty fleet maneuvers and open sea-battles against Pelopidas, but in the second Punic War he was defeated by the sinking of an armed frigate. With his ships he wandered from Athens to Hain Mamre, bought Caledonian grapes and pomegranates there, and conquered the Beduins. He besieged the Acropolis with gun-boats and had the Persian garrisons put to the stake as living torches. The succeeding Pope Gregory VII... eh...Nero, followed his example and because of him all the Athenians, all the Roman-Germanic-Celtic tribes who did not favor the priests,

were burned by the Druids on Corpus Christi Day as a sacrifice to the Sun-God, Baal. That is the Stone Age, Spearheads made of bronze.

(Bleuler 1911/1950, p. 15)

Bleuler recognized that these two "performances ... are amazingly similar" despite "diametrically different" clinical pictures. Bleuler's analyses of these stories included his assessment that,

These two performances indicate a moderate degree of schizophrenic association disturbance. ... In these patients, the most important determinant of the associations is completely lacking --- the concept of purpose. It looks as though ideas of a certain category (in the first case pertaining to the Orient, in the second, to data of ancient history) were thrown into one pot, mixed, and subsequently picked out at random, and linked with each other by mere grammatical form or other auxiliary images. Still, certain sequences of the ideas are more closely linked to each other by some sort of common thread which, however, proves too loose to provide a logically useful connection (Fleet-maneuvres – sea battle – armed frigate; Acropolis – Persian garrison – burning – living torches – Nero; priests – Druids – Corpus Christi Day – Sun-God Baal, etc.).

(Bleuler 1911/1950, p. 16)

See Chap. 13 for a detailed discussion of why these examples of "schizophrenic thought," according to Bleuler, are actually examples of distractibility, flight of ideas, and racing thoughts specific to mania and therefore diagnostic of a bipolar disorder. In Chap. 13, a manic patient was able to explain his apparent blocking by filling in his thoughts that he experienced but did not have time to verbally express because of his racing thoughts. That Bleuler's second patient was "still able to work and still full of ambitions" is consistent with bipolar disorder.

Grandiosity, evident in the psychotic statement below, is overlooked by Bleuler with regards to indications of mania:

A hebephrenic [schizophrenic] demanded his release from the hospital by petitioning the Government as follows: "You are invited to carry out my release and to announce this fact in public notices in the newspapers of May, 1905. Otherwise you will be discharged from your position in accordance with my traditional rights. You may continue to exercise your offices until the new election. Respectfully ...."

(Bleuler 1911/1950, p. 18)

Bleuler further discusses "the course of the associations" of his patients with schizophrenia as follows:

... the patients [with schizophrenia] may loose themselves in the most irrelevant side-associations, and a uniform chain of thought does not come about. (Bleuler 1911/1950, p. 18)

All the indicated disturbances [loose associations] may range from a maximum which corresponds to complete confusion, to a minimum which may be hardly noticeable.

(Bleuler 1911/1950, p. 21)

Many [schizophrenic] patients complain that they must think too much, that their ideas chase each other in their heads. They themselves "thought-overflow" (because they cannot hold anything in their minds), of "pressure of thoughts," of "collecting of thoughts," because too much seems to come to mind at one time.

(Bleuler 1911/1950, p. 32)

6.3 Selected Quotes from Bleuler's Textbook, *Dementia Praecox*... 105

The range of severity of manic distractibility, racing thoughts, and flight of ideas noted by Bleuler above, but misattributed to the thinking of schizophrenia, is consistent with the range of severity observed across a spectrum of manic patients. Some manic patients, with only mild distractibility, have been able to connect apparently unrelated thoughts when asked, that is, the case described in Chap. 13. Bleuler did recognize some connectivity between apparently unrelated thoughts of at least a few of his "schizophrenic" patients when he said,

> The emergence of an idea without any connection with a previous train of thought, or without any external stimulus, is ... so foreign to normal psychology that one is obliged to look even in the patient's seemingly most far-fetched ideas, for the associative path originating in a previous concept or in an external stimulus. In this way, it may be possible in some, through not in all cases, to demonstrate the connecting links. Still, in a sufficient number of cases, we will succeed in pointing out several of the main directions along which the derailment of thoughts took place.
>
> (Bleuler 1911/1950, pp. 22–23) (Chap. 13)

Bleuler assigns "pressure of thoughts" which he said can continue for years, as a symptom of schizophrenia, not mania, in contrast to current belief (Bleuler 1911/1950, p. 32). He quoted another patient who he apparently misdiagnosed with schizophrenia:

> In my mind there ran like an endless clockwork, a compulsive, torturing, uninterrupted chain of ideas.
>
> (Bleuler 1911/1950, p. 33)

Under the subheading titled "Affectivity," Bleuler stated that,

> ... [the schizophrenic] psychosis became "chronic" when the affects began to disappear. Many schizophrenics in the later stages cease to show any affect for years and even decades at a time. ... indifference seems to be the external sign of their state; an indifference to everything – to friends and relations, to vocation or enjoyment, ... to good fortune or to bad. "I don't care the least, one way or another," is what a [schizophrenic] patient ... said. ... Patients consciously and deliberately isolate themselves ....
>
> (Bleuler 1911/1950, p. 40)

This description is consistent with chronic psychotic depression (Swartz and Shorter 2007).

Bleuler's description of labile and/or inappropriate affect is also consistent with psychotic depression. In this section, Bleuler described a "hebephrenic"/disorganized schizophrenic patient whose symptoms seem consistent with a rapid cycling bipolar patient:

> A hebephrenic was under impending sentence for some violation of the law. He was slightly euphoric, considered himself lucky to have come to the hospital for medical care. He praised the paintings (bad ones) on the wall, did not want to be transferred to a better ward because the patients in his ward were so nice. After being transferred to the new ward, he berated and cursed his old ward endlessly. During a slight fever (and occasionally without any discernible cause) he became depressed, cried like a child that he was going to die. This same reaction showed itself for the most insignificant reasons; for example, when he related how reluctant his father had been to pay the small semi-annual tuition fee for him. If someone

said anything which displeased him, he would become excited, threatening, shattered objects nearby, threw money away in his rage, beat up his wife. In spite of this liability of affect with a mild manic mood, the schizophrenic affect disturbance was quite clear. ... In this well-educated and polite man there was complete loss of his sense of social tact.

(Bleuler 1911/1950, p. 44)

Bleuler continued in his descriptions of "schizophrenic behavior:" "Far more striking than the quick changes of affect ... are the unprovoked mood swings and variations; ..."

(Bleuler 1911/1950, p. 45)

Bleuler continued "It is indeed striking how early those feelings that regulate social intercourse among people are blunted. ... Often there is not a trace of modesty left, even in [schizophrenic] patients who are otherwise relatively not too deteriorated. ... They will masturbate openly. A patient, an intelligent high school student, writes to his mother as follows: "Dear Mother, Come to see me as soon as possible. I must know how old you were the night my father made me."

(Bleuler 1911/1950, p. 49)

These patients' statements and moods are consistent with mania (Chap. 13).

In the next subheading titled "Ambivalence," Bleuler discussed another of his fundamental symptoms he said was diagnostic of schizophrenia. As an example of "affective ambivalence," Bleuler gave examples such as,

1) ... simultaneously [having] pleasant and unpleasant feelings, 2) ... the husband both loves and hates his wife. ... 3) She suffers the most intense anxiety that they are going to shoot her and yet she constantly begs the attendant to shoot her, ... 4) Another [schizophrenic patient] verbigerates, "You devil, you angel, you devil, you angel." (She is referring here to her lover.) ... 5) ... the [schizophrenic] patient wishes to eat and does not wish to eat. ... 6) One [schizophrenic] patient, ... was bitterly conscience-stricken because once, in his youth, he had committed fellatio on a young boy. Yet in later years he persistently, and with crude violence attempts to commit fellatio on other patients. 7) The "voices" advise him to drown himself and in the very same sentence, ... they scornfully berate him for wishing to drown himself.

(Bleuler 1911/1950, pp. 53, 54)

In this author's opinion, the examples of ambivalence given above from Bleuler's book may not warrant any diagnosis. Some of the examples are compatible with a mood disorder such as suicidal ideations in the context of psychotic depression, or in other cases, the comments could be within a normal range of ambivalence.

Bleuler did recognize that the functions of: "orientation, ... sensation, memory, consciousness and mobility are not directly disturbed."

The fourth "A" of Bleuler's fundamental symptoms was "Relation to Reality: Autism" discussed in a subsequent subsection. Bleuler understood the term autism to mean,

"... the loss of the sense of reality or the detachment from reality, together with the relative and absolute predominance of the inner life [of delusions], ..." He also said, "To a considerable extent, reality is transformed through illusions and largely replaced by hallucinations ..."

In summary, autism or autistic thinking means psychotic thinking or psychosis that is nondisease specific.

6.3 Selected Quotes from Bleuler's Textbook, *Dementia Praecox*... 107

Table 6.5 Selected quotes from *Dementia Praecox or the Group of Schizophrenias* (E. Bleuler 1911/1950) attributed to schizophrenia but diagnostic of a psychotic mood disorder

Quote no.	Page no.	Selected quotes	Current author's comments
1	14, 28	Bleuler associated loose associations with schizophrenia. He said "… we know of two disturbances peculiar to schizophrenia—pressure of thoughts, that is, a pathologically increased flow of ideas, and the particularly characteristic 'blocking'" (p. 14) "A patient wrote, 'The capital heavens not only stand over the parish house in Wil, but also over America, South Africa, Mexico, McKinley, Australia.' …" (p. 28).	Loose associations, tangentiality and blocking are rather explained by the distractibility and defective selective attention mechanism specific to manic thought processing (Chap. 13 of the current book).
2	32	"Pure 'pressure of thoughts' can continue for years [in schizophrenia] … Many patients complain that they must think too much, that their ideas chase each other in their heads. They themselves speak of 'thought-overflow' (because they cannot hold anything in their minds), of 'pressure of thoughts' of 'collecting of thoughts,' because too much seems to come to mind at one time…. There is a pathological pressure of ideas…. 'In my mind there ran like an endless clockwork a compulsive, torturing, uninterrupted chain of ideas… What ideas, what images have tumbled around in my head!.'"	These descriptions by Bleuler and the statements of patients themselves are diagnostic of the defect in manic thought processing, not a separate disease.
3	39	"In manic phases of schizophrenia, flight of ideas [of schizophrania] is added to the typically schizophrenic association disturbances. In depressive episodes, we find inhibition of thinking and disturbances of association brought about by abnormal affective reactions."	It is time to make the 180° transition from Bleuler's beliefs that symptoms of mania and depression can exist in schizophrenia to the understanding that symptoms of mania and/or depression define a mood disorder in psychotic patients.
4	40, 41	Bleuler believed that schizophrenia was characterized by "emotional deterioration" that he defined as "the disappearance of affect…. indifference seems to be the external sign of their state; an indifference to everything- to friends and relations, to vocation or enjoyment…. to good fortune or to bad. 'I don't care the least, one way or the other,…'. … A hebephrenic [schizophrenic] talks about his father's death: 'Since I was home…. I went to the funeral and was happy, however, that it was not I who was being buried; I am buried alive now.' … the patients consciously and deliberately isolate themselves…"	Rather than symptoms of another disease, Bleuler's descriptions and the patients' statements are diagnostic of psychotic depression.

(continued)

Table 6.5 (continued)

Quote no.	Page no.	Selected quotes	Current author's comments
5	73	"A [schizophrenic] patient may have sat around for years in a demented euphoria, uttering nothing but the most banal phrases; then all of a sudden he may take part in every kind of work and appear recovered in every respect."	This description of marked changes in mood and behavior is characteristic of a bipolar switch and not a different disease.
6	93	"More advanced cases [of schizophrenia] show the habit of collecting all sorts of objects, useful as well as useless, with which they would fill their apartments so that there was hardly room to move around. Ultimately this collecting mania becomes so utterly senseless that their pockets are always crammed full of pebbles, pieces of wood, rags and all kinds of other trash."	This description of OCD/hoarding points to Bleuler's misconceptions about his disease of schizophrenia encompassing myriad psychiatric syndromes.
7	96, 97, 115	Bleuler believed that auditory hallucinations or "voices" were pathognomonic of schizophrenia. He said, "The 'voices' are the means by which the megalomaniac realizes his wishes, the religiously preoccupied achieves his communication with God and the angels; the depressed are threatened with every kind of catastrophe; the persecuted curse night and day.... the 'voices' threaten, curse, criticize... the persecutor or heavenly figures.... are hallucinated: paradise, hell, a castle,.... 'The talking machine is going all the time.' The patient is 'wired for sound?' He is at 'war.'"	Bleuler did not recognize the mood congruency of voices. Many of his quotes indicate depression or mania. The "talking machine" and being "wired for sound" are symptoms of mania and racing thoughts.
8	117–119	Bleuler believed delusions also defined schizophrenia. He said, "The persecutory delusion is the most frequently met of all the well known types of delusional content. 'There is no kind of human corruption by which one has not sinned against me.... ' Poison has been put into the patient's food, the air, the water, in the wash-basin, the clothes."	Psychotic depression may cause delusions of sin which encourage delusions of persecution that explain the persecutory delusional symptoms misattributed by Bleuler to schizophrenia (Lake 2008b).

6.3 Selected Quotes from Bleuler's Textbook, *Dementia Praecox*... 109

9	119–120	"The delusion of grandeur concerns itself very little with either facts, feasibility or the conceivability of the fulfillment of human desires. ... The patient has 'as much money as there are snow-flakes on the ground.' He is going to be King of England. A palace of gold and precious stones is being built for him... Another patient... claims that 'since he is the Lord, all the gold and silver in the world is at his disposal.' ... He is going to invent 'a perpetual motion machine,' 'become a soldier and conquer the world.' He also possesses a remedy against spinal cord diseases. He can fly;...."	Such descriptions of delusions of grandeur from psychotic patients are specific to mania and a psychotic bipolar disorder.
10	120, 121	Bleuler also believed religious delusions were diagnostic of schizophrenia. "In the religious sphere, the patient is a prophet or even God and as such he has brought to the earth all the carriages in which men now ride. A woman patient 'is Christ the Lord of the world'. She is the 'Highest Good.' ... She is the Savior's Housekeeper, the Bride of Christ, 'the five-hundredth Messiah, God's Golden Book and must be rewarded.' ... A schizophrenic was able to save a lady from sickness by masturbating while thinking of her, and so forth."	Delusional religiosity speaks to grandiosity and mania rather than a separate disease. Modest hypersexuality does not define any psychotic disorder, but when occurring in psychotic patients, it suggests mania.
11	147	Bleuler described the speech of schizophrenia. "The impulse to speak has frequently undergone a change. Many patients talk a great deal, often indeed continuously ... their thoughts are transformed into speech, without relation to the environment. ... Many patients are constantly uttering chains of words; they talk but do not say anything..... Conversely, there are other patients who will not talk at all (mutism)."	These two patterns of speech in psychotic patients warrant a diagnosis of a psychotic mood disorder and not a different disorder.
12	223, 224	Bleuler attributed confusion and incoherence to schizophrenia. He said, "Most disturbances of association, if sufficiently pronounced, lead to confusion. ... The patients speak completely disconnectedly, often in half-broken sentences. They are quite restless and constantly busy doing something, but their activities lack purpose and are not carried through to the end,...."	This description is consistent with the hyperactivity of mania and the inability to complete one project before starting another.

6.4 Bleuler's Accessory Symptoms: Hallucinations and Delusions Embraced as Diagnostic of Schizophrenia

In Chapter II, Bleuler addressed "The Accessory Symptoms." Bleuler correctly recognized that,

> It is primarily the accessory phenomenon which make his [the patient's] retention at home impossible, or it is they which make the psychosis manifest and give occasion to require psychiatric help.

Bleuler listed eight accessory symptoms, two of which he divided into multiple subtypes (Table 6.1). Bleuler said in his first subsection on "Hallucinations,"

> Characteristic of schizophrenic hallucinations is the preference for the auditory sphere … Almost every schizophrenic who is hospitalized hears "voices," occasionally or continually. … The patients hear blowing, rustling, humming, shooting, thundering, music, crying, laughing, whispering, talking. They can see individual objects, landscapes, animals, human beings, and every other possible figure. … The usual occurrence is that the "voices" threaten, curse, criticize and console in short sentences or abrupt words; that the persecutor or heavenly figures, certain kinds of animals, fire or water and also some desire or hoped for situation are hallucinated: paradise, hell, a castle, a robbers cave is seen; that … poison … is tasted in food; that a poisonous vapor or a wonderfully glorious perfume surrounds the patient. They feel the passion of love or all kinds of torture that can be affected by physical means on their abused bodies. … The "voices" are the means by which the megalomaniac realized his wishes, the religiously preoccupied achieves his communication with God and the Angels; the depressed are threatened with every kind of catastrophe; the persecuted curse day and night. … The voices not only speak to the patient, but they pass electricity through his body, beat him, paralyze him, take his thoughts away. … Threats and curses form the main and most common content of these "voices." Day and night they come from everywhere – from the walls, from above and below, from the cellar and the roof, from heaven and from hell, from near and far.
>
> (Bleuler 1911/1950, pp. 94–97)

The passages above are suggestive of grandiose, erotic, threatening, and punishing hallucinations, consistent with psychotic mood disorders.

Bleuler's next subsection was "Delusions" where he discussed:

> The persecutory delusion is the most frequently met of all the well-known types of delusional content. "There is no kind of human corruption by which one has not sinned against me," said one of our paranoids. These patients are driven from their jobs by calumny and, particularly, by every kind of nasty chicanery. They are assigned especially hard work; their materials are ruined, all kinds of defamatory or otherwise injurious insinuations are made against them. Before a patient entered a village, his visit would be heralded and he would then be berated by all the people. They wanted to send him to Siberia, to enslave him. Two whores lived across the street from him; and each time that he sat down to his meal they called out such disgusting things that he could put nothing into his mouth. He has been robbed. The attendants and other patients wear his clothing. He is used as a lavatory.
>
> Schizophrenics in a more lucid state consider themselves to be the victims of a certain "gang of murderers" with whom the patients connect every difficulty they encounter. The Freemasons, the Jesuits, … their fellow-employees, mind-readers, "spiritualists," enemies invented *ad hoc*, are constantly straining every effort to annihilate or at least torture and frighten the patients. Wherever the patients find themselves they are exposed to those hostile forces, be it that their enemies in person pursue the patient from place to place and hide

6.4 Bleuler's Accessory Symptoms: Hallucinations and Delusions Embraced...

> in the walls, in the next room, in the cellar, in the very air; be it that these hostile forces observe and note his every action and thought by means of "mountain-mirrors," or by electrical instruments and influence him by means of mysterious apparatus and magic. ...
>
> Rather than being concerned about the technique of the tortures, the patient seeks more often to find some reason as to why so much trouble is being taken to do all this to him. There are people who are jealous of him, who fear his commercial or sexual competition, or who out of meanness, out of pleasure in torturing, out of inquisitiveness or for some other private purposes, use him for experiments. ...
>
> The delusions of being poisoned is also a very common one. Poison has been put into the patient's food, the air, the water, in the wash-basin, the clothes. It is injected into them from afar, through the mouth and other body orifices. The patient was given "first rate hydrochloric acid, hair-bread, and urine to eat." Besides the poison, all sorts of utterly disgusting ingredients are mixed in his food. The soup was made with footbath water; liquid manure is pumped into his stomach. ...
>
> The delusion of grandeur concerns itself very little with either facts, feasibility or the conceivability of the fulfillment of human desires. ...The patient has a talent for mathematics; he will fill in the gaps of his education and become a great mathematician. His father has a fine business and he will soon be rich. A prominent lady is in love with him; she sends him a box of cigars every day. However, for the most part this thirst for grandeur of some kind transcends all bounds. The patient has "as much money as there are snow-flakes on the ground." He is going to be the King of England. A palace of gold and precious stones is being built for him. The Lord is his only master. He has cured all these poor souls in the hospital. ...
>
> In the religious sphere, the patient is a prophet or even God; ... A woman patient "is Christ and the Lord of the World." She is the "Highest Good." ... She is the Savior's housekeeper, the Bride of Christ, "the five hundredth Messiah, God's Golden Book and must be rewarded." The [schizophrenic] patient is like God ... as everything which she even dares to think comes to pass at once. In women, these religious, grandiose ideas usually have an erotic character. ...
>
> A male patient believes that every woman, who strikes his fancy, is in love with him. Women give birth to 150 children every night. A sterile woman was examined as to her pelvic organs by a doctor and a policeman, both admiring her "talents." ...
>
> A hebephrenic [patient] is "son of the financier G., that is Napoleon."
>
> (Bleuler 1911/1950, pp. 117–123)

The examples of patients' hallucinations and delusions given above are entirely compatible with psychotic thought but are not disease specific. The paranoid, grandiose, and erotic hallucinations and delusions have become more recognized as mood congruent and are accounted for by psychotic mania or psychotic depression (Chap. 12) (Lake 2008b).

Bleuler listed "Speech and Writing" as another accessory symptom of schizophrenia where he said:

> The impulse to speak has frequently undergone a change. Many patients talk a great deal, often indeed continuously. ... Their thoughts are transformed into speech, without relation to the environment. Or such a relation may be entirely one-sided, as when a patient asks a question ... but shows no need for an answer; he gives us no time for one, nor does he listen. The presence of a person often serves as a stimulus to mere speech activity, ... Many patients are constantly uttering chains of words; they talk but do not say anything.
>
> Conversely, there are other patients who will not talk at all (mutism). ...
>
> To a large extent, inappropriate figures of speech are employed, ... "I was the patience of Christ," ... a patient "owns a branch office of God," which means that she has the right to coin money. ... A patient complains that she is not "selling," she thus identifies amorous

with business activity, ... [another female patient used the term] "vaccination while being mounted" and [a male patient used the term] "to perform holy vaccination" both to designate coitus." Another example is "... Mr. S. has been promenading in figures of speech" which means that Mr. S. was mentioned during a conversation.

The schizophrenic construction of new word combinations is of course well-known. They are, indeed, partly comprehensible but only rarely occur with the usual rules of language. ... Another patient is "be-millioned," that is, she had received millions. ... "I am England" means "England belongs to me;" "I am the son," is equivalent to "I am the Lord and Creator of the Sun."

(Bleuler 1911/1950, pp. 147–153)

Bleuler gave numerous examples of schizophrenia patients' writings that commonly have a grandiose and a manic flavor to them as do the examples given just above. Flight of ideas, pressure of speech, loose erotic associations, and new words are suggestive of manic thought (Chap. 13). Another example Bleuler gave for schizophrenia was,

Centraleurope andt centraleuropera No. 3258 Ernest Gisler Troth also the key to Mr. Minister Dr. Daiser DDiv, etc., etc. Standdenbank pprr p. 96 or letter-post 3 vvia Imperially andt Royally also Imperially Royally business Titt, Rheinau. Mo work Badd goodd 3/8 Herr dr. N. C. 30/7 Bern 27/7AD 28/7 short 30/7 3/8 Aa 1906 Datum. Tthey pay on presentation of a receipt Frcs 8 thousandd in banknotes also Titt. ...

[According to Bleuler] Summing up, the piece of writing goes something like this: We, the Emperor of Central Europe, E. no. 3251 wed to Miss Gisler (whereby the right to be free was given), Possessor and Lord of the bank through which we satisfy our needs by using postal-notes, and owner of the factory in Rheinau, issue the following decree:

"You, or the Bernese Central Bank are to pay on demand on the presentation of a note, 8000 francs in cash plus 10 percent. ..."

[Bleuler continued] Words are formed into perfectly correct sentences whose purpose, however, is unintelligible. ...It is not unusual for a piece of writing to founder in a mire of uncontrolled associations.

(Bleuler 1911/1950, pp. 154–156)

A similar dialogue is examined in Chap. 13 with a suggested mechanism of a sensory gating defect in manic thought processing.

Bleuler discussed his ideas about depression in schizophrenia under the subheading of "Melancholic Conditions." Here he said,

The melancholic symptom triad of depressive affect, inhibition of thinking and of action is one of the most frequent acute disturbances in schizophrenia. ...

... depressed schizophrenics can laugh about their own melancholic delusions and behavior. ... the [depressed schizophrenic] patient groans, laments, repeats the same thing a thousand times: that his head ought to be knocked off, that he wants to go home, that he is the worst of men, that he is going straight to hell – but with all this, he goes on doing any number of things which cannot be explained by the depression. He tears his shirt, his bedclothes, scratches not only himself but also the wall; leaves his bed a hundred times, hinders and disturbs the attendants in their care of the other patients, smears his feces, smashes dishes, etc. He makes brutal attempts at suicide by ramming his head against a wall, jumping out of bed head-first on the floor; inflicting all kinds of mutilations on himself. ... The refusal of food is quite common; nevertheless the use of the feeding tube is not always necessary. ...

Delusions and especially hallucinations are rarely absent. Threatening and accusing voices, poisonous vapors, electrical currents, and fire are often perceived. The patients

6.4 Bleuler's Accessory Symptoms: Hallucinations and Delusions Embraced...

believe they are tortured in every conceivable way. They are being killed; their children's eyes pierced, they are forced to spend the night in subterranean torture chambers. They are handed over to the other patients to be torn to pieces; they have committed every earthly sin; they have ruined and rendered their dearest ones miserable and unhappy.

(Bleuler 1911/1950, pp. 208, 209)

Psychotic depression, either bipolar or unipolar, is the most likely diagnosis for these patients (Swartz and Shorter 2007).

Bleuler's next subheading was titled "Manic Conditions." Similar to Bleuler's assignment of melancholic conditions to schizophrenia, he also diagnosed patients with classic symptoms of mania as having schizophrenia. He referred to such patients as "schizophrenic manics" and characterized them as follows:

The patients delight in all kinds of silly tricks, stupid and bad jokes. These pranks are quite typical of hebephrenics. They make silly puns and jokes; tease, laugh at everything and everyone in their family, ridicule the most cherished human values, etc. These patients curse, fume, label everything with a nickname, stick out their tongues, roll their eyes, speak loudly and in bizarre tones, gesticulate a great deal, exaggerate, caricature. Their speech becomes inappropriate, snappy. They turn somersaults, stand on their heads, twist themselves like snakes, declaim, sing, pray. Day and night, every and all unpleasant little habits are practiced; they are destructive, scream and smear. Outbursts of wild rage are even more common in these people than in the usual type of manic; much rarer are the transient shifts to tearful sadness. The frenzies may set in without any apparent cause or occasion. In many of these cases one sees very little of euphoria. ... Manic schizophrenics may also be incommunicative, almost mute. In general, they do little to enter into relationships with their environment; they close their eyes, in some cases continuously for weeks or months at a time. Distractibility may be absent for short periods or at all times. Those patients go through their tricks, speeches, gyrations, quite oblivious to their surroundings. Often the flight of ideas is mixed with confused schizophrenic associations; indeed, the former may be completely concealed by these schizophrenic associations. ...

Although these people show the flight of ideas and euphoric-like moods, make plans and shower us with letters, one never succeeds in getting them to undertake any task or work. ...

When delusions are present, they are usually transitory, and of a persecutory or grandiose character. ...Yet particularly, ideas of persecutions are often continually maintained; the same can be said for the erotic ideas.

(Bleuler 1911/1950, pp. 210, 211)

Each of these signs and symptoms that Bleuler attributes to schizophrenia is actually characteristic of mania and depression, that is, bipolar disorder. Notable examples are: silly jokes, pranks, laughter, cursing, hyperactivity (pressure of activity), lack of a need for sleep, destructiveness, wild rage, transient shifts to tearful sadness, flight of ideas, confused associations, euphoric moods, excessive letter writing, persecutory, erotic, or grandiose delusions.

Bleuler's next subheading was "Catatonic Conditions" in which he associated catatonic schizophrenia with euphoria, flight of ideas, and pressure of activity that cycled with melancholic symptoms. He noted that:

Some mute patients will answer in writing or they may even spontaneously fill whole pages with writing. ...

The hyperkinetic cases ... are constantly in motion without really doing anything (pressure of activity, "flight of activity" ...). They clamber about, move around, shake the branches of trees in the garden, hop over the beds, bang on the table 20 times, and then on the wall; ... They cry, sing, verbigerate, laugh, curse, scream and spit all over the room. They grimace, showing sadness, happiness or horror. ... In stuporous cataleptic individuals, vague lifeless movements predominate. ...

A number of these patients [catatonic schizophrenics] are manifestly manic (with demonstrable flight of ideas); others are melancholic; still others are irritable, anxious, or feel themselves persecuted.

(Bleuler 1911/1950, pp. 211–214)

These descriptions of catatonic schizophrenia are entirely compatible with mania and depression, severe with psychotic and catatonic features and not a new diagnosis.

Another subheading under the "Accessory Symptoms" was "Confusion, Incoherence." Here, Bleuler discussed concepts of manic defective thinking but attributes such to schizophrenia (Chap. 13). He said:

Most disturbances of association, if sufficiently pronounced, lead to confusion. Special attention has to be given to these confusional states which are a direct consequence of the fragmentation of the association. This type of incoherence represents an acute syndrome in almost all cases [of schizophrenia]. The patients speak completely disconnectedly, often in half-broken sentences. They are quite restless and constantly busy doing something, but their activities lack purpose and are not carried through to the end, even such simple actions as leaving a room.

(Bleuler 1911/1950, pp. 223, 224)

Section II is *titled "The Subgroups"* of schizophrenia (Table 6.3). Bleuler added his subtype of simple schizophrenia to the Kraepelinian subtypes of catatonia, hebephrenia (disorganized), and paranoid.

Bleuler first discussed "The Paranoid Group" of schizophrenic patients:

The patients do not feel as they used to [feel] anymore; ... Then come "suspicions," notions that they are destined ... to this or that. They refer completely indifferent events to themselves. ... Gradually, but also quite suddenly, the delusions of reference attain full credibility and certainty. School children run after them; ... It is clear enough that they despise and insult him. Someone "calls out" after him that he has done nasty things with small children, that he masturbates, that he steals. ... Even the newspaper reports contain more or less concealed illusions to him. The minister's sermon is directed at him. The patient changes his dwellings, his jobs, but everywhere there is whispering about him. Wherever he turns, signs and signals point at him. People ... play tricks on him; ... He is given only the worse, the hardest work. ... There is a conspiracy; ... One day he hears how they are talking about him; then they ... call him nasty names, curse, reproach, scorn him. ... Finally, the patient becomes violent, turns on his tormentors. He clouts somebody on the ear or shoots, or creates a disturbance, especially at night. He does not dare to leave his quarters and lives there in peculiar disorder, filth, and hunger. He is then seized and brought to the hospital. After some time, he becomes more sociable; he begins to do a certain amount of work. Ultimately he can be released, but without any essential improvement in his delusional ideas.

(Bleuler 1911/1950, pp. 227–229)

See Chaps. 12 and 13 for explanations of how such paranoia is generated by psychotic manic grandiosity and psychotic depressive guilt. In keeping with these writings of Bleuler, even today violence and murders by psychotic individuals are typically attributed to schizophrenia by the media rather than bipolar disorders (Sect. 15.5).

6.4 Bleuler's Accessory Symptoms: Hallucinations and Delusions Embraced...

Bleuler described cycling relapses in these patients he diagnosed with paranoid schizophrenia. He discussed hallucinations and delusions that he said were characteristic of patients with paranoid schizophrenia:

> During the night an angel, Christ, or God appears to show the patient A New Way. In the persecuted, there is often a period of hallucinatory excitement lasting several hours or even several days, frequently combined with marked confusion and disorientation. On some occasion, ... he has become convinced of his own greatness, or of the evilness of his persecutors. Such revelations are found in the case histories of most delusional schizophrenics. ...
>
> The many litigious schizophrenics belong to this group [paranoid]. A young woman had charge of a physician's household. Perhaps he really did make some erotic advances to her. In any event, she imagined that he had promised to marry her. She demanded that he fulfill his promise and marry her; she made all sorts of scenes, difficulties, and unpleasantnesses, and he finally had to dismiss her. She carried her complaints to the courts, always of the opinion that she had and could prove all her allegations. Then she lodged a complaint against the judge himself because he had not found in her favor. She became more and more confused, could not work. Lawyers got most of her possessions in the course of the many lawsuits. She was judged to be mentally ill by a board of experts, she filed a complaint against the expert testimony, etc. From time to time, she managed to spend a year outside the hospital although never without difficulty....
>
> The delusions both of grandeur and eroticism show essentially the same variations as do the delusions of persecution. The [schizophrenic] patients believe that they are loved by persons of a higher social standing than themselves. In the main, the patients wish to give these persons an opportunity to communicate with them. They heap curses and vilification on their lovers and occasionally transfer their affections to still other persons who are then treated in the same way. The megalomaniac patients [with schizophrenia] have made marvelous inventions; they are prophets, philosophers, world-reformers, who, only in relatively exceptional instances, are able to collect followers because they are, after all, often too confused, behave far too badly, far too awkwardly to really impress others.
>
> (Bleuler 1911/1950, pp. 230, 231)

Such descriptions of grandiosity and erotic delusions suggest the diagnosis of mania and bipolar disorder. Litigiousness is compatible with manic hyperactivity with some retention of focus although it is inappropriate. In this case, Bleuler does not report the patients' sleep patterns directly, but he describes manic behavior occurring "day and night" and "... hallucinatory excitement lasting several hours or even several days ...." One might expect that his litigious female patient busied herself all night writing legal briefs for her case. Another possible diagnosis for this woman is a delusional disorder (DSM-IV-TR 297.1), the erotomanic type, described in the DSM-IV-TR as having "delusions that another person, usually of higher status, is in love with the individual."

Bleuler detailed his own addition to the subtypes of schizophrenia under the subheading of "Schizophrenia Simplex."

> This group is rarely found in hospitals but outside it is as common as any of the other forms. In private practice, we often see it, indeed as frequently in the relatives who bring the patients as in the patients themselves. On the lower levels of society, the simple schizophrenics vegetate as day laborers, peddlers, even as servants. They are also vagabonds and hoboes as are other types of schizophrenics of mild grade. On the higher levels of society, the most common type [of simple schizophrenia] is the wife (in a very unhappy role, we can say), who is unbearable, constantly scolding, nagging, always making demands but

never recognizing duties. Her family never considers the possibility of illness, suffers for many years a veritable hell of annoyances, difficulties, unpleasantnesses from the "mean" woman. They usually employ every possible means to conceal the true state of affairs in the home from the prying eyes of the outside world. The possibility of keeping the anomaly secret is facilitated by the fact that many of these patients still manage to conduct themselves in an entirely unobtrusive way. Frequently one is veritably forced to keep the situation secret from the world at large because there are many people who readily step in and defend these women who themselves know how to play the role of injured and persecuted innocence. …

Furthermore, there are many simple schizophrenics among eccentric people of every sort who stand out as world saviors and world reformers, philosophers, writers and artists, beside the "degenerated" and deteriorated. …

These cases diagnosed with simple schizophrenia are offered by Bleuler as classic examples but are rather better examples of the subjective, sexist, overinclusiveness of Bleuler's concept of schizophrenia. Additional vignettes from Bleuler are given below:

A teacher, who had done very well in school, goes to Romania as a tutor because he was unable to find a teaching position immediately after graduation. He remains there some eight years but in the end permits himself to be cheated out of his salary by his employers. He returns home penniless. He seeks employment as a teacher, substitutes in various places, but for years is unable to find a permanent position. Finally, a tiny village appoints him to a permanent teaching job only to dismiss him after six months because of inefficiency. He tries another canton with no better success. Given one position which he might have been able to retain permanently, he suddenly leaves without reason and without notice or consideration for others. Naturally, he was always in very poor financial straits; got into debt and mortgaged his pension under rather unfavorable conditions for himself; pawned most of his belongings. All this he did with the idea that circumstances would somehow change since up to now it was only this or that which was merely accidently lacking. If someone would only advance him some money, he was quite certain that he would then be able to find a position and then everything would easily be straightened out once more. That he himself was to blame for his bad luck and difficulties, he did not suspect at all, despite many efforts to give him insight. Finally he bombards the government officials with demands for his "rights" in which demands he mixes a good bit of cursing and insults, etc. He proceeds to insult and injure those who had given him financial credit.

Multiple short-term jobs, getting into debt, bombarding government officials with demands for his rights mixed with curses are consistent with the poor decisions, grandiosity, hyperactivity, and irritability of mania and depression. Bleuler continued,

Another type with marked irritability: A normal, intelligent girl marries at twenty and lives happily for more than five years. Very gradually she becomes irritable, gesticulates while talking, her peculiarities continue to increase; she cannot keep a servant anymore; she is constantly quarrelling with her neighbors. Within her own family group, she has developed into an unbearable domestic tyrant who knows no duties, only rights. She is unable to manage the household or do the housework any more because she makes all kinds of silly, stupid, and useless purchases and is proving herself utterly impractical.

"Silly, stupid, and useless purchases" are also typical of the poor judgment and spending sprees of mania.

6.4 Bleuler's Accessory Symptoms: Hallucinations and Delusions Embraced...

If we examine some individuals more closely, we often tend to suspect the presence of simple schizophrenia without, however, being able to make a definite diagnosis at the given time; but very often, after days or years, our suspicions can be confirmed. Thus, there is no doubt that many simple schizophrenics are at large whose symptoms are not sufficiently pronounced to permit the recognition of mental disorder.

Such mild cases are often considered to be "nervous" or "degenerated" individuals, etc. But if we follow the anamnesis of those who are admitted to the hospital in later years because of an exacerbation of their difficulties, a criminal charge, a pathological drinking bout or some such episode, we can usually find throughout the entire past history of the individual mildly pathological symptoms which in the light of their recent illness unquestionably have to be considered as schizophrenic.

(Bleuler 1911/1950, pp. 236–239)

Bleuler's discussion above again demonstrates his broad, subjective, over-inclusiveness of his concept of schizophrenia.

Section III was titled, "The Course of the Disease." Under the subheading of "The Temporal Course," Bleuler said that, "It is impossible to describe all the variations which the course of schizophrenia may take." He then gave some examples of different courses of his cases that he diagnosed with schizophrenia:

(1) Housekeeper: markedly religious. Was melancholic for many months during puberty. A voice whispered to her what she was to write in a letter. Then for the next ten years, "the very model of young maidenhood," very devoted, tractable and conscientious. Then a manic condition which lasted for many years with foolish, silly, erotic, and religious delusions. Later she was again able to resume work.

(2) A female factory worker: Was manic for several weeks shortly after her first menses. Then well, but irritable, seclusive, withdrawn; she felt she was being mocked, laughed incessantly. At age twenty-one, silly manic delusions; was released as "cured." She remained well until age twenty-three. Then, confused religious delusions, but again improved. However, she was no longer able to hold her job. After about five years, gradual elaboration of a hallucinatory, confusional state; agitated, even in the hospital; she is no longer able to do any work.

(3) Farmer: Insomniac since age twenty-five. At age twenty-eight, a twilight state lasting several months. "Cured" overnight. Was "well" till age thirty; but at the funeral of a neighbor who had committed suicide, he became very excited and agitated. After he met an old sweetheart of his, he became dull, mute, refused food for several days. At age thirty-one, his sweetheart wrote him a letter which he read. Thereupon a sudden, severe, depressed catatonic state, improved after a year; released as able to work. One year later, suicide. …

(4) Woman: Was in a mental hospital at age ten. At age twenty, following a rape, she is "crazy." Then recovers and is apparently well. At age seventy-one, she is again a patient in a mental institution.

(5) Woman: depressive catatonia after puberty. Then considered as well. Marries and has children. Then in her 70th year, melancholic schizophrenic episode.

(6) Physician: Neurasthenia at twenty-nine. Then at thirty-one after typhoid fever, catatonic. At forty-seven, apparently "cured." He then resumes his practice, marries. Has been well for the past two years.

(Bleuler 1911/1950, pp. 147–148)

Bleuler used the vignettes given above as well as others as typical examples of the various courses of schizophrenia. Bleuler diagnosed all of them with schizophrenia, each with a specific subtype. Vignettes one, two, and three have episodes of both mania and depression. The farmer, vignette three, suicided. Suicide is primarily associated with severe depression. A diagnosis of schizophrenia is doubtful in vignettes four and five because they were hospitalized at 71 and 70 years of age, respectively; vignette five was apparently severely depressed. Vignette six, the physician, may have suffered "catatonia" as a result of his typhoid fever rather than schizophrenia.

Under subsection C "The Termination of the Disease: 1. Death," Bleuler gave several organic causes of death in patients he had diagnosed with schizophrenia. For example, he said,

> The immediate causes [of death in schizophrenia] may be cerebral pressure due to cerebral edema or increased cerebrospinal fluid: metabolic disturbances (including auto-intoxications) and cerebral paralysis as seen in catatonic or epileptiform attacks.
>
> (Bleuler 1911/1950, p. 254)

Such causes of death raise questions as to whether the psychotic or other symptoms utilized by Bleuler to diagnose schizophrenia were actually due to an organic disease, negating the diagnosis of schizophrenia or any functional psychosis.

Many of Bleuler's statements from Section IV, "Schizophrenia in Conjunction with Other Psychoses" and Section V, "The Concept of Disease," further support the contention that Bleuler misdiagnosed schizophrenia in cases having organic diseases capable of causing psychotic symptoms. Bleuler discussed making the diagnosis of schizophrenia in patients with cretinism, senile dementia, brain tumors, general paresis, alcoholism, obsessive-compulsive states, epilepsy, fever deliria, Wernicke's psychoses, hysteria, "nervous persons," and "masturbation insanity." However, in Section V, Bleuler did acknowledge that,

> Yet we cannot exclude the possibility that certain mild organic disturbances bring forth symptom complexes which we now designate as Dementia Praecox. It is possible, furthermore, that some kind of intoxication, for instance, by alcohol, may bring about similar clinical pictures.
>
> (Bleuler 1911/1950, p. 279)

Despite this statement, Bleuler's belief that schizophrenia overruled organic diseases was expressed later in Section V on pages 282, 288, and 289 when he said,

> Chronic alcohol-paranoia has frequently been diagnosed by others; I, however, have not yet seen such a patient, who gave me even the slightest reason to see in him anything other than an ordinary schizophrenic who also drank. …
>
> …schizophrenia, itself, also predisposes to delirium tremens.
>
> I have also seen alcoholic hallucinosis develop on the basis of schizophrenia. …
>
> Obviously almost all of Wernicke's "motility psychoses" are also schizophrenias.
>
> Of the chronic diseases, all those designated as dementing types, primary and secondary dementias, etc., belong to our disease [schizophrenia], as well as the greater portion of the paranoias of other writers. …
>
> Bleuler continued saying that, "A large number of women whom I considered schizophrenics passed for hysterically insane in other places whereby it was implied that the insanity was somehow or other a further development of the hysteria …"

6.4 Bleuler's Accessory Symptoms: Hallucinations and Delusions Embraced...

> "Nervous" persons, too, whose conversations are often confused, who refuse nourishment and exhibit delusions of jealously, are, as far as our experience goes, neither neurasthenics nor narcoleptics, but [schizophrenic] catatonics.
>
> Many, although not all, of the very severe form of compulsive conditions, of folie du doute ..., and of impulsive behavior undoubtedly belong to schizophrenia ... These clinical pictures termed pyromania, kleptomania, etc., are sometimes schizophrenics.
>
> The masturbation insanity described by various authors must obviously be included in schizophrenia.
>
> (Bleuler 1911/1950, pp. 288–289)

Such statements clarify Bleuler's belief that his disease, schizophrenia, subsumed many other diseases and conditions and lead to skepticism of his ideas in general. Bleuler's aggressive overinclusiveness of the use of his diagnosis of schizophrenia may have involved self-image. Yet, it is his concepts presented in his 1911 book that have influenced academic psychiatry more than any other individual with regard to the diagnoses of functionally psychotic patients.

Bleuler discounted the diagnostic value of manic and depressive symptoms:

> "Combinations of schizophrenia with melancholia and mania or with manic depressive psychosis ... have not yet been demonstrated with any certainty." However, he then said, "Manic and melancholic symptoms are so common in our [schizophrenic] patients that we must assume that they [manic and melancholic symptoms] are usually released by the [schizophrenic] disease process itself, and thus are part of the schizophrenia."
>
> (Bleuler 1911/1950, p. 268)

In Section V, "The Concept of Disease," Bleuler said,

> Dementia Praecox comprises the majority of psychoses here-to-fore designated as functional.

Based on the bulk of Bleuler's writings, the interpretation of Bleuler's concept of schizophrenia has been that schizophrenia accounts for all functional psychoses. Bleuler criticized,

> "... many German as well as foreign authors ..." for continuing to separate "... acute and chronic hallucinatory paranoia, amentia, and confusion mentale ..." from schizophrenia. He said, "The establishment of the Dementia Praecox concept has brought clarity and order to this confusion [of classification]. The Kraepelinian Dementia Praecox is an actual disease concept. The concept includes symptoms which occur only and always in Dementia Praecox. Thereby the disease group is provided with concrete delimitations."

Bleuler likened schizophrenia to the role played by syphilis that was proved to be the etiology of what had been considered to be many different diseases. He mistakenly anticipated that a pathophysiology would be discovered for schizophrenia that would also be common to many other chronic dementing diseases, both functional and organic.

Quite the opposite of Bleuler's prediction, no pathophysiology has been documented despite major expenditures of time and money, and in fact, schizophrenia has no unique diagnostic symptoms not also found in documented cases of psychotic bipolar and unipolar disorders. In a footnote, Bleuler references Kraepelin's doubt of his dichotomy and adds that, "... I cannot follow him in that direction and maintain my position [that schizophrenia is distinct from Manic-Depressive Insanity] ...." (Bleuler 1911/1950, pp. 271, 278–279).

Section VI was titled "Diagnosis." In the first subsection titled, "General Remarks," Bleuler revealed again how indiscriminately he gave a diagnosis of schizophrenia;

> As in every other disease, the symptoms must have reached a certain degree of intensity if they are to be of any diagnostic value. Yet in milder cases of schizophrenia we find a number of prominent manifestations, which strongly fluctuate within the limits of what is regarded, if not as healthy, at least as "not mentally ill." Character anomalies, indifference, lack of energy, unsociability, stubbornness, moodiness, the characteristic for which Goethe could only find the English word, "whimsical," hypochondriacal complaints, etc., are not necessarily symptoms of an actual mental disease; they are, however, often the only perceptible signs of schizophrenia. It is for this reason that the diagnostic threshold of schizophrenia is higher than that of any other disease; and it is because of this that latent cases are such a common occurrence.

(Bleuler 1911/1950, p. 294)

6.5 Functional Psychosis Does Not Equal Schizophrenia

Bleuler stated on page 304 of his book that a diagnosis of schizophrenia must be made when functional psychotic symptoms were present:

> All the phenomena of manic-depressive psychosis may also appear in our disease [schizophrenia]; the only decisive factor is the presence or absence of schizophrenic symptoms [psychosis]. Therefore, neither a state of manic exaltation nor a melancholic depression, nor the alternation of both states has any significance for the diagnosis. Only after careful observation has revealed no schizophrenic features, may we conclude that we are dealing with a manic-depressive psychosis.

Although Bleuler certainly did not intend for schizophrenia to be limited to psychotic patients, after the publication of the DSM-III in 1980, it was his accessory symptoms of hallucinations and delusions, the fundamental symptom of a disturbance of affect and the subtypes of paranoid, disorganized, and catatonic that came to define schizophrenia. These subtypes doubled as diagnostic criteria. These same diagnostic criteria of schizophrenia continue in the DSM-5 draft proposal despite the elimination of the subtypes as subtypes, (but not as diagnostic criteria). Bleuler's most impactful legacy has been making a diagnosis of schizophrenia in any functionally psychotic patient.

6.6 Conclusions

It is important to note that Bleuler's book, like those of Kraepelin, was based on his observations and opinions of his inpatients' behavior, dialogue, and letters. It is not that Bleuler's observations were inaccurate; in fact, his writings give valuable insights into the psychotic behaviors, thoughts, and writings expressed by his mentally ill

6.6 Conclusions

inpatients around the turn of the nineteenth century. His descriptions are typical of a similar patient population today. Where Bleuler erred was in his opinion that certain psychotic and nonpsychotic thoughts and behaviors constituted a disease different from manic-depressive insanity, more specifically, his disease, schizophrenia. His investment in schizophrenia became his life's work. In keeping with his bias of enhancing the diagnosis of schizophrenia, Bleuler broke the tradition of Hecker, Kahlbaum, Kraepelin, and others who had considered only young, psychotic, and chronic patients for the diagnosis of dementia praecox or schizophrenia. Bleuler diagnosed schizophrenia in patients of any age, with or without psychotic symptoms and with or without a chronic, deteriorating course.

His book may have influenced academic psychiatry in the USA as much or more than any other textbook and thus all of the mental health professions. It was required reading in many psychiatry residency training programs through the 1970s. Bleuler's fundamental and accessory symptoms became diagnostic criteria in the DSMs, and his other signs and symptoms were also thought suggestive if not diagnostic (Tables 2.5, 6.1, 6.3, and 6.4). Bleuler's concepts about schizophrenia are still found in current textbooks, the DSM-IV-TR, the draft of the DSM-5 (Tables 2.5 and 3.4), and the ICD-10. Sometimes of more importance than what the physician actually wrote has been the interpretations of his or her meaning; more specifically, which statements have been chosen to emphasize in teaching in some cases have obscured the original authors' ambivalence. Kraepelin's reversal of his dichotomy later in his career is a good example of choosing to emphasize the dichotomy versus his question of whether schizophrenia was different from psychotic mood disorders. With regard to Bleuler's writings, academic psychiatry focused on his accessory symptoms, hallucinations, delusions, disorganization, and catatonia, as diagnostic of schizophrenia. This is still evident in the DSM-5 draft proposal. Although this was not Bleuler's core message, the equation of functional psychosis to schizophrenia has remained ingrained among mental health professions and others. Bleuler actually stated on page 13 of his text that,

> As far as we know, the fundamental symptoms are characteristic of schizophrenia, while the accessory symptoms [hallucinations and delusions] may also appear in other types of illness [bipolar disorders]. (Table 6.2)

Rather, Bleuler's core emphasis was the widespread prevalence of schizophrenia among nonpsychotic, nonchronic cases of eccentricity of any age. Reflecting the absence of demarcation between normal and some of Bleuler's nonpsychotic patients with schizophrenia, Szasz said, "There is, in short, no such thing as schizophrenia" (Szasz 1976).

Most striking about Bleuler's text is the prevalence of manic and depressive symptoms in patients he diagnosed with schizophrenia (Table 6.5). He believed that many signs and symptoms now considered indicative or diagnostic of a psychotic mood disorder were diagnostic of schizophrenia. An attempt at a reversal or at least a modification of this dogma occurred in 1933 with the publication by Jacob Kasanin discussed in the next chapter.

Bleuler was unlucky to have chosen to rename and focus upon dementia praecox rather than manic-depressive insanity.

Chapter 7
Jacob Kasanin (1897–1946) and Schizoaffective Disorder

> *Schizo-Affective Psychosis: Fact or Fiction?* [title of article]
> ... support for the adoption of some widely agreed upon epithet to describe this state [schizoaffective disorder] is indicated.... at least a subgroup of these psychoses [schizoaffective disorder] has a definite relationship to the major affective disorders. An old proverb reads; "A person with a bad name is already half-hanged." This may well be the case with the term schizoaffective disorder.
>
> (Procci 1976)

> *There is no demarcation between schizoaffective disorder and psychotic mood disorders... Without inter-rater reliability in DSM-IV [for] schizoaffective disorder, there could be no validity. If there is no validity, why are we using it?... Schizoaffective disorder seems an entity 'beyond necessity.'*
>
> (Swartz 2002b)

> *Taken together, there is growing evidence that a substantial proportion of etiological factors is shared between schizophrenia and bipolar disorder.... In summary, the historical starting point of the concept of schizoaffective disorder is not valid anymore.... The task forces for new versions of the DSM-and ICD-diagnostic systems and manuals... would be badly advised if they would just continue the historical and current concepts of schizoaffective disorder into the future.*
>
> (Maier et al. 2006)

7.1 Introduction

Jacob Kasanin was born in Slavgorod, USSR, in 1897. He migrated to the USA in 1915 and graduated from the University of Michigan with an M.D. in 1921 and an M.S. in Public Health in 1926. He served as Senior Research Associate at Boston

Psychopathic Hospital and as the Director of the Department of Mental Hygiene of the Federated Jewish Charities in Boston. One of his research interests was the study of the functional psychoses in children. In 1931, he became the Clinical Director of the Rhode Island State Hospital where he was supported by a research grant from the Rockefeller Foundation to study schizophrenia. He published his famous paper in the *American Journal of Psychiatry* in 1933 titled "The Acute Schizoaffective Psychoses," after reading it at the 88th Annual Meeting of the American Psychiatric Association in Philadelphia, PA, in May/June of 1932. He later became the Director of the Department of Psychiatry at the Michael Reese Hospital in Chicago from 1936 to 1939. The importance of this new diagnosis was that it rejoined schizophrenia and bipolar disorder after almost a half century of separateness.

7.2 Schizoaffective Disorder Contradicts the Concepts of Kraepelin and Bleuler About Schizophrenia

Kraepelin's dichotomy and psychiatry's interpretation of Bleuler's concept that hallucinations and delusions were pathognomonic of schizophrenia regardless of a predominance of mood disturbance dominated the mental health field from the early 1900s through the 1980s and beyond. This was despite Kasanin's 1933 introduction of the term "acute schizoaffective psychoses" (Kasanin 1933). Schizoaffective disorder challenged Bleuler's assertion that psychosis means schizophrenia and Kraepelin's dichotomy that two separate diseases account for severe mental illness. Schizoaffective disorder connected schizophrenia and bipolar disorder and recognized the diagnostic significance of mood symptoms in psychotic patients. Although Kasanin said that Kraepelin's classification,

> "… was simple and empirically extremely useful, because it allowed the institutional physician to orient himself quickly in his case and even give a prognosis,…" he added that, "On the other hand, its very rigidity, together with the underlying concept of an immutable disease process in dementia praecox was quite detrimental to the field of psychiatry, …"

(Kasanin 1933)

Kasanin seemed to question the zone of rarity between schizophrenia and bipolar disorder when he said,

> It is the problem of the psychiatrist as a scientist to discover general laws which hold true of a large number of patients and a principle of classification must be found with establishment of definite differential criteria. The problem is extremely difficult. It took almost one hundred years to crystallize out the disease concept of general paresis and even then when the objective diagnostic criteria were established, it was found that mistakes in diagnosis reached as high as 50 percent. In the so-called functional psychoses, the problem is still unsolved.

(Kasanin 1933)

In his article, he summarized the cases of nine hospitalized psychotic patients initially diagnosed with dementia praecox or schizophrenia. The Kasanin patients suffered from hallucinations and/or delusions (i.e., were psychotic), but he thought

7.3 Schizoaffective Disorder Merges Schizophrenia and Psychotic Mood Disorders

Table 7.1 DSM-IV-TR diagnostic criteria for schizoaffective disorder (Modified for brevity)[a]

A. Uninterrupted period of illness during which major depression, mania, or a mixed episode is concurrent with symptoms that meet criterion A for schizophrenia[b,c] (see below).
B. During some period of this illness, there have been delusions and/or hallucinations for at least 2 weeks with an absence of prominent[b] mood symptoms.
C. Symptoms that meet criteria for mood episode are present for a substantial[b] portion of the total duration of active and residual periods of illness.
D. Substances and general medical conditions are excluded.

[a]Abbreviated format without change in meaning or substance
[b]Underlines added by author for emphasis
[c]Criterion A for schizophrenia: characteristic symptoms: patient must have two symptoms during a 1-month (active) phase (except as noted below):
1. Delusions
2. Hallucinations
3. Disorganized speech (frequent derailment, incoherence)
4. Grossly disorganized or catatonic behavior
5. Negative symptoms (affective flattening, alogia, and avolition)

Note: Only one symptom is required if delusions are bizarre or hallucinations are a voice commenting on one's behavior/thoughts, or if two or more voices are conversing with each other.

they were different from the typical patient diagnosed with schizophrenia because they had distinct and prominent manic and/or depressive symptomatology, had had an acute onset of symptoms, active social lives and healthy premorbid personalities, only brief periods of psychosis lasting weeks to a few months, and recovered to lead successful lives. These patients had outcomes better than patients typically diagnosed with schizophrenia but worse than those then considered acceptable for a mood disorder diagnosis. He concluded that they differed enough from "classical" schizophrenia, as described by Kraepelin (1913, 1919) and Bleuler (1911/1950), that a compromising diagnostic name was needed. Today, Kasanin's patients would likely be diagnosed with a psychotic mood disorder, that is, unipolar or bipolar disorder, severe with psychotic features. However, the universality of Bleuler's concept probably prevented the more radical shift to the diagnosis of a psychotic affective/mood disorder. This would have prevented the introduction of an additional diagnosis that has become obsolete as such patients are now usually considered by most to suffer from psychotic mood disorders (Sects. 7.6 and 7.7). The current DSM-IV-TR diagnostic criteria are given in Table 7.1 and are similar to those in the proposed DSM-5.

7.3 Schizoaffective Disorder Merges Schizophrenia and Psychotic Mood Disorders

The concept of schizoaffective disorder linked schizophrenia with mood disorders, and this encouraged comparative studies that have progressively resulted in a closing of the conceptual gap between schizophrenia and psychotic mood disorders (Fig. 3.1). Although schizoaffective disorder was initially considered a diagnosis for patients who suffered symptoms and a course in between patients with typical schizophrenia and classic (nonpsychotic) bipolar, such patients diagnosed with schizoaffective disorder likely represent an intermediate level of severity and chronicity between chronic psychotic mood disorders and classic (nonpsychotic) mood disorders.

The naming of schizoaffective disorder may have been one of the first shifts in the concept about the diagnosis of psychotic patients away from Bleuler's view that 100% of psychotic patients have schizophrenia and toward the recognition of psychotic mood disorders. The "schizo" prefix of schizoaffective disorder was maintained in keeping with the misconception that hallucinations and/or delusions were disease specific for schizophrenia. At that time, for Dr. Kasanin, prominent mood symptoms only warranted an intermediary diagnosis. However, outside of Dr. Kasanin's realm of influence and for 50 years at least, such patients were usually diagnosed with schizophrenia because they suffered from hallucinations and/or delusions. Bleuler's (1911) and later Schneider's (1959) concepts dominated the field especially in the USA.

7.4 Examples of Psychotic Mood Symptoms from Kasanin's Cases

Kasanin "… personally studied …" nine patients who were described as follows: all were diagnosed with dementia praecox or schizophrenia, all were in their 20s and 30s, in excellent physical health, had average to superior intelligence, had a precipitating factor, "… got a good deal of satisfaction out of life.," were "… keen, ambitious, forward, some of them rather seclusive, others quite sociable. … were very sensitive, critical of themselves, introspective, very unhappy and preoccupied with their own conflicts, problems, …." Most striking were symptoms of mania and depression in these psychotic patients diagnosed with schizophrenia. Kasanin said of his nine cases that, "The psychosis is usually ushered in by a latent depression and a certain amount of rumination going on for some time …." Specific examples from his paper are:

> Patient #1 was a 21-year-old clerk who took a job in New York City believing that "… he was picked out for a big success in the financial world." He became delusional and suicidal after losing his job and scheduling surgery to remove his deformed thumb. "The patient spent his two weeks salary riding in taxies" because he felt his death was imminent. Upon admission to the psychiatric unit, he said that "Things began to look rather gloomy in his place of employment." He said he began to have ideas of suicide and "Then all of a sudden a "biblical" saying flashed into his mind, … He felt that God or the Supreme Being was in some way putting the thought into his head and that he was to commit suicide and that he was going to die."
>
> Patient #3 was a 33-year-old married male who, in the weeks before his psychotic episode and admission to the hospital, became "… markedly preoccupied with his troubles; he had much less to say than usual and he was particularly glum. His appetite became poor and he slept badly at night. … He felt he was grossly inadequate. Then suddenly on Thanksgiving day he became very talkative on religious matters. … He felt that God and the Devil were having a great struggle with regard to his conversion … He talked continually about the Bible. … Several times during [Thanksgiving] day he got down on his knees and prayed and stated that a spirit had come over him. He was restless and slept little during the night." He expressed delusional guilt over "… having stolen a cake of soap. I brought it home without paying for it." This man previously had not been particularly religious.

Patient #4 was a 42-year-old businessman who "A week before admission ... suddenly began to talk about religion, said that God appeared to him, became very excited and on the day of admission showed the family a razor, ..." This patient's family history was positive for suicide and depression. This patient who had "... never cared for religion before. ... suddenly began to talk about religion. ... God appeared to him and had chosen him to do certain things. ... the patient said that he was going to reform everybody and insisted that the whole family should go to church on Sunday mornings. ... He lay awake nights thinking of what God told him to do." During the first week of hospitalization, "The mood changed from an initial elation to a mild depression...."

Patient #8 was a 20-year-old male laborer who "... was sent to the hospital by his family because about two weeks before admission he became overactive, exhibited queer behavior and spoke a great deal about his theories of life...." At work, "... the patient began to talk a great deal and ... began to sing very loudly. Quite suddenly he declared that he was going on the stage or else would join a professional baseball team. ... He sent a telegram to a Boston baseball team ... asking the manager for a position. He told his family that he was going to make a great deal of money ... He slept very poorly and was very restless at night. A week before the admission he went to one of the Harvard physicians and offered his body for scientific purposes ... He was quite excited for several days and spoke a great deal about scientific experiments on his brain and the cure of insanity. ... Finally he became so excited that he was taken to the outpatient department from which he was referred to the house."

(Kasanin 1933)

In these cases, the religiosity, grandiosity, increased activities and speech, and poor judgment along with cycles of depression are suggestive of a bipolar disorder, severe with psychotic features, rather than any other disorder.

7.5 Schizoaffective Disorder Ignored for 30 Years But Then Flourished

Schizoaffective disorder became firmly established as a recognized subtype of schizophrenia with the publication in 1952 of the first DSM. The DSM-I (APA, DSM 1952) and the DSM-II (APA, DSM 1968) defined "schizoaffective schizophrenia" as the "category for patients showing a mixture of schizophrenic symptoms and pronounced[1] elation or depression." Two subtypes were described: excited and depressed. Despite the centrality of mood symptoms, schizoaffective disorder was defined as a subtype of schizophrenia, not a subtype of mood disorders. The placement of schizoaffective disorder in the current and future DSMs and in textbook chapters on schizophrenia reflects the influence of Bleuler and later Schneider and inhibited the consideration of schizoaffective disorder and schizophrenia as psychotic mood disorders. The current DSM-IV-TR diagnostic criteria are given in Table 7.1.

The next notation to "schizoaffective psychoses" following Kasanin's appears to have occurred in 1943 when Cobb used this term in his textbook to include both schizophrenia and manic-depressive illness under one diagnosis, implying that these

---

[1] Underlined by author for emphasis.

Table 7.2 PubMed literature cites of schizoaffective disorder (SAD)

Total # articles citing SAD—29,766

Total # articles with SAD in title—619

Year	Articles citing SAD	Articles with SAD in title	Year	Articles citing SAD	Articles with SAD in title
1949	0	0	1980	516	10
1950	1	0	1981	493	11
1951	0	0	1982	579	10
1952	1	0	1983	510	18
1953	1	1	1984	589	23
1954	2	0	1985	575	13
1955	0	0	1986	558	9
1956	1	0	1987	495	11
1957	0	0	1988	548	21
1958	2	0	1989	574	22
1959	1	0	1990	583	27
1960	1	0	1991	539	19
1961	2	1	1992	555	18
1962	4	0	1993	545	17
1963	0	0	1994	585	14
1964	17	0	1995	563	17
1965	289	0	1996	613	14
1966	435	0	1997	587	19
1967	606	0	1998	623	22
1968	674	1	1999	719	27
1969	639	1	2000	731	23
1970	642	0	2001	771	31
1971	568	1	2002	757	35
1972	536	0	2003	964	27
1973	535	0	2004	907	47
1974	520	4	2005	1,084	48
1975	554	1	2006	1,516	43
1976	477	0	2007	1,781	48
1977	485	4	2008	1,843	46
1978	542	1	2009	1,690	60
1979	585	14	2010	1,478	51

two diseases were linked or the same disease (Cobb 1943). Schizoaffective disorder became a very popular diagnosis beginning in the late 1960s. An index of the acceptance and clinical popularity of schizoaffective disorder is reflected by the number of cites in the scientific literature (Table 7.2). Based on a PubMed literature search for articles citing schizoaffective disorder, the diagnosis was little used in the literature between the mid-1930s and the mid-1960s despite its description in 1933 and inclusion in the DSM from 1952 (Figs. 3.2, 7.1), likely reflecting the dominant concept

7.5 Schizoaffective Disorder Ignored for 30 Years But Then Flourished

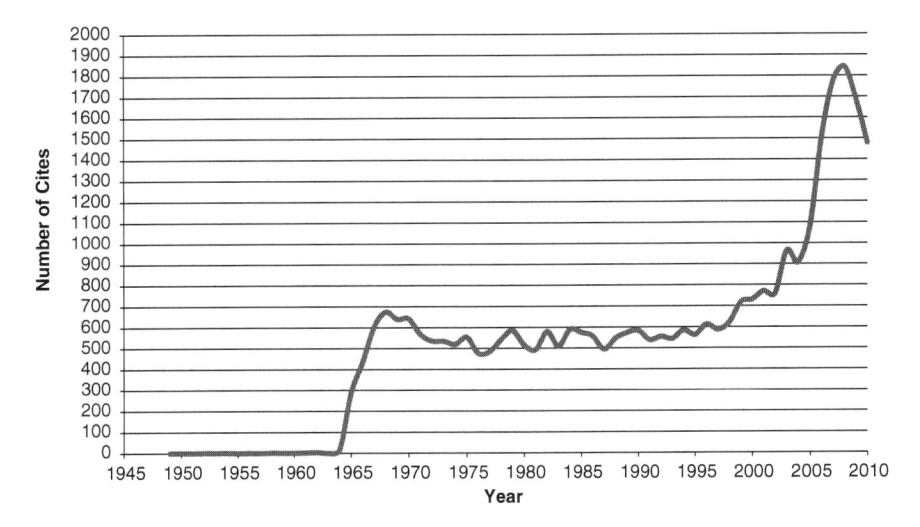

Fig. 7.1 PubMed literature cites of schizoaffective disorder

Although named in 1933 (Kasanin) and used by Cobb in 1943, the diagnosis of schizoaffective disorder did not begin to appear in the literature until the mid to late 1960s. Figure 7.1 presents the number of PubMed cites in the scientific literature as an index of the popularity of the use of the diagnosis in clinical practice. The number of literature cites seemed to have plateaued between 1970 and 2000. A clear increase in the number of cites began in 2000 that increased through 2008 before declining. Some of the increase in number of cites between 2005 and 2009 are explained by publications concluding that schizoaffective disorder is invalid as a disease different from a psychotic mood disorder

that psychosis was schizophrenia. The number of PubMed cites sharply increased in 1965 and 1966, plateaued or decreased slightly in the 1970s, and remained stable until 1999 when the number of papers about schizoaffective disorder increased substantially again through 2008 (Table 7.2, Fig. 3.2). The decrease in the 1970s may reflect the influence of a number of publications that questioned the validity of schizoaffective disorder and schizophrenia (Table 7.3) (Kendell and Gourlay 1970b; Fowler et al. 1972; Carlson and Goodwin 1973; Abrams and Taylor 1976a; Szasz 1976; Procci 1976; Pope and Lipinski 1978; Brockington and Leff 1979).

After almost 80 years, schizoaffective disorder remains firmly established in the psychiatric nomenclature as demonstrated by the continued diagnosis and treatment of patients and lectures and publications about schizoaffective disorder. The literature on schizoaffective disorder is extensive. Since 2000, there have been at least 12,906 articles published that refer to schizoaffective disorder, and the trend was upwards through 2008 (Table 7.2). This is somewhat misleading since several of these recent articles question the validity of schizoaffective disorder as a disorder different from a psychotic mood disorder and recommend its elimination (Table 7.3) (Maier et al. 1993; Taylor and Amir 1994; Kendler et al. 1995; Dieperink and Sands 1996; Harrow et al. 2000; Maj et al. 2000; Swartz 2002b; Averill et al. 2004; Lake and Hurwitz 2006a, b, 2007a, b; Maier et al. 2006; Vollmer-Larsen et al. 2006).

Table 7.3 Selected quotes discounting the validity of schizoaffective disorder: schizoaffective disorder is a psychotic mood disorder; there is no schizoaffective disorder

Quote no.	Journal (year)	Author(s)	Field of study	Selected quotes of summary/conclusions	Results
1	AGP (1976)	Procci	Review	"Schizoaffective psychosis: fact or fiction?" [article title]. "… support for the adoption of some widely agreed upon epithet to describe this state [schizoaffective disorder] is indicated …. at least a subgroup of these psychoses [schizoaffective disorder] has a definite relationship to the major affective disorders. An old proverb reads: 'A person with a bad name is already half-hanged.' This may well be the case with the term schizoaffective disorder."	Schizoaffective disorder invalid
2	Psycho Med (1979)	Brockington and Leff	Clinical symptoms	"Their mutual concordance [8 definitions of schizoaffective disorder] is very low, mean 0.19, showing that there is very poor agreement about the meaning of the term schizoaffective disorder at present."	Schizoaffective disorder invalid
3	BJP (2000)	Harrow et al.	Clinical symptoms/ outcome	"Schizoaffective disorder outcome was better than schizophrenia outcome and poorer than outcome for psychotic affective disorders…. The results could fit a symptom dimension view of schizoaffective disorder course."	Continuum/ ambivalent
4	J Affect Disord (2000)	Maj et al.	Clinical symptoms	"The Cohen's kappa was 0.22 for diagnosis of schizoaffective disorder, 0.71 for that of manic episode and 0.82 for that of major depressive episode…. The inter-rater reliability of the DSM-IV criteria for schizoaffective disorder is not satisfactory."	Schizoaffective disorder invalid
5	Eur Psychiatr (2001)	Benabarre et al.	Clinical symptoms/ epidemiology/ prognoses	"The results reaffirmed that, from the standpoints of demographics, clinical features and prognosis, schizoaffective disorder bipolar type can be classified as a phenotypic form at an intermediate point between bipolar I disorder and schizophrenia…. although cross-sectional symptoms were closer to the schizophrenia spectrum, the course of the illness resembled more that of bipolar patients, resulting in an intermediate outcome."	Continuum/ ambivalent
6	Psychiatr Times (2002b)	Swartz	Review	"… There is no demarcation between schizoaffective disorder and psychotic mood disorders…. Without inter-rater reliability in DSM-IV [for] schizoaffective disorder, there could be no validity. If there is no validity, why are we using it?… Schizoaffective disorder seems an entity 'beyond necessity.'"	Schizoaffective disorder invalid
7	Psychiatr Quart (2004)	Averill et al.	Epidemiology/ clinical symptoms	"Although several differences were found in symptom severity across domains, no symptom was identifiable associated with the diagnosis of schizoaffective disorder and the diagnosis was unstable over time, thereby bringing into question the validity of schizoaffective disorder as a diagnostic entity."	Schizoaffective disorder invalid

7.5 Schizoaffective Disorder Ignored for 30 Years But Then Flourished

8	*Acta Psychiatr Scand* (2004)	Jager et al.	Clinical symptoms and long-term outcome	"... With respect to the long-term outcome, ICD-10 schizoaffective disorder had a prognosis similar to that of affective disorders."	Similar/overlap
9	*Acta Psychiatr Scand* (2006a)	Maier et al.	Editorial	"Taken together, there is growing evidence that a substantial proportion of etiological factors is shared between schizophrenia and bipolar disorder.... In summary, the historical starting point of the concept of schizoaffective disorders is not valid anymore.... The task forces for new versions of the DSM-and ICD-diagnostic systems and manuals... would be badly advised if they would just continue the historical and current concepts of schizoaffective disorders into the future."	Similar/overlap/ schizoaffective disorder invalid
10	*Acta Psychiatr Scand* (2006)	Vollmer-Larsen et al.	Clinical symptoms	"No patients fulfilled the schizoaffective disorder lifetime diagnosis according to DSM-IV criteria.... A moratorium on the clinical use of the schizoaffective disorder diagnosis is suggested."	Schizoaffective disorder invalid
11	*Psychiatr Res* (2006b)	Lake and Hurwitz	Review	"We suggest that the trend begun by Dr. Kasanin be extended to what we believe is a logical conclusion, i.e., the functional psychoses are psychotic mood disorders; there is no schizoaffective disorder (or schizophrenia)."	Schizoaffective disorder invalid
12	*Curr Opin Psychiatr* (2007b)	Lake and Hurwitz	Review	"Patients diagnosed with Schizoaffective Disorder likely suffer from a psychotic Mood Disorder. The diagnosis of Schizoaffective Disorder, which can result in substandard treatment, should be eliminated from the diagnostic nomenclature."	Schizoaffective disorder invalid

7.6 Schizoaffective Disorder Is a Compromise Diagnosis

By the 1970s and 1980s in many clinical environments, patients with hallucinations and/or delusions plus disturbances of mood received the diagnosis of schizoaffective disorder rather than the more traditional diagnosis of schizophrenia (Figs. 3.1 and 3.2). Initially, in the 1970s, schizoaffective disorder was diagnosed primarily in psychotic patients with prominent mood symptoms and those with mood congruent hallucinations and delusions (Fig. 3.2). This change in the pattern of the diagnoses of psychotic patients represented some movement in the concept of the cause of psychosis away from schizophrenia and toward psychotic mood disorders (Fig. 3.1). Clinically, schizoaffective disorder has been broadly embraced as a "diagnostic compromise," covering both schizophrenia and mood disorders. The diagnosis of schizoaffective disorder has been used when the physician is unsure if the psychotic patient with a disturbance of mood suffers from schizophrenia or a psychotic mood disorder. Doubt about the correct diagnosis commonly occurs when a psychotic patient presents with mood symptoms but has a past history of inpatient admissions with the diagnosis of schizophrenia. Schizoaffective disorder appears to solve this diagnostic dilemma but may not serve such patients well with respect to their pharmacological management and other aspects of their lives. By the 1980s and 1990s, the schizoaffective diagnosis was given to more psychotic patients with mood incongruent, bizarre psychoses, and a chronic deteriorating course who previously would have been diagnosed with schizophrenia (Fig. 3.2). More recently, psychotic patients with mood symptoms and mood-congruent or mood-incongruent psychoses began to be diagnosed with psychotic mood disorders (Figs. 3.1 and 3.2). Bruijnzeel and Tandon (2011) state that, "In fact, almost one third of patients with psychotic symptoms currently [2011] receive a diagnosis of schizoaffective disorder in many mental health care systems." The current author hopes this is an overestimation since the basic DSM diagnostic criteria appear flawed.

7.7 Flawed Diagnostic Criteria for Schizoaffective Disorder

Some authors contend that the DSM-IV-TR (APA, DSM 2000) (and DSM-5) diagnostic criteria A and B that establish schizoaffective disorder as a disease separate from a psychotic mood disorder are flawed. (Table 7.1) The DSM criterion A for the diagnosis of schizoaffective disorder depends on two parts: Part 1: the presence of a major depressive, a manic, or a mixed episode, that is, a mood disorder, that is concurrent with Part 2: the presence of at least two of the five core diagnostic symptoms that "meet criterion A for the diagnosis of Schizophrenia" (hallucinations, delusions, disorganization of speech and behavior, catatonia, and the "negative symptoms"). (Table 7.1) The first flaw in the DSM definition of schizoaffective disorder involves Part 2 of criterion A that justifies the "schizo" preface of schizoaffective disorder. When schizoaffective disorder was defined, developed, and established, these five DSM, criterion A symptoms (for schizophrenia) were considered disease specific and diagnostic of schizophrenia (Table 2.5). The "schizo" of schizoaffective disorder depends or builds upon the presumption of the disease specificity of these symptoms and is only warranted if these criterion A symptoms do define and are unique for schizophrenia. These criterion A symptoms for schizophrenia are not disease specific and only define "psychotic" but not any specific disorder. A rewording of criterion A for schizoaffective disorder is needed: instead of "symptoms that meet criterion A for Schizophrenia," substitute "psychotic," the equivalent of "hallucinations, delusions, disorganization, catatonia, negative symptoms." This updated translation then states: Part 1: the presence of a major depressive, a manic, or a mixed episode and Part 2: the presence of "psychotic" symptoms. Therefore, what criterion A, (as well as C and D) for schizoaffective disorder really define is a psychotic affective/mood disorder (Table 7.1) and not a separate disorder.

Criterion B for schizoaffective disorder was likely added to "secure" schizoaffective disorder as a disease separate from a severe mood disorder with psychotic features (Table 7.1). Criterion B for schizoaffective disorder may be flawed in two ways (Lake and Hurwitz 2006a, 2007b). First, criterion B attempts to differentiate schizoaffective disorder from a psychotic mood disorder based on the occurrence of "at least a 2-week" period at any time during the illness, when hallucinations and/or delusions are present, but "prominent mood symptoms" are absent. There are no scientific data and little logic that support naming a separate disorder based on such a 2-week period of psychosis in the absence of "prominent mood symptoms." What if only "subtle" or mild mood symptoms are present during the 2 weeks? How scientifically grounded is the distinction between "prominent" and "nonprominent" mood symptoms? Even if there are no observable mood symptoms at all during some 2-week period when psychotic symptoms are present, "prominent" mood symptoms have occurred (by criterion A), and according to criterion C, symptoms of a mood disturbance must be "present for a substantial portion of the total duration" of the illness (Table 7.1). Severe bipolar disorders satisfying rigorous criteria can reach such psychotic proportions that mood incongruent hallucinations and delusions overshadow and obscure mood symptoms for weeks to months at a time (Carlson and Goodwin 1973; Post 2010).

The second flaw of criterion B for a diagnosis of schizoaffective disorder is that even if there were supportive scientific data that such a 2-week period of psychosis without "prominent" mood symptoms warranted naming a new disease, the reliability of eliciting the existence of such a 2-week period from an acutely psychotic patient may be no better than chance. There is also considerable variation and subjectivity in eliciting psychotic versus mood symptoms depending upon the emphasis of the questions asked by the interviewing physician. Such variability is reflected by the data of Brockington et al. (1979) and Maj et al. (2000) discussed below.

Criterion D excludes physical or organic causes for schizoaffective disorder, which is also equally compatible with the diagnosis of a mood disorder. Criteria A, C, and D of the diagnostic criteria for schizoaffective disorder are entirely compatible with a diagnosis of a psychotic mood disorder and not a separate disease (Table 7.1). Continuing to base the existence of a separate disease on such unreliable history and nondata-based criteria leads to skepticism of the validity of schizoaffective disorder as a diagnosis and invites criticism of psychiatry for lacking scientific grounding.

In addition to the flaws in the diagnostic concepts of schizophrenia and schizoaffective disorder detailed above, schizoaffective disorder appears to have no validity as a disease as judged by Maj's and Brockington's calculations of the Cohen's kappa (0.22 and 0.19, respectively) for the interrater reliability for diagnosing schizoaffective disorder, in contrast to the kappas for mania and major depression, 0.71 and 0.82 respectively (Brockington and Leff 1979; Brockington et al. 1979, 1980a, b; Maj et al. 2000). As noted by Swartz (2002b),

> ... without interrater reliability, Schizoaffective Disorder has no validity and if there is no validity, why are we using it?

The diagnostic criteria for both schizoaffective disorder and schizophrenia are flawed because they depend on the outdated concept of the disease specificity of their diagnostic symptoms and course. Without specific and unique diagnostic criteria, these disorders lack a scientific basis as medical disorders. In contrast, the diagnostic criteria are disease specific for bipolar disorder (Chap. 4) Bipolar disorder is scientifically grounded and has a high interrater reliability. Hallucinations and delusions are not used as diagnostic criteria for bipolar disorder but are only used as "specifiers," that is, "with psychotic features," that indicate level of severity (Tables 2.3, 2.4, 7.1) (APA, DSM-IV-TR 2000). Several authors have recommended that schizoaffective disorder be eliminated (Table 7.3) (Abrams and Taylor 1976a; Procci 1976; Brockington and Leff 1979; Maier et al. 1993, 2006; Taylor and Amir 1994; Kendler et al. 1995; Dieperink and Sands 1996; Harrow et al. 2000; Maj et al. 2000; Swartz 2002b; Averill et al. 2004; Maier 1992, 2006; Lake and Hurwitz 2006b, 2007; Vollmer-Larsen et al. 2006). It is predicted that most, if not all, functionally psychotic patients will be determined to have some symptoms of a disturbance of mood and despite the severity of their psychotic symptoms and chronicity of the course, will eventually receive diagnoses of psychotic mood disorders (Table 3.5; Figs. 3.1 and 3.2).

Despite the above (Table 7.3), the DSM-5 draft proposal appears to maintain the diagnosis of schizoaffective disorder essentially unchanged except for a trivial rewording from the DSM-IV-TR of criterion C:

> Symptoms that meet criteria for a major mood episode are present for a substantial portion of the total duration of the active and residual portion of the illness.

Criterion C from the proposed DSM-5 reads:

> A major mood episode is present for the majority (50%) of the total duration of the illness.

Bruijnzeel and Tandon (2011) imply that this change will improve the reliability of the diagnosis of schizoaffective disorder with this change when they said:

> In the current DSM-5 proposal, an effort is made to improve reliability of this condition by providing more specific criteria reconceptualizing it as a longitudinal and not a cross-sectional diagnosis. ... the most significant change is proposed in Criterion C of schizoaffective disorder.

The consensus recommendations from the authors who have written about the poor reliability of the diagnosis (Table 7.3) are a more radical but logical change, that is, elimination. Minor changes suggested for the DSM-5 made in criterion "A: The Characteristic Symptoms" for schizophrenia upon which the DSM diagnosis for schizoaffective disorder depends and the change to criterion C for schizoaffective disorder fall far short of any chance for "improving reliability" of schizoaffective disorder.

7.8 Conclusions

Schizoaffective disorder, introduced in 1933 by Dr. Jacob Kasanin, represented an early, major change in the concept about the diagnoses of psychotic patients, away from the beliefs of E. Bleuler, that is, that hallucinations, delusions, disorganization, and catatonia define schizophrenia, and toward the recognition of a significant role for mood disorders. Schizoaffective disorder established a connection between schizophrenia and mood disorders, traditionally considered mutually exclusive, a connection that has strengthened progressively toward the diagnostic unity of all three disorders. Schizoaffective disorder enabled the development of the continuum concept, leading to the same disease idea put forth in this book. A basic tenet of medicine holds that if discrepant symptoms can be explained by one disease instead of two or more, it is likely there is only one disease. The scientific justification for schizoaffective disorder and schizophrenia as disorders distinct from a psychotic mood disorder has been substantially questioned.

The "schizo" prefix in schizoaffective disorder rests upon the presumption that the diagnostic symptoms for schizophrenia are disease specific. They are not, since patients with severe mood disorders can evince any or all of the "schizophrenic" symptoms that mean "psychotic" symptoms and not any specific disease. These data and a very low interrater reliability for schizoaffective disorder suggest that the concepts of schizoaffective disorder and schizophrenia as valid diagnoses are flawed. Clinically, schizoaffective disorder remains popular because it encompasses both schizophrenia and a psychotic mood disorder when there is a diagnostic question.

Dr. Kasanin was a visionary and brave to break with the established dogma that hallucinations and/or delusions meant schizophrenia. He did initiate an early move away from this concept of Bleuler so widely accepted by the mental health professions in the USA. For Kasanin to have diagnosed such patients in 1933 as "psychotic affectives" may have been too great a leap, although today his patients would likely be diagnosed as suffering from a psychotic mood disorder. He probably did not intend to create the diagnostic quagmire that schizoaffective disorder has become. It is suggested that the trend begun by Dr. Kasanin be extended to what seems a logical conclusion, that is, the functional psychoses are psychotic mood disorders; there is no schizoaffective disorder or schizophrenia. Based on the proposed DSM-5, this may not happen; maybe in the DSM-6?

Chapter 8
Kurt Schneider (1887–1967): First- and Second-Rank Symptoms, Not Pathognomonic of Schizophrenia, Explained by Psychotic Mood Disorders

> ... these symptoms [Schneider's First-Rank Symptoms] which he [Schneider] considers [pathognomonic of schizophrenia] occur in 1/4 of the cohort of manic-depressive patients.
>
> (Carpenter et al. 1973)
>
> These results confirm previous findings that FRSs [Schneider's First-Rank Symptoms] are not specific to schizophrenia and suggest in addition that a dimension of nuclear psychotic experiences of developmental origin extends across categorically defined psychotic disorders.
>
> (Gonzalez-Pinto et al. 2003)

8.1 Introduction

Kurt Schneider was born in 1887 in Crailsheim, Kingdom of Wurttemberg. He went to medical school in Berlin and Tubingen. After serving in World War I, he obtained his postgraduate qualification in psychiatry. In 1931, he became the director of the Psychiatric Research Institute in Munich, previously founded by Kraepelin. He served as an army doctor during World War II and in 1946 took the chair as professor of psychiatry and neurology at the University of Heidelberg, School of Medicine where he became dean. He retired in 1955. Schneider was influenced by Kraepelin and Karl Jaspers who developed the school of "phenomenology."

Schneider's major textbook *Clinical Psychopathology* was updated five times and translated to English by Ms. M. W. Hamilton in 1959. Professor Anderson at the Royal Infirmary, Manchester, England wrote the preface to *Clinical Psychopathology* and said that Schneider "… for more than 40 years, was one of the outstanding figures in European Psychiatry" and exerted a "… profound influence on psychiatric thinking" (Schneider 1959, preface). Schneider's book had a major influence upon Academic Psychiatry in the USA as well as in Europe. He essentially reinforced the concept of Bleuler that schizophrenia was a valid disease different from bipolar disorders.

Table 8.1 K. Schneider's "pathognomonic" first- and second-rank symptoms of schizophrenia

First-rank symptoms[a]:
Hearing one's thoughts spoken aloud
Hearing voices arguing about oneself[b]
Hearing voices commenting on one's actions[b]
Having bodily sensations imposed from outside
Having one's thoughts/feelings inserted or withdrawn by external sources
Having one's thoughts broadcast
Having delusional perceptions
Second-rank symptoms[a]:
Other disorders of perception[c]
Sudden delusional ideas
Perplexity[c]
Depressive and euphoric mood changes[d]
Feelings of emotional impoverishment[c,d]
"… and several others as well"[c]

[a]None of these symptoms alone or any combination are disease specific, and they occur frequently in severe mood disorders with psychotic features.
[b]Either of these two symptoms are recognized as pathognomonic alone in the DSM-IV-TR since the presence of either by itself satisfies criteria under "NOTE" in section A, characteristic symptoms of schizophrenia.
Criterion A for schizophrenia—characteristic symptoms—patient must have two symptoms during a 1-month (active) phase (except as noted below):
1. Delusions
2. Hallucinations
3. Disorganized speech (frequent derailment, incoherence)
4. Grossly disorganized or catatonic behavior
5. Negative symptoms (affective flattening, alogia and avolition)
NOTE: Only one symptom is required if delusions are bizarre or hallucinations: [Are of] a voice commenting on one's behavior/thoughts or if two or more voices are conversing with each other
[c]Possibly not indicative of any mental illness
[d]Suggestive of a mood disorder

Analogous to Bleuler's fundamental and accessory symptoms, Schneider developed his own first- and second-rank symptoms that he taught were pathognomonic of schizophrenia (Table 8.1). His first-rank symptoms became widely accepted as pathognomonic of schizophrenia. As had Bleuler, Schneider minimized the diagnostic importance of disturbances of mood and wrote that the presence of hallucinations and/or delusions, encompassing his first-rank symptoms, mandated the diagnosis of schizophrenia. The longevity of the impact of Schneider's first-rank symptoms is demonstrated by their continuing influence 50 years after their publication. According to the DSM-IV-TR, at least two of his first-rank symptoms are still considered diagnostic of schizophrenia (Tables 2.5 and 8.1). Because of this substantial influence of Schneider, his book is excerpted below to show the reader that many of the signs and symptoms Schneider believed diagnostic of schizophrenia are actually accounted for by psychotic mood disorders.

8.2 Selected Quotes From Schneider's Textbook *Clinical Psychopathology* (1959); Bleuler's Concept Reinforced: Psychosis Means Schizophrenia

In the first chapter titled "Classification of Clinical Material and Definition of Illness," Schneider differentiated functional versus organic psychosis, postulating a somatic origin for all psychoses, but for the functional group, no abnormality could yet be identified. This concept continues today. Schneider apparently recognized the incongruity of Kraepelin's terminology of his dichotomy of dementia praecox and manic-depressive insanity in that manic-depressive insanity means insanity or psychosis (Table 2.7). Bleuler did not seem to be concerned when he said that manic-depressive insanity could not be psychotic or the diagnosis would be schizophrenia. Schneider's dichotomy of his functional disorders was "cyclothymia" and "schizophrenia" (Table 8.2). Schneider's "cyclothymia" replaces manic-depressive insanity or bipolar disorder and clarifies the absence of psychosis or even severe incapacitating symptoms although patients with the diagnosis of cyclothymia were apparently hospitalized. His use of cyclothymia rather than manic-depressive insanity is consistent with Bleuler's view that functional psychosis was not necessary for, but when present, mandated the diagnosis of schizophrenia despite symptoms of a mood disturbance; mood disorders, considered to be cyclothymia by Schneider, could not be psychotic. As with Kraepelin, there must have been at least some ambivalence in Schneider's mind when he admitted that,

… cyclothymic mania may be difficult to differentiate from schizophrenia.

(Schneider 1959, p. 90).

Schneider's cyclothymia is in keeping with our current definition that cyclothymia has a mild symptom profile absent of psychosis, but he used cyclothymia to encompass all mood disorders. Based on the current concept of the diagnostic importance of mood symptoms, Schneider, like Kraepelin and Bleuler before him, mistakenly overemphasized the diagnostic importance of hallucinations and delusions (Table 8.3).

In support of Kraepelin's (initial) and Bleuler's ideas of a dichotomy, Schneider believed that schizophrenia was different from, more severe than, more important than, and clearly more prevalent than cyclothymia or bipolar disorder. Schneider wrote that schizophrenia was discriminated from cyclothymia (bipolar) based upon its "persisting state" as opposed to cyclothymia's "episodic nature." However later in his book, Schneider minimized course of illness as diagnostic when he said the

Table 8.2 Schneider's dichotomy

- Schizophrenia
- Cyclothymia

NOTE: By using cyclothymia instead of manic-depressive insanity as Kraepelin had, Schneider strongly supports Bleuler's contention that there could be no psychotic mood disorder because psychosis meant schizophrenia

Table 8.3 Relevant quotes from *Clinical Psychopathology* (K. Schneider 1959)

Quote no.	Page no.	Selected quotes	Current author's comments
1	14	"In contrast to Cyclothymic, Schizophrenic presents a diagnosis with a wide and undefined area in which to play and there is a natural tendency to include any a-typical case within the motley schizophrenic cluster. For this reason few cases are left ultimately undefined."	Schneider's broad approach to the diagnosis of schizophrenia parallels that of Bleuler, allowing an overbroad spectrum of people to receive the diagnosis of schizophrenia.
2	90	"Cyclothymic depression provides a basis from which in daily practice we can differentiate fairly reliably the various forms of schizophrenia. The same can scarcely be said of cyclothymic mania."	Schneider implies that the differentiation between schizophrenia and mania is "unreliable."
3	91	"From these schizophrenic types [catatonic, paranoid] there are at times transitions to types of cyclothymic depression and types of cyclothymic mania, but much more often to the latter."	In suggesting "transitions" from schizophrenia to depression and mania, Schneider obscures a dichotomy, that is, differences between schizophrenia and bipolar disorders.
4	92	"… psychiatric diagnosis must be based on the presenting situation, not on the course taken by the illness."	This approach allows an immediate diagnosis of schizophrenia when organic causes of psychosis are ruled out regardless of course. Schneider appeared to contradict himself as shown in the quote below.
5	93	"As a rule, schizophrenic symptoms have an unfavorable, if erratic course, while with cyclothymic symptoms, complete remission of the existing phase can be expected."	Schneider implies that the course of schizophrenia can be "erratic" overlapping with mood disorders. Bipolar disorders are now accepted as having the potential for a chronic, nonremitting, noncycling deteriorating course.
6	96	"… sometimes it is hopelessly difficult to ascertain for certain whether [an] hallucination has occurred or not … there are patients who have no hallucinations but will answer in the affirmative when questioned about hearing voices; on closer inquiry, it transpires that they have not meant unreal but actual voices."	Although this is wise advice, it has typically not been followed, and schizophrenia has been erroneously diagnosed.
7	96	"Certain modes of hearing voices are of special diagnostic importance for assuming a schizophrenia: hearing one's own thoughts (or thoughts being audible), voices conversing or arguing with one another and voices that keep up a running comment on the patient's behavior."	Although these first-rank symptoms have been amply discounted as disease specific, the presence of one such auditory hallucination allows the fulfillment of criterion A for the diagnosis of schizophrenia (Tables 2.5 and 8.1).
8	97	"A schizophrenic woman speaking of electrical influences said, 'The electricity works of the whole world are directed onto me.'"	Despite the grandiosity of this statement, the diagnosis was schizophrenia, not mania.
9	98	"Thought-blocking is a nonspecific and universally common symptom. Shy, embarrassed people will show it, … The true picture is thus often obscured and leads to mistakes in diagnosis. It is hard to go wrong with the gross, painful thought-blocking that takes place in cyclothymic depression with its classic accompaniment of profound, almost physical melancholia and severely retarded movement."	Despite this statement by Schneider, thought blocking became accepted as a sign of schizophrenia, not a mood disorder.

8.2 Selected Quotes From Schneider's Textbook *Clinical Psychopathology* (1959)… 141

10	104	"Compulsive states … sometimes appear in cyclothymic phases and at the beginning of Schizophrenia."	This quote implies overlap of obsessive-compulsive disorder, a mood disorder, and a schizophrenia, and such overlap leads to doubt of the validity of schizophrenia as a separate disease.
11	104–106	"Delusional perception belongs … to disturbances … of thought. It is always a schizophrenic symptom … on rare occasions, it may occur with epileptic twilight states, toxic psychoses, and morbid, cerebral changes, as indeed can all symptoms that are schizophrenic …. Where there is delusional perception we are always dealing with schizophrenic psychosis.…"	Although confusion between organic and functional psychosis, specifically schizophrenia, is evident, Schneider concludes that "delusional perception" means schizophrenia regardless of the possibility of an organic disorder.
12	108	"However, there are cases where we have to suppose some schizophrenic psychosis simply on the basis of bizarre, fantastic, crazy notions and the context in which they are elaborated."	This statement is overinclusive and leads to skepticism of the validity of Schneider's concepts overall as noted by his second-rank symptoms (Table 8.1).
13	114	"An exceptional ego inflation, the quality of annihilation of all that is gone before, the aura of revelation, the blinding illumination or black finality are certainly qualities very suggestive of a schizophrenic delusional notion.…"	Although Schneider recognized that these "are not impeccable criteria and can equally attend the notions of normal … people," these symptoms are currently considerably more suggestive of mania and depression than any other disease.
14	118	"Only really experienced clinicians will risk taking weak rapport as an important, sometimes decisive, factor in diagnosing schizophrenia."	"Weak rapport" should not hold any diagnostic importance in the current author's opinion.
15	120	"Here is another example [of alien control]: a schizophrenic student said, 'I cannot respond to any suggestion; thousands and thousands of wills work against me.'"	Again, the symptom of grandiosity does not appear to be considered of diagnostic relevance in this case.
16	133	"Among the many abnormal modes of experience that occur in schizophrenics, there are some which we put in the first-rank of importance, … because they have this special value in helping us to determine the diagnosis of schizophrenia as distinct from non-psychotic abnormality or from cyclothymia."	Schneider's influence upon Academic Psychiatry and the DSM has been substantial and long-lasting as demonstrated by the ability to diagnose schizophrenia with the presence of one of his first-rank symptoms despite data invalidating his first-rank symptoms as disease specific.
17	134–135	"Among [the Second-Rank Symptoms of Schizophrenia] are other hallucinations, delusional notions, perplexity, depressed and elated moods, experiences of flattened feeling, and so on. … Symptoms of first-rank importance do not always have to be present for a diagnosis [of schizophrenia] to be made; at least, we cannot rely on their being continuously there to observe. We are often forced to base our diagnosis on the symptoms of second-rank importance, occasionally and exceptionally on mere disorders of expression alone, provided these are relatively florid and numerous."	Schneider enables the diagnosis of schizophrenia based on his second-rank symptoms that include "… perplexity, depressed and elated moods …, and so on." He supports Bleuler's concept that neither psychosis nor chronicity of course is necessary for the diagnosis of schizophrenia.
18	135	"In cyclothymia [bipolar disorder], there seem at present to be no known symptoms of first-rank importance, nothing of which we can say, if this is present, then so is cyclothymia."	In sharp contrast to Schneider's impression, the diagnostic criteria for mania and thus bipolar disorders are detailed, specific, and have a high interrater reliability (Tables 2.3, 2.4, and 3.1).
19	143	"Let me repeat that cyclothymia and schizophrenic can only be distinguished as types in principal."	Schneider seems ambivalent about clear differences between these disorders.

presenting symptoms, that is, his own first-rank symptoms, called for the diagnosis of schizophrenia regardless of course, even one of cycles of mania and depression. Schneider's emphasis on schizophrenia versus cyclothymia can be found on pages 5 and 6 of his book. For example, out of 1,647 patients from the State Hospital at Muenchen Schwabing between 1932 and 1936, 941 were diagnosed with schizophrenia and 166 were diagnosed with cyclothymia (Schneider 1959, pp. 12–13). Schneider said that,

> In contrast to Cyclothymia, Schizophrenia presents a diagnosis with a wide and undefined area in which to play and there is a natural tendency to include any a-typical case within the motley schizophrenic cluster. For this reason few cases are left ultimately undefined.

The predominance of schizophrenia over mood disorders was generally accepted among mental health professionals between the late nineteenth century and the 1990s, and Schneider's work reinforced and promoted this belief.

Schneider eluded to a current issue of how one's training effects the differential diagnosis between schizophrenia and mood disorders when he said that the diagnosis depends upon "… what we are accustomed to call a Schizophrenia or a Cyclothymia." The diagnosis "… depends wholly on the clinical standpoint adopted at the time." This infers that it is the training of the diagnostician that influences the decision between schizophrenia and bipolar in psychotic patients (Schneider 1959, p. 14). Schneider's and Bleuler's perspectives, which is that the presence of psychotic symptoms means schizophrenia, influenced the curriculum in Academic Psychiatry for several generations and continues to do so at some academic medical centers.

Chapter 6, titled "Cyclothymia and Schizophrenia," is the most extensive and important chapter of Schneider's book, extending 56 pages. In it, he addressed several important issues and took a conservative stance as to overdiagnosis, but these conservative ideas have not been as influential as his writings that schizophrenia was defined by certain hallucinations and delusions. Schneider addressed one of the primary causes of misdiagnosis today. He said,

> There are no demonstrable, concrete symptoms to add up or put together as in a physical diagnosis [for the diagnosis of psychiatric disorders]. Instead, we have to assess statements and evaluate the patient's behavior and bearing. … Clinical diagnosis often seems to precede inquiry and the symptoms tend to get evaluated in the light of it. Thus, if the investigator presupposes a schizophrenia, expressions such as "disjointed," "lack of affect," etc., will crop up without fail and perhaps wrongly.

Although Schneider warned against a hasty diagnosis of schizophrenia, it is clear that Schneider believed "disjointed" and "lack of affect" suggested schizophrenia, and the premature diagnosis of schizophrenia has frequently been the case in psychotic patients (Pope and Lipinski 1978). In this chapter, Schneider also emphasized the importance of identifying organic causes of psychosis. He stated that "… the delirious patient may give a picture that strongly suggests a schizophrenic state." He mentioned general paresis of the insane, epilepsy, trauma, infection and parasitic infection as having a potential for being misdiagnosed as schizophrenia. Neither of these critical points have been part of Schneider's legacy.

In keeping with both Kraepelin and Bleuler, Schneider felt that schizophrenia was a group of disorders, and he discussed simple, catatonic, paranoid, and hebephrenic schizophrenia. He disagreed with Kraepelin when he minimized the diagnostic importance of the course of the illness when he said,

> ... psychiatric diagnosis must be based on the presenting situation, not on the course taken by the illness.

Despite this, Schneider stated in the same paragraph that,

> As a rule, schizophrenic symptoms have an unfavorable, if erratic, course, while with cyclothymia symptoms, complete remission of the existing phase can be expected.

8.3 Schneider's First- and Second-Rank Symptoms of Schizophrenia Reflect Obsolescence but Remain in the DSM and ICD

It is in Chap. 6 of his book where Schneider enumerated his famous "first- and second-rank symptoms of schizophrenia" (Table 8.1). These special "symptoms" have been the most memorialized aspect of Schneider's work. Schneider himself did not list his "symptoms" in table form so that subsequent authors have extracted them. A summary is found on pages 133–135 of Schneider's book.

Schneider discussed "disturbances of perception" as the core of his first-rank symptoms. He said:

> "... the most important disturbances for psychiatric diagnosis are the false perceptions or hallucinations." He defined a "hallucination" as "something which in fact is not there [that] is seen, heard, smelt, tasted or bodily felt." He emphasized that, "... sometimes it is hopelessly difficult to ascertain for certain whether hallucination has occurred or not." He noted, "...that there are patients who have no hallucinations but will answer in the affirmative when questioned about hearing voices; on closer inquiry, it transpires that they have not meant unreal but actual voices."

Another source of false positive reports of auditory hallucinations, in the current author's experience, is patients' misinterpretations of their thoughts as "voices." Despite Schneider's warnings, mental health professionals have tended to overdiagnose psychosis and schizophrenia, in part due to his insistence that the diagnosis of schizophrenia be made when the presence of any of his sometimes quite subjective and disease nonspecific first- and second-rank symptoms can be justified (Table 8.1).

On page 96, Schneider addressed his views of the diagnostic importance of certain auditory hallucinations, encompassing first-rank symptom numbers one, two, and three, probably the most critical of his first-rank symptoms. He said,

> Certain modes of hearing voices are of special diagnostic importance for assuming a schizophrenia: hearing one's own thoughts (or thoughts being audible), voices conversing or arguing with one another and voices that keep up a running comment on the patient's behavior.

It should be noted from the DSM that normally two or more of the "characteristic symptoms" from criterion A of schizophrenia are needed for the diagnosis, but the presence of only one of these auditory hallucinations of Schneider's first-rank symptoms ("a voice keeping up a running commentary on the person's behavior or thoughts or two or more voices conversing with each other") essentially allows a diagnosis of schizophrenia (Tables 2.5 and 8.1). Despite the more recent observations by several authors that such auditory hallucinations are disease nonspecific and in fact are predominately explained by psychotic mood disorders, this misconception continues to cause the misdiagnosis of schizophrenia (Carpenter et al. 1973; Goodwin 1989; Post 1992; Pini et al. 2001). The DSM-5 draft proposal due for completion in 2013 appears to drop references to any of Schneider's first-rank symptoms likely because they do commonly occur in psychotic mood disorders. This seems a modest concession, given the disease nonspecificity of the remaining diagnostic criteria for schizophrenia (Table 2.5).

Schneider gave examples of patients' statements that he thought warranted the diagnosis of schizophrenia:

> A schizophrenic woman, for instance, replied to the questions about hearing voices with the answer, "I hear my own thoughts. I can hear them when everything is quiet." A schizophrenic man said, "When I try to think, my head gets full of noise; it's as if my brain were in an uproar with my thoughts." Another schizophrenic heard his own voice night and day, like a dialogue, one voice always arguing against the other. A schizophrenic woman heard a voice say, whenever she wanted to eat, "Now she is eating, here she is munching again," or when she patted the dog, she heard, "What is she up to now, fondling the dog:"....
>
> (Schneider 1959, p. 86)

These examples seem arbitrary in even concluding the presence of a psychosis and are certainly disease nonspecific if not suggestive of obsessive-compulsive disorder or the racing thoughts of mania ("… my head gets full of noise; … it's as if my brain were in an uproar with my thoughts.").

"Somatic" hallucinations such as caused by "various devices, rays, suggestion, hypnotic influence, etc., frequently of a sexual nature," were considered "of extreme importance in the diagnosis of schizophrenia."

This has become first-rank symptom number four known as delusional ideas of influences. Schneider gave case vignettes of direct quotes from several of his patients that he interpreted as diagnostic of schizophrenia:

> A schizophrenic woman speaking of electrical influences said, "The electricity works of the whole world are directed on to me."… Another [schizophrenic] woman described her bodily feelings as a "sort of intercourse as if a man was really there. He was not there of course, nobody was there. I was quite alone but it was as if a man was with me, as though we were having intercourse… that is what I felt."
>
> (Schneider 1959, p. 97)

In this author's opinion, assuming that these cases were inpatients and generally dysfunctional, the descriptions are more likely suggestive of psychotic mania. In the first example (just above), the patient seems a bit grandiose believing "The electricity works of the whole world…" were focused on her. In the last example of the woman who said she experienced feelings like intercourse, there is the suggestion of the hypersexuality common to mania.

8.3 Schneider's First- and Second-Rank Symptoms... 145

Schneider next addressed disturbances of thinking accurately discounting "blocking" as specific for schizophrenia saying that,

> "Shy, embarrassed people will show it, ..." and that "thought-blocking [also] takes place in cyclothymic depression with its classic accompaniment of ... severely retarded movement."

It should be noted that, despite this statement by Schneider, subsequent investigators have opined that thought blocking is specific to schizophrenia. Schneider did attribute "interruption of thought" as specific to schizophrenia. He also attributed "flight of ideas" to "pseudomanic schizophrenia." This is another example of the dominance of schizophrenia over mood disorders in light of the established association of mania and "flight of ideas." Pseudomanic schizophrenia is likely psychotic mania. He elaborated on "schizophrenic flight of ideas" attributing "... units of thought stream, linked partly by sound matching and partly by association with external stimuli" and "thinking [that] does not connect adequately with what has preceded it..." to schizophrenia when these examples of "flight of ideas" and tangentiality are symptoms of mania (Lake 2008a, b) (Chaps. 12 and 13). He correctly discussed some overlap "among normal people" saying that "There are those who are naturally scatter-brained...." Schneider then said that,

> "Thought-withdrawal as well as interruption of thought is a particularly important sign for the diagnosis of Schizophrenia ..." especially "... when it is recounted that 'other people' are taking the thoughts away."

Schneider addressed first-rank symptom numbers five and six on page 100 (Schneider 1959). "On the same level as thought-withdrawal [in importance for diagnosing schizophrenia, are] thought-intrusion and expropriation of thoughts [or] diffusion of thoughts." These phenomena are now referred to as "thought broadcasting."

> "Interruption of thought is illustrated by a schizophrenic woman who said, 'When I want to hang on to my thoughts, they break off.' A schizophrenic man stated that his thoughts were 'taken from me years ago by the parish council.' They had constantly 'robbed' him of all his thoughts; 'it takes them three days.'" Other examples are: a schizophrenic shirt-maker who, "... at times ... could not calculate at all [because] ... she had to think thoughts she did not want to think, evil thoughts. She attributed all this to being hypnotized by a priest. ... A schizophrenic shop-keeper said, 'People see what I am thinking; you could not prove it but I just know it is so. I see it in their faces; it would not be so bad if I did not think such unsuitable things – swine or some other rude word...' Another schizophrenic woman said that when she was younger her father could hear her thoughts and rightly took them away from her."
>
> (Schneider 1959, pp. 100, 101)

Mania and obsessive-compulsive disorder, not schizophrenia, more likely explain Schneider's examples. Schneider invoked both "thought-withdrawal and thought intrusion" in these cases, but these thoughts suggest flight of ideas, grandiosity, and obsessions about "unacceptable or sinful" hypersexual thoughts. About "compulsive thinking" in schizophrenia, Schneider said,

> Compulsive states ... sometimes appear ... at the beginning of Schizophrenia.
>
> (Schneider 1959, p. 104)

Obsessive-compulsive disorder has subsequently been considered as part of a schizophrenic picture but severe obsessive-compulsive disorder can become so disabling as to be misdiagnosed as schizophrenia so that the association of obsessive-compulsive disorder with schizophrenia translates to severe obsessive-compulsive disorder that causes dysfunctionality (Chap. 13) (Lake 2008b).

Schneider next addressed first-rank symptom number seven, that is, delusions, dividing them into "two major forms:" delusional perception and delusional notion. He said that:

> "... delusional perception ... almost always carries great import, is urgent and personal, a sign or a message from another world. It is as if some 'loftier reality' spoke through the perception ..." He clarified that, "delusional perception belongs therefore, not to disturbances of perception but to those of thought. It is always a schizophrenic symptom, ..." Schneider acknowledged that, "... on rare occasions, it may occur with epileptic twilight states, toxic psychoses and morbid, cerebral changes ..." Yet he added that, "Where there is delusional perception, we are always dealing with schizophrenic psychosis ..."

(Schneider 1959, pp. 105–107)

The flavor of Schneider's descriptions above is one of grandiosity suggesting mania.

As examples of a type of "delusional perception" are ideas of reference that Schneider believed meant schizophrenia:

> A schizophrenic man had three strangely significant experiences with dogs and described the last as follows: "A dog lay in wait for me as he sat on the steps of a Catholic convent. He got up on his hind legs and looked at me seriously. He then saluted with his front paw as I approached him." ... A schizophrenic woman told the following tale: "My son is under the spell of a blacksmith who has hypnotized him. I had just visited my boy in Koeln and as I stood below the station a woman came up and said the train was up there. ... In the train sat a man and I thought he was trying to influence me; he looked so oddly at me, I thought, 'What a queer creature;' I thought he was the blacksmith. He must have dyed his hair, as he had been fair.... I am sure he had me already under his spell. ... A week ago I went to the doctor and sat in the waiting room; there was a stranger there; he could have been the smith; I should have got his name and address."

(Schneider 1959, p. 105)

Ideas of reference do not necessarily mean any disorder but can suggest a psychotic process. They are disease nonspecific and typically contain a flavor of grandiosity indicating mania. A worthwhile question in such cases is "What is the meaning to you of the dog's or the blacksmith's interactions with you?" This answer can reveal grandiosity. A history of recent insomnia with increased energy is also productive for consideration of mania.

Schneider then discussed delusional notions:

> By a delusional notion we mean notions such as those of religious or political eminence, or of having special gifts, or of being persecuted or loved, and so on.

(Schneider 1959, p. 107)

Such "notions" also indicate grandiosity but Schneider clarified that they "...are of far less significance for the diagnosis of schizophrenia [than are delusional perceptions]."

Schneider gave an example of a misdiagnosis of paranoid schizophrenia based on the misassumption of a delusion:

> A girl, for example, was diagnosed as a paranoid schizophrenic because she alleged a count was concerned about her and was keeping his eye on her. Actually, this was the truth as the count, with whom she had grown up and by whom she had had a child when she was 18 years old, constantly inquired about her and her child.
>
> (Schneider 1959, p. 108)

Schneider did not clarify whether this patient was hospitalized because of the misidentification of a delusion.

Schneider said that,

> However, there are cases where we have to suppose some schizophrenic psychosis simply on the basis of bizarre, fantastic, crazy notions and the context in which they are elaborated.

Thus, the idea that "bizarre, fantastic, crazy" delusions were pathognomonic of schizophrenia solidified Bleuler's teachings and influenced psychiatry for decades.

Another example of possible manic grandiosity or narcissism that Schneider interpreted as schizophrenia was given on page 112 of his book when he said,

> Thus, a schizophrenic man may think that the crown engraved on his christening fork had betokened aristocratic descent.

Continuing with this theme of Schneider's interpretation of mood disturbances as schizophrenia, he warned that,

> An exceptional ego inflation, the quality of annihilation of all that has gone before, the aura of revelation, the blinding illumination or black finality are certainly qualities very suggestive of a schizophrenic delusional notion; ... yet, they are not impeccable criteria and can equally well attend the notions of normal, psychopathic, or psychotic people.
>
> (Schneider 1959, p. 114)

Despite Schneider's warnings, some of his followers have been quick to diagnose schizophrenia.

Schneider also attributed symptoms explained by depression as signs of schizophrenia although with less confidence. For example, he said that,

> The terms "lack of feeling," "blank," and "unresponsive" have traditionally but incorrectly been applied almost exclusively to schizophrenic patients and we should use them with reluctance.

Schneider was more certain about the absence of or even

> ... weak rapport as an important, sometime decisive factor in diagnosing schizophrenia.

He equated "inadequacy of feeling response" and "shallowness of feeling" as symptoms of schizophrenia. Schneider clarified that,

> Only really experienced clinicians will risk taking weak rapport as an important, sometimes decisive, factor in diagnosing schizophrenia.
>
> (Schneider 1959, p. 118)

In this author's opinion, such "symptoms" are too subjective to ever be considered as "decisive" for any diagnosis. In contrast to Bleuler, Schneider correctly did not emphasize "ambivalence of feeling" as pathognomonic of schizophrenia.

Schneider wrote that "... certain disturbances of the sense of identity are highly specific for schizophrenia" (Schneider 1959, p. 120). He defined "disturbances of identity" as involving "thought-withdrawal and the influencing of thought, feeling, impulse (drive), and will." He said,

> If I find thought-withdrawal in a psychosis of no known somatic base, there is only an agreed convention that I then call this psychosis a schizophrenia.

Schneider discussed "depersonalization and derealization" as symptoms of schizophrenia. These symptoms have been demonstrated to be nondisease specific.

Schneider expanded his discussion of his first-rank symptoms on page 133. He said that,

> Among the many abnormal modes of experience that occur in schizophrenics, there are some which we put in the first rank of importance, ... because they have this special value in helping us to determine the diagnosis of schizophrenia as distinct from non-psychotic abnormality or from cyclothymia.

He emphasized again that "these symptoms of first-rank importance" are pathognomonic of schizophrenia, listing them as follows:

> "... audible thoughts, voices heard arguing, voices heard commenting on one's actions, the experience of influences playing on the body (somatic passivity experiences), thought-withdrawal and other interferences with thought, diffusion of thought, delusional perception and all feelings, impulses (drives), and volitional acts that are experienced by the patient as the work or influence of others. When any of these modes of experience is undeniably present and no basic somatic illness can be found, we may make the decisive clinical diagnosis of schizophrenia." Schneider next recognized that, "Any one of these signs, however, may sometimes occur in psychotic states that arise from a known physical illness: alcoholic psychoses, ... epileptic twilight states, the psychoses of anemia, and other symptomatic psychoses, as well as a number of diverse morbid cerebral processes."
>
> (Schneider 1959, pp. 133, 134)

Schneider did not recognize that psychotic mood-disordered patients can exhibit one or all of his first- and/or his second-rank symptoms. Schneider clarified that,

> Symptoms of first-rank importance do not always have to be present for a diagnosis [of schizophrenia] to be made; at least, we cannot rely on their being continuously there to observe. We are often forced to base our diagnosis on the symptoms of second-rank importance, occasionally and exceptionally on mere disorders of expression alone, provided these are relatively florid and numerous. ...
>
> Schizophrenic symptoms of first-rank importance have a decisive weight beyond all others in establishing a differential [diagnosis] between schizophrenia and cyclothymia, and must have undisputed precedence when it comes to the allocation of the individual case.
>
> (Schneider 1959, pp. 134, 135)

By this, Schneider meant that his symptoms of second-rank importance can be diagnostic of schizophrenia and that his symptoms of first-rank importance do not have to be present continuously. Schneider's second-rank symptoms are given in Table 8.1 and are especially disease nonspecific such as number three "perplexity" and number six "and several others [symptoms] as well." Numbers four and five are actually symptoms of mania and depression rather than any other disease (Table 8.1).

In contrast to schizophrenia, Schneider said that,

> In cyclothymia [bipolar disorder], there seem at present to be no known symptoms of first-rank importance, nothing of which we can say, if this is present, then so is cyclothymia.

In this author's view, the data, especially the history of bipolar disorder (Chaps. 3 and 4), demonstrate disease-specific symptoms in contrast to a lack of disease-specific symptoms for schizophrenia (Tables 2.3, 2.4, 2.5). Examples are Schneider's first- and second-rank symptoms that are nonspecific and, in fact, accounted for by psychotic mood disorders (Cardno et al. 2002; Carpenter et al. 1973; Crichton 1996; McGuffin et al. 1982; Pini et al. 2001).

8.4 Conclusions

Although Schneider emphasized the error of rushing to a diagnosis of schizophrenia based on a preconceived bias, his writings led to that very result of the overdiagnosis of schizophrenia. His warning was expressed on page 144 when he said,

> At no time, however, should the investigator hurriedly force what he has observed into whatever conceptual mold he may have had in hand. ... Most mistaken diagnoses have come about for this very reason, that there has been too great a hurry to overlay the actual observations with some technical terminology.

He also warned against missing an organic etiology in a psychotic patient diagnosed with schizophrenia.

Schneider believed that the presence of any of his first-rank symptoms meant the diagnosis of schizophrenia despite a cycling course between episodes of mania and depression. In making his diagnosis, he emphasized presenting symptoms and de-emphasized the course of the illness, even a cycling course. His lasting impact on psychiatry is demonstrated by the retention for 50 years of at least two of his first-rank symptoms in our primary source of psychiatric diagnoses, the DSM. This is despite considerable data from the 1970s that found Schneider's first-rank symptoms common in psychotic mood-disordered patients. By 2013 with the expected publication of the DSM-5, all remnants of the first-rank symptoms may be history.

His use of "cyclothymia" rather than manic-depressive insanity reinforced Bleuler's ideas that psychotic symptoms rule out a mood disorder. Like Bleuler's accessory symptoms, Schneider's first-rank symptoms were disease nonspecific and are explained by psychotic mood disorders in the vast majority of functional psychotic cases according to Pini et al. (2001).

Like Bleuler's fundamental symptoms, Schneider's second-rank symptoms allowed, if not encouraged, the indiscriminate diagnosis of schizophrenia among the nonmentally ill and mood-disordered populations. Schneider's emphasis on the diagnosis of schizophrenia in all functionally psychotic patients regrettably has had a major influence on mental health professionals leading to the misdiagnosis of schizophrenia in thousands if not tens or hundreds of thousands of psychotic patients. The negative impact of such a misdiagnosis is discussed in Chap. 15.

Chapter 9
Concepts of Schizophrenia and Bipolar Disorder in the 1950s and 1960s

> *These observations [of schizophrenic and manic-depressive cases] could be expressed graphically by viewing the cases of functional mental illness in terms of a spectrum: ...*
>
> (Beck, 1967)
>
> *[Winokur et al.] recorded the prevalence of symptoms in 100 directly observed manic episodes. ...[They note that] delusions (persecutory, passivity, sexual, religious, and depressive), hallucinations, posturing, and symbolism may occur in mania even though these features are often considered symptoms of schizophrenia.*
>
> (Winokur et al. 1969)

9.1 Introduction

A history of the differential diagnoses of psychotic disorders from BCE through the anticipated publication of the DSM-5 in 2013 is revealing with regard to how the concept of a dichotomy between schizophrenia and bipolar disorder developed, a concept that is now losing support. This chapter focuses on relevant events that occurred in the 1950s and 1960s. The evolution of the concepts of schizophrenia, the major mood disorders and their interrelationships is reviewed from the DSM-I (APA, DSM 1952) through the DSM-II (APA, DSM 1968) in this chapter. The emphasis is on data that show similarities and overlap between the diagnoses of schizophrenia and psychotic mood disorders.

Several factors coalesced during this time period to increase the predominance of the diagnosis of schizophrenia in functionally psychotic patients (Table 9.1). The influences of Kraepelin (1919), Bleuler (1911), and later Schneider (1959) dominated academic psychiatry and the mental health professions in the USA as compared to Europe and especially the UK (Sect. 9.6). The discovery of the striking effectiveness of chlorpromazine (Thorazine) in psychotic patients, the equation of psychotic symptoms with schizophrenia, and the misunderstanding that chlorpromazine and subsequent

Table 9.1 Events in the 1950s and 1960s that promoted schizophrenia and demoted bipolar disorders

Event	Impact on the diagnoses of schizophrenia and bipolar disorder
Chlorpromazine (Thorazine) developed and prescribed for schizophrenia	Increase in the diagnosis of schizophrenia, not bipolar disorder
Electroconvulsive therapy used to treat schizophrenia	Increase in the diagnosis of schizophrenia, not bipolar disorder
Lithium use delayed due to serious adverse effects, including deaths. As an element, it could not be patented and was not profitable for pharma	Decreased diagnoses and focus on bipolar disorders
Primary/functional psychoses equated with schizophrenia	Increase in the diagnosis of schizophrenia, not bipolar disorder
DSM-I and II promoted schizophrenia	Increase in the diagnosis of schizophrenia, not bipolar disorder
NIMH funding much greater for schizophrenia than bipolar disorders	Increase in the diagnosis of schizophrenia, not bipolar disorder
The pharmaceutical industry focused on antipsychotic/antischizophrenia medications, not mood-stabilizing drugs	Increase in the diagnosis of schizophrenia, not bipolar disorder
Schizophrenia recognized by the media, politicians, and the public as common, debilitating, expensive, and warranting government assistance	Funding and research focus on schizophrenia, not bipolar disorders
Severe functional mental illness portrayed in the media as schizophrenia, not mania	Increase in the diagnosis of schizophrenia, not bipolar disorder
K. Schneider published his book titled *Clinical Psychopathology* with his pathognomonic first-rank symptoms of schizophrenia; he supported Bleuler's concept of psychosis equals schizophrenia	Increase in diagnosis, funding, research, publications, grant applications, conferences, and lectures on schizophrenia, not mood disorders
Academic psychiatry in the USA embraced the teachings of Kraepelin, Bleuler, and Schneider emphasizing schizophrenia	Increase in diagnosis, funding, research, publications, grant applications, conferences, and lectures on schizophrenia, not mood disorders

antipsychotic drugs were antipsychotic/antischizophrenia medications boosted the diagnosis of schizophrenia in psychotic patients. The delay of the use of lithium in bipolar patients and the absence of any other effective treatment inhibited the diagnosis of bipolar disorders. More patients with diagnoses of schizophrenia meant an enormous cost for treatment and maintenance that was attributed to the disease called schizophrenia. Schizophrenia gained the reputation of a common, chronic, lifelong, disabling, and expensive disease requiring government care. The numbers of patients with the diagnosis of schizophrenia increased and government and pharmaceutical attention on causes and more effective treatments followed. This meant more federal grant money and pharmaceutical funding for research on schizophrenia, resulting in increased numbers of diagnoses, publications, lectures, meetings, books, and grant proposals on schizophrenia. This cycle continued, and increased for many decades, well into the 1990s and 2000s especially for numbers of publications (Fig. 9.1) but probably not for the number of diagnoses of schizophrenia by the 1980s and 1990s (Fig. 3.2).

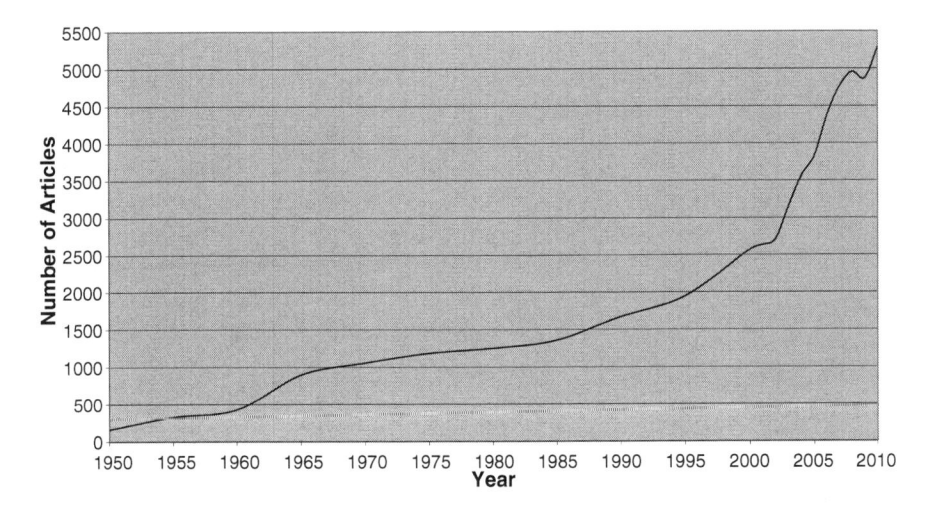

Fig. 9.1 PubMed literature cites of schizophrenia/schizophrenic
The number of articles written about schizophrenia as recorded by PubMed in the 1950s and 1960s, if not also in the 1970s and 1980s, was expected to be higher. This may be an artifact involving overlooked recordings by PubMed during these early years. The rate of increase in cites per year increases steadily from 1970 to 1990 when the rate of increase sharply rises. From the year 2000, the number of cites more than doubled to 2010. This doubling is paralleled by cites of schizophrenia in titles of articles

Adding skepticism to the validity of schizophrenia were large cross-international variations in the frequency of diagnoses of schizophrenia and bipolar disorder. These data derived from diagnostic comparison studies between psychiatrists in the USA and the UK as well as studies over time in the USA. The DSM-I and II were published during this time period and although both referenced the potential for psychosis in mood disordered patients, schizophrenia continued to be defined by psychotic symptoms as well as much more broad nonpsychotic symptoms (Tables 6.1 and 6.4). The timing of Schneider's publication in 1959, 48 years after Bleuler's book, seemed to be especially influential in reinforcing psychiatry's interpretation of Bleuler's concept that hallucinations and delusions meant schizophrenia.

9.2 The Effectiveness of New "Antipsychotic/Antischizophrenia" Medications in the 1950s Increased the Acceptance of Schizophrenia as a Bona Fide Disease

According to Wikipedia, chlorpromazine (Thorazine) was synthesized in 1950, possessed specific antipsychotic action, and was the prototype for the subsequent large class of phenothiazine drugs developed to treat schizophrenia, not bipolar disorders:

> The introduction of chlorpromazine into clinical use has been described as the single greatest advance in psychiatric care, dramatically improving the prognosis of patients in psychiatric hospitals worldwide ... and was one of the driving forces behind the deinstitutionalization movement.

In 1933, in search for improved antihistamine drugs, the French pharmaceutical company, Laboratories Rhone-Poulenc, synthesized promethazine, a pronounced sedative and an improved antihistaminic. It was used successfully in patients undergoing surgery in France. In December of 1950, chlorpromazine, a derivative of promethazine, was developed and found to induce indifference to aversive stimuli in rats. It was distributed for testing in patients in 1951 and successfully used as an anesthetic booster in surgical patients as it was reported to be "… the best drug to date in calming and reducing shock, …." It was noted to cause hypothermia and suggested it may induce "artificial hibernation." Of interest, it was said that psychiatrists were reluctant to use chlorpromazine initially, but on January 19, 1952, it was given to a 24-year-old psychotic manic inpatient, "… who responded dramatically" and was able to be discharged. Results from a first clinical trial conducted at the Hospital Sainte-Anne in Paris on 38 psychotic patients mostly diagnosed with schizophrenia were published in 1952 showing a dramatic response:

> … treatment with chlorpromazine went beyond simple sedation with patients showing improvements in thinking and emotional behavior.

(Wikipedia 2011)

Rhone-Poulenc licensed chlorpromazine to Smith, Kline and French in the USA, now GlaxoSmithKline, and by 1954, it was being broadly used in the USA to treat schizophrenia, mania, and other psychotic disorders. The use of chlorpromazine and subsequent drugs of this type is credited with emptying psychiatric hospitals in the USA, a movement that has been compared to that of penicillin treatment of infectious diseases. In 1955, there were 558,992 psychiatric inpatients; by 1970, 337,619; by 1980, 150,000; and by 1990, between 110,000 and 120,000 inpatients. Most of these inpatients were diagnosed with schizophrenia.

Chlorpromazine was widely used so that by 1964 some 50 million people worldwide had taken it. The use of chlorpromazine largely replaced the use of electroconvulsive therapy (ECT), psychosurgery, and insulin shock therapy for schizophrenia. Its popularity declined in the late 1960s as newer drugs were developed. It was the chlorpromazine molecule that enabled the discovery of tricyclic antidepressants.

Schizophrenia was equated with psychoses. Chlorpromazine and subsequent antipsychotic drugs became known as antipsychotic/antischizophrenia medications because they were designed and developed by many different pharmaceutical companies to treat schizophrenia because schizophrenia offered the largest patient base for sales. Although chlorpromazine was effective in psychotic mood disordered patients, most psychotic patients were diagnosed with schizophrenia, not a mood disorder, and the drug was much less effective in nonpsychotic mood disordered patients (Fig. 11.1). The effectiveness in schizophrenia was emphasized as opposed to mood disorders, and that led to the increased diagnosis of schizophrenia since clinicians tend to diagnose disorders for which they have effective treatments. This led to increased pharmaceutical focus on developing new antipsychotic/antischizophrenia medications, government support for research in schizophrenia, increased attention to schizophrenia by academic psychiatry and more publications, seminars, meetings, and grant proposals on schizophrenia (Fig. 9.1). All of the antipsychotic drugs, from chlorpromazine through the current atypicals, are effective in treating psychoses, but since psychosis had been equated with schizophrenia, the effectiveness of "antipsychotic/antischizophrenia" medications in psychotic patients led to the conclusion that schizophrenia was the correct diagnosis. The promotion of clinical trials to test new antipsychotic/antischizophrenia medications required the recruitment of patients diagnosed with schizophrenia by clinician-researchers. This served as a substantial bias to make the diagnosis of schizophrenia among psychotic patient populations because clinical studies usually pay per patient recruited and treated. There have been more than two dozen "antipsychotic/antischizophrenia" medications introduced worldwide and each required substantial funding for development, animal, and human trials. New antipsychotic drugs continue to be released, marketed, and promoted. Recent examples include paliperidone palmitate (Invega Sustenna) from Ortho-McNeil-Janssen Pharmaceuticals, Inc., lurasidone (Latuda) from Dainippon Sumitomo Pharma Co. (Sunovion Pharmaceuticals Inc. is the US subsidiary) and iloperidone (Fanapt) from Novartis Pharmaceuticals Corp. Regrettably and despite the fact that the first report of the efficacy of chlorpromazine occurred in a psychotic manic patient, the antipsychotics became known as antipsychotic/antischizophrenia medications that greatly supported the validity of schizophrenia.

For the atypical antipsychotics, there has been a recent broadening of targeted mental health populations other than those with schizophrenia by the producer pharmaceuticals. This effort for sales may represent a shrinking market of patients with schizophrenia for both clinical trials and sales. Examples of some of the other targeted conditions include major depression, bipolar disorders, anxiety disorders, sleep disorders, and childhood and adolescent disorders such as ADD, ADHD, and autism. Some pharmaceutical companies have sustained large FDA-imposed fines for some of these marketing practices.

9.3 Electroconvulsive Therapy (ECT) Initially Used to Treat Schizophrenia

According to Wikipedia, agents producing seizures were used to treat psychotic psychiatric conditions as early as the sixteenth century. In 1785, seizure induction was documented as therapeutic in psychotic patients in the London Medical Journal. In 1934, the Hungarian neuropsychiatrist, Ladislas J. Meduna used convulsive therapy to treat schizophrenia, the pervasive diagnosis for psychotic patients at that time, because he mistakenly believed that schizophrenia and epilepsy were antagonistic disorders. To induce seizures, he initially used camphor and later, metrazol. Metrazol convulsive therapy was used worldwide by 1937 when the first international meeting on convulsive therapy was held in Switzerland. In 1937, the Italians Ugo Cerletti and Lucio Bini used electricity (electroconvulsive therapy, ECT) as a substitute for metrazol to produce seizures in patients. For this they were nominated but did not win the Nobel Prize. By 1940, ECT was introduced in both the UK and the USA, and through the 1940s and 1950s, the use of ECT became widespread. Although ECT is now known as effective specifically in severe depression, it was initially used during the 1940s, 1950s, and 1960s in the treatment of patients diagnosed with schizophrenia. Some of the effectiveness of ECT in these patients with "schizophrenia" may have been due to the misdiagnosis of psychotically depressed patients as having schizophrenia. As above, positive therapeutic effects of ECT in patients diagnosed with schizophrenia led to increased diagnoses of schizophrenia. Even the widespread negative portrayal of ECT in the popular media such as Ken Kesey's novel and movie, *One Flew Over the Cuckoo's Nest*, where ECT was used as an instrument of punishment and terror, gave support to schizophrenia as a bona fide disease because the patient was thought to have schizophrenia.

9.4 The National Institute of Mental Health (NIMH) and the Pharmaceutical Industry Focused on Schizophrenia Rather Than Mood Disorders

Hundreds of millions if not billions of dollars have been invested in research on schizophrenia by the NIMH and pharmaceutical companies. During these decades, it was schizophrenia that was considered to be the most severe, chronic, incapacitating, and prevalent of the severe mental illnesses. Federal grant money was made available to study schizophrenia. This fueled research and clinical and academic emphasis on schizophrenia, not mood disorders. The number of publications on schizophrenia has been impressive (Table 9.2; Fig. 9.1).

Table 9.2 PubMed literature cites of schizophrenia/schizophrenic

Year	Number of citations Anywhere in article	Title only
1950	160	109
1955	328	204
1960	427	294
1965	897	390
1970	1,057	403
1975	1,186	491
1980	1,252	544
1985	1,359	568
1990	1,671	741
1995	1,948	1,009
2000	2,574	1,386
2001	2,637	1,449
2002	2,713	1,493
2003	3,155	1,696
2004	3,563	1,896
2005	3,827	2,108
2006	4,381	2,366
2007	4,764	2,570
2008	4,955	2,595
2009	4,872	2,532
2010	5,278	2,877
Totals	53,004	27,721

9.5 The Use of Lithium in Bipolar Patients Was Delayed in the USA

According to Wikipedia, lithium was first used in the nineteenth century to treat gout because laboratory studies showed that lithium could dissolve uric acid crystals. Apparently, because excess uric acid in the nineteenth century was thought to be involved with manic and depressive disorders, lithium was used to treat mania from the 1870s, at least in New York and in Denmark. This treatment was isolated and short-lived due to at least two factors: (1) the pharmaceutical industry was reluctant to invest in an element drug that could not be patented and (2) reports of severe side effects and deaths from the prescription of lithium salts as a substitute for sodium in patients with hypertension. This practice of using lithium in hypertension was discontinued in 1949 when there was a ban on the sale of lithium in the USA.

The effectiveness of lithium in mania was rediscovered in Australia by John Cade who published his results in 1949. Cade was studying patients with schizophrenia and thought uric acid might play a role in causing symptoms of schizophrenia. He needed a soluble urate salt and used lithium urate, finding it to cause tranquilization in rodents. Cade discovered that the effect was caused by the lithium ion and proved the effectiveness of lithium in controlling mania in chronically hospitalized patients (Cade 1949). The low therapeutic index of lithium and the reports of deaths due to lithium prevented acceptance by the rest of the world. Clinical trials in the 1960s and 1970s by Mogens Schou (1968, 1979) and Poul Baastrup (1964) from Denmark and Sam Gershon (Gershon and Yuwiler 1960) and Fred Goodwin (1989; Carlson and Goodwin 1973) in the USA proved lithium could be effectively used to treat mania safely. The FDA approved lithium for the treatment of bipolar disorders in 1970, but lithium did not become widely used for bipolar disorders in the USA until the mid- to late 1970s.

The effective use of chlorpromazine (Thorazine) to treat schizophrenia from the 1950s and the absence of an effective treatment for bipolar disorders until the mid-1970s greatly skewed the diagnosis of psychotic patients toward schizophrenia and away from bipolar in the USA but less so in the UK.

9.6 Discrepancies in Diagnostic Comparisons Between the USA and the UK

Kramer (1961) reported that in 1957 schizophrenia was diagnosed in the USA in over 22% of first admissions in contrast to less than 11% for all primary mood disorders combined. Comparative figures for the UK in 1956 were about 14% for schizophrenia and 33% for bipolar disorders. The overall cross-national difference was nearly fivefold (Pope and Lipinski 1978). Kramer (1961) reported that a bipolar disorder was diagnosed nine times as often in the UK compared to the USA. These data prompted further comparisons which found that psychiatrists in the USA diagnosed schizophrenia commonly and bipolar disorders rarely in comparison to psychiatrists in the UK (Kramer et al. 1969; Cooper et al. 1972; Edwards 1972). Cooper et al. (1972) examined 250 consecutive psychiatric admissions at each of two hospitals, one in New York and one in London. An international panel using detailed structured interviews arrived at "project diagnoses" for all 500 patients and compared these diagnoses to the "local diagnoses" actually made at each of the two hospitals. In the New York hospital, the "local diagnosis" of schizophrenia was more than eight times as frequent as the diagnosis of a bipolar disorder. This was in sharp contrast to both the "project diagnoses" and the "local diagnoses" by London psychiatrists who found a ratio of 1:1 for schizophrenia to bipolar disorder. In London, schizophrenia accounted for 34% of admission diagnoses compared to 65% of admissions in New York. For mania alone, 22 New York patients were so diagnosed by the International Panel, but of these, only one patient (4.5%) was diagnosed with mania by New York psychiatrists; 20 of these 22 cases (91%) were diagnosed with schizophrenia in New York. A second study similarly compared diagnostic practices at nine other New York hospitals versus nine other London area hospitals. This study revealed that schizophrenia was diagnosed by New York psychiatrists 12 times as often as all major mood disorders and 100 times as often as mania. Discounting alcoholic and organic psychoses, schizophrenia accounted for 82% of all of the New York admissions (Pope and Lipinski 1978). Pope and Lipinski (1978) concluded that, "… it seems likely that undue reliance on 'schizophrenic' symptoms led the New York centers to grossly over-diagnose schizophrenia at the expense of MDI [manic-depressive insanity or bipolar disorder]." Results did not change significantly when other European countries were compared to the USA or other states in the USA were studied.

These comparison studies emphasize the greater influence that Bleuler and Schneider had upon academic psychiatry in the USA versus that in the UK and other European countries. Although the data do not prove incorrect diagnostic practices in the USA, Pope and Lipinski (1978) certainly believed that this was the case.

Further inconsistencies occurred over decades in the frequency of the diagnosis of schizophrenia in the USA. For example, Kuriansky et al. (1974) reviewed case records from the New York State Psychiatric Institute between 1932 and 1970. Between 1932 and 1941, 28% of all patients were diagnosed on admission as having schizophrenia; between 1947 and 1956, the percent of admission diagnoses of schizophrenia was 77%, decreasing to about 50% by 1970. In contrast, the diagnosis of schizophrenia at the Maudsley Hospital in London was almost stable at 20% between 1938 and 1978 (Pope and Lipinski 1978). Similarly, demonstrating a fluid increase in the percentage of admission diagnoses of schizophrenia in the USA were data from the Manhattan State Hospital showing that schizophrenia and bipolar disorders were diagnosed about equally in 1928 and 1929, but by 1938, schizophrenia was diagnosed four times as often (Hoch and Rachlin 1941). Such variability in the diagnosis of schizophrenia cross-nationally and over time within the USA raises a question of the validity of the diagnosis of schizophrenia.

9.7 Overlap of Diagnostic Symptoms Between Schizophrenia and Psychotic Mood Disorders from the Diagnostic and Statistical Manual for Mental Disorders-I (DSM-I) and the DSM-II

In contrast to most medical and surgical specialties where diagnostic criteria are based on objective and often quantifiable pathophysiology such as blood tests or X-rays, the diagnosis of psychiatric disorders continues to depend on subjective assessments based on patients' self-reported experiences, their observed behaviors, and the testimonies of patients' significant others; no objective laboratory or imaging tests are available except to rule out most organic/physical causes of psychotic and other presenting symptoms. As a result, the psychiatric diagnosis can vary according to what questions are asked and the interpretation of patients' answers. These variables depend upon the education, beliefs, and biases of the diagnostician to a greater extent than when an objective basis for diagnosis is available. Standardized classifications and diagnostic criteria have been critical to the advancement of psychiatric diagnoses. The current author has changed from an earlier bias toward diagnosing schizophrenia (Lake et al. 1980) to one of diagnosing a mood disorder in functionally psychotic patients (Lake 2010a, b).

Attempts to classify psychiatric and especially psychotic disorders began in earnest in the mid-1800s. Prior to this, manic-depressive insanity could be considered the only functional psychotic disease; there was no dementia praecox or schizophrenia (Chap. 3). Angst (2002) cited the historical review of Kahlbaum (1863) who he said "… summarized about 30 different systems of classification from Plater (1625), considered to be the founder of medical and psychiatric classification, [all the way] to Morel (1851)." Between the mid-nineteenth and mid-twentieth centuries, the absence of objective findings stimulated individual mental health professionals to create their own idiosyncratic, redundant, and often confusing names and diagnostic criteria for various psychiatric syndromes and subtypes based on their observations and interpretations. The concepts of the neuroses and the schizophrenias were developed during this period. In an attempt to rectify these problems and to increase consensus for a set of common psychiatric disorders and diagnostic criteria, an early classification system was developed in the 1930s that led to the first DSM, the DSM-I (APA, DSM 1952). No other series of publications on diagnostics has had as great an influence on psychiatry, the mental health and legal professions, the media, and the public. From at least the 1960s, most graduating medical doctors and other mental health professionals have owned one. It has been through these diagnostic manuals that schizophrenia and bipolar disorder have been codified. Details from the seven editions of the DSM are valuable as they reveal increasing overlap between the diagnostic criteria for schizophrenia and mood disorders. Apparently, DSM sections on schizophrenia and bipolar disorders are written by separate experts in their respective fields, and the similarities and overlaps have not been adequately addressed as to their implications of a relationship between these disorders that have been considered mutually exclusive of one another. This section highlights similarities of diagnostic symptoms from the first and second editions of the DSM. The overlap suggests the elimination of the two disease concept and the Kraepelinian dichotomy. The DSM-I and II maintained Bleuler's fundamental symptoms and his simple subtype as diagnostic of schizophrenia.

9.7.1 The DSM-I (APA, DSM 1952)

In 1951, George N. Raines, MD, Chairman, Committee on Nomenclature and Statistics, wrote the foreword for the first DSM. His foreword gives an excellent summary of the development of the DSMs. He wrote that,

> The development of a uniform nomenclature of disease in the United States is comparatively recent. In the late twenties, each large teaching center employed a system of its own origination, no one of which met more than the immediate needs of the local institution. Despite their local origins, for lack of suitable alternatives, these systems were spread in use throughout the nation, ordinarily by individuals who had been trained in a particular center, [and] hence had become accustomed to that special system of nomenclature. Modifications in the transplanted nomenclatures immediately became necessary, and were made as expediency dictated. There resulted a polyglot of diagnostic labels and systems, effectively blocking communication and the collection of medical statistics. In late 1927, the New York Academy of Medicine spearheaded a movement out of this chaos towards a nationally accepted standard nomenclature of disease. In March, 1928, the first National Conference on Nomenclature of Disease met at the Academy; this conference was composed of representatives of interested governmental agencies and of the national societies representing the medical specialties. A trial edition of the proposed new nomenclature was published in 1932, and distributed to selected hospitals for a test run. Following the success of these tests, the first official edition of the Standard Classified Nomenclature of Disease was published in 1933, and was widely adopted in the next two years. Two subsequent revisions have been made, the last in 1942. The nomenclature in this manual [DSM-I] constitutes the section on Diseases of the Psychobiologic Unit from the Fourth Edition of the Standard Nomenclature of Diseases and Operations, 1952.
>
> Prior to the first edition of the Standard, psychiatry was in a somewhat more favorable situation regarding standardized nomenclature than was the large body of American medicine. The Committee on Statistics of the American Psychiatric Association (then the American Medico-psychological Association) had formulated a plan for uniform statistics in hospitals for mental disease which was officially adopted by the Association in May, 1917. This plan included a classification of mental disease which, although primarily a statistical classification, was usable in a limited way as a nomenclature. The National Committee for Mental Hygiene introduced the new classification and statistical system in hospitals throughout the country, and continued to publish the "Statistical Manual for the Use of Hospitals for Mental Diseases" through the years. The Committee on Nomenclature and Statistics of the American Psychiatric Association collaborated with the National Committee in this publication. With approval of the Council, and by agreement with the National Committee for Mental Hygiene (now the National Association for Mental Health), the Mental Hospital Service of the American Psychiatric Association now assumes responsibility for future publication of the Statistical Manual, which has been re-titled, "Diagnostic and Statistical Manual for Mental Disorders," and is presented here in its first edition.

With the publication of the DSM-I (APA, DSM 1952), schizophrenia was given broad acceptance as the disease described by Eugene Bleuler in 1911. The DSM-I basically divided "psychotic disorders" into "affective reactions" and "schizophrenic reactions" (Tables 2.7 and 9.3). Even though "psychotic reactions" that included delusions and hallucinations were noted to occur in severe mania and depression, the schizophrenic reactions became defined by psychosis and other symptoms and could include "affective disturbances in varying degrees and mixtures." For example, under the diagnosis of "manic-depressive reactions" it was written, "These groups comprise the psychotic reactions which fundamentally are marked by severe mood swings, and a tendency to remission and recurrence. Various accessory symptoms such as illusions, delusions, and hallucinations may be added to the fundamental affective alteration. Manic depressive reaction is synonymous with the term manic depressive psychosis. The reaction will be further classified into the appropriate one of the following types: manic, depressed, or other."

The other major mood disorder with potential for psychosis was "psychotic-depressive reaction." A description of these patients from the DSM-I is given below:

> These patients are severely depressed and manifest evidence of gross misinterpretation of reality, including, at times, delusions and hallucinations. This reaction differs from the manic depressive reaction, depressed type, principally in (1) absence of history of repeated depressions or of marked cyclothymic mood swings, (2) frequent presence of environmental precipitating factors. This diagnostic category will be used when a "reactive depression" is of such quality as to place it in the group of psychoses....

Although the DSM-I section on the affective reactions recognized the potential for psychoses, Bleuler's idea that psychosis meant schizophrenia regardless of mood disturbances prevailed in clinical settings.

Following the "affective reactions" were the "schizophrenic reactions" (Table 9.3). There were nine different schizophrenic reactions described in the DSM-I. The overall description was as follows:

> This term [schizophrenic reaction] is synonymous with the formerly used term dementia praecox. It represents a group of psychotic reactions characterized by fundamental disturbances in reality testing, relationships and concept formations, with affective, behavioral, and intellectual disturbances in varying degrees and mixtures. The disorders are marked by a strong tendency to retreat from reality, by emotional disharmony, unpredictable disturbances in stream of thought, regressive behavior, and in some, by a tendency to "deterioration." The predominant symptomatology will be the determining factor in classifying such patients into types.

Notable in the DSM-I is that "schizophrenic reaction, schizoaffective type" is included under the "schizophrenic reactions" and its description was as follows:

> This category is intended for those cases showing significant admixtures of schizophrenic and affective reactions. The mental content may be predominantly schizophrenic, with pronounced elation or depression. Cases may show predominantly affective changes with schizophrenic-like thinking or bizarre behavior. The prepsychotic personality may be at variance, or inconsistent, with expectations based on the presenting psychotic symptomatology. On prolonged observation, such cases usually prove to be basically schizophrenic in nature.

The overlap and similarities between the above descriptions of the "affective" versus the "schizophrenic reactions" were apparently overlooked. "Affective disturbances"

Table 9.3 DSM-I (APA, DSM 1952) classifications of the primary/functional psychotic reactions

DSM no.	Name of disorder	Description
796	Involutional psychotic reaction	"… psychotic reactions characterized most commonly by depression occurring in the involutional period, without previous history of manic depressive reaction, … The reaction tends to have a prolonged course… characterized chiefly by depression and others chiefly by paranoid ideas."
x10	**Affective reactions**	"These psychotic reactions are characterized by a primary, severe, disorder of mood, with resultant **disturbance of thought and behavior**, in consonance with the affect."
x11	Manic-depressive reaction, manic type	"… characterized by elation or irritability, with over-talkativeness, flight of ideas, and increased motor activity."
x12	Manic-depressive reaction, depressed type	"… cases with outstanding depression of mood and with mental and motor retardation and inhibition; … Perplexity, stupor or agitation may be prominent symptoms, …."
x13	Manic-depressive reaction, other	"… cases with marked mixtures of the cardinal manifestations of the above two phases (mixed type), or those cases where continuous alteration of the two phases occur (circular type). Other … varieties … included here [are] … (manic stupor or unproductive mania)… ."
x14	Psychotic-depressive reaction	"… evidence of **gross misinterpretation of reality**, including, at times, **delusions and hallucinations**. … [There is an] absence of history of repeated depressions or of … mood swings, [and the] frequent presence of environmental precipitating factors. … [i.e.,] a 'reactive depression'."
x20	**Schizophrenic reactions**	"… a group of psychotic reactions characterized by fundamental disturbances in reality relationships and concept formations with **affective, behavioral, and intellectual disturbances** in varying degrees and mixtures. … **emotional disharmony, unpredictable disturbances in stream of thought**,… and in some, by a tendency to 'deterioration'."
x21	Schizophrenic reaction, simple type	"… reduction in external attachments and interests and impoverishment of human relationships … involves adjustment on a lower psychobiological level of functioning, usually accompanied by apathy and indifference … manifests an increase in severity of symptoms over long periods, usually with apparent mental deterioration,…."
x22	Schizophrenic reaction, hebephrenic type	"… shallow, inappropriate affect, unpredictable giggling, silly behavior and mannerisms, delusions, … hallucinations, and regressive behavior."
x23	Schizophrenic reaction, catatonic type	"… conspicuous motor behavior, exhibiting either marked generalized inhibition (stupor, mutism, negativism and waxy flexibility) or excessive motor activity and excitement. … may regress to a state of vegetation."

(continued)

9.7 Overlap of Diagnostic Symptoms Between Schizophrenia... 163

Table 9.3 (continued)

DSM no.	Name of disorder	Description
x24	Schizophrenic reaction, paranoid type	"… **delusions of persecution, and/or of grandeur**, ideas of reference, and often hallucinations. … unpredictable behavior, … attitude of hostility and aggression. **Excessive religiosity** … with or without delusions of persecution. There may be an **expansive delusional system of omnipotence, genius, or special ability**."
x25	Schizophrenic reaction, acute undifferentiated type	"… confusion of thinking and turmoil of emotion, … Very often … accompanied by an **pronounced affective coloring of either excitement or depression**."
x26	Schizophrenic reaction, chronic undifferentiated type	"… mixed symptomatology … includes … 'latent,' 'incipient,' and 'pre-psychotic' schizophrenic reactions."
x27	Schizophrenic reaction, schizoaffective type	" … significant admixtures of schizophrenic and affective reactions. …."
x28	Schizophrenic reaction, childhood type	"… schizophrenic reactions occurring before puberty. ….."
x29	Schizophrenic reaction, residual type	"… after a … schizophrenic reaction, have improved sufficiently to be able to get along in the community, but who continue to show recognizable residual disturbance of thinking, affectivity, and/or behavior."
x30	**Paranoid reactions**	"… persistent delusions, generally persecutory or grandiose … [with] consistent … emotional responses and behavior …."
x31	Paranoia	"… extremely rare. … an intricate, complex, and slowly developing paranoid system, often logically elaborated after a false interpretation of an actual occurrence … the patient considers himself endowed with superior or unique ability. … normal stream of consciousness, without hallucinations and with relative intactness and preservation of the remainder of the personality, in spite of a chronic and prolonged course."
x32	Paranoid state	"… paranoid delusions. … lacks the logical nature of systematization seen in paranoia; yet it does not manifest the bizarre fragmentation and deterioration of the schizophrenic reactions. It is likely to be of a relatively short duration, thought it may be persistent and chronic."

are noted as a characteristic of schizophrenia. This description of schizophrenia, especially "affective symptoms" as well as each of the other symptoms is compatible with psychotic mood disorders. This overlap of symptoms between psychotic mood disorders and schizophrenia continued through each edition in the DSM including the current DSM-IV-TR (Chap. 11). A disturbance of affect has been considered a core symptom of schizophrenia since Bleuler (1911) published his four fundamental symptoms. Variously described as blunted, flat, inappropriate, or restricted, through seven DSM editions over six decades, a disturbance of affect has and will continue to be associated with schizophrenia as in the DSM-5 (proposed for 2013) as opposed to being restricted to the affective or mood disorders.

9.7.2 The DSM-II (APA, DSM 1968)

The DSM-II was prepared by the Committee on Nomenclature and Statistics of the APA and published by the APA in 1968. In the foreword, it was written that,

> The first edition of the Manual (1952) made an important contribution to U.S. and, indeed, world psychiatry. It was reprinted twenty times through 1967 and distributed widely in the U.S. and other countries. Until recently, no other country had provided itself with an equivalent official manual of approved diagnostic terms. DSM-I was also extensively, though not universally, used in the U.S. for statistical coding of psychiatric case records. In preparing this new edition, the Committee has been particularly conscious of its usefulness in helping to stabilize nomenclature in textbooks and professional literature.

The wide distribution of the DSM-I led to the wide acceptance of its contents, including the dichotomy and schizophrenia as a valid disease.

In the DSM-II mental illness was basically divided into two groups, the neuroses and the psychoses; the latter being further subdivided broadly into the schizophrenias including schizoaffective disorder, manic-depressive insanity (bipolar disorder), and the paranoid states, with schizophrenia the dominant disease of the four (Table 9.4; Figs. 3.1 and 3.2).

Significant changes from the DSM-I to the DSM-II included the elimination of "reaction" after schizophrenia and affective psychoses that were renamed "major affective disorders." The number of possible subtypes of schizophrenia increased to 13 (Table 9.4). The focus on schizophrenia is suggested by the large increase of subtypes. There was no specification for length of time a patient had to suffer symptoms. Schizophrenia was described as

> … a group of disorders manifested by characteristic disturbances of thinking, mood and behavior.

The inclusion of "disturbances … of mood" as a symptom of schizophrenia reinforced the misconception of Bleuler from 1911 that schizophrenia could have any symptom of a mood disorder, but mood disorders could not have symptoms of schizophrenia, that is, psychosis. The DSM-II emphasized that schizophrenia is

> … **a thought** disorder to be distinguished from the major Affective illnesses which are dominated by **a mood** disorder. (Chap. 13)

"Schizophrenia, simple type" was retained and described as,

> This psychosis is characterized chiefly by a slow and insidious reduction of external attachments and interests and by apathy and indifference leading to impoverishment of interpersonal relations, mental deterioration, and adjustment on a lower level of functioning.

This subtype, subsequently eliminated (APA, DSM-III 1980), allowed the misdiagnosis of patients suffering from chronic depression and social problems. It sharply increased the population susceptible to a misdiagnosis of schizophrenia giving credence to the validity of schizophrenia.

Table 9.4 DSM-II (APA, DSM 1968): The neuroses and the psychoses not attributed to physical conditions listed previously

DSM no.	Disorder
• *The neuroses*	
300	Neuroses
300.0	Anxiety neurosis
300.1	Hysterical neurosis
300.13	Hysterical neurosis, conversion type
300.14	Hysterical neurosis, dissociative type
300.2	Phobic neurosis
300.3	Obsessive-compulsive neurosis
300.4	Depressive neurosis
300.5	Neurasthenic neurosis (neurasthenia)
300.6	Depersonalization neurosis
300.7	Hypochondriacal neurosis
300.8	Other neurosis
300.9	Unspecified neurosis
• *The psychoses*	
295	Schizophrenia
295.0	Schizophrenia, simple type
295.1	Schizophrenia, hebephrenic type
295.2	Schizophrenia, catatonic type
295.23	Schizophrenia, catatonic type, excited
295.24	Schizophrenia, catatonic type, withdrawn
295.3	Schizophrenia, paranoid type
295.4	Acute schizophrenic episode
295.5	Schizophrenia, latent type
295.6	Schizophrenia, residual type
295.7	Schizophrenia, schizoaffective type
295.73	Schizophrenia, schizoaffective type, excited
295.74	Schizophrenia, schizoaffective type, depressed
295.8	Schizophrenia, childhood type
295.90	Schizophrenia, chronic undifferentiated type
295.99	Schizophrenia, other [and unspecified] types
296	Major affective disorders (affective psychoses)
296.0	Individual melancholia
	Manic-depressive illnesses (manic-depressive psychoses)
296.1	Manic-depressive illness, manic type (manic-depressive psychosis, manic type)
296.2	Manic-depressive illness, depressed type (manic-depressive psychosis, depressed type)
296.3	Manic-depressive illness, circular type (manic-depressive psychosis, circular type)
296.33	Manic-depressive illness, circular type, manic
296.34	Manic-depressive illness, circular type, depressed
296.8	Other major affective disorder (affective psychosis, other)
296.9	[Unspecified major affective disorder]
	[affective disorder not otherwise specified]
	[manic-depressive illness not otherwise specified]
297	Paranoid states
297.0	Paranoia
297.1	Involutional paranoid state (involutional paraphrenia)
297.9	Other paranoid state
298	Other psychoses
298.0	Psychotic-depressive reaction (reactive depressive psychosis)

9.8 The Timing of Schneider's Book (1959) Supported Schizophrenia

The timing of Schneider's publication, 48 years after that of Bleuler, may have been such that his overlapping concepts were especially reinforcing of those of Bleuler. Without Schneider's book, it is possible that Bleuler's bias toward schizophrenia may have faded after a half century. Rather, Schneider's teachings that certain auditory hallucinations and delusions were pathognomonic of schizophrenia were close enough to the beliefs of Bleuler that both men's ideas bolstered each other's (Chaps. 6 and 8). Schneider's first- and second-rank symptoms of schizophrenia paralleled if not essentially copied Bleuler's accessory and fundamental symptoms of schizophrenia.

9.9 Conclusions

During these decades, schizophrenia achieved wide recognition as a common, severe, chronic, incapacitating, treatment-intensive, and expensive mental illness among mental health professions, physicians in general, the public, the media, and politicians. Federal and pharmaceutical funding flowed to clinical and basic science researchers in schizophrenia in an effort to discover causes and treatments. Comparatively speaking, only modest to minimal support was focused on mood disorders that were thought to be less common, less chronic, less severe, and less treatable. Several factors occurred during these times that furthered this discrepancy between attention to schizophrenia versus mood disorders (Table 9.1). The success of the "antipsychotic/antischizophrenia" medications, ECT, and the delay of the use of lithium in the USA contributed to government, pharmaceutical, academic, and clinical focus on schizophrenia. That this emphasis on schizophrenia may have become excessive in the USA was supported by comparative cross-national studies between the USA and the UK of the frequency of the diagnosis of schizophrenia versus that of bipolar disorder. The publication of Schneider's work in 1959 had substantial influence as he essentially affirmed the teachings of Bleuler and increased focus on schizophrenia.

The evolution of the DSMs from 1952 through the DSM-5 (APA, DSM 2013) shows remarkable overlap in the clinical descriptions and signs and symptoms across the sections of schizophrenia and bipolar disorder (Chaps. 10 and 11). The knowledge that some bipolar and unipolar depressed patients suffered psychosis was clearly presented in the DSM-I (APA, DSM 1952) and even before in the Standard Classified Nomenclature of Disease (1933). Despite this, academic psychiatry in the USA followed the teachings of Bleuler and Schneider and emphasized that psychosis, even in mood-disturbed patients, indicated the diagnosis of schizophrenia, not a psychotic mood disorder.

Chapter 10
Changing Concepts in the 1970s and 1980s: The Overlap of Symptoms and Course Between Schizophrenia and Psychotic Mood Disorders

> ... the results of this further analysis do not lend support to the view that schizophrenic and affective psychoses are distinct entities. ... as most of American psychiatrists do, by glossing over the affective symptoms and regarding the illness as a form of schizophrenia ....
>
> (Kendell & Gourlay 1970b)
>
> ... the schizophrenic syndrome is a non-specific clinical entity which can be symptomatic ... of manic-depressive psychosis ... particularly the manic phase ...
>
> (Ollerenshaw 1973)
>
> Some factors involved in manic and schizophrenic thought pathology are similar. There may be a general psychosis factor that cuts across psychotic diagnoses ... hospitalized manics are as thought disordered as schizophrenics ... The results support formulations that thought disorder is not unique to schizophrenia.
>
> (Harrow et al. 1982)
>
> Our findings do not fully support the present classification system, and suggest that its emphasis on hallucinations and delusions is overvalued. ...our analyses repeatedly yielded a single discriminate function, indicating that... schizophrenics and affectives can be represented on a continuous distribution of clinical features representing a single underlying process.
>
> (Taylor and Amir 1994)

10.1 Introduction

During these two decades, the number of publications that reported overlap and similarities in phenomenology between patients diagnosed with schizophrenia and psychotic mood disorders increased progressively. Also, by inference, these works questioned the Kraepelinian dichotomy and the validity of schizophrenia as a disease separate from psychotic mood disorders. There were at least 25 publications, one of which reviewed 166 other publications prior to 1978 (Pope and Lipinski 1978). However, this literature that documented the occurrence of hallucinations, delusions, disorganization, and chronicity in severe mood disordered patients appeared to have minimal, if any, impact upon academic psychiatry or the subsequent DSM's attention to the redundant diagnostic criteria between schizophrenia and psychotic mood disorders. Psychoses and chronicity continued to be considered diagnostic of schizophrenia despite being common in psychotic mood disorders. The works of several of these authors are summarized in this chapter and in selected quotes that are given in Tables 1.1 and 10.1.

As judged by the number of PubMed cites, the increased frequency of the diagnosis of schizoaffective disorder in the mid-to-late 1960s through the 1990s signaled a shift away from diagnosing all functionally psychotic patients with schizophrenia and at least toward diagnosing psychotic patients with mood symptoms as suffering from mood disorders (Table 7.2). A substantial literature during these decades suggests that schizoaffective disorder is a psychotic mood disorder and not a separate disease (Chap. 7).

In the 1960s, Beck (1967, 1972) proposed the concept of a spectrum between schizophrenia and manic depression. The concept of a spectrum implies a relationship between both ends of the severity spectrum of psychotic symptoms and a single disorder. A spectrum contradicts the Kraepelinian dichotomy. The spectrum idea has been broadly endorsed from the 1980s by Crow and others (Sects. 10.9 and 11.7).

Two DSMs, the DSM-III (APA, DSM 1980) and the DSM-III-R (APA, DSM 1987), were published during these decades.

10.2 Symptoms and Course of Schizophrenia Observed in Severe Bipolar Patients: The Early Reports

In addition to 2,000 years of individual case reports of psychotic bipolar patients (Table 3.1), several authors published their observations of large groups of bipolar patients in the predrug era which allowed a more accurate record of the natural history of the untreated condition (Kraepelin 1921; Rennie 1942; Lundquist 1945; Astrup et al. 1959). In over 300 bipolar patients across all studies, over half were reported to have hallucinations, delusions, and/or confusion. At least six major textbooks published in the 1960s also noted the presence of psychotic symptoms in severe depression and mania (Carlson and Goodwin 1973).

In the 1970s, several authors initiated a second generation of doubt regarding the Kraepelinian dichotomy after earlier skepticism expressed by Specht (1905), Kraepelin (1920), and Kasanin (1933). There were over two dozen publications in respected psychiatric journals that challenged the dichotomy and the prevalence and indirectly the validity of schizophrenia by recognizing substantial overlap and similarities of presenting psychotic symptoms and chronic courses between patients

Table 10.1 Selected quotes showing overlap and similarity of symptoms and course between schizophrenia and psychotic mood disorders from the 1970s and 1980s and before

Quote no.	Journal (year)	Author(s)	Field of study	Selected quotes of summary/conclusions	Results
1	*AJP* (1942)	Rennie	Prognosis	"The material for this paper consists of 208 cases of manic-depressive reactions … Nearly half the series (99 cases) had delusion material as part of their psychoses. Overwhelmingly the delusions are paranoid in nature. … Forty-five of these patients were hallucinated. … as follows: conversed with God; … people talking through stomach; … saw and heard God and angels; saw snake coming to her; … God's voice; … saw God; … Other behavior … included … wetting and soiling on the floor, self-exposure; stupor …; smearing, naked; gruesome interests; tantrums, confabulations; blocking … Seventy-nine percent had recurrences … Chronic cases … 7.7%. … The unfavorable depressions may develop a schizophrenic picture. Deterioration may occur in depression. … Attacks tend to become prolonged as they recur … shortening the course in subsequent attacks."	Similar/overlap
2	*Acta Psychia Neurol Scand* (1945)	Lundquist	Prognosis and course	"… discussed the symptoms of confusion and hallucinations occurring during the acute phase of the first manic episode … the duration of untreated manic episodes was shorter in patients with confusion [and unrelated] to the presence of hallucinations" (Carlson and Goodwin 1973).	Similar/overlap
3	*Acta Psychia Neurol Scand* (1959)	Astrup et al.	Review	"…151 cases … with affective psychoses … have been personally reexamined … 19 cases have taken a chronic course, [about 13%] and 13 of these were found to be atypical schizophrenias, … Factors indicating a less favorable prognosis are: … Paranoid traits, … Depersonalization, … Absence of hallucinations, … more than 2 psychotic periods."	overlap

(continued)

Table 10.1 (continued)

Quote no.	Journal (year)	Author(s)	Field of study	Selected quotes of summary/conclusions	Results
4	*Depression: Clin Exp Theor Aspects* (1967)	Beck	Book	"These observations could be expressed graphically by viewing the cases of functional mental illness in terms of a spectrum: at one end are the pure manic-depressive cases with a good prognosis; and at the other are the pure schizophrenic cases with a poor prognosis. In between are varying blends of these disorders (the schizo-affective cases) with a fair prognosis."	Continuum
5	*Manic-Depressive Illness* (1969)	Winokur et al.	Book	They "… recorded the prevalence of symptoms in 100 directly observed manic episodes. … [they note that] delusions (persecutory passivity, sexual, religious, and depressive), hallucinations, posturing, and symbolizism may occur in mania even though these features are often considered symptoms of schizophrenia" (Carlson and Goodwin 1973).	Similar/overlap
6	*BJP* (1970b)	Kendell and Gourlay	Review (symptoms, psychotic features)	"… the results of this further analysis do not lend support to the view that schizophrenic and affective psychoses are distinct entities. … as most of American psychiatrists do, by glossing over the affective symptoms and regarding the illness as a form of schizophrenia …."	Schizophrenia and bipolar similar
7	*AGP* (1970)	Lipkin et al.	Response to lithium trial	"Acute manic episodes may be mistaken for acute paranoid reactions [and misdiagnosed as paranoid schizophrenia]. … several cases of recurrent psychotic episodes previously diagnosed as paranoid … schizophrenia … which on reexamination … appeared to us to be recurrent manic-depressive illness … and have responded to … lithium.…"	Schizophrenia and bipolar similar
8	*AGP* (1972)	Fowler et al.	Review (symptoms, psychotic features)	"The Validity of Good Prognosis Schizophrenia" [title of article]; "… family studies do not validate good prognosis schizophrenia as schizophrenia and suggest that most good prognosis cases are variants of affective disorder. … the presence or absence of an affective syndrome is of considerably more diagnostic importance than schizophrenic symptoms."	Schizophrenia and bipolar similar

9	BJP (1972)	Mendlewicz et al.	Heredity	"... in manic patients with a positive family history of affective disorder.... almost half have been previously misdiagnosed as schizophrenic.... [likely] the result of a higher incidence of psychotic symptoms during mania and therefore the tendency to misdiagnose schizophrenia in patients with more psychotic manias" (Carlson and Goodwin 1973).	Schizophrenia and bipolar similar
10	AGP (1973)	Carpenter et al.	Clinical symptoms	"... these symptoms [FRSs] which he [Schneider] considers [pathognomonic of schizophrenia] occur in 1/4 of the cohort of manic-depressive patients."	Schizophrenia and bipolar similar
11	AGP (1973)	Carlson and Goodwin	Clinical symptoms (psychotic features)	"... during acute episodes of mania, with between 50% and 80% of patients showing evidence of psychotic symptoms. ... at the peak of their manic episodes [patients] became grossly psychotic with disorganized thoughts, extremely labile affect, delusions, hallucinations, and brief ideas of reference."	Schizophrenia and bipolar similar
12	BJP (1973)	Ollerenshaw	Review (symptoms)	"... the schizophrenic syndrome is a non-specific clinical entity which can be symptomatic ... of manic-depressive psychosis ... particularly the manic phase ... as well as schizophrenia itself."	Schizophrenia and bipolar similar
13	AGP (1974)	Abrams et al.	Review (symptoms, psychotic features)	"... many patients whose conditions are diagnosed as paranoid schizophrenia actually suffer from an affective illness ...."	Paranoid schizophrenia same as psychotic bipolar
14	AJP (1974)	Taylor et al.	Review (symptoms, family history, and treatment response)	"... many patients receiving the diagnosis of acute schizophrenia actually suffer from an affective illness and rarely satisfy rigorous criteria for schizophrenia."	Acute schizophrenia same as psychotic bipolar
15	AGP (1975)	Guze et al.	Clinical symptoms (psychotic features)	"... overall incidence of psychosis in patients with bipolar disorder is as high as 50% ... both inpatient and outpatient populations are considered."	Schizophrenia and bipolar similar

(continued)

Table 10.1 (continued)

Quote no.	Journal (year)	Author(s)	Field of study	Selected quotes of summary/conclusions	Results
16	AGP (1976)	Procci	Review (symptoms, family history, and treatment response)	"Schizo-Affective Psychosis: Fact or Fiction?" [title of article] "… support for the adoption of some widely agreed upon epithet to describe this state [schizoaffective disorder] is indicated. … at least a subgroup of these psychoses [schizoaffective disorder] has a definite relationship to the major affective disorders. An old proverb reads; 'A person with a bad name is already half-hanged.' This may well be the case with the term schizoaffective disorder."	Schizoaffective disorder invalid; schizophrenia and bipolar similar
17	BJP (1976)	Szasz	Editorial	"There is, in short, no such thing as schizophrenia."	Schizophrenia invalid
18	AGP (1976)	Tsuang et al.	Clinical symptoms	"… we have shown that the 85 atypical schizophrenics resembled much more the bipolars than the schizophrenics. From this, we conclude that a diagnosis of schizophrenia should not be made solely on the basis of schizophrenic symptoms. It is concluded that great care should be taken in diagnosing schizophrenia in a patient who also has manic symptoms."	Schizophrenia and bipolar similar/overlap
19	AGP (1976a, b)	Abrams and Taylor	Clinical symptoms	"We found that a majority of patients admitted with one or more catatonic signs had diagnosable affective illness, most frequently mania."	Schizophrenia and bipolar similar/overlap
20	AGP (1978)	Pope and Lipinski	Review (symptoms, family history, and treatment response)	"It seems likely that the findings summarized in this review [i.e., that many schizophrenics are actually misdiagnosed mood disordered patients] have not been adequately acknowledged by many modern American diagnosticians. The over diagnosis of schizophrenia and under diagnosis of bipolar disorder is a particularly serious problem in contemporary America. There are no known pathognomonic symptoms for schizophrenia, nor even any cluster of symptoms, …. to be valid in diagnosing schizophrenia. The non-specificity of 'schizophrenic' symptoms brings into question all research that uses them as the primary method of diagnosis."	Schizophrenia invalid

10.2 Symptoms and Course of Schizophrenia Observed... 173

21	*Psycho Med* (1979)	Brockington and Leff	Clinical symptoms	"... there is very poor agreement about the meaning of the term schizo-affective psychosis ... but [our findings] highlight a striking overlap with mania. This may well reflect the difficulty of the diagnostic separation of mania from schizophrenia ...."	Schizoaffective disorder invalid; schizophrenia and bipolar similar; continuum
22	*BJP* (1979)	Brockington et al.	Clinical symptoms	"Kraepelin's hypothesis that the functional psychoses consists of two distinct disease entities receives some support from our findings, but there is still no compelling evidence that the universe of psychotic patients falls naturally into these two groups."	Schizophrenia and bipolar similar/ overlap; ambivalent
23	*Psycho Med* (1980a)	Brockington et al.	Clinical symptoms	"They [schizophrenia and manial] have a number of properties in common, including heritability, response to neuroleptics and the tendency to post-psychotic depression. In the area of psychotic phenomena such as delusions, hallucinations and passivity phenomena, the overlap is almost complete."	Schizophrenia and bipolar similar/ overlap
24	*Psycho Med* (1980b)	Brockington et al.	Clinical symptoms	"Depressed Patients with Schizophrenic or Paranoid Symptoms" [article title] "These findings are not easily reconciled with Kraepelin's two entities principle but suggest a continuum of outcome between schizophrenia and unipolar depressive psychosis."	Schizophrenia and psychotic mood disorders similar/overlap
25	*AGP* (1982)	Harrow et al.	Review (psychotic features)	"Some factors involved in manic and schizophrenic thought pathology are similar. There may be a general psychosis factor that cuts across psychotic diagnoses. ... hospitalized manics are as thought disordered as schizophrenics ...; The results support formulations that thought disorder is not unique to schizophrenia."	Schizophrenia and bipolar similar

(continued)

Table 10.1 (continued)

Quote no.	Journal (year)	Author(s)	Field of study	Selected quotes of summary/conclusions	Results
26	*Hosp Community Psych* (1983)	Pope	Clinical symptoms	"The presence of putative 'schizophrenic' symptoms is no longer held to be valuable in distinguishing between manic–depressive illness and schizophrenia. … To misdiagnose schizophrenia as bipolar rarely does harm; to misdiagnose bipolar disorder as schizophrenia may adversely affect a patient's entire future."	Schizophrenia and bipolar similar/overlap
27	*Psych Clinics NA* (1986)	Doran et al.	Review (symptoms)	"Further studies assessing the validity of the diagnostic systems for schizophrenia may have to rely on features other than cross-sectional symptoms and longitudinal course. Such characteristics as pharmacologic responsivity and genetic transmission and the development of biologic markers may be the prospective cornerstones for validating the diagnosis of schizophrenia."	Ambivalent
28	*AJP* (1986)	Grossman et al.	Clinical symptoms (psychotic features)	"… 30% of the manic patients showed severe positive thought disorder 2–4 years after hospitalization."	Schizophrenia and bipolar similar
29	*Br J Clinic Psycho* (1988)	Bentall et al.	Clinical	"One possible reason for this lack of progress [in discovering the aetiology of schizophrenia] is that schizophrenia is not a valid object of scientific enquiry. Data from published research (mainly carried out by distinguished psychiatrists) are reviewed casting doubt on: (i) the reliability, (ii) the construct validity, (iii) the predictive validity, and (iv) the aetiological specificity of the schizophrenia diagnosis."	Schizophrenia invalid
30	*J Clin Psych* (1989)	Goodwin	Clinical course	"… 17% of the total population [with severe mood disorders] were truly treatment resistant and did not recover at all …"	Schizophrenia and bipolar similar

10.2 Symptoms and Course of Schizophrenia Observed...

diagnosed with schizophrenia and those with severe bipolar or unipolar disorders (Tables 1.1, 10.1). Examples are Winokur et al. (1969), Kendell and Gourlay (1970a, b), Beck (1967, 1972), Fowler et al. (1972), Mendlewicz et al. (1972), Carlson and Goodwin (1973), Carpenter et al. (1973), Ollerenshaw (1973), Taylor et al. (1974), Abrams et al. (1974), Guze et al. (1975), Abrams and Taylor (1976a, b), Procci (1976), Tsuang et al. (1976), and Pope and Lipinski (1978). As detailed below, these authors and others documented that severely psychotic bipolar patients can suffer bizarre, mood-incongruent hallucinations and nonsystematized paranoid delusions and gross disorganization of thought and of behavior, (Procci 1976; Harrow et al. 1982, 1995; Grossman et al. 1986; Bentall et al. 1988; Goodwin 1989; Kendler 1991; Taylor 1992; Tohen et al. 1992; Taylor and Amir 1994; Dieperink and Sands 1996; Kendler et al. 1998; Moller 2003; Ketter et al. 2004; Korn 2004; Murray et al. 2004; Craddock and Owen 2005; Hafner et al. 2005; Maier et al. 2006; Lake and Hurwitz 2006a, 2007a; Goodwin and Jamison 2007; Lake 2008a, b) catatonia,(Kruger and Braunig 2000; Carroll et al. 2005; Fink and Taylor 2006) the "negative symptoms" (when depressed), (Swartz 2002a; Belmaker 2004; Post 2007; Swartz and Shorter 2007; Schloesser et al. 2008) Schneider's "pathognomonic" first- and second-rank symptoms, (Carpenter et al. 1973; Crichton 1996; Peralta and Cuesta 1999; Cardno et al. 2002; Gonzalez-Pinto et al. 2003) and a chronic, deteriorating, treatment-resistant, nonremitting course (Carlson and Goodwin 1973; Pope 1983; Goodwin 1989; Brockington 1992; Post 1992, 2007, 2010; Harrow et al. 1995; Jager et al. 2004; Belmaker 2004; Lake and Hurwitz 2006b).

Several of the authors were British, and even some of the American authors who shared some skepticism about schizophrenia published in the British literature. Schizophrenia was more fully embraced in the USA than in Great Britain, where bipolar was emphasized in psychotic patients (Sect. 9.6). For example, Kendell and Gourlay (1970a, b), from The Institute of Psychiatry, The Maudsley Hospital, in patients with mixed symptomatology, pointed out that,

> "... most American psychiatrists ... gloss over the affective symptoms and regard the illness as a form of schizophrenia differing in no significant respect from other schizophrenias." They continued to explain that, "What is a depressive illness with paranoid symptoms in one centre [in the U.K.] is paranoid schizophrenia with depressive symptoms in another [in the U.S.], and so on." They recognized that, "... once the existence of patients who are intermediate both in symptomatology and prognosis is conceded, the traditional concept of Manic-Depressive Illness and Schizophrenia as distinct disease entities becomes open to question." Although their initial results were equivocal, follow-up data presented in an addendum led to the conclusion that, "... the results of this further analysis do not lend support to the view that schizophrenic and affective psychoses are distinct entities."

Fowler et al. (1972), from Washington University, School of Medicine, reported that,

> "... family studies do not validate good prognosis schizophrenia as schizophrenia and suggest that most good prognosis cases are variances of affective disorder." They emphasized that, "... the presence or absence of an affective syndrome is of considerably more diagnostic importance than schizophrenic symptoms."

Mendlewicz et al. (1972), from the New York State Psychiatric Institute, reported that almost half of their manic patients (with a positive family history of affective disorder) had been misdiagnosed as having schizophrenia. Ollerenshaw (1973) published his article in the British Journal of Psychiatry while he was a senior registrar at Powick Hospital, Worcester, Great Britain. He concluded that,

> Certain similarities between the course of "acute schizophrenia" and the course of manic-depressive psychoses are indicated. ...The schizophrenic syndrome is a non-specific clinical entity which can be symptomatic ... of manic-depressive psychosis – particularly the manic phase ...

He believed that schizophrenia should be a diagnosis of exclusion, made only after organic causes and manic-depressive psychosis are ruled out. This is opposite of the teachings of Bleuler and Schneider.

Goodwin and many colleagues, while at the NIMH, Bethesda, MD, admitted, studied, and followed for months to decades classic bipolar patients (Carlson and Goodwin 1973; Goodwin and Jamison 2007). They documented that many of their hospitalized bipolar patients suffered severe acute manic episodes characterized by bizarre behavior, hallucinations, paranoia, confusion, and extreme dysphoria (Table 10.2). During such severe "Stage III" intervals, patients were so psychotic that the classic manic or depressive symptoms were obscured by the psychotic symptoms sometimes for weeks to months. They reported that 70% of their inpatients experienced such psychotic episodes, where

> "Thought processes that earlier had been only difficult to follow now became incoherent and a definite loosening of associations was often described. The illusions were bizarre and idiosyncratic; hallucinations were present in six [of 20] patients; disorientation to time and place was observed in six patients during this stage [without an organic etiology]; and three patients also had ideas of reference." Carlson and Goodwin (1973) said that, "Despite symptoms that might have otherwise prompted a diagnosis of schizophrenia, patients appeared clearly manic both earlier in the course and later as the episode was resolving."

These early observations have been substantiated in other bipolar patient populations by many other researchers.

Also from the NIMH, Carpenter et al. (1973) discounted Schneider's first-rank symptoms as pathognomonic of schizophrenia because the symptoms were present in 25% of their cohort of manic-depressive patients. Nor did the first-rank symptoms relate to the duration or outcome of the illness. More recent studies have concurred with their findings, and the percent of psychotic mood disordered patients with first-rank symptoms seem considerably higher than 25% (Cardno et al. 2002; Gonzalez-Pinto et al. 2003). Carpenter may have justifiably influenced the proposed elimination of the diagnostic relevance of the first-rank symptoms from the DSM-5 draft.

The SUNY, Stony Brook, NY group, (Taylor and Abrams 1973, 1975; Abrams et al. 1974; Taylor et al. 1974) concluded that about 50% of psychotic patients admitted to the hospital with diagnoses of "acute" or paranoid schizophrenia actually suffered from "an affective illness." They explained this discrepancy based on

> "... the mistaken belief that certain phenomena often associated with schizophrenia [hallucinations and delusions] did not occur in affective disorders, and that more intensive investigation of paranoid schizophrenics might disclose a high proportion of patients suffering from affective illness." Abrams et al (1974) concluded, "... that many individuals receiving the diagnosis of paranoid schizophrenia are actually suffering from mania, ..."

Table 10.2 Classical and "atypical" symptoms in 20 manic patients (adapted from Carlson and Goodwin 1973)

Symptoms	Patients manifesting symptoms, %
Hyperactivity	100
Extreme verbosity	100
Pressure of speech	100
Grandiosity	100
Manipulativeness	100
Irritability	100
Euphoria	90
Mood lability	90
Hypersexuality	80
Flight of ideas	75
Delusions	75
Sexual	(25)
Persecutory	(65)
Passivity	(20)
Religious	(15)
Assaultiveness of threatening behavior	75
Distractibility	70
Loosened associations	70
Fear of dying	70
Intrusiveness	60
Somatic complaints	55
Some depression	55
Religiosity	50
Telephone abuse	45
Regressive behavior (urinating or defecating inappropriately; exposing self)	45
Symbolization or gesturing	40
Hallucinations (auditory and visual)	40
Confused	35
Ideas of reference	20

They questioned, "… the validity of the widely prevalent diagnostic label of paranoid schizophrenia, as used by a sample of New York psychiatrists." Taylor et al (1974) said that, "Fifty years after its introduction by Bleuler, acute schizophrenia remains a diagnostic label without a disease." Taylor and Abrams (1973) "… noted that their manic patients, all previously diagnosed as schizophrenic, frequently demonstrated symptoms classically associated with schizophrenia (e.g., first-rank symptoms, auditory hallucinations)." They concluded that "… cardinal signs of mania were diagnostically decisive even in the presence of such phenomena."

Lipkin et al. (1970) reached similar conclusions, warning that many psychotic manic patients might be misdiagnosed as having acute or paranoid schizophrenia. Abrams and Taylor (1976a, b) found even more misdiagnoses of catatonic schizophrenia reporting that over 67% had a psychotic mood disorder and not schizophrenia. More recent reviews of such research support these conclusions (Lake and Hurwitz 2006a, b; Lake 2008b).

Procci (1976) published a survey of the literature regarding schizoaffective disorder concluding that "... at least a subgroup of the psychoses has a definite relationship to the major affective disorders." Procci clearly disparaged the use of schizoaffective disorder as a diagnosis when he compared it to an old proverb:

> "A person with a bad name is already half-hanged;" and when he recommended an "... epithet to describe this state [schizoaffective disorder] is indicated."

He noted that several authors appeared to endorse a spectrum between patients diagnosed with schizophrenia and those with mood disorders. Others have concluded that patients diagnosed with schizoaffective disorder actually have a psychotic mood disorder (Lake and Hurwitz 2006b, 2007a, b; Aries and Hurwitz 2010).

Tsuang et al. (1976), from the University of Iowa, College of Medicine, reported that 80% of patients diagnosed with,

> "... atypical schizophrenia ... had suffered one or more manic symptoms at index admission." They warned "... that great care should be taken in diagnosing schizophrenia in a patient who also has manic symptoms" because "... when they actually have a bipolar affective disorder [they] will not have an opportunity to benefit from this [lithium] treatment."

Pope (1983) certainly concurred.

10.3 Thomas S. Szasz

Szasz (1976) at the SUNY, Upstate Medical Center, Syracuse, NY, published in the British Journal of Psychiatry his scathing attack upon the validity of schizophrenia. He contrasted the differences between the discovery of the causes of syphilitic paresis and other infectious diseases with the descriptions by Kraepelin and Bleuler of schizophrenia without any pathophysiology. Szasz said,

> "In other words, Kraepelin and Bleuler did not discover [dementia praecox and schizophrenia] the diseases for which they are famous; they invented them." He continued by saying that Bleuler "... subtly redefined the criterion of disease from histopathology to psychopathology --- that is, from abnormal bodily structure to abnormal personal behavior."

Szasz stressed the overlap of applicability of the "inclusion criteria" for schizophrenia to nonpsychiatric, mentally healthy populations. He said that,

> "The names of psychiatric diseases were henceforth the unquestioned and unquestionable proofs of the existence of such diseases ...." He felt that, "It [schizophrenia] is the greatest scientific scandal of our scientific age. ... There is, in short, no such thing as schizophrenia. Schizophrenia is not a disease, but only the name of an alleged disease."

His 1976 publication may have influenced the elimination of simple schizophrenia from the DSM-III (APA, DSM 1980). There is a large literature on the occurrence of hallucinations and delusions among the normal population (Bentall et al. 1988; Bentall and Fernyhough 2008; Smith 2002; Moynihan et al. 2002).

The current author does not concur with the Szaszian idea that functional psychotic illness does not exist; rather that schizophrenia is a psychotic mood disorder.

10.4 Harrison G. Pope and Joseph F. Lipinski

Pope and Lipinski (1978) from McLean Hospital and Harvard Medical School, Boston, MA, published their famous paper titled, "Diagnosis in Schizophrenia and Manic-Depressive Illness" as an "original article" in the Archives of General Psychiatry. They reviewed 166 publications and concluded that,

> "…classical 'schizophrenic' symptoms, including many types of hallucinations, delusions, catatonic symptoms, and Schneiderian first rank symptoms, are reported in 20%-50% of well-validated cases of manic-depressive illness… [and that] most so-called schizophrenic symptoms, taken alone and in cross-section, have remarkably little, if any, demonstrated validity in determining diagnosis, prognosis, or treatment response in psychosis. … There are no known pathognomonic symptoms for schizophrenia, nor even any clusters of symptoms, … as yet adequately demonstrated to be valid in diagnosing schizophrenia…. In the United States, particularly, overreliance on such symptoms alone results in over-diagnosis of schizophrenia and under-diagnosis of affective illnesses, particularly mania. … This compromises both clinical treatment and research." In fact, Pope and Lipinski questioned the validity of "all research" on Schizophrenia based on the non-specificity of "schizophrenic symptoms." They also said that, "The chronically confused state of research of schizophrenia may partially be owed to an illusory faith in the significance [of the diagnostic] symptoms [for Schizophrenia] …"

Pope (1983) again discounted diagnostic symptoms of schizophrenia saying that,

> "The presence of putative 'schizophrenic' symptoms is no longer to be held to be valuable in distinguishing between manic-depressive illness and schizophrenia." He emphasized that, "To misdiagnose schizophrenia as bipolar disorder rarely does harm; to misdiagnose bipolar disorder as schizophrenia may adversely affect a patient's entire future."

10.5 I.F. Brockington

Brockington and colleagues, initially from the Department of Psychiatry, University Hospital of South Manchester, UK, and later at the Illinois State Psychiatric Institute, Chicago, IL, addressed similarities between patients diagnosed with schizophrenia and psychotic mood disorders and essentially discounted schizoaffective disorder as a valid disease saying that,

> "… there is very poor agreement about the meaning of the term 'schizo-affective' at present." They concluded that their data showed that there is not only "… a relatively low concordance between definitions of schizo-affective psychosis, but highlighted a striking overlap with mania." (Brockington and Leff 1979) Although Brockington et al (1979) found "some support" for Kraepelin's dichotomy, they said that, "… there is still no compelling evidence that the universe of psychotic patients falls naturally into these two groups."

They suggested a shift from the concept of Bleuler to one emphasizing the presence of manic symptoms determining the diagnosis even in the presence of paranoia, hallucinations, and delusions. They said that schizophrenia and mania

> ... have a number of properties in common, including heritability, response to neuroleptics and the tendency to post-psychotic depression. ... In the area of psychotic phenomena such as delusions, hallucinations and passive phenomena, the overlap [of symptoms between schizophrenia and psychotic mood disorders] is almost complete.

They concluded that their patients meeting criteria for "schizomanic" psychosis should mostly be regarded as manic:

> This conclusion should lead to some revision of present ideas on the incidence and diagnosis of mania.

(Brockington et al. 1980a)

Brockington et al. (1980b) also looked at depressed patients with "schizophrenia" or paranoid symptoms. They said that,

> These results therefore give no support to the hypothesis that the "functional psychoses" can be divided into 2 main disease entities (Kraepelin's "two entities principle"). ... but suggest a continuum of outcome between schizophrenia and unipolar depressive psychosis.

10.6 Martin Harrow, Linda Grossman, Marshall Silverstein, Jay Himmelhoch, and Herbert Meltzer

Meltzer et al., from the Illinois State Psychiatric Institute, The Michael Reese Hospital and Medical Center and the University of Chicago, Chicago, IL, compared thought pathology between "manic and schizophrenic patients" (Harrow et al. 1982; Grossman et al. 1986). They found that,

> "The data indicate that [1] most hospitalized manics are severely thought disordered; [2] hospitalized manics are as thought disordered as schizophrenics ... [5] even after the acute phase, some manics show severe thought pathology." Upon two to four year post-hospitalization follow-up, "... 30% of the manic patients showed severe positive thought disorder ...." They concluded that, "The results support formulations that thought disorder is not unique to schizophrenia. Some factors involved in manic and schizophrenic thought pathology are similar. There may be a general psychosis factor that cuts across psychotic diagnoses."

10.7 Reports from the NIMH

Doran et al. (1986) from the NIMH published a review on the differential diagnosis of schizophrenia and psychotic mood disorders. They admitted that,

> "Despite this longevity [of knowledge about] ... the syndrome we at present call 'schizophrenia,' ... the rapid scientific advancement in our century, and the biologic movement in psychiatry, we continue to struggle with delineating the important features of this mental

illness [schizophrenia]." They concluded that, "Future studies assessing the validity of diagnostic systems for schizophrenia may have to rely on features other than cross-sectional symptoms and longitudinal course."

Also at the NIMH, Goodwin (1989) documented the prevalence of psychotic features and the occurrence of a chronic treatment-resistant course. He reported that in a two-year follow-up posthospitalization for an acute bipolar episode of mania or depression, over 50% had not recovered or stayed euthymic. He said that,

> ... 17% of the total population [of bipolar inpatients on his NIMH unit] were truly treatment-resistant and did not recover at all, ...

He counted as "the poor-outcome group" some 40% of his total sample. He found that lithium was equally effective in bipolar and unipolar disorders and that the antidepressants increased cycling in both groups. Lithium would generally not be prescribed for psychotic bipolar manic or depressed patients misdiagnosed with schizophrenia or unipolar depression. In fact, one study suggested that lithium is contraindicated in schizophrenia (Shopsin et al. 1971). These data emphasize the importance of correct diagnoses among psychotic patients.

10.8 Richard P. Bentall

Bentall and colleagues (1988), from the Department of Psychiatry, New Medical School, Liverpool, UK, seemed to be of a similar opinion of that of Szasz (1976). They said that,

> ... little of certainty has been found out about the etiology of the hypothesized schizophrenia disease process. One possible reason for this lack of progress is that schizophrenia is not a valid object of scientific inquiry. Data from published research (mainly carried out by distinguished psychiatrists) are reviewed casting doubt on: (i) the reliability, (ii) the construct validity, (iii) the predictive validity, and (iv) the etiological specificity of the schizophrenic diagnosis.

Their arguments make a persuasive case for abandoning the concept of schizophrenia as a valid disease and eliminating it altogether from the DSM-5.

10.9 An Introduction to the Continuum Concept

In contrast to the initial concept of a dichotomy by Kraepelin, later Kraepelin appeared to recognize overlap and to conceptualize a relationship between schizophrenia and bipolar disorder as a continuum without a sharp line of demarcation. The very nature, naming and embracement of schizoaffective disorder from 1933 as a disease concept speak to a continuum of severity between schizophrenia and mood disorders. Several authors, including Beck (1967, 1972), Brockington et al. (1980b), Crow (1986, 1990a, b), and Taylor (1992), have stated more forcefully than Ketter et al. (2004), their beliefs that the psychotic diseases, traditionally called schizophrenia, schizoaffective disorder, and psychotic mood disorders represent a spectrum of severity. This author interprets this spectrum/continuum or "dimensionally similar" concept to be consistent with the hypothesis of a single disease process with a wide spectrum of severity as has Crow, but this idea is extended to speculate that this single disease process is a mood disorder that can vary from mild to blatantly psychotic (Tables 11.1, 11.13, 11.14; Figs. 3.1, 11.3) (Brockington and Leff 1979; Brockington et al. 1979; Lake and Hurwitz 2006a, b, 2007a, b). This idea of a "continuum" has been revised recently by Crow (1986, 1990a, b, 2010).

Kraepelin's later idea of overlap, suggestive of a continuum, had little or no impact and was greatly overshadowed by his and Bleuler's emphasis on the predominance of schizophrenia over bipolar disorders and the dichotomy. Bleuler and Schneider minimized and subjugated mood symptoms to their very broad symptoms of "schizophrenia." Bleuler's teachings that psychosis mandates, but is not necessary for a diagnosis of schizophrenia overshadowed the late questions by Kraepelin as well as the many other descriptions in the literature spread over 2,000 years of bipolar patients exhibiting hallucinations, delusions, and chronicity (Table 3.1). See Sect. 11.7 for a fuller discussion of the continuum idea.

10.10 Overlap and Similarities Between Schizophrenia and Mood Disorders from the DSM-III (APA, DSM 1980) and the DSM-III-R (APA, DSM 1987)

10.10.1 The DSM-III (APA, DSM 1980)

The DSM-III was published in 1980 with the aim of providing "... diagnostic criteria to improve the reliability of diagnostic judgments." Also new to the DSM-III was "... the inclusion of decision trees to aid the clinician in understanding the organization and the hierarchical structure of the classification." There were five axes designated by roman numerals to allow a "multiaxial evaluation":

> For some diagnoses ..., beginning with the DSM-III (APA, DSM 1980) there was an attempt to replace subjective observations and opinions with available scientific data as the basis for subtypes and diagnostic criteria. This led to substantial changes in the DSM-III regarding the neuroses and the schizophrenias. Recognizing that the diagnosis of neurosis was confusing, misunderstood, socially stigmatizing and lacking a scientific basis, the DSM-III eliminated the term "neurosis" from the official nomenclature and either dropped or reorganized and renamed its subtypes.
>
> (Lake and Hurwitz 2007a)

Schizophrenia was listed as the "schizophrenic disorders" and the number of subtypes dropped to five. The most significant change was the elimination of Bleuler's subtype of "simple schizophrenia" that almost, but not quite, restricted schizophrenia to a psychotic process. The core diagnostic symptomatology for the five subtypes remained essentially unchanged, with various delusions, hallucinations, or incoherence including "blunted, flat, or inappropriate affect ... catatonic or disorganized behavior." The retention of Bleuler's core fundamental symptom, that is, a disturbance of affect, as diagnostic of schizophrenia still allowed an abundance of misdiagnoses of schizophrenia because of its subjectivity. Also needed for the diagnosis of schizophrenia in the DSM-III was "Deterioration from a previous level of functioning...." and "Continuous signs of the illness for at least six months at some time during the person's life..." The time requirement, deterioration, the reduction of the number of subtypes, and the elimination of simple schizophrenia would seem to have been an effort to restrict the diagnosis of schizophrenia. The six-month time requirement may have been instituted because of misdiagnoses of schizophrenia that were based on an acute psychosis of only hours or days potentially due to organic causes or an acute psychotic mood disorder. However, the addition of the need for six months of illness and a deterioration from a previous level of function in no way separated schizophrenia from a severe mood disorder since a substantial percent of severe mood disorders fulfill these criteria.

The influence of Schneider is apparent in the DSM-III diagnostic criteria for the schizophrenic disorders (Chap. 8). Schizoaffective disorder was moved out of the section on schizophrenia where it was listed as a subtype in the DSM-II to the section titled "Psychotic Disorders, Not Elsewhere Classified" in the DSM-III. The movement of schizoaffective disorder suggests a conceptual movement toward diagnosing psychotic patients with mood symptoms away from schizophrenia if not toward the mood disorders section.

The affective disorders with a potential for psychosis were called "major affective disorders" and included bipolar disorders and major depression. Diagnostic criteria were detailed. A fifth digit to the diagnostic code allowed the designation of a major affective disorder "with psychotic features." Under this description of psychotic features in affective disorders, according to the DSM-III, there could be "... gross impairment in reality testing, as when there are delusions or hallucinations, or grossly bizarre behavior ... or depressive stupor (the individual is mute and unresponsive)." Before the DSM-III, mood-incongruent and bizarre delusions or hallucinations meant schizophrenia, not a mood disorder. In the DSM-III for the affective disorders, the diagnostician was asked to specify whether the psychotic features were mood-congruent or mood-incongruent. Also requested for the diagnosis of an affective disorder was a rule out of both the dominance of a "preoccupation with a mood-incongruent delusion or hallucination or bizarre behavior" when the affective syndrome was not present. In other words, an affective disorder could be diagnosed in the presence of mood-incongruent hallucinations or delusions such as persecutory delusions, thought insertion, thought broadcasting, and delusions of control and in the presence of "bizarre behavior," as long as these occurred during the affective syndrome. Despite this, the diagnosis of schizophrenia over a major affective disorder was typically dictated by the presence of "... a mood-incongruent delusion or hallucination ..." or "... bizarre behavior ..." whether an affective syndrome was present or not.

These additions to the DSM-III under mood disorders certainly overlap with criteria that were supposedly diagnostic of schizophrenia but there were no adjustments to the criteria for schizophrenia in light of this overlap.

10.10.2 The DSM-III-R (APA, DSM 1987)

The DSM-III-R was published in 1987 with "... its provision of diagnostic criteria to improve the reliability of diagnostic judgments." Schizophrenia remained largely unchanged from the DSM-III with five subtypes. However, one subtle change appeared to upgrade the diagnostic value of mood symptoms. Under diagnostic criterion A (3) for schizophrenia, hallucinations of a voice must not have content with any "... apparent relationship to depression or elation..." This necessity for mood incongruency for the diagnosis of schizophrenia would seem to indicate some movement toward diagnosing psychotic patients with mood symptoms as suffering from mood disorders in sharp opposition to the teachings of Bleuler and Schneider. In general, however, mental health professionals continued to diagnose functionally psychotic patients with schizophrenia. For example, in this same section, an auditory hallucination of "... a voice keeping up a running commentary on the person's behavior or thoughts, or two or more voices conversing with each other ..." warranted the diagnosis of schizophrenia as per Schneider's first-rank symptoms (Table 8.1). Schneider's first-rank symptoms usually trumped mood congruency of the auditory hallucination so that even if a first-rank symptom was mood-congruent, the diagnosis would likely be schizophrenia.

Under the DSM-III-R section titled "Mood Disorders," instead of "Affective Disorders," psychotic features could be either "mood-congruent or mood-incongruent ..." Persecutory delusions, thought insertion, and delusions of being controlled, as well as catatonic symptoms are given as potential features of psychotic mood disorders. These symptoms were previously and continue to be considered diagnostic of schizophrenia, not mood disorders. Thus, catatonia has continued as both a diagnostic symptom of schizophrenia and as a potential feature of psychotic mood disorders from the DSM-III-R even through the proposed DSM-5 due in 2013. For schizophrenia, catatonia is a diagnostic criterion and a major subtype until 2013; while for the mood disorders, catatonia is not used for the diagnosis but is a potential feature, thus accentuating the disease nonspecificity of the diagnostic criteria for schizophrenia (Chap. 12). Schizoaffective disorder remained in the section titled "Psychotic Disorders, Not Elsewhere Classified" and was not moved under the mood disorders.

10.11 Conclusions

The 1970s and 1980s were remarkable for the number of investigators from different sites, especially in the USA and the UK, who reported considerable overlap in symptoms and course between patients diagnosed with schizophrenia and psychotic mood disorders. The review by Pope and Lipinski (1978) was thorough and they, as others, essentially questioned the validity of schizophrenia as different than a psychotic mood disorder. Szasz (1976) discounted schizophrenia as a disease at all.

10.11 Conclusions

Bentall et al. (1988) appeared to agree. Crow (2010) has presented additional data to support his idea of a continuum between schizophrenia and mood disorders that he initially discussed in 1986 and 1990. This continuum theory has been widely embraced and implies a single disease, not two (Tables 3.1, 11.13; Figs. 3.1, 3.2, 11.3).

From 1980 and the publication of the DSM-III, the mood disorders were recognized to involve psychotic or "grossly bizarre behavior." The DSM-III-R (APA, DSM 1987) added the possible mood disorder features such as catatonia, mood-incongruent or persecutory delusions, thought insertion, and delusions of control. There have been no corresponding adjustments to the DSM sections on schizophrenia from the DSM-III through the proposed DSM-5 (APA, DSM 2013) to accommodate the overlapping additions to the mood disorders sections of symptoms supposedly diagnostic of schizophrenia but potentially present in psychotic mood disorders.

Even more remarkable has been the absence of substantial impact of these reports of similarities in symptoms upon academic psychiatry, textbooks of psychiatry and psychology, the mental health professions in general and therefore the public and the media. Despite the consistency of findings of no disease-specific diagnostic criteria for schizophrenia, Departments of Psychiatry via the DSMs have continued to teach students and residents that schizophrenia is defined by hallucinations, delusions, disorganization, catatonia, and a chronic deteriorating course and is distinct from psychotic mood disorders. This speaks to the remarkable impact of Kraepelin, Bleuler, and Schneider. The beliefs of these psychiatrists that schizophrenia was a bona fide illness separate from psychotic mood disorders overwhelmed the contradictory literature from BCE until about 1850 and from the 1970s and 1980s. Even though the preliminary publication of proposed changes for the DSM-5 recommends deletion of the subtypes of schizophrenia, schizophrenia and schizoaffective disorder continue to be recommended as bona fide diseases.

Chapter 11
Changing Concepts in the 1990s, 2000s, and 2010s: More Overlap and Similarities

> *Our findings do not fully support the present classification system, and suggest that its emphasis on hallucinations and delusions is overvalued. ... our analyses repeatedly yielded a single discriminate function, indicating that ... schizophrenics and affectives can be represented on a continuous distribution of clinical features representing a single underlying process.*
>
> (Taylor & Amir 1994)
>
> *In this study of more than 2 million Swedish families, we found evidence of a substantial genetic association between schizophrenia and bipolar disorder. ... These results challenge a nosological dichotomy between schizophrenia and bipolar disorder and are consistent with a reappraisal of these disorders as distinct diagnostic entities.*
>
> (Lichtenstein et al. 2009)
>
> *Several studies ... provide compelling evidence that genetic susceptibility and, by implication, elements of the underlying pathogenetic mechanisms are shared between bipolar disorder and schizophrenia. ... genome-wide association studies (GWAS) have demonstrated the existence of common DNA variants (single nucleotide polymorphisms) that influence risk of both schizophrenia and bipolar disorder.*
>
> (Craddock and Owen 2010b)

11.1 Introduction

In addition to more clinical reports of overlapping phenomenology, an expanding number of recent, comparative, basic science, and preclinical studies from various US and UK laboratories found surprising similarities between patients diagnosed with schizophrenia and bipolar disorder (Table 11.1). Over 150 studies from the 1990s and 2000s were reviewed that either compared some aspects of the two

Table 11.1 Summary of areas of overlap between schizophrenia and mood disorders

Area of study	See Table No.
Clinical studies: signs, symptoms, and course (from 1990s and 2000s)	11.2
Brain metabolic and neurochemical studies	11.3
Brain imaging studies	11.4
Epidemiological studies	11.5
Psychopharmacological studies	11.6
Heritability and family studies	11.7
Molecular genetic studies	11.8
Neurocognitive, selective attention, and insight studies	11.9
Studies supporting a continuum not a dichotomy	11.13

diagnoses and/or supported bipolar disorder as a bona fide disorder. Some of these comparative studies are summarized with selected authors' quotes in Tables 11.2, 11.3, 11.4, 11.5, 11.6, 11.7, 11.8, 11.9, and 11.13.

Table 11.2 addresses clinical overlap and similarities from publications in the 1990s and 2000s. Additional tables of quotes are divided into seven groups according to the type of basic science or preclinical study: (1) brain metabolic/neurochemical (Table 11.3), (2) brain imaging (Table 11.4), (3) epidemiological (Table 11.5), (4) psychopharmacological (Table 11.6), (5) heritability and family (Table 11.7), (6) molecular genetic studies (Table 11.8), and (7) neurocognitive, selective attention, and insight (Table 11.9). These areas of similarities and overlap are listed in Table 11.1. The selected quotes of conclusions from these tables are revealing in their consistency across a breadth of disciplines (Tables 11.3, 11.4, 11.5, 11.6, 11.7, 11.8, 11.9). If schizophrenia and psychotic mood disorders are in fact different, such overlap would not occur, even from selected studies.

Most suggestive of the present unitary hypothesis, that is, that schizophrenia represents the most severe cases on the severity continuum for psychotic bipolar disorders and is not a separate disease, are results from selected molecular genetic studies that indicate susceptibility overlap for psychosis in patients diagnosed with schizophrenia and psychotic bipolar disorders (Table 11.8) (Crow 1990a, b; Taylor and Amir 1994; Asherson et al. 1998; Cardno et al. 1999, 2002; Detera-Wadleigh et al. 1999; Berrettini 2000, 2001, 2003a, b; Valles et al. 2000; Blackwood et al. 2001; Maziade et al. 2001, 2005; Ujike et al. 2001; Badner and Gershon 2002; Bailer et al. 2002; Hattori et al. 2003; Potash et al. 2003; Hodgkinson et al. 2004; Macgregor et al. 2004; Park et al. 2004; Schumacher et al. 2004; Shifman et al. 2004; Craddock and Owen 2005; Craddock et al. 2005; Funke et al. 2005; Green et al. 2005; Hamshere et al. 2005; Schulze et al. 2005; Craddock and Owen 2010a, b).

Support for the idea of a continuum has grown, and quotes from studies are cited in Table 11.13. A continuum suggests one disorder with a broad spectrum of severity.

Table 11.2 Selected quotes from clinical studies showing overlap of signs and symptoms comparing schizophrenia and psychotic mood disorders from the 1990s and 2000s

Quote no.	Journal (year)	Author(s)	Field of study	Selected quotes of summary/conclusions	Results
1	J Clin Psychiatr (1990)	Pope et al.	Clinical symptoms	"This hypothesis would argue that on occasion a few individuals may display malignant forms of affective disorder that eventually pursue a chronic course, where affective symptoms become less prominent and where chronic psychotic symptoms, including bizarre delusions and auditory hallucinations, dominate the clinical picture. Such individuals will clearly meet DSM-III-R criteria for schizophrenia, but this diagnosis may be misleading. In particular, such patients, if presumed schizophrenic, might be less likely to receive a trial of agents effective in the treatment of affective disorders."	Overlap/similar
2	AGP (1990)	Tohen et al.	Clinical symptoms (course)	"During the 4-year follow-up, only 28% of the sample [of bipolar patients] remained in remission … the results suggest that … current treatment regiments have limited ability to prevent relapse in many bipolar patients."	Similar
3	AGP (1991)	Kendler	Review (symptoms, psychotic features)	"—Mood-incongruent psychotic affective illness is a distinct subtype of affective illness — diagnostic validators tend to support this the second (of four) viewpoints—"	Similar
4	Europe Psy (1992)	Brockington	Clinical symptoms	"It is important to loosen the grip which the concept of 'schizophrenia' has on the minds of psychiatrists. Schizophrenia is an idea whose very essence is equivocal, a nosological category without natural boundaries, a barren hypothesis."	Schizophrenia invalid
5	AJP (1992)	Post	Clinical symptoms (course)	"This formulation highlights the critical importance of early intervention in the illness [bipolar disorders] in order to prevent malignant transformation to rapid cycling, spontaneous episodes, and refractoriness to drug treatment" [possibly leading to a misdiagnosis of schizophrenia].	Similar

(continued)

Table 11.2 (continued)

Quote no.	Journal (year)	Author(s)	Field of study	Selected quotes of summary/conclusions	Results
6	AJP (1992)	Taylor	Review	"Future research should focus on factors that may reveal overlap between schizophrenia and affective disorder---".	Similar (continuum) /ambivalent
7	Can J Psychiatr (1994)	Lapierre	Review (symptoms and family history)	"---there is no compelling evidence to indicate a common pathophysiology for schizophrenia and bipolar disorder."	Different/dichotomy
8	Schizophrenia Bull (1995)	Harrow et al.	Clinical symptoms (psychotic features)	"The study results question the views of several major theorists on the importance, persistence, and prognostic significance of delusions in schizophrenia."	Similar (continuum /ambivalent
9	Psychiatr Ann (1996)	Dieperink and Sands	Review/symptoms (psychotic features)	"Psychosis is prevalent in bipolar disorder---. When differentiating from schizophrenia and schizoaffective disorder, presenting signs and symptoms are usually not helpful---".	Similar
10	Biol Psychiatr (2000)	Berrettini	Review (epidemiology, family and molecular genetics)	"Are Schizophrenic and Bipolar Disorders Related?..." [article title] "Schizophrenic and bipolar disorders are similar in several epidemiologic respects, including age at onset, lifetime risk, course of illness, worldwide distribution, risk for suicide, gender influence, and genetic susceptibility.... our nosology will require substantial revision during the next decade, to reflect this shared genetic susceptibility, as specific genes are identified."	Similar
11	J Affect Disord (2000)	Maj et al.	Clinical symptoms	"The Cohen's kappa was 0.22 for diagnosis of SAD, 0.71 for that of manic episode and 0.82 for that of major depressive episode.... The inter-rater reliability of the DSM-IV criteria for SAD is not satisfactory."	Schizoaffective Disorder invalid
12	BJP (2000)	Harrow et al.	Clinical symptoms/ outcome	"SAD outcome was better than SZ outcome and poorer than outcome for psychotic affective disorders.... The results could fit a symptom dimension view of SAD course."	Continuum/ ambivalent

13	Benabarre et al. *Eur Psychiatr* (2001)	Clinical symptoms/ epidemiology/ prognoses	"The results reaffirmed that, from the standpoints of demographics, clinical features and prognosis, SAD bipolar type can be classified as a phenotypic form at an intermediate point between bipolar I disorder and schizophrenia.... although cross-sectional symptoms were closer to the schizophrenia spectrum, the course of the illness resembled more that of bipolar patients, resulting in an intermediate outcome."	Continuum/ ambivalent
14	Pini et al. *AJP* (2001)	Insight	"Patients with schizophrenia … do not differ from patients with bipolar disorder …. The lack of significant differences [in insight] between patients with schizophrenia and patients with bipolar disorder was not a result of low statistical power."	Similar
15	Swartz *Psych Times* (2002a, b)	Clinical symptoms	"Apathetic major depression with catatonic features [catatonic depression], completely overlaps with schizophrenia and schizophreniform disorder [depending on duration]."	Similar
16	Gonzalez-Pinto et al. *Schiz Res* (2003)	Clinical symptoms	"These results confirm previous findings that FRSs are not specific to schizophrenia and suggest in addition that a dimension of nuclear psychotic experiences of developmental origin extends across categorically defined psychotic disorders."	Continuum
17	Kendell and Jablensky *AJP* (2003)	Review	"Diagnostic categories defined by their syndromes should be regarded as valid only if they have been shown to be discrete entities with natural boundaries that separate them from other disorders.... Unfortunately, once a diagnostic concept such as schizophrenia --- has come into general use, it tends to become reified. That is, people too easily assume that it is an entity of some kind that can be evoked to explain the patient's symptoms and whose validity need not be questioned."	Similar/overlap

(continued)

Table 11.2 (continued)

Quote no.	Journal (year)	Author(s)	Field of study	Selected quotes of summary/conclusions	Results
18	Psych News (2003)	Rosack	Editorial/review	"A common molecular pathway may lead to variations in dopamine dysfunction that manifests as either schizophrenia or bipolar disorder, tying the two disorders together as 'chemical cousins.'"	Similar
19	Acta Psych Scand (2004)	Jager et al.	Clinical symptoms and long-term outcome	"… With respect to the long-term outcome, ICD-10 SAD had a prognosis similar to that of affective disorders."	Similar/overlap
20	Medscape Psych Mental Health (2004)	Korn	Review	"Schizophrenia and Bipolar Disorder: An Evolving Interface" [article title] "---there is increasing evidence of connections between the two disorders; --- It is also becoming increasingly evident that there are many similarities. --- in family studies, genetic analysis, common symptoms complexes, psychopharmacologic responses, as well as other areas."	Similar
21	Schiz Res (2004)	Murray et al.	Review (cognitive)	"Finally, following the onset of illness, common factors are likely to underlie the deterioration in brain structure in cognitive and social function, which can occur in both illnesses" [SZ and BP].	Overlap/ambivalent
22	Encephale (2005)	Azorin et al.	Clinical symptoms/ review	"Current data tend to favor the ranging of the disorder within a unitary spectrum of functional psychosis the diathesis of which could be activated by an episode of mood disorder."	continuum/ ambivalent
23	Schiz Res (2005)	Hafner et al.	Review	"The high frequency of depressive symptoms at the prepsychotic prodromal stage and their increase and decrease with the psychotic episode suggests that depression in SZ might be the expression of an early, mild stage of the same neurobiological process that causes psychosis."	Similar/ambivalent
24	J Affect Disord (2005)	Nardi et al.	Clinical symptoms	"Schizobipolar disorder patients have demographic, clinical and therapeutic features similar to bipolar I patients and data support its definite inclusion in the bipolar spectrum group."	Schizoaffective disorder is bipolar

25	AJP (2006)	Fink and Taylor	Clinical symptoms	"Catatonia is more frequently associated with mania, melancholia and psychotic depression than it is with schizophrenia."	Overlap
26	Curr Psychiatr (2006a)	Lake and Hurwitz	Review	"Three disorders - schizophrenia, schizoaffective disorder and psychotic bipolar disorder - have been evoked to account for the variance in severity in psychotic patients, but psychotic bipolar disorder expresses the entire spectrum."	Similar/same
27	Curr Psychiatr (2006a)	Lake and Hurwitz	Clinical symptoms	"Evidence supports the idea that functional psychoses are predominately… if not entirely … caused by psychotic mood disorders."	Similar/same
28	Psychiatr Res (2006b)	Lake and Hurwitz	Review	"We conclude that the data overall are compatible with the hypothesis that a single disease, a mood disorder, with a broad spectrum of severity, rather than three different disorders, accounts for the functional psychoses."	Similar
29	Curr Opin Psychiatr (2006)	Maier et al.	Review	"….the validity of the diagnostic distinction between schizophrenia and bipolar disorder is increasingly challenged…. The diagnostic split between schizophrenia and bipolar disorder is unable to define distinct etiological and/or pathophysiological entities."	Similar/overlap
30	Manic-Depressive Illness (2007)	Goodwin and Jamison	Book	"It can be seen… that delusions were present in 12–66% of bipolar depressive episodes and in 44–96% of manic episodes."	Similar
31	Curr Opin Psychiatr (2007a)	Lake and Hurwitz	Review	"The concept of schizoaffective disorder promoted the coalescence of schizophrenia and bipolar eroding the Kraepelinian Dichotomy. A wide array of comparative data showing similarities and overlap led to the prediction of an end to the Kraepelinian Dichotomy, inviting the conclusion that a single disease (mood disorders) explains all the functional psychoses."	Similar/same

(continued)

Table 11.2 (continued)

Quote no.	Journal (year)	Author(s)	Field of study	Selected quotes of summary/conclusions	Results
32	*Neuropsych Disorder Treat* (2007b)	Lake and Hurwitz	Review	"Like the neuroses, there is stigma, confusion and misunderstanding about the condition called schizophrenia, resulting in substantial negative impact on bipolar patients misdiagnosed as having schizophrenia. The psychoses, including the schizophrenias, likely are explained by a single disease, psychotic bipolar disorder, that has demonstrated a wide spectrum of severity of symptoms and chronicity of course, not traditionally recognized."	Schizophrenia is a psychotic mood disorder
33	*Psychotic Depression* (2007)	Swartz and Shorter	Book	"There is a whole concept of major psychiatric illness as a single disease process, suggesting that schizophrenia might be the chronic untreated form of psychotic depression and of psychotic mixed manic-depressive states." (pg 19)	Similar/same
34	*Schiz Bull* (2008a)	Lake	Review	"Comparative clinical and recent molecular genetic data find phenotypic and genotypic commonalities lending support to the idea that paranoid schizophrenia is the same disorder as psychotic bipolar. Mania explains paranoia when grandiose delusions that one's possessions are so valuable that others will kill for them. Similarly, depression explains paranoia when delusional guilt convinces patients they deserve punishment."	Similar/same
35	*Schiz Bull* (2008b)	Lake	Review	"The zone of rarity between schizophrenia and psychotic mood disorders is blurred because severe disorders of mood are also disorders of thought. This relationship calls into question the tenet that schizophrenia is a disease separate from psychotic mood disorders."	Similar/same

36	*Eup Arch Psych Clin Neurosci* (2008)	Muller and Schwarz	Psychoneuroimmunology	"In recent years, not only new research in the fields of psychopathology and clinical outcome, but also findings of biological markers in the areas of neurophysiology, neuroendocrinology, psychoneuroimmunology, genetics or psychopharmacology show a big overlap between both groups of disorders.... By means of findings from the field of psychoneuroimmunology and inflammation it will be shown that different pathological mechanisms in depression and schizophrenia may lead to the same final common pathway of information.... the Kraepelinian dichotomy still has a significant value from a biologic-psychiatric point of view."	Schizophrenia and depression are different; Kraepelinian dichotomy supported
37	*Encephale* (2009)	Demily et al.	Review	"... symptoms associated with the diagnosis of schizophrenia can be associated with psychotic mood disorders: hallucinations and delusions (50%) disorganized speech and behavior (all patients with moderate to severe mania or mixed episode), negative symptoms (all patients with moderate to severe depression). The social and job dysfunction may be due to disturbances in the volitional system in patients with schizophrenia or severe bipolar disorder.... In this way, it has been suggested that psychotic symptoms may be distributed along a continuum that extends from schizophrenia to psychotic mood disorders with increasing level of severity.... Likewise, common factors can explain cognitive and social disorders in psychosis."	Continuum
38	*Neuropsychopharmacology* (2009)	Fischer and Carpenter	Opinion: Kraepelinian dichotomy	"... the boundary between the two major psychoses [schizophrenia and psychotic mood disorders] is porous. Hallucinations, delusions, and disordered thoughts are observed in both.... The most robust symptomatic distinctions between schizophrenia and non-schizophrenia psychotic diagnostic classes were restricted affect, poor rapport and poor insight."	Schizophrenia and psychotic mood disorders different; recommend two separate syndromes

(continued)

Table 11.2 (continued)

Quote no.	Journal (year)	Author(s)	Field of study	Selected quotes of summary/conclusions	Results
39	*Psychiatr Ann* (2010a)	Lake	Editorial/review	"The validity of schizophrenia and schizoaffective disorder are questioned on the basis of the non-specificity of their diagnostic criteria noted in the literature since the 1970's."	Schizophrenia and schizoaffective disorder invalid
40	*Psychiatr Ann* (2010b)	Lake	Review	"… it may be time to consider retiring the historic diagnosis of schizophrenia, as occurred with the neuroses [in 1980]. The concept put forward in this work, if accurate, is of discipline-altering impact."	Schizophrenia the same as a psychotic mood disorder
41	*Psychiatr Ann* (2010c)	Lake	Review	"Because there are established endophenotypic [clinical, genetic, cognitive] differences between psychotic and non-psychotic mood disordered patients, the 'dichotomy' may be between psychotic and non-psychotic mood disordered patients and not schizophrenia."	Schizophrenia is a psychotic mood disorder
42	*Psychiatr Ann* (2010)	Post	Clinical symptoms/review	"Patients with otherwise classic courses of bipolar illness, with discrete episodes and well intervals can, never the less, look indistinguishable from those with schizophrenia during an acute manic psychosis. …They [psychotic manic patients] were extremely disorganized and psychotic…. Auditory and visual hallucinations would often also be present. Extremely regressed behavior, such as smearing or eating feces, occurred…. Many patients with bipolar illness go through a progressively deteriorating course of incomplete symptom resolution between episodes and acquire a dysthymic interval between episodes of increasing severity, often accompanied by increasing degrees of cognitive dysfunction."	Similar
43	*Psychiatr Ann* (2010)	Swartz	Clinical symptoms/review	"The standard of clinical practice makes it too easy to diagnose schizophrenia when psychotic depression should apply. … The drama of psychosis can hide depression… Over diagnosing schizophrenia is a defensive action not just for the psychiatrist, but for the institution and its administration… [because] diagnosing schizophrenia lowers the bar of expectations completely…. tardive psychosis classified as schizophrenia is reliably caused by antipsychotic drugs."	Schizophrenia similar to psychotic depression

11.2 Additional Reviews of Clinical Overlap and Similarities

Several authors in the 1990s and 2000s continued to add their observations of overlap and similarities in clinical presentations and course between patients diagnosed with schizophrenia and those with psychotic mood disorders (Kendler 1991; Brockington 1992; Post 1992, 2010; Taylor 1992; Harrow et al. 1995; Dieperink and Sands 1996; Berrettini 2000; Swartz 2002a, b; Gonzalez-Pinto et al. 2003; Kendell and Jablensky 2003; Rosack 2003; Korn 2004; Murray et al. 2004; Azorin et al. 2005; Hafner et al. 2005; Nardi et al. 2005; Fink and Taylor 2006; Lake and Hurwitz 2006a, b; Maier et al. 2006; Goodwin and Jamison 2007; Lake and Hurwitz 2007a, b; Swartz and Shorter 2007; Lake 2008a, b; Lake 2010a, b). Most reviews (Kendler 1991; Taylor 1992; Taylor and Amir 1994; Dieperink and Sands 1996; Berrettini 2000; Swartz 2002a, b; Kendell and Jablensky 2003; Moller 2003; Rosack 2003; Korn 2004; Murray et al. 2004; Azorin et al. 2005; Hafner et al. 2005; Lake and Hurwitz 2006a, b; Maier et al. 2006; Lake and Hurwitz 2006a, b; Swartz and Shorter 2007; Lake 2008a, b; Craddock and Owen 2010a, b; Lake 2010a, b) concluded that there is substantial overlap and similarities, but at least two reviews (Lapierre 1994; Fischer and Carpenter 2009) said that schizophrenia is a disease separate from bipolar disorder. Some reviews were ambivalent (Harrow et al. 1995; Ketter et al. 2004; Murray et al. 2004; Azorin et al. 2005).

Long-term observations of classic bipolar patients published during the 1990s and 2000s substantiated earlier reports in revealing that hallucinations, delusions, disorganization, and catatonia are common in severe mood disorders (Tohen et al. 1990; Kendler 1991; Dieperink and Sands 1996; Pini et al. 2001; Swartz 2002a, b; Gonzalez-Pinto et al. 2003; Hafner et al. 2005; Nardi et al. 2005; Fink and Taylor 2006; Goodwin and Jamison 2007; Lake and Hurwitz 2007a, b; Swartz and Shorter 2007; Lake 2008b). Further and most critical, some of these long-term follow-up studies of classic cycling bipolar patients showed the potential for deterioration into a chronic, downhill, noncycling, treatment-resistant, dysfunctional state (Pope et al. 1990; Pope and Yurgelun-Todd 1990; Tohen et al. 1990; Post 1992, 2010; Harrow et al. 1995; Goodwin and Jamison 2007). Such a course has mistakenly been considered pathognomonic of schizophrenia.

The occurrence of psychosis and chronicity in mood-disordered patients essentially eliminates any specificity to the DSM diagnostic criteria for schizophrenia, raising the question of its validity.

11.3 Overlap and Similarities from Basic Science and Preclinical Studies Comparing Schizophrenia and Mood Disorders

The following subheadings summarize selected comparative studies grouped according to the area of research: (1) brain metabolic/neurochemical, (2) brain imagining, (3) epidemiological, (4) psychopharmacological, (5) family and

Table 11.3 Selected brain metabolic and neurochemical studies comparing schizophrenia and psychotic mood disorders

Quote no.	Journal (year)	Author(s)	Field of study	Selected quotes of summary/conclusions	Results
1	Neuropsychopharmacology (1989)	Cohen et al.	Brain metabolic	"Evidence for Common Alterations in Cerebral Glucose Metabolism in Major Affective Disorders and Schizophrenia." [article title] "Regional glucose metabolic rates -- measured in affectively disordered patients during the performance of auditory discrimination -- are similar to those previously observed in schizophrenia."	Similar
2	AJP (1995)	Pearlson et al.	Neurochem	"--like schizophrenic patients, patients with psychotic bipolar disorder have elevations of D2 dopamine receptor B-max values---. Elevations in dopamine receptor values thus may occur in psychiatric states that are characterized by psychotic symptoms rather than being specific to schizophrenia."	Similar/overlap
3	BJP (1996)	al-Mousawi et al.	Brain metabolic	"Abnormal patterns of metabolism could be determined in decreasing order, in schizophrenia, mania and depression."	Continuum
4	Brain Res Bull (2001)	Knable et al. (from the Stanley Foundation)	Neurochem/brain metabolic	"Schizophrenia was associated with the largest number of abnormalities, many of which are also present in bipolar disorder."	Similar/overlap
5	Neuropsychopharmacology (2002)	McCullum-Smith and Meador-Woodruff	Brain metabolic/neurochem	"These results [decreased expression of excitatory amino acid transporters 3 and 4 transcripts in the striatum] --extend the body of evidence implicating abnormal glutamatergic neurotransmission in schizophrenia and mood disorders."	Similar/overlap
6	PNAS (2003)	Koh et al.	Neurochem	"The present study supports the hypothesis that schizophrenia and bipolar disorder may be associated with abnormalities in dopamine receptor-interacting proteins."	Similar
7	The Lancet (2003)	Tkachev et al.	Neurochem	"Our study also showed similar expression changes to the schizophrenia group in bipolar brains.... The high degree of correlation between the expression changes in schizophrenia and bipolar disorder provide compelling evidence for common pathophysiological pathways that may govern the disease phenotypes of schizophrenia and bipolar affective disorder."	Similar

| 8 | *AGP* (2004) | Woo et al. | Neurochem | "The density of gamma-aminobutyric acid interneurons that express the NMDA NR(2A)SUBUNIT appears to be decreased in SZ and BP." | Similar/ overlap |
| 9 | *Neuropsycho-pharmacology* (2006) | Marx et al. | Neurochem | "A number of neuroactive steroids act at an inhibitory $GABA_A$ and excitatory NMDA receptors and demonstrate neuroprotective and neurotrophic effects. Neuroactive steroids may therefore be candidate modulators of the pathophysiology of schizophrenia and bipolar disorder, and relevant to the treatment of these disorders." | Similar |

heritability, (6) molecular genetics, and (7) neurocognitive, selective attention, and insight (Table 11.1).

11.3.1 Brain Metabolic and Neurochemical Studies

As early as 1989, Cohen et al. (1989) found similarities in cerebral glucose metabolism across patients diagnosed with schizophrenia and major mood disorders (Table 11.3). Elevations of D_2 dopamine receptor values did not distinguish between psychotic bipolar patients and those diagnosed with schizophrenia, supporting the contention of differences between psychotic and nonpsychotic bipolar patients and overlap and unity across psychotic bipolar and schizophrenia (Pearlson et al. 1995). Commonalities of abnormal patterns of brain metabolism and neurochemistry occurred across patients diagnosed with schizophrenia, mania, and depression with decreasing abnormalities from schizophrenia to mood disorders (al-Mousawi et al. 1996; Knable et al. 2001; McCullum-Smith and Meador-Woodruff 2002; Tkachev et al. 2003; Koh et al. 2003; Woo et al. 2004). Marx et al. (2006) implicated neuroactive steroids as modulators of the pathophysiology of both schizophrenia and bipolar disorder.

11.3.2 Brain Imagining Studies

Patients diagnosed with schizophrenia were initially contrasted to nonpsychiatric control groups, and significant abnormalities in those diagnosed with schizophrenia were reported, giving support to the Kraepelinian dichotomy and the validity of schizophrenia. In the late 1990s, research began to compare groups diagnosed with schizophrenia versus bipolar disorders, and reports of differences were found (Pearlson et al. 1997; Hirayasu et al. 1998; Altshuler et al. 2000). Other laboratories reported some similar structural abnormalities in temporal horn volume (Roy et al. 1998), thalamic abnormalities (Dasari et al. 1999), small left hippocampal volumes (Velakoulis et al. 1999), and other asymmetries (Bilder et al. 1999). Other structural brain abnormalities, especially involving the basal ganglia and white matter were similar between patients diagnosed with bipolar disorder and schizophrenia, while abnormalities involving gray matter appeared to differ (Osuji and Cullum 2005; Borkowska and Rybakowski 2001; Sweeney et al. 2000; Chambers and Perrone-Bizzozero 2004) (Table 11.4).

Certainly other studies, not reviewed here, have found differences, but some of the differences reported might be explained by the misdiagnosis of psychotic mood patients with schizophrenia and the existence of brain structural differences between psychotic and nonpsychotic mood-disordered patients. Mood disorders vary widely in severity and chronicity which might account for structural brain differences among patients with mood disorders.

Table 11.4 Selected brain imagining studies comparing schizophrenia and psychotic mood disorders

Quote no.	Journal (year)	Author(s)	Field of study	Selected quotes of summary/conclusions	Results
1	Biol Psychiatr (1997)	Pearlson et al.	Imaging	"Schizophrenic but not bipolar patients had an alteration of normal posterior superior temporal gyrus asymmetry. ---left anterior STG and right amygdala were smaller than predicted in schizophrenia but not bipolar disorder. Left amygdala was smaller and right anterior STG larger in bipolar disorder but not schizophrenia."	Different/supports a dichotomy
2	AJP (1998)	Hirayasu et al.	Imaging	"Both the patients with schizophrenia and those with affective psychosis had significant left-less-than-right asymmetry of the posterior amygdala-hippocampal complex. These findings suggest that temporal lobe abnormalities are present ---for schizophrenia and that low volume of the left posterior superior temporal gyrus gray matter is specific to schizophrenia compared with affective disorder."	Different/supports a dichotomy/ambivalent
3	Biol Psychiatr (1998)	Roy et al.	Imaging	"Temporal Horn Enlargement is Present in Schizophrenia and Bipolar Disorder" [article title]; "... this structural abnormality [increased temporal horn volume] does not differentiate the structural neuropathology of schizophrenia from that of bipolar disorder."	Similar
4	Int J Psychophys (1999)	Bilder et al.	Imaging	"These asymmetries.... all showed the same diagnostic group effect.... The findings state a 'continuum' rather than a 'diagnostic specificity' hypothesis, and suggest that reduction of normal hemispheric asymmetries may mark a neurodevelopment factor for major mental illnesses...."	similar/continuum
5	Psych Res (1999)	Dasari et al.	Imaging	"... thalamic abnormalities reported in adult schizophrenic and bipolar patients are also observed in adolescent patients. Our findings also add to the evidence implicating the thalamus in the pathophysiology of schizophrenia and bipolar disorder."	Similar
6	AGP (1999)	Velakoulis et al.	Imaging	"---the finding of smaller left hippocampal volume in patients with first-episode schizophrenia and affective psychosis does not support the prediction that smaller hippocampi are specific to schizophrenia."	Similar/overlap
7	Biol Psychiatr (2000)	Altshuler et al.	Imaging	"The results suggest differences in affected limbic structures in patients with schizophrenia and bipolar disorder."	Different/supports a dichotomy

11.3.3 Epidemiological Studies

Early epidemiological data indicating schizophrenia and bipolar disorder "breed true" were one of the strongest supports of the two diseases model, but more recent data have discounted the "breed true" results (Lichtenstein et al. 2009) (Sect. 11.3.5). Other epidemiological literature raised questions about the validity of schizophrenia from the 1980s and before (Sect. 9.6). Examples are early cross-cultural comparisons of the prevalence of the diagnoses of schizophrenia and bipolar disorder between the USA and the UK showing substantial differences (Kramer 1961; Kramer et al. 1969; Cooper et al. 1972; Edwards 1972; Pope and Lipinski 1978). Other studies in the USA over time also revealed marked differences in the percent of psychotic patients diagnosed with schizophrenia (Hoch and Rachlin 1941; Kuriansky et al. 1974; Pope and Lipinski 1978). The titles of two more recent articles are additional examples: "Where Have All the Catatonics Gone?" (Mahendra 1981) and "Is Schizophrenia Disappearing?" (Der et al. 1990). Stoll et al. (1993) reported a threefold decrease in the diagnosis of schizophrenia between 1976 and 1989 that was parallel to a fourfold increase in diagnoses of major mood disorders (Fig. 3.2). These data can be interpreted as a shift away from the concept that psychosis equals schizophrenia and toward the recognition that mood-disordered patients suffer psychotic symptoms. Extrapolated further, these data suggest that the diagnosis of schizophrenia is a misdiagnosis of a psychotic mood disorder (Figs. 3.1 and 3.2) (Table 11.5).

Core epidemiological characteristics are strikingly similar between bipolar and schizophrenic disorders, suggesting a consideration that they are a single disease. For example, both are common, chronic, lifelong illnesses affecting approximately 1% (for psychotic bipolar) of the population worldwide. Average age of onset of both are typically from late adolescence to early adulthood. Onset occurs less frequently in prepubertal children or after the age of 50. According to Berrettini (2003a, b), both, "… have similar age-at-onset distributions. … [Both] describe psychotic disorders that often assume episodic courses of illness (with partial to complete remissions and clear exacerbations)." The sexes are equally affected and the risk for suicide in both disorders is reported to be substantial. Both respond to some of the atypical antipsychotic drugs (Tohen et al. 2003). Substantial familial aggregation for both disorders in the families of patients with schizophrenia and bipolar disorder has been demonstrated (Lichtenstein et al. 2009). Molecular linkage studies found overlapping susceptibility at several gene sites (Berrettini 2003a, b; Craddock and Owen 2005, 2010a, b).

Such overlap in epidemiological characteristics points to a single disease. Since the DSM and the ICD diagnostic criteria for schizophrenia are consistent between the USA and the UK and have not changed significantly in the USA since the DSM-III (1980), such variability in the prevalence of the diagnosis of schizophrenia both between the USA and the UK and within the USA suggests doubt as to the validity of schizophrenia.

11.3 Overlap and Similarities from Basic Science...

Table 11.5 Selected epidemiological studies comparing schizophrenia and psychotic mood disorders

Quote no.	Journal (year)	Author(s)	Field of study	Selected quotes of summary/conclusions	Results
1	Psychol Med (1981)	Mahendra	Epidemiology	"Where Have All The Catatonics Gone?" [article title]	Compatible
2	The Lancet (1990)	Der et al.	Epidemiology	"Is Schizophrenia Disappearing?" [article title]	Compatible
3	AJP (1993)	Stoll et al.	Epidemiology (shifts in diagnostic frequencies)	"Schizophrenia diagnoses decreased from a peak of 27% in 1976 to 9% in 1989 (a threefold decrease), and diagnoses of major affective disorders rose from a low of 10% in 1972 to 44% in 1990 (a fourfold increase).—Although a real decrease in new cases of schizophrenia may have occurred, this effect was probably minor and dominated by a larger shift of such diagnoses to affective categories."	Compatible
4	Biol Psychiatr (2000)	Berrettini	Review (epidemiology, family and molecular genetics)	"Are Schizophrenic and Bipolar Disorders Related? ..." [article title]; "Schizophrenic and bipolar disorders are similar in several epidemiologic respects, including age at onset, lifetime risk, course of illness, worldwide distribution, risk for suicide, gender influence, and genetic susceptibility... our nosology will require substantial revision during the next decade, to reflect this shared genetic susceptibility, as specific genes are identified."	Schizophrenia and bipolar similar
5	NeuroMolecular Med (2004)	Berrettini	Epidemiology	"BPD and SZ share common multiple epidemiological characteristics, consistent with the hypothesis that the two groups share some risk factors [and] ... some genetic susceptibility."	Schizophrenia and bipolar similar

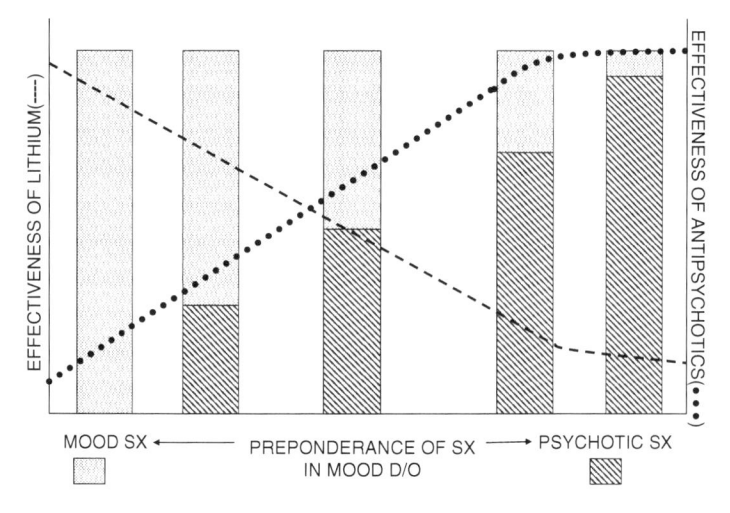

Fig. 11.1 Bipolar responsivity to lithium and antipsychotics along two axes

The ineffectiveness of lithium in severely psychotic patients (mis)diagnosed with schizophrenia may be better understood when bipolar symptom severity is viewed as occurring along two axes: one for psychotic symptoms and the other for mood symptoms. Lithium stabilizes mood but is not an antipsychotic so the beneficial effects of lithium in bipolar disorders are most obvious in classic (nonpsychotic) bipolar patients with a preponderance of mood symptoms that are not obscured by psychotic symptoms. Lithium should seem less effective or ineffective acutely in psychotic bipolar patients whose psychotic symptoms overwhelm their mood symptoms, possibly explaining the reported ineffectiveness of lithium in patients (mis)diagnosed with schizophrenia but who really have psychotic mania or depression. The typical antipsychotic drugs are effective antipsychotics but less effective or ineffective in stabilizing mood and are most useful at the severe end of the psychosis severity axis, that is, in psychotic bipolar patients traditionally called "schizophrenic," intermediate in "schizoaffective" (mood disorders with a moderate degree of psychotic features) and least effective in classic, nonpsychotic mood disorders

11.3.4 Psychopharmacological Studies

The documented differences in therapeutic responsivity to lithium versus the typical antipsychotics between patients diagnosed with schizophrenia versus bipolar disorders have been cited as evidence for two separate diseases. Although most studies reported that lithium is ineffective in patients diagnosed with schizophrenia, there are data that suggest that lithium is effective in schizophrenia (Gershon and Yuwiler 1960; Prien et al. 1972; Small et al. 1975; Wagemaker et al. 1985; Atre-Vaidya and

Taylor 1989). However, the apparent ineffectiveness of lithium in severely psychotic patients (mis)diagnosed with schizophrenia may be better understood when bipolar symptom severity is viewed as occurring along two axes: one for psychotic symptoms and the other for mood symptoms (Fig. 11.1). Lithium stabilizes mood but is not an antipsychotic, so the beneficial effects of lithium in bipolar disorders are most obvious in classic (nonpsychotic) bipolar patients with a preponderance of mood symptoms that are not obscured by psychotic symptoms. Lithium should seem less effective or ineffective acutely in psychotic bipolar patients whose psychotic symptoms overwhelm their mood symptoms, possibly explaining the reported ineffectiveness of lithium in patients (mis)diagnosed with schizophrenia but who really have psychotic mania or depression. The effectiveness of lithium in "schizoaffective disorder," considered here as a moderately psychotic mood disorder, is, as expected, intermediate between its benefits in nonpsychotic mood disorders and schizophrenia (Prien et al. 1972; Pope and Lipinski 1978; Procci 1976; Wagemaker et al. 1985; Korn 2004), but at least one study reported a worsening of symptoms by lithium in schizoaffective disorder (Johnson 1970). These data invite the hypothesis that the lithium-resistant patients diagnosed with schizophrenia may actually suffer from psychotic mood disorders (Atre-Vaidya and Taylor 1989). A few recent studies find valproate (Depakote), an established mood stabilizer, to be an effective adjuvant in patients diagnosed with schizophrenia (Citrome et al. 2000; Casey et al. 2003; Ketter et al. 2004), suggesting the patients might actually suffer from psychotic bipolar disorder (Table 11.6).

The typical neuroleptics are effective antipsychotics but less effective or ineffective in stabilizing mood and are most useful at the severe end of the psychosis severity axis, that is, in psychotic bipolar patients, traditionally called "schizophrenic," intermediate in "schizoaffective" (mood disorders with a moderate degree of psychotic features) and least effective in classic, nonpsychotic mood disorders (Fig. 11.1). When the effectiveness of lithium and the typical antipsychotics in bipolar disorder is considered as occurring along psychosis and mood symptom spectra, the pharmacological responses are compatible with a single disease.

Some evidence suggests that the atypicals are effective in both schizophrenia and bipolar disorders both with and without psychotic features (Yatham 2003; Mason 2004; Tohen et al. 2004), a point in favor of only one disorder (Moller 2003; Korn 2004; Ketter et al. 2004). Further support for unity are some similar neurotransmitters implicated as abnormal in patients with either diagnosis such as dopamine, norepinephrine, serotonin, and gamma-aminobutyric acid; both disorders are similarly aggravated by stimulants (Moller 2003).

Table 11.6 Selected psychopharmacological studies comparing schizophrenia and psychotic mood disorders

Quote no.	Journal (year)	Author(s)	Field of study	Selected quotes of summary/conclusions	Results
1	J Neuropsycho (1960)	Gershon and Yuwiler	Psychopharmacology	"In acute schizophrenic excitements, ---, lithium administration results in control of the psychomotor over-activity and behavioral disturbances and in addition often produces complete disappearance of all symptoms."	Overlap
2	AGP (1972)	Prien et al.	Psychopharmacology	"---both treatments (lithium and chlorpromazine (Thorazine)) showed a significant reduction in affective and schizophrenic behavior. The possibility that lithium carbonate may have neuroleptic properties is considered---".	Similar
3	S Med J (1985)	Wagemaker et al.	Psychopharmacology	"Responders to lithium treatment are found in all three diagnostic categories [schizophrenia, schizoaffective and bipolar disorders]."	Similar/ overlap
4	J Clin Psychiatr (1989)	Altre-Vaidya and Taylor	Psychopharmacology	"---as affectively ill patients and some schizophrenics respond to the same biological treatments [lithium]; diagnostic criteria need further refinement or the two disorders share a common pathophysiology."	Similar/ overlap
5	Psychiatr Serv (2000)	Citrome et al.	Psychopharmacology	"The adjunctive use of valproate nearly tripled from 1994 to 1998 among patients with a diagnosis of schizophrenia. --- Controlled clinical trials are needed to examine the adjunctive use of mood stabilizers, in particular valproate, among patients with schizophrenia."	Similar
6	Neuropsychopharmacology (2003)	Casey et al.	Psychopharmacology	"Treatment with divalproex in combination with an atypical antipsychotic agent resulted in earlier improvements in a range of psychotic symptoms among acutely hospitalized patients with schizophrenia."	Similar
7	J Clin Psychopharmacol (2003)	Yatham	Psychopharmacology	"The results of several clinical trials suggest that atypical antipsychotics --- are effective for the treatment of acute mania, and open label studies suggest that atypical antipsychotics may have long-term mood-stabilizing effects."	Similar

8	*BJP* (2004)	Tohen et al.	Psychopharmacology	"Patients taking olanzapine added to lithium or valproate experienced sustained symptomatic remission, but not syndromic remission, for longer than those receiving lithium or valproate monotherapy."	Similar
9	*Ann Clin Psychiatr* (2004)	Masan	Psychopharmacology	"This review focuses on risperidone, olanzapine, quetiapine, and ziprasidone and provides evidence that these drugs demonstrate activity against manic episodes of bipolar disorder when used as adjunctive therapy and possibly as monotherapy ---."	Similar
10	*J Affect Disord* (2004)	Baethge et al.	Psychopharmacology	"The results of the study show that lithium and carbamazepine appear to be highly effective in treating patients with SAD [schizoaffective disorder]."	Similar/overlap

11.3.5 Family and Heritability Studies

For decades the Kraepelinian dichotomy and thus the validity of schizophrenia was supported by heritability studies indicating that schizophrenia and bipolar disorders "breed true" (Tsuang et al. 1980; Kendler et al. 1993), although some families were reported in which there were cases of both schizophrenia and bipolar disorder (Pope and Yurgelun-Todd 1990). First-degree relatives of patients diagnosed with schizophrenia did have an increased incidence of schizophrenia and bipolar and unipolar disorders (Gershon et al. 1988; Maier et al. 1993); this seemed to be true for psychotic mood disorders among relatives of probands diagnosed with schizophrenia (Kendler et al. 1993). Probands with schizoaffective disorder had an increased incidence of schizophrenia and bipolar and unipolar disorders in their offspring (Rice et al. 1987). However, as recently as 2000, Berrettini (2000) summarized the heritability literature by saying, "Despite numerous carefully conducted investigations, no family study of schizophrenia reports increased risk for bipolar disorders among first-degree relatives of schizophrenia probands; however, the first-degree relatives of schizophrenia probands and the first-degree relatives of bipolar disorder probands are at increased risk for schizoaffective disorder and recurrent unipolar depression disorders." More recent data contradict this statement having reported an increase of bipolar-disordered patients in families with schizophrenia, as well as the converse (see below) (Table 11.7).

The study by Cardno et al. (2002) is recent and rigorously controlled. Results of their studies of 77 monozygotic and 89 same-sex dizygotic twin pairs indicated "significant genetic correlations" between these two diagnoses. The authors concluded that,

> Heritability estimates for schizophrenia, schizoaffective disorder, and mania are substantial and similar.

These studies by Cardno et al. (1999, 2002) and Valles et al. (2000) support the common conclusion that psychosis is inherited in support of only one disorder. The Maudsley triplets are another early example since they were genetically identical and two had a lifetime diagnosis of schizophrenia, while the third, a lifetime diagnosis of bipolar disorder (McGuffin et al. 1982).

The idea that it is psychosis that is inherited irrespective of which diagnosis the patients are given is increasingly supported (Crow 1990a, b; Kendler et al. 1993, 1998; Taylor and Amir 1994; Cardno et al. 1999, 2002; Valles et al. 2000; Schurhoff et al. 2003). For example, Valles et al. (2000) demonstrated that relatives of probands with psychotic, but not nonpsychotic, bipolar disorder have an increased risk of schizophrenia. They also showed the converse, that is, relatives of probands with schizophrenia have an increased risk of psychotic, but not nonpsychotic, bipolar disorder. They concluded that psychosis may be a nonspecific indicator of illness severity and is certainly not disease-specific for schizophrenia. More specifically, paranoid delusions seem to be inherited across diagnoses. Schurhoff et al. (2003) said that,

> Delusional proneness appears to be an inherited predisposition common to both Schizophrenia and Bipolar Disorder.

11.3 Overlap and Similarities from Basic Science... 209

Table 11.7 Selected heritability and family studies comparing schizophrenia and psychotic mood disorders

Quote no.	Journal (year)	Author(s)	Field of study	Selected quotes of summary/conclusions	Results
1	J Clin Psychiatr (1990)	Pope and Yurgelun-Todd	Genetic (heritability)	"… the authors encountered two pedigrees in which schizophrenic individuals had first-degree relatives with bipolar disorder… This hypothesis would argue that on occasion a few individuals may display malignant forms of affective disorder that eventually pursue a chronic course where affective symptoms become less prominent and where chronic psychotic symptoms, including bizarre illusions and auditory hallucinations, dominate the clinical picture. Such individuals will clearly meet DSM-III-R criteria for schizophrenia, but this diagnosis may be misleading. In particular, such patients, if presumed schizophrenic, might be less likely to receive a trial of agents effective in the treatment of affective disorders."	Overlap
2	AGP (1993)	Kendler et al. (the Roscommon family study)	Genetic (heritability)	"The familial liability to schizophrenia predisposes to psychosis, and especially mood-incongruent psychosis, when affectively ill. ---these results do not support the hypothesis that, ---schizophrenia and affective illness are on a single etiologic continuum."	Different/ambivalent
3	AGP (1993)	Maier et al.	Genetic (heritability)	"The schizophrenic and bipolar disorders were transmitted independently ---. These data suggest that there could be a familial relationship between the predispositions to schizophrenia and to major depression."	Ambivalent
4	AGP (1998)	Kendler et al. (the Roscommon family study)	Genetic (heritability)	"The familial vulnerability to psychosis extends across several syndromes, being most pronounced in those with schizophrenia-like symptoms. The familial vulnerability to depressive and manic affective illness is somewhat more specific."	Continuum
5	AGP (1999)	Cardno et al.	Genetic (heritability)	"Heritability estimates for schizophrenia, schizoaffective disorder, and mania were substantial and similar."	Similar

(continued)

Table 11.7 (continued)

Quote no.	Journal (year)	Author(s)	Field of study	Selected quotes of summary/conclusions	Results
6	*Schiz Res* (2000)	Valles et al.	Genetic (heritability)	"Our results suggest that the transmission of psychosis is not disorder-specific. Bipolar illness characterized by a high familial loading is associated with increased risk of schizophrenia in the relatives.... at the severest extreme of the affective spectrum, an overlap exists between familial liability to schizophrenia and bipolar disorder. This may be indicative of a degree of correlated liability and/or a continuum of severity between bipolar illness and schizophrenia."	Similar/ overlap
7	*AJP* (2002)	Cardno et al.	Genetic (heritability)/twin study	"… there is a degree of overlap in the genes contributing to RDC schizophrenic, schizoaffective and manic syndromes."	Similar
8	*Schiz Res* (2002)	Maier et al.	Genetic (heritability)	"Thus, our findings support the hypothesis that psychotic, as well as affective disorders, aggregate in families of individuals with schizophrenia."	Similar/ overlap
9	*J Affect Disord* (2003)	Kelsoe	Genetic (heritability)	"—the same genes may predispose to a variety of phenotypes ranging from schizoaffective disorder to cyclothymic temperament."	Similar (continuum) / ambivalent
10	*AJP* (2003)	Schurhoff et al.	Genetic (heritability)	"Delusional proneness appears to be an inherited predisposition common to both schizophrenia and bipolar disorder."	Similar/ overlap
11	*AGP* (2005)	Laursen et al.	Genetic (heritability)	"We found that the risk of SAD was equally strongly associated with SZ and BP among first-degree relatives."	Continuum/ ambivalent
12	*Arch Gen Psychiatr* (2009)	Van Snellenberg et al.	Heritability	"This meta-analysis provides direct evidence for familial coaggregation of schizophrenia and BD, a finding that argues against the view that these disorders are entirely discrete diagnostic entities. Rather, a continuum model is supported"	Similar/ overlap/ continuum
13	*Lancet* (2009)	Lichtenstein et al.	Genetic heritability	"In this study of more than 2 million Swedish families, we found evidence of a substantial genetic association between schizophrenia and bipolar disorder. … These results challenge nosological dichotomy between schizophrenia and bipolar disorder and are consistent with a reappraisal of these disorders as distinct diagnostic entities."	Similar/overlap

Schulze et al. (2005) concurred that,

> These data suggest that bipolar affective disorder with persecutory delusions… overlaps with schizophrenia. The genetic overlap… hints at a weakness of specificity of the current classification systems,…

The above data suggest at least a partial overlap in familial susceptibility for bipolar and schizophrenia disorders. More recent data from the largest family study of the two disorders ever conducted have convincingly dismissed the long-held idea that schizophrenia and bipolar disorders "breed true" (Lichtenstein et al. 2009). About 40,000 probands with two hospitalizations for schizophrenia and another 40,000 patients with two hospitalizations for bipolar disorder were studied in Sweden. Lichtenstein et al. (2009) found an increased incidence of both illnesses in family members of either type of proband.

That patients diagnosed with schizophrenia "breed" psychotic bipolar and the converse invites the suggestion that these conditions could be one and the same. It is the propensity for psychosis that is heritable in mood-disordered patients. That schizophrenia and psychotic bipolar disorder crossbreed destroys a cornerstone support for the Kraepelinian dichotomy and the validity of schizophrenia as a separate disorder. Given the duplicity of the diagnostic criteria between psychotic bipolar and schizophrenia, assuming psychotic mood in place of "schizophrenia" may be reasonable and fulfills the tenant of Ockham's razor (Fig. 11.2).

11.3.6 Molecular Genetic Studies

Molecular genetic studies compel the consideration of only one disease, not two (Table 11.8). Examples are results from genetic linkage studies showing overlap reviewed recently by Craddock et al. (2005, 2006), Craddock and Owen (2005, 2010a, b), Hamshere et al. (2005), Berrettini (2000, 2001, 2003), and Park et al. (2004). In a recent review, Craddock and Owen (2010a) summarize the comparative genetic literature showing overlap under the headings of (1) family studies, (2) twin studies, (3) linkage studies of schizophrenia and bipolar disorder, (4) genome-wide association studies, and (5) linkage and association studies of schizoaffective disorder. Crow (2007) concisely explained linkage studies as,

> The search for linkage is the attempt to locate predisposing genes by identifying sites (polymorphisms) in the genome at which sequence variations (alleles) travel with illness within families that have more than one affected member. It is thus a method of locating a disease-inducing gene at a specific site on a particular chromosome.

For example, systematic, whole-genome linkage studies of patients diagnosed with schizophrenia and bipolar disorder show several chromosomal regions with sequence variations in common which is consistent with shared susceptibility genes. Direct molecular genetic support for a substantial genetic overlap between the two disorders derive from recent large-scale genome-wide association studies in which thousands of individuals diagnosed with schizophrenia and bipolar disorders

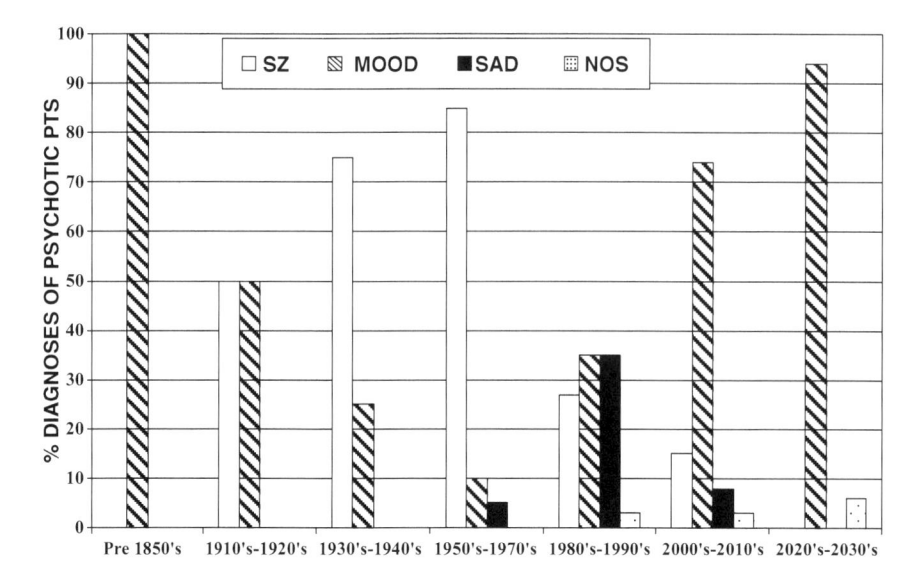

Fig. 11.2 Estimated diagnoses of functionally psychotic patients over 2000 years

Abbreviations: SZ schizophrenia, SAD schizoaffective disorder, BP bipolar disorder, MOOD psychotic mood disorder, NOS psychosis not otherwise specified (for the purpose of this graph, NOS includes unrecognized organic causes)

Before the 1850s, manic-depressive insanity was the only disease still today considered to be functional that was diagnosed in psychotic patients cycling from depressions to manias and back. There were other diseases considered functional such as "general paresis of the insane" but which organic causes have been determined. There was no dementia praecox or schizophrenia until the latter half of the nineteenth century.

By the 1910s and 1920s, the influences of Kraepelin and Bleuler caused the rapid increase in the diagnosis of schizophrenia over manic-depressive insanity in psychotic patients so that their ratio was approximately 50/50.

By the 1930s and 1940s, schizophrenia may have been diagnosed in 75% of functionally psychotic patients versus 25% for manic-depressive insanity.

By the 1950s through the 1970s, the frequency of the diagnosis of schizophrenia had increased even further to approximately 85% compared to 10% for manic-depressive insanity. Schizoaffective disorder had begun its impressive increase.

In the 1980s and 1990s, schizoaffective disorder became very popular, possibly topping both schizophrenia and bipolar disorder in the diagnosis of psychotic patients. Psychosis Not Otherwise Specified may have comprised a small percentage of psychotic patients' diagnoses.

By the 2000s and 2010s, psychotic bipolar disorders are even more recognized and schizophrenia along with schizoaffective disorder diagnoses decreased toward zero. A continuation of this trend suggests a ratio similar to the pre-1850s with psychotic mood disorders accounting for the vast majority of functionally psychotic patients.

By 2020, schizophrenia and schizoaffective disorder may have been eliminated, and about 94% of functionally psychotic patients will be diagnosed with a psychotic mood disorder. About 6% may be diagnosed with a psychotic disorder NOS while organic causes and mood symptoms are sought.

have been studied for hundreds of thousands of common DNA variance (single-nucleotide polymorphisms) spread across the genome (Craddock and Owen 2005, 2010a, b). These studies demonstrate common DNA variance that increases the risk of diagnoses of both schizophrenia and bipolar disorders. Examples of specific risk loci include ZNF804A and CACNA1C. Thus Craddock and colleagues concluded that,

> ... there is evidence for overlap in the identity of genes showing gene-wide association signals in genome-wide association studies of schizophrenia and bipolar disorder. Perhaps more compellingly, there is strong evidence that the aggregate polygenic contribution of many alleles of small effect to susceptibility for schizophrenia also influences susceptibility to bipolar disorders.
>
> (Moskvina et al. 2009; The International Schizophrenia Consortium 2009)

At least one rare but specific genetic translocation between chromosomes 1 and 11 from a large Scottish family study is reported to increase the risk of psychiatric disorders including schizophrenia, bipolar disorder, major depressive disorder, and alcohol abuse (Blackwood et al. 2001).

Although there remain several susceptibility loci reported to be unique to either schizophrenia or bipolar disorder, increasing focus on psychotic bipolar disorder has revealed increasing similarities and overlap. Some reports of loci said to be unique to schizophrenia may be flawed. Research focused initially on patients diagnosed with schizophrenia compared with controls, not psychotic bipolar patients. Susceptibility genes identified from patients diagnosed with schizophrenia but not from controls were assumed to be unique to schizophrenia, but with subsequent research on psychotic bipolar patients, overlap and similarities have emerged (Berrettini 2000, 2001, 2003a, b; Park et al. 2004; Craddock et al. 2005; Hamshere et al. 2005). Specific examples of this phenomenon are (1) the D-amino acid oxidase activator [DAOA/(G72)/G30] on chromosome 13q22-34 that was initially linked to schizophrenia (Chumakov et al. 2002) but subsequently found by at least five independent studies to be linked to bipolar disorders (Badner and Gershon 2002; Hattori et al. 2003; Schumacher et al. 2004; Craddock et al. 2005; Green et al. 2005) and (2) the DISC-1 locus at 1q42 that was perhaps prematurely named "Disrupted In Schizophrenia-1" since it was first associated with patients diagnosed with schizophrenia without testing bipolar patients (Millar et al. 2000; Devon et al. 2002). Similarly to the DAOA/G30 site, more recent data from several labs suggest linkage of DISC-1 to bipolar and schizoaffective pedigrees (Millar et al. 2000; Blackwood et al. 2001; Hodgkinson et al. 2004; Macgregor et al. 2004; Hamshere et al. 2005).

Another interpretation of such results of exclusivity (other than there are two diseases) invokes the idea that it is psychosis (or no psychosis) that is heritable in mood-disordered patients as indicated by the data noted above (Crow 1990a, b; Cardno et al. 1999, 2002; Valles et al. 2000; Schurhoff et al. 2003; Ketter et al. 2004; Schulze et al. 2005). Loci isolated in psychotic bipolar patients (potentially misdiagnosed with schizophrenia) may be absent in nonpsychotic bipolar patients and such data misinterpreted as indicative of two disorders.

Table 11.8 Selected molecular genetic studies comparing schizophrenia and psychotic mood disorders

Quote no.	Journal (year)	Author(s)	Field of study	Selected quotes of summary/conclusions	Results
1	*Mol Psychiatr* (1998)	Asherson et al.	Review (molecular genetics)	In summary: "It is therefore possible that a broad phenotype including unipolar depression, bipolar disorder, schizoaffective disorder and schizophrenia when accompanied by significant affective symptoms can result from mutations within a gene in this region" [chromosome 4p]. "The dopamine D5 receptor gene lies within the region identified by the linkage studies and is therefore a major candidate for the putative disease gene."	Similar/overlap
2	*PNAS* (1999)	Detera-Wadliegh et al.	Review (molecular genetics)	"By comprehensive screening of the entire genome, we ... gained evidence for the overlap of susceptibility regions for bipolar disorder and schizophrenia."	Similar/overlap
3	*Bipolar Disord* (2001)	Berrettini	Review (molecular genetics)	"Two of these regions [18p11 and 22q11] (implicated repeatedly in bipolar disorders) are also implicated in genome scans of schizophrenia, suggesting that these two distinct nosological categories may share some genetic susceptibility."	Similar
4	*Am J Hum Genetics* (2001)	Blackwood et al.	Review (molecular genetics)	"The results of karyotypic, clinical and ERP investigations of this family suggest that the recently described genes DISC1 and DISC2, which are directly disrupted by the breakpoint on chromosome 1, may have a role in the development of a disease phenotype that includes schizophrenia as well as unipolar and bipolar affective disorders."	Similar/overlap
5	*Nature* (2001)	Maziade et al.	Review (molecular genetics)	"Our results suggest that both specific and common susceptibility loci must be searched for in SZ and BP."	Similar/overlap
6	*Psychiatr Res* (2001)	Ujike et al.	Review (molecular genetics)	"There were no significant differences in the CAG repeat number of longer or shorter alleles among the four diagnostic groups---."	Similar
7	*Mol Psychiatr* (2002)	Badner and Gershon	Genetics (molecular)	"We found the strongest evidence for susceptibility loci on 13q and 22q for bipolar disorder, and on --- 13q and 22q for schizophrenia."	Similar/overlap
8	*Biological Psychiatr* (2002)	Bailer et al.	Molecular genetics	"We detected a potential susceptibility locus for bipolar disorder and schizophrenia on chromosome 3q. .... Our data suggests shared loci for schizophrenia and bipolar affective disorders and are consistent with the continuum model of psychosis."	Similar/overlap/continuum

11.3 Overlap and Similarities from Basic Science... 215

9	*Am J Med Genetics* (2003a)	Berrettini	Review (molecular genetics)	"... there are five genomic regions for which evidence suggests shared genetic susceptibility of BPD and SZ.... Family and linkage studies are consistent with the concept that SZ and BPD share some genetic susceptibility. Multiple regions of the genome, including 18p11, 13q32, 22q11, 10p14, and 8p22, represent areas with potential BPD/SZ shared genetic susceptibility."	Similar
10	*World Psychiatr* (2003b)	Berrettini	Molecular genetics	"Family and linkage studies are consistent with the concept that SZ and BPD share some genetic susceptibility. Multiple regions of the genome, including 18p11, 13q32, 22q11, 10p14 and 8p22, represent areas with potential BPD/SZ shared genetic susceptibility.... it will be necessary to develop a new, genetically based nosology, in which this overlap is accurately represented."	Similar/overlap
11	*Am J Hum Genetics* (2003)	Hattori et al.	Molecular genetics	"Taken together with the earlier report, this is the first demonstration of a novel gene(s) (G72/G30 genes), --- independently associated with both bipolar illness and schizophrenia."	Similar/overlap
12	*AJP* (2003)	Potash et al.	Molecular genetics	"--- 10 families with psychotic bipolar disorder demonstrate suggestive linkage to two chromosomal regions, 13q31 and 22q12, which are in or near regions previously implicated in both bipolar disorder and schizophrenia. --- these overlapping phenotypes may be most closely associated with the putative susceptibility loci."	Similar/overlap
13	*Am J Hum Genetics* (2004)	Hodgkinson et al.	Molecular genetics	"Multiple haplotypes contained within four haplotype blocks extending between exon 1 and exon 9 are associated with schizophrenia, schizoaffective disorder, and bipolar disorder. These data support the idea that these apparently distinct disorders have at least a partially convergent etiology and that variation at the DISC1 locus predisposes individuals to a variety of psychiatric disorders."	Similar/overlap
14	*Mol Psychiatr* (2004)	Macgregor et al.	Molecular genetics	"These results, together with results from a number of other recent studies, stress the importance of the 1q42 region in susceptibility to both BPAD and SCZ."	Similar/overlap

(continued)

Table 11.8 (continued)

Quote no.	Author(s)	Journal (year)	Field of study	Selected quotes of summary/conclusions	Results
15	Mansour et al.	Genes Brain Behav (2004)	Molecular genetics	"Modest associations with SNPs at ARNTL (BmaL1) and TIMELESS genes were observed in the BP 1 samples.... Associations with TIMELESS and PERIOD3 were also detected in the Pittsburg SZ/SAD group."	Overlap
16	Park et al.	Mol Psychiatr (2004)	Molecular genetics	"Our results suggest that BP in conjunction with psychosis is a potentially useful phenotype that may: ... cast light on the genetic relationship between BP and schizophrenia."	Similar/overlap
17	Schumacher et al.	Mol Psychiatr (2004)	Molecular genetics	"The association of variation at G72 with schizophrenia as well as BPAD provides molecular support for the hypothesis that these two major psychiatric disorders share some of their etiologic background."	Similar/overlap
18	Shifman et al.	Am J Med Genet B Neuropsych Genet (2004)	Molecular genetics	"We suggest that polymorphisms in the COMT gene may influence susceptibility to both diseases [bipolar and schizophrenia] ...."	Similar/overlap
19	Craddock et al.	J Med Genetics (2005)	Review (molecular genetics)	"Increasing evidence suggests an overlap in genetic susceptibility across the traditional classification system that dichotomized psychotic disorders into schizophrenia or bipolar disorder, most notably with findings at DAOA(G72), DISC1, and NRG1.—we can expect that over the coming years molecular genetics will catalyze a re-appraisal of psychiatric nosology as well as providing a path to understanding the pathophysiology." [of bipolar and schizophrenia].	Similar
20	Fawcett	AJP (2005)	Editorial	"... of the [eleven] chromosome loci found for the transmission of schizophrenia and bipolar disorder, eight have been found to overlap ...."	Similar
21	Funke et al.	Behav Brain Funct (2005)	Molecular genetics	"Our results support the view that COMT variation provides a weak genetic predisposition to neuropsychiatric disease including psychotic [schizophrenic] and affective disorders."	Similar/overlap
22	Green et al.	AGP (2005)	Molecular genetics	"Our findings suggest that neuregulin 1 plays a role in influencing susceptibility to bipolar disorder and schizophrenia and that it may exert a specific effect in the subset of functional psychosis that has manic and mood-incongruent psychotic features."	Similar/overlap

11.3 Overlap and Similarities from Basic Science...

23	*AGP* (2005)	Hamshere et al.	Molecular genetics	"Our linkage findings strongly support the existence of loci that influence susceptibility across the functional psychosis spectrum. The DISC1 gene lies within 2.5 mega bases of our peak marker on chromosome 1q42 and has been previously implicated in schizophrenia, bipolar disorder, and, recently, schizoaffective disorder."	Similar/overlap
24	*Mol Psychiatr* (2005)	Kohn and Lerer	Molecular genetics	"Taking a topographic approach, we identify five loci of positive findings on chromosome 6q and suggest that each may harbor gene(s) that confer susceptibility to SZ or BP or may modify their onset or clinical course."	Similar/overlap
25	*Mol Psychiatr* (2005)	Maziade et al.	Molecular genetics	"— our data support the following trends: (i) results from several genome scans of SZ and BP in different populations tend to converge in specific genomic regions and (ii) some of these susceptibility regions may be shared by SZ and BP, whereas others may be specific to each. The present results support the relevance of investigating concurrently SZ and BP within the same study and have implications for the modeling of genetic effects."	Similar/overlap
26	*Am J Hum Genet* (2005)	McQueen et al.	Molecular genetics	"Our results establish genome-wide significance to BP on chromosomes 6q and 8g, which provides solid information to guide future gene-finding efforts that rely on fine-mapping and association approaches."	Similar
27	*AJP* (2005)	Schulze et al.	Molecular genetics	"These data suggest that bipolar affective disorder with persecutory delusions ... overlaps with schizophrenia. The genetic overlap between schizophrenia and bipolar affective disorder hints at a weakness of specificity of the current classification systems, which are based merely on clinical symptoms."	Similar/overlap
28	*Schiz Bull* (2006)	Craddock et al.	Molecular genetics	"In particular, the pattern of findings emerging from genetic studies shows increasing evidence for an overlap in genetic susceptibility across the traditional classification categories - including association findings at *DAOA (G72)*, *DTNBP1 (dysbindin)*, *COMT*, *BDNF*, *DISC1*, and *NRG1*. The emerging evidence suggests the possibility of relatively specific relationships between genotype and psychopathology. For example, *DISC1* and *NRG1* may confer susceptibility to a form of illness with mixed features of schizophrenia and mania...."	Similar/overlap

(continued)

Table 11.8 (continued)

Quote no.	Journal (year)	Author(s)	Field of study	Selected quotes of summary/conclusions	Results
29	AGP (2006)	Williams et al.	Review (molecular genetics)	"We found a similar pattern of association in bipolar cases and in schizophrenia cases in which individuals had experienced major mood disorder.... our results imply that variation at the DAOA/G30 locus influences susceptibility to episodes of mood disorder across the traditional bipolar and schizophrenia categories."	Similar/overlap
30	World Psychiatr (2007)	Craddock and Owen	Molecular genetics	"Recent molecular genetic findings have demonstrated very clearly the inadequacies of the dichotomous view, and highlighted the importance of better classifying cases with both psychotic and affective symptoms. ... If psychiatry is to translate the opportunities offered by new research methodologies, we must move in a classificatory approach that is worthy of the 21st century."	Similar/overlap
31	AJP (2007)	Crow	Review (molecular genetics)	"Epigenetic variation associated with chromosomal rearrangements that occurred in the hominid lineage and that relates to the evolution of language could account for predisposition to SZ and SAD and BP and failure to detect such variation by standard linkage approaches."	Continuum/similar/overlap
32	AJP (2007)	Goes et al.	Molecular genetics	"The 13q21-33 finding supports prior evidence of bipolar disorder/schizophrenia overlap in this region, while the 2p11-q14 findings is, in the authors' knowledge, the first to suggest that this schizophrenia linkage region might also harbor a bipolar disorder susceptibility gene."	Similar/overlap
33	Schiz Bull (2007)	Owen et al.	Molecular genetics	"However, recent findings emerging from genetic studies show increasing evidence for an overlap in genetic susceptibility across the traditional binary classification of psychosis [the Kraepelinian Dichotomy]. Moreover, the emerging evidence suggests the possibility of relatively specific relationships between genotype and psychopathology. For example, variation in Disrupted in Schizophrenia I (DISCI) and Neuregulin 1 (NRGI) may confer susceptibility to a form of illness with mixed features of schizophrenia and mania. ... It is important to note that this widely held notion [Kraepelinian Dichotomy] is incorrect."	Similar/overlap

11.3 Overlap and Similarities from Basic Science... 219

34	*Schiz Bull* (2009)	Craddock et al.	Molecular genetics	"We conclude that if psychiatry is to translate the opportunities offered by new research methodologies. we must finally abandon a 19th-century dichotomy and move to a classificatory approach that is worthy of the 21st century."	Similar/overlap
35	*Hum Genetics* (2009)	O'Donovan et al.	Molecular genetics	"The ZNF804A and CACNA1C loci appear to influence risk for both disorders, a finding that supports the hypothesis that schizophrenia and BD are not etiologically distinct. In the case of schizophrenia, a number of rare copy number variants have also been detected that have fairly large effect sizes on disease risk, and that additionally influence risk of autism, mental retardation and other neurodevelopmental disorders. The existing findings point to some likely pathophysiological mechanisms but also challenge current concepts of disease classification."	Similar/overlap
36	*Psychiatr Ann* (2010a)	Craddock and Owen	Molecular genetics	"Several studies published in the past decade (particularly in the past five years) provide compelling evidence that genetic susceptibility, and by implication, some elements of the underlying pathogenetic mechanisms, are shared between bipolar disorder (BD) and schizophrenia. ... specific risk loci, [include] ZNF804A ... and CACNA1C ..."	Similar/overlap
37	*BJP* (2010b)	Craddock and Owen	Molecular genetics	"Several studies ... provide compelling evidence that genetic susceptibility and, by implication, elements of the underlying pathogenetic mechanisms are shared between bipolar disorder and schizophrenia. ... genome-wide association studies (GWAS) have demonstrated the existence of common DNA variants (single nucleotide polymorphisms) that influence risk of both schizophrenia and bipolar disorder."	Similar/overlap

11.3.7 Neurocognitive, Selective Attention, and Insight Studies

Initial studies of cognitive function compared patients diagnosed with schizophrenia to normal controls, and positive findings appeared to imply that schizophrenia is a bona fide entity (Toulopoulou et al. 2007) (Table 11.9). When psychotic manic and depressed patients were subsequently studied with regard to their cognitive functions, milder but quantitatively similar defects were reported, supporting the idea of endophenotypic similarities (Table 11.9; Chap. 13) (Rund et al. 1992; Sweeney et al. 2000; Borkowska and Rybakowski 2001; Kerr et al. 2003; Schretlen et al. 2007; Hurwitz and Aires 2010). The data of Osuji and Cullum (2005) showed that cognitive defects in bipolar patients directly correlated with the severity of the condition, that is, greater defects with early onset, more episodes and chronicity of the mood disorder. Quraishi and Frangou (2002) reported that although bipolar patients in remission outperformed patients diagnosed with schizophrenia on most cognitive measures, this difference disappeared when the bipolar patients were acutely symptomatic. Like schizophrenia, Bipolar-I patients showed moderate to severe impairments on tests of episodic memory, specific executive functions, and attentional and processing speed tasks (Glahn et al. 2007). Traditionally considered indicative of schizophrenia, a significant proportion of bipolar patients failed to regain premorbid levels of functioning even after the resolution of major affective symptoms, with neuropsychological impairment persisting even during euthymia (Suwalska et al. 2001; Zubieta et al. 2001; Martinez-Aran et al. 2004a, b; Robinson and Ferrier 2006).

Hurwitz and Aires (2010) recently reviewed evoked response potential studies from patients diagnosed with schizophrenia and bipolar disorders. Such subclinical abnormalities have been referred to as endophenotypes and include P50 gating and P300 amplitude measurements. "Endophenotypes are least common in the normal population, more common in clinically normal subjects with psychiatrically ill relatives, and most common in the mentally ill" (Hurwitz and Aires 2010). They said that such studies were initially conducted in patients diagnosed with schizophrenia. Such results supported the validity of schizophrenia and the dichotomy. However, Hurwitz and Aires (2010) reported that subsequent research on patients with psychotic bipolar disorders demonstrated similar abnormalities. They concluded that "This argues for a single disease with a broad spectrum of severity."

Premorbid impairment in visual spatial reasoning was similar in patients subsequently diagnosed with bipolar disorder or schizophrenia (Oltmanns 1978; Rund et al. 1992; Sereno and Holzman 1996; Addington and Addington 1997; van Os et al. 1997; Politis et al. 2004; Olincy and Martin 2005; Tiihonen et al. 2005). Abnormalities in memory increased the chances of psychosis in general, leading to diagnoses of both bipolar disorder and schizophrenia (McIntosh et al. 2005). Rund et al. (1992) found "… no differences between the two patient sub-groups [bipolar and schizophrenia]…" with regard to the neurocognitive tests they used. Attentional performance and insight were similar across diagnoses (Pini et al. 2001). These data can be interpreted to indicate that the spectrum of severity of cognitive defects can be explained by mood disorders alone.

Table 11.9 Selected cognitive function, selective attention, and insight studies comparing schizophrenia and psychotic mood disorders

Quote no.	Journal (year)	Author(s)	Field of study	Selected quotes of summary/conclusions	Results
Cognitive function					
1	Acta Psych Scand (1992)	Rund et al.	Cognitive function	"There were no differences [in vigilance defects] between the two patient subgroups [BP and SZ], either on the number of correct hits [on the CPT] or on commission errors [SAT]. Neither CPT nor SAT deficit, thus, seem to be specific schizophrenic characteristics."	Similar
2	AGP (1997)	Van Os et al.	Cognitive function	"The findings give credence to the suggestion that affective disorder, especially its early-onset form, is preceded by impaired neurodevelopment."	Similar
3	Biol Psychiatr (2000)	Sweeney et al.	Cognitive function	"Neuropsychological findings ... indicate widely distributed deficits in cognitive domains subserved by temporal, parietal, and frontostriatal systems in bipolar patients during mixed/manic states of illness."	Similar
4	Bipolar Disord (2001)	Borkowska and Rybakowski	Cognitive function	"A higher degree of cognitive dysfunction connected with frontal lobe activity during an acute depressive episode was found in bipolar comparative with unipolar depressed patients. These results may corroborate other findings pointing to ... some similarities between bipolar illness and schizophrenia."	Similar/overlap
5	Psychiatr Poland (2001)	Suwalska et al.	Cognitive function	"... patients with bipolar disorder do not make full recovery between episodes of illness and the neuropsychological dysfunction may persist beyond these episodes. ... the results of the patients with affective disorders with psychotic features were comparable with those of schizophrenics. Recent studies point to an association between decreased prefrontal cortex volume and cognitive disturbances. Attention is focused on hippocampus volume as well, since it is associated with cognitive defects in bipolar."	Similar
6	Psychiatr Res (2001)	Zubieta et al.	Cognitive function	"BP patients ... demonstrate reductions in specific cognitive domains [verbal learning, executive functioning and motor coordination] even after prolonged asymptomatic phases. Scores on tests of executive functioning were negatively correlated with the number of episodes of mania and depression. Some of these deficits appear to be associated with a more severe course of illness and poorer social and occupational functioning."	Similar/overlap
7	J Affect Disord (2002)	Quraishi and Frangou	Cognitive function	"Remitted bipolar disorder patients out-perform stable schizophrenics on most cognitive measures but this advantage disappeared when they were acutely symptomatic. Symptomatic bipolar disorder patients have widespread cognitive abnormalities. Trait related deficits appear to be present in verbal memory and sustained attention. Executive function and visual memory may be also affected at least in some recovered bipolar disorder patients."	Similar

(continued)

Table 11.9 (continued)

Quote no.	Journal (year)	Author(s)	Field of study	Selected quotes of summary/conclusions	Results
8	J Affect Disord (2003)	Kerr et al.	Cognitive function	"Bipolar affective disorder patients often show cognitive deficits that are similar to those found in schizophrenia patients. Theory of mind defects are found in currently symptomic bipolar patients. These findings add to a growing evidence that common mechanisms may contribute to bipolar affective disorder and schizophrenia."	Similar
9	Neurochem Res (2004)	Chambers and Perrone-Bizzozero	Cognitive/neurodevelopmental	"Female subjects with SZ and BP exhibited decreased myelination in the hippocampal formation. … Our results demonstrate an interaction between gender, mental illness, and myelination, and may be related to cognitive defects seen in SZ and BP."	Similar/overlap
10	AJP (2004a)	Martinez-Aran et al.	Cognitive function	"A poor performance was observed in all bipolar groups regarding executive function and verbal memory in relation to the healthy comparison subjects. These cognitive difficulties, especially related to verbal memory, may help explain the impairment regarding daily functioning, even during remission."	Similar/overlap
11	Bipolar Disord (2004b)	Martinez-Aran et al.	Cognitive function	"Results provide evidence of neuropsychological impairment in euthymic bipolar patients, … suggesting verbal memory and executive dysfunctions. Cognitive impairment seems to be related to a worse clinical course and poor functional outcome."	similar/overlap
12	BJP (2005)	McIntosh et al.	Cognitive/neurodevelopmental	"Abnormalities of memory appear to be related to an increased liability to psychosis in general."	Overlap/ambivalent
13	Psych Clinics of North Am (2005)	Osuji and Cullum	Cognitive function	"Bipolar disorder is often associated with cognitive defects that tend to be present regardless of mood state. Greater impairment tends to be seen in BP patients who are older, have an early onset of the disease, and suffer a more severe course of illness. … cognitive defects are present early in patients with BP disorder and may be cumulative, showing an association with the number of episodes [particularly depressed] over time. Cognitive defects in BP disorder may share some common characteristics with those seen in patients with SZ, although the latter tend to show much greater and generalized cognitive impairment. … deficits in executive function, episodic memory, sustained concentration, and, to a lesser extent, visio spatial skills seem to be the most consistent areas of impairment in BP disorder. Just as neuroimaging anomalies have been well documented in BP disorder, structural brain abnormalities have been noted in BP disorder, most commonly involving the basal ganglia or white matter. Specific comparisons of cerebral atrophy and ventricular size between patients with SZ and BP have not been definitive, …"	Similar/ambivalent
14	AJP (2005)	Tiihonen et al.	Cognitive function	"These results indicate that premorbid visual spatial reasoning is impaired in bipolar disorder and schizophrenia … This suggests that a subtle neurodevelopmental aberration is involved in the etiology of bipolar disorder and schizophrenia."	Similar

15	*Bipolar Disord* (2006)	Robinson and Ferrier	Review/cognitive function	"… a large proportion of [BP] patients failed to regain premorbid levels of functioning after the resolution of major affective symptoms. … BP patients exhibit neuropsychological impairment that persists even during the euthymic state, which may be a contributory factor to poor psychosocial outcome."	Similar
16	*Biol Psychiatr* (2007, Epub)	Glahn et al.	Cognitive function	"Bipolar I patients overall showed moderate impairments on tests of episodic memory and specific executive measures …. and moderate to severe defects on attentional and processing speed tasks. … Bipolar I patients with a history of psychosis were impaired on measures of executive functioning and spatial working memory compared with bipolar patients without history of psychosis. Defects in attention, psychomotor speed and memory appear to be part of the broader disease phenotype in patients with bipolar disorder."	Similar
17	*Biol Psychiatr* (2007)	Schretlen et al.	Cognitive function	"Patients with bipolar disorder suffer from cognitive defects that are milder but qualitatively similar to those of patients with schizophrenia. These findings support the notion that schizophrenia and bipolar disorder show greater phenotypic similarity in terms of the nature than severity of their neuropsychological defects."	Similar
18	*Psychiatr Ann* (2010)	Hurwitz and Aires	Evoked response potential	"The most replicated ERP findings in schizophrenia research were subsequently sought and found in psychotic bipolar disorder. P50 gating was first described in schizophrenia and subsequently demonstrated in psychotic bipolar disorder. … This argues for a single disease with a broad spectrum of severity."	Similar
Selective attention and insight					
1	*J Abnormal Psychology* (1978)	Oltmanns	Selective attention	"… distraction interferes with schizophrenics' and manics' information processing [similarly]…; problems in selective attention seems to be more closely related to thought disorder than to diagnostic categories."	Similar
2	*Schiz Res* (1996)	Sereno and Holzman	Selective attention	"The somewhat similar pattern of behavior of schizophrenic and affective disorder subjects suggests that abnormal spatial selective attentional processes may not be specific to schizophrenia."	Similar
3	*Schiz Res* (1997)	Addington and Addington	Selective attention	"There were no differences [in visual attention] between the schizophrenic and the bipolar subjects."	Similar
4	*AJP* (2001)	Pini et al	Insight	"Patients with schizophrenia …. do not differ from patients with bipolar disorder. … The lack of significant differences [in insight] between patients with schizophrenia and patients with bipolar disorder was not a result of low statistical power."	Similar
5	*Compreh Psychiatr* (2004)	Politis et al.	Selective attention	"No significant differences were found on attentional performance between the psychotic depressed patients and those with schizophrenic disorder."	Similar
6	*AJP* (2005)	Olincy and Martin	Auditory evoked potential	"This defect [diminished suppression of the P50 auditory evoked potential] may represent a common psychological mechanism associated with the vulnerability to psychosis in people with bipolar illness as well as in people with schizophrenia."	Similar

11.4 Overlap and Similarities Between Schizophrenia and Mood Disorders in the DSM from the DSM-IV (APA, DSM 1994) Through the DSM-5 (APA, DSM Proposed 2013)

Prior to the DSM-IV (APA, DSM 1994), all four prior editions of the DSM made clear that manic-depressive reactions, affective disorders, or mood disorders could be marked with psychotic features including hallucinations and delusions. Despite this redundancy with the diagnostic criteria for schizophrenia, the severity of psychosis and chronicity of course continued to be used to justify the diagnosis of schizophrenia. Such redundancy between "diagnostic" symptoms of schizophrenia and potential features of mood disorders continued with the DSM-IV published in 1994 and the DSM-IV-TR published in 2000 (Table 11.10). Another major confounding overlap was the addition of course chronicity to the mood disorders with the DSM-IV (Table 2.4). Recognition that mood disorders could be psychotic and chronic would seem to have eliminated the two major differentiating features of schizophrenia and raised concern about its validity. Many, if not most, functionally psychotic patients do have symptoms of a mood disturbance that may be either obscured by flagrant psychotic symptoms, subtle or overlooked due to the misconception that psychosis means schizophrenia (Chap. 12).

11.4.1 The DSM-IV (APA, DSM 1994)

The DSM-IV published in 1994 stated that, "One of the most important features [of the DSM-IV] ... is its provision of diagnostic criteria to improve the reliability of diagnostic judgments." The "characteristic symptoms" diagnostic of schizophrenia changed very little from the DSM-III-R to the DSM-IV. Disorganized speech and behavior were added to replace "incoherence or marked loosening of associations." Also added was the term "negative symptoms, i.e., affective flattening, alogia or avolition." These modified "flat or grossly inappropriate affect" from the DSM-III-R. More attention to Schneider's first-rank symptoms was given since "... only one Criterion A Symptom is required instead of two if delusions are bizarre or hallucinations consisted of a voice keeping up a running commentary on the person's behavior or thoughts, or two or more voices conversing with each other." Otherwise, the DSM-IV required at least two of the criterion A "characteristic symptoms" for the diagnosis of schizophrenia (Table 2.5). Social/occupational dysfunction, duration, and subtypes remained largely unchanged in the DSM-IV from the DSM-III-R. Bizarre delusions of schizophrenia were redundant with the potential psychotic feature of bizarre delusions in the DSM chapter on "Mood Disorders." The "negative symptoms" of schizophrenia were redundant with the symptoms of severe depression.

The Mood Disorders were divided into three parts in the DSM-IV: (1) mood episodes, (2) mood disorders, and (3) specifiers (Table 2.4). The "chronic specifier" was indicated when major mood symptoms were "... met continuously for at least the past two years." The "severity/psychotic ... specifier" allowed the mood disorders

11.4 Overlap and Similarities Between Schizophrenia... 225

Table 11.10 Overlap and similarities in the DSM-IV-TR (2000) diagnostic criteria between schizophrenia and psychotic mood disorders

Date	DSM no.	Symptoms diagnostic of schizophrenia	Symptoms commonly present in a psychotic mood disorder	Comments
2000	DSM-IV-TR	Delusions	With psychotic features: delusions, hallucinations (Table 2.4)	Both potentially with psychoses to include mood incongruent delusions and hallucinations.
		Hallucinations	Mood incongruent hallucinations, persecutory delusions, thought insertion or broadcasting, delusions of control	Delusions and hallucinations in both frequently paranoid and persecutory that are explained by psychotic mania causing delusional grandiosity or psychotic depression causing delusional guilt.
		Disorganized speech (derailment or incoherence)	Flight of ideas, racing thoughts, pressure of speech, distractibility [leading to derailment, disorganized speech and incoherence]	Derailment, loose associations, disorganized and incoherent speech are common to psychotic mania due to a defective sensory filter.
		Grossly disorganized or catatonic behavior	[Can have] catatonic and [grossly disorganized] behavior	Disorganized and catatonic behaviors are consistent with psychotic mania and stuporous depression.
		Negative symptoms (affective flattening, alogia, avolition)	[Severe depression causes affective flattening, alogia and avolition]	Severely depressed patients are mute (alogia), have flat affects and no motivation (avolition).
		Symptoms for at least 6 months	[Can have] symptoms for two years or more	Psychotic mood disorders can become chronic, persistent, treatment resistant without further cycling for life.
		Marked deterioration in function	Diminished ability to think or concentrate cause significant ... impairment in social, occupational or other important areas of functioning [i.e., a marked deterioration]	Cycling or chronic psychotic mood disorders cause marked dysfunctionality typically far below premorbid function.
		Organic causes including drugs—ruled out	Organic causes including drugs—ruled out	Identical for both disorders.

Table 11.11 Proposed for DSM-5 (2013): the subtypes eliminated as subtypes but retained as diagnostic criteria[a]

Subtypes of schizophrenia proposed for elimination in the DSM-5	Subtypes of schizophrenia retained as diagnostic criteria	Comments
Paranoid subtype, that is, delusions, hallucinations	Delusions, hallucinations	For mood disorders hallucinations and delusions are not diagnostic but are frequent in severe cases.
Disorganized subtype	Disorganized speech	Disorganization of behavior and speech are very common to psychotic mania.
Catatonic subtype	Catatonia	The literature suggests that catatonia is far more frequent in patients diagnosed with psychotic mood disorders than any other psychiatric condition.

[a]Thus eliminating the subtypes of schizophrenia will have negligible effect on either the diagnosis of schizophrenia or the number of patients misdiagnosed; prior diagnoses of schizophrenia will not need to be reassessed except to drop the subtype.

to be indicated as "severe with psychotic features: delusions or hallucinations," to be further specified as mood-congruent or mood-incongruent psychotic features. Another specifier, the "catatonic features specifier" allowed catatonia to be used with severe mood disorders (Table 2.4). The description of the detailed signs and symptoms of catatonia in the "Mood Disorders" chapter is identical to that in the chapter on "Schizophrenia" (Table 12.3). Despite these additional redundancies, no parallel adjustments were made to the diagnostic criteria of schizophrenia.

Schizoaffective disorder was moved with the section on "Psychotic Disorders Not Otherwise Classified," a separate section from that on schizophrenia in the DSM-III-R, and back into the section titled "Schizophrenia and Other Psychotic Disorders." This change represents a movement back toward Bleuler and Schneider and away from the idea that psychotic mood disorders account for schizoaffective disorder and schizophrenia.

11.4.2 The DSM-IV-TR (APA, DSM 2000)

In the "Introduction" of the DSM-IV-TR, the current DSM, it is stated that, "It should be noted that an evidenced-based text revision of the DSM-IV was published in 2000 … as DSM-IV-TR …" The subtypes of schizophrenia remained unchanged as did the criterion A "characteristic symptoms." Retained is the ability to diagnose schizophrenia with a single criterion A symptom when that symptom is one of Schneider's first-rank symptoms (Table 8.1). Schizoaffective disorder remains in the chapter titled "Schizophrenia and Other Psychotic Disorders" and not in the chapter titled "Mood Disorders." The redundancies between the DSM diagnostic symptoms of schizophrenia and the potential features of severe mood disorders remain substantial and are carried into the DSM-5 (Tables 11.10 and 11.11).

11.4.3 The DSM-5 (APA, DSM Proposed 2013)

The seventh edition of the DSM (DSM-5) is currently under development and available for public review (Bruijnzeel and Tandon 2011). Its scheduled publication is in May 2013. The work group is recommending that the subtypes of schizophrenia, dating to the 1850s, not be included in the DSM-5 (Chap. 12). Also apparently eliminated will be the ability to fulfill criterion A, the characteristic symptoms of schizophrenia, with one of Schneider's first-rank symptoms. Schizophrenia itself is apparently being retained with essentially the same diagnostic criteria redundant with the DSM features of chronic psychotic mood disorders (Tables 2.5, 11.10, and 11.11). In the proposed revision, updated May 17, 2010, the core diagnostic characteristic symptoms for schizophrenia continue to be (1) delusions, (2) hallucinations, (3) disorganized speech, (4) catatonia, and (5) negative symptoms, that is, restricted affect or avolition/asociality (Tables 11.11, 12.1, 12.3, and 12.9). Criteria B, C, D, and E are similar to those in the DSM-IV-TR and are redundant with the characteristics of severe mood disorders (Tables 2.3, 2.4, and 2.5). Schizoaffective disorder appears to have been retained in the chapter on "Schizophrenia and Other Psychotic Disorders" despite suggestions from several authors that schizoaffective disorder be dropped from the DSM-5 because such patients appear to have psychotic mood disorders and not any other disorder (Table 7.3) (Procci 1976; Swartz 2002b, 2004; Lake and Hurwitz 2006b, 2007b). The only changes for schizoaffective disorder scheduled for the DSM-5 are trivial (Sect. 7.7) (Bruijnzeel and Tandon 2011).

Dropping the subtypes of schizophrenia is a substantial change in the concept of schizophrenia because, for about 150 years, schizophrenia could not stand on its own but required a subtype. Still, the subtypes of schizophrenia double as diagnostic symptoms that are not being dropped (Table 11.11). The five core "characteristic symptoms" for a diagnosis of schizophrenia, under proposal for retention in the DSM-5, are all more prevalent in psychotic mood disorders than in any other disorder (Tables 3.5 and 11.11) (Pini et al. 2001).

The addition of nine dimensions in the proposed DSM-5 (Table 11.12) is a change in the concept of schizophrenia (Bruijnzeel and Tandon 2011). What is striking about these nine dimensions is their applicability to mood disorders, especially depression. Numbers 7 and 8 are "Depression" and "Mania." Numbers 1 through 3 are the positive symptoms, displayed by most, if not all, psychotic mood-disordered patients. Dimension numbers 4 through 7 and 9 are classic dimensions disturbed in major depression. Rating these dimensions on a 0–4 scale will yield valuable clinical information but is appropriate for the mood disorders rather than any other disease. The mindset appears to continue the obsolete idea that hallucinations and delusions determine a diagnosis of schizophrenia despite the presence of mania and/or depression at any point in the course of the disease.

Although there are proposed changes in the "Mood Disorders" chapter of the DSM-5, none have substantial impact upon the focus of this book.

Table 11.12 Proposed for DSM-5 (2013): nine dimensions of "schizophrenia" are more applicable to psychotic mood disorders[a,b]

1. Delusions
2. Hallucinations
3. Disorganization
4. Restricted emotional expression
5. Avolition/asociality
6. Impaired cognition
7. Depression
8. Mania
9. Psychomotor symptoms

[a]Change to DSM-5: add nine dimensions, which will be assessed on a 0–4 scale cross-sectionally, with severity assessment based on past month (major change)
[b]All of these nine dimensions proposed for schizophrenia are quite applicable to psychotic mood disorders, especially 7 and 8 making the disease of schizophrenia redundant to psychotic mood disorders.

11.5 Psychotic Depression Accounts for Many Patients Diagnosed with Schizophrenia

Because the positive and negative symptoms of schizophrenia are core symptoms of psychotic depression, the historical relationship of psychotic depression to schizophrenia is relevant. Although psychotic depression, paranoia, and suicide were recognized as characteristics of mood disorders for 2,000 years (Table 3.1), they became associated with schizophrenia due to the influences of Bleuler (1911), Schneider (1959), and their followers based on the belief that psychosis meant schizophrenia. There was a marked decrease in the prevalence of the diagnosis of psychotic depression and a parallel increase in schizophrenia in hospitalized patients through the first three quarters of the twentieth century (Figs. 3.2 and 15.7). Swartz and Shorter (2007) found that the rate of the diagnosis of psychotic depression in one hospital decreased from 75% in 1892 to 39% in 1942/3 and to 30% in 1981/2 while the rate of the diagnosis of schizophrenia increased.

There have been conflicting ideas about the association of paranoia with both depression and schizophrenia (Kraepelin 1921; Brockington et al. 1980b). In 1921 Kraepelin described "paranoid depression," but typically, such patients have been diagnosed with schizophrenia (Doran et al. 1986). Kraepelin placed paranoid psychosis as a core subtype of schizophrenia as did Bleuler and subsequent generations of psychiatrists, editions of the DSM, and textbooks of psychiatry. Some examples of the inappropriate subordination of psychotic depression to schizophrenia are: (1) The "negative symptoms" (alogia, avolition, affective flattening or restricted affect, and asociality) that are held in the DSM as diagnostic of schizophrenia, not depression (Table 2.5). These negative symptoms of schizophrenia are common to severe depression, are disease nonspecific, and do not warrant continuing as a diagnostic criterion for schizophrenia or any other disease. (2) The diagnosis of "postschizophrenic depression," as justified by McGlashan and Carpenter (1976) and that remains in the ICD as a subtype of schizophrenia. "Postschizophrenic depression" is most likely psychotic depression in partial remission of the psychotic symptoms rather than a separate disease (Brockington et al. 1980b; Swartz and Shorter 2007). The DSM has not embraced "postschizophrenic depression" as has the ICD. Symptoms of depression can be obscured by psychotic symptoms and not become evident until the psychosis begins to remit, potentially leading to the misconception of postschizophrenic depression (Carlson and Goodwin 1973; Post 1992). Sands and Harrow (1994) reported that over 50% of patients previously hospitalized with psychotic depression were likely psychotic at a year posthospitalization but were only "subsyndromally" depressed, likely leading to misdiagnoses of schizophrenia. (3) Schizoaffective disorder, depressed subtype, was reported to share more characteristics with schizophrenia (psychosis and poor prognosis) than with bipolar disorder (Coryell et al. 1984). However, severe depression in established bipolar or unipolar patients can stop cycling, become chronically psychotic with an irritable, dysphoric mood, and treatment resistant with persistent cognitive defects and dysfunctionality (Carlson and Goodwin, 1973; Post 1992, 2007; Pierson et al. 2000; Bearden et al. 2001; Chambers and Perrone-Bizzozero 2004; Glahn et al. 2004; McIntosh et al. 2005; Tiihonen et al. 2005; Weiser et al. 2005; Goodwin and Jamison 2007). The poor prognosis of psychotic depression with "negative symptoms of schizophrenia" may be the explanation for the misdiagnosis of schizophrenia in such patients. (4) Hafner et al. (2005) reported that the lifetime prevalence of depression was 83% in patients diagnosed with schizophrenia at their first admission. Other data concluded that depression is the most common premorbid sign for a subsequent diagnosis of schizophrenia (psychosis), but it seems likely that depression is the risk factor for psychotic depression that can deteriorate to a chronic course as part of a severe mood disorder (Hafner et al. 2005; Weiser et al. 2005; Maier et al. 2006). Demonstrating the misconception that psychosis means schizophrenia rather than psychotic depression, Hafner et al. (2005) said,

> Showing considerable overlap in symptoms and functional impairment at their initial stages, schizophrenia and unipolar depression became clearly distinguishable with the emergence of psychotic symptoms [they assumed to be schizophrenia, not psychotic depression].

Suicide may be increased in psychotically depressed patients misdiagnosed with schizophrenia because patients with the diagnosis of schizophrenia may not receive appropriate antidepressants, mood-stabilizing medications, or ECT. The suicide rate in psychotic depression may approach 20%, and 40% of patients with a diagnosis of psychotic depression died from all causes within 15 years of their admission to a hospital (Vythilingam et al. 2003). Depression with psychotic features (either unipolar or bipolar) seems the appropriate diagnosis in such patients described above.

11.6 C.M. Swartz and E. Shorter (2007)

In 2007 Swartz and Shorter published their textbook titled *Psychotic Depression*. They documented that patients with psychotic depression can manifest each and every symptom given in the current DSM as diagnostic of schizophrenia (Table 2.5). For example, patients with psychotic depression can exhibit delusions, hallucinations, disorganized speech to include frequent derailment and incoherence, grossly disorganized or catatonic behavior, affective flattening, alogia, and avolition (the last three are termed the "negative symptoms" of schizophrenia). They noted that at least 50% of major mood-disordered patients suffer psychotic symptoms. These symptoms comprise criterion A, characteristic symptoms of schizophrenia, two or more of which, when "… present for a significant portion of time during a 1-month period…" warrant the diagnosis of schizophrenia according to the DSM. Criteria B and C for a diagnosis of schizophrenia, that is, social/occupational dysfunction and duration, are also documented to frequently occur in patients with psychotic depression. Swartz and Shorter (2007) emphasized the relationship of paranoid delusions to severe depression rather than schizophrenia (Tables 3.1 and 3.2). They credited others such as the London physician, James Sims, with linking melancholia or severe depression with paranoid delusions in 1799 (Chap. 3). Beck (1967, 1972) also connected severe depression and paranoid delusions and spoke of a spectrum of severity linking schizophrenia and mood disorders (Table 11.13, Quote 3). Swartz and Shorter (2007, p 19) therefore appeared to question the validity of schizophrenia as separate from a psychotic mood disorder (Table 11.2, Quote 33).

11.7 The Development and Implications of the Continuum Concept

The idea of a "continuum" between patients diagnosed with schizophrenia and a mood disorder contradicts and eliminates the concept of the Kraepelinian dichotomy. A continuum between schizophrenia and mood disorders implies a single disease and raises doubt about the validity of schizophrenia as separate from psychotic mood disorders. Doubt focuses upon schizophrenia rather than bipolar disorders because of the absence of disease-specific diagnostic criteria for schizophrenia as discussed in Chap. 4. Although major advances toward endorsing the continuum theory occurred primarily after the late 1980s, there were earlier references to doubt about the validity of the dichotomy.

Prior to the designation of dementia praecox or schizophrenia as separate from manic-depressive insanity or bipolar disorder, which occurred in the latter half of the nineteenth century, there was no dichotomy (Table 15.7; Fig 11.2). Although Kraepelin is credited with establishing "The Dichotomy" between schizophrenia and bipolar disorder around

11.7 The Development and Implications of the Continuum Concept

Table 11.13 Selected quotes supporting the continuum theory of a single disease encompassing schizophrenia and mood disorders

Quote no.	Journal (year)	Author(s)	Field of study	Selected quotes of summary/conclusions	Results
1	*Themes Variations Eur Psychiatr* (1920/1974)	Kraepelin	Book	"It is becoming increasingly clear that we cannot distinguish satisfactorily between these two illnesses (dementia praecox/schizophrenia and manic-depressive insanity/bipolar) and this brings home the suspicion that our formulation of the problem may be incorrect."	Similar/continuum
2	*AJP* (1933)	Kasanin	Clinical symptoms	He first used "schizoaffective disorder" to diagnose a group of nine patients with symptoms of both schizophrenia and bipolar disorder. "These groups [schizophrenia and bipolar disorders] are so general and contain such a large number of heterogeneous cases with different clinical pictures that it is no wonder that the experimental results are quite worthless. I doubt very much if experimental research in Psychiatry will ever yield any results unless we deal with fairly homogeneous groups."	Similar/continuum
3	*Depression Clin Exp Theoret Aspects* (1967)	Beck	Book	"These observations could be expressed graphically by viewing the cases of functional mental illness in terms of a spectrum: at one end are the pure manic-depressive cases with a good prognosis; and at the other are the pure schizophrenic cases with a poor prognosis. In between are varying blends of these disorders (the schizo-affective cases) with a fair prognosis."	Continuum
4	*BJP* (1970b)	Kendell and Gourlay	Clinical symptoms	"[Upon a reanalysis of the data] ... The overall distribution of scores no longer has a predominate trimodal profile and does not differ significantly from a normal distribution ... At all events the results of this further analysis do not lend support to the view that schizophrenic and affective psychosis are distinct entities."	Similar/continuum
5	*Psychol Med* (1980b)	Brockington et al.	Clinical symptoms	"These findings are not easily reconciled with Kraepelin's two entities principle but suggest a continuum of outcome between schizophrenia and unipolar depressive psychosis."	Continuum

(continued)

Table 11.13 (continued)

Quote no.	Journal (year)	Author(s)	Field of study	Selected quotes of summary/conclusions	Results
6	BJP (1986)	Crow	Review (genetics)	"Three observations challenge Kraepelin's binary view of the functional psychosis: a bimodal distribution of the clinical features of manic-depressive illness and schizophrenia has not been demonstrated; affective illness appears to predispose to schizophrenia in later generations; and 'schizoaffective' illnesses cannot be separated in family studies from either of the prototypical psychoses. The alternative concept is that psychosis is a continuum extending from unipolar, through bipolar affective illness and schizoaffective psychosis to typical schizophrenia, with increasing degrees of defect."	Continuum
7	BJP (1990a)	Crow	Review (genetics)	"It must be assumed that these diseases (schizophrenia and affective illnesses) are genetically related. ...that the psychoses represent a continuum of variation at a single genetic locus."	Same/continuum
8	Acta Psychiatr Scand (1990b)	Crow	Review (molecular genetics)	"The recurrent psychoses ...manic depressive illness and schizophrenia, ...may be distributed along a continuum that extends from unipolar depressive illness through bipolar and schizoaffective psychosis to schizophrenia with increasing severities of defect state. It is proposed that this continuum rests on a genetic base ....such variation relates to changes at a single genetic locus."	Same/continuum
9	AGP (1993)	Maier et al.	Family study	"The most significant finding is the increased risk of UP [unipolar, MDD] depression in the relatives of SCZ [schizophrenia] probands. This finding violates the predictions of a simple dichotomous model of SCZ and affective disorders."	Continuum
10	Compreh Psychiatr (1994)	Taylor and Amir	Review (clinical symptoms)	"Our findings do not fully support the present classification system, and suggest that its emphasis on hallucinations and delusions is overvalued. ... our analyses repeatedly yielded a single discriminate function, indicating that ...schizophrenics and affectives can be represented on a continuous distribution of clinical features representing a single underlying process."	Similar/continuum

11.7 The Development and Implications of the Continuum Concept

11	*Schiz Res* (2003)	Gonzalez-Pinto et al.	Clinical symptoms	"These results confirm previous findings that FRSs are not specific to schizophrenia and suggest in addition that a dimension of nuclear psychotic experiences of developmental origin extends across categorically defined psychotic disorders."	Continuum
12	*J Clin Psychiatr* (2003)	Moller	Review	"Bipolar Disorder and Schizophrenia: Distinct Illnesses or a Continuum" [article title]; "Family and twin studies suggest hereditary overlap between the two disorders.... Certain susceptibility markers appear to be located on the same chromosomes.... [the two] also demonstrate some similarities in neurotransmitter dysfunction. ... A conceptual case can be made for a relationship between schizophrenia and bipolar disorder. ... the Kraepelinian dichotomy between bipolar disorder and schizophrenia may be gradually succumbing to a theory of disease overlap and continuum."	Similar/continuum
13	*J Psychiatr Res* (2004)	Ketter et al.	Review	"Psychotic bipolar disorders have characteristics such as phenomenology, biology, therapeutic response and brain imaging findings suggesting both commonalities with and dissociations from schizophrenia.... Taken together, these characteristics are in some instances most consistent with a dimensional view, with psychotic bipolar disorders being intermediate between non-psychotic bipolar disorders and schizophrenia spectrum disorders. However, in other instances, a categorical approach appears useful."	Continuum/ ambivalent
14	*J Med Genetics* (2005)	Craddock et al.	Review (molecular genetics)	"Increasing evidence suggests an overlap in genetic susceptibility across the traditional classification system that dichotomized psychotic disorders into schizophrenia or bipolar disorder, most notably with findings at DAOA(G72), DISC1, and NRG1. ---we can expect that over the coming years molecular genetics will catalyze a re-appraisal of psychiatric nosology as well as providing a path to understanding the pathophysiology" [of bipolar and schizophrenia].	Similar

(continued)

Table 11.13 (continued)

Quote no.	Journal (year)	Author(s)	Field of study	Selected quotes of summary/conclusions	Results
15	BJP (2005)	Craddock and Owen	Molecular genetics	"Now molecular genetic studies are beginning to challenge and will soon, we predict, overturn the traditional dichotomous view. … The Kraepelinian dichotomy has been useful for 100 years. Now it is time to move on."	Similar/continuum
16	SZ Bull (2006)	Craddock et al.	Molecular genetics	"… current genetic findings suggest that rather than classifying psychosis as a dichotomy, a more useful formulation may be … a spectrum of clinical phenotypes with susceptibility conferred by overlapping sets of genes."	Similar/continuum
17	Encephale (2009)	Demily et al.	Review	"… symptoms associated with the diagnosis of schizophrenia can be associated with psychotic mood disorders: hallucinations and delusions (50%) disorganized speech and behavior (all patients with moderate to severe mania or mixed episode), negative symptoms (all patients with moderate to severe depression). The social and job dysfunction may be due to disturbances in the volitional system in patients with schizophrenia or severe bipolar disorder. … In this way, it has been suggested that psychotic symptoms may be distributed along a continuum that extends from schizophrenia to psychotic mood disorders with increasing level of severity. … Likewise, common factors can explain cognitive and social disorders in psychosis."	Continuum
18	Psychiatr Ann (2010)	Crow	Review	"My hypothesis, therefore, is that this mechanism is a source of variation that specifically relates to cerebral asymmetry and language. Herein lies the variation, not only of the continuum of psychosis but other aspects of human diversity."	Similar
19	Psychiatr Ann (2010a)	Craddock and Owen	Review	"Time will tell as to whether this will be most usefully achieved by using multiple overlapping 'categorical' domains of psychopathology or multiple dimensions. The clinical need is for an optimal balance of simplicity and clinical utility. Of course, the traditional dichotomy is simple - and this perhaps explains its persistence, despite increasingly questioned clinical usefulness."	Continuum/ambivalent

11.7 The Development and Implications of the Continuum Concept

1900, he later recanted (Table 11.13, Quote 2; Table 15.7) (Kraepelin 1920/1974). Kraepelin's reversal was ignored for over 50 years. As noted by Crow (2010),

> But such was the power of a simple binary classification [the Kraepelinian Dichotomy] that a century of clinicians, textbook writers, and examiners adopted the system with uncritical enthusiasm and regardless of the reservations of its progenitor.

In 1933 Kasanin named schizoaffective disorder as a compromise or intermediary diagnosis between schizophrenia and nonpsychotic bipolar disorder. Although he may have been unaware of his linking the two major disorders, his schizoaffective disorder diagnosis certainly facilitated consideration of a continuum rather than a dichotomy (Chap. 7).

In his 1967 book about depression, Beck directly referred to "a spectrum" between manic-depressive and schizophrenia cases (Table 11.13, Quote 3). Kendell and Gourlay (1970a, b) reported a unimodal distribution of symptoms from patients diagnosed with schizophrenia and bipolar disorder after a reanalysis of their data (Table 11.13, Quote 4). Their data contradicted the Kraepelinian dichotomy and suggested a continuum. Angst et al. (1979, 1983) and Gershon et al. (1982) concluded from their family genetic studies of schizophrenia, schizoaffective disorder, and bipolar disorders that the three could exist on a continuum rather than distinct disorders. Brockington et al. (1980b) deduced from their studies of family history, response to treatment, and outcome of patients presenting with both depression and schizophrenia or paranoid symptoms that these disorders formed a continuum and not a dichotomy (Table 11.13, Quote 5). Over a decade later, Maier et al. (1993) came to the same conclusion of a continuum between major depression and schizophrenia. Taylor and Amir (1994), from the Chicago Medical School, confirmed the impressions of Kendell and Gourlay (1970a, b) in concluding that the clinical features of patients diagnosed with schizophrenia and mood disorders fall on a continuum rather than a dichotomy. Moller (2003) also embraced the continuum versus the dichotomy. Ketter et al. (2004) were ambivalent in their conclusions in considering a spectrum versus a categorical approach. Craddock and colleagues firmly dismissed the dichotomy in several publications which also acknowledged genetic similarities and overlap (Craddock 2005; Craddock and Owen 2005, 2010a, b; Craddock et al. 2005, 2006) (Table 11.13, Quotes 14–16, 19).

It was Tim Crow who may be best known for embracing and developing the continuum theory. Crow (2010) published an article titled, "The Continuum of Psychosis -- 1986–2010" in which he outlined his thought processes over the decades that have concluded that one disease explains the functional psychoses. Crow was quoted in a 1987 Lancet editorial saying that,

> "... he [Crow] suggests that psychotic illness should be regarded not as separate disease entities but as a single illness with a spectrum of symptoms...." Crow has proposed "... a theory that encompasses the origins of language and the speciation process [that] could account for the diverse phenomena of psychosis."
>
> (Crow 2010) (Table 11.13, Quotes 6–8, 18)

Figures 3.1 and 11.3 suggest the original versus a current concept of the continuum or dimensional theory.

ORIGINAL CONTINUUM CONCEPT

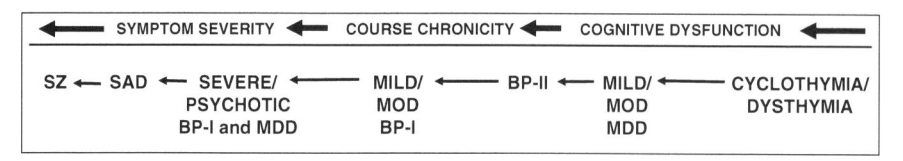

← SYMPTOM SEVERITY ←	COURSE CHRONICITY ←	COGNITIVE DYSFUNCTION ←
SZ ← SAD ← SEVERE/ ← PSYCHOTIC BP-I and MDD	MILD/ ← BP-II ← MOD BP-I	MILD/ ← CYCLOTHYMIA/ MOD DYSTHYMIA MDD

CURRENT CONTINUUM CONCEPT

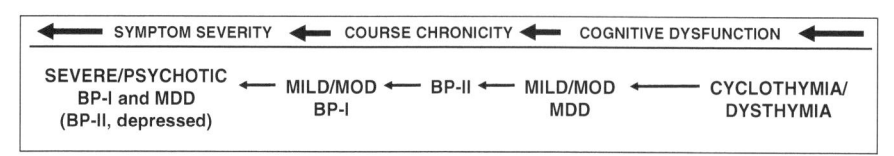

← SYMPTOM SEVERITY ←	COURSE CHRONICITY ←	COGNITIVE DYSFUNCTION ←
SEVERE/PSYCHOTIC BP-I and MDD (BP-II, depressed)	← MILD/MOD ← BP-II ← BP-I	MILD/MOD ← CYCLOTHYMIA/ MDD DYSTHYMIA

Fig. 11.3 Continuum/dimensional concept explained by mood disorders: the original versus the current concept

The original continuum concept could be conceived as encompassing seven groups of disorders based on severity and prognosis.

A simplified concept eliminates schizoaffective disorder (SAD) and schizophrenia (SZ) as redundant with severe/psychotic mood disorders to include bipolar-I and major depressive disorder (MDD). Bipolar-II is shown as intermediate in severity and chronicity, but this is misleading because the depressive episodes in bipolar-II can become psychotic and chronic. As such bipolar-II is shown in parenthesis at the most severe end of the spectrum based on its depressive phase.

Abbreviations: *SZ* schizophrenia, *SAD* schizoaffective disorder, *BP-I* bipolar disorder, *type I*, *BP-II* bipolar disorder, type II, *MDD* major depressive disorder, *MOD* moderate

11.8 Conclusions

Fischer and Carpenter (2009) clarified the one versus two disease theories by saying that,

> … the paramount issue is whether the two diagnostic classes [schizophrenia and psychotic mood disorders] comprise one heterogeneous disorder with an artificial boundary or two disorders with overlapping features.

Carpenter and colleagues support the latter. The flaw in the cornerstone of the concept of schizophrenia as a distinct condition is its dependence on the early twentieth century belief that psychosis and chronicity uniquely define schizophrenia as "the disorder of thought." Also held as especially indicative of the validity of schizophrenia and the dichotomy of two diseases has been the (mis)perceptions for decades that (1) families with schizophrenia and bipolar disorder "bred true,"(2) there was a differential responsivity to certain medications, (3) specific cognitive defects were unique to schizophrenia, (4) specific genetic sequence variations linked only to schizophrenia, (5) the "deficit syndrome" and "negative symptoms" were unique to schizophrenia, and (6) "the massive volume of literature [on schizophrenia]" was too large for schizophrenia to be invalid. A definitive answer is inhibited by several factors: (1) the absence of specific pathophysiology for either condition; (2) the observation that in established bipolar patients, psychotic symptoms can mask and draw

11.8 Conclusions

Table 11.14 Differences between schizophrenia and psychotic mood disorders resolved by one disorder

A. Early concept
• Classic SZ and classic BP (nonpsychotic BP): different and breed true
○ SZ breeds SZ, not classic (nonpsychotic) BP
○ Classic(nonpsychotic) BP breeds classic BP, not SZ
B. Recent findings
• There is chronic, psychotic BP
• Classic (nonpsychotic BP) and psychotic BP are different based on psychosis
○ DAOA/G30 associates with "SZ" and psychotic BP
• Valles et al. (2000):
○ "SZ" breeds Psychotic BP, not classic (nonpsychotic) BP
○ Psychotic BP breeds "SZ"
○ Nonpsychotic BP breeds BP, not "SZ"
• Crow
○ Psychosis is inherited irrespective of diagnosis
C. Current speculations
• SZ is psychotic BP
• There is no SZ
• Psychotic BP and classic (nonpsychotic) BP generally breed true
○ Psychotic BP breeds primarily psychotic BP, not nonpsychotic BP
○ Classic (nonpsychotic) BP breeds primarily classic BP

Abbreviations: SZ schizophrenia, *BP* bipolar disorder

attention away from mood symptoms leading to a misdiagnosis of schizophrenia or schizoaffective disorder; (3) the accepted concept of two diseases, not one for over a century, generating bias in the interpretation of comparative studies; (4) the perpetuation of the dichotomy by the DSMs, ICDs, and textbooks; and (5) the influence of many academic leaders in the field of psychiatry who support schizophrenia as a valid disease distinct from psychotic mood disorders and thus the dichotomy.

The heterogeneity in results from family studies of "classic schizophrenic" patients (read psychotic patients) versus "classic bipolar patients" (read nonpsychotic) is resolved if the "schizophrenia" and "schizoaffective disorder" patients are actually misdiagnosed, psychotic bipolar patients. There are genetic differences between "classic" (nonpsychotic) bipolar and psychotic bipolar patients that can be misinterpreted as differentiating schizophrenia from bipolar disorder (Tables 11.7, 11.8, and 11.14). The third conclusion of Pope and Lipinski (1978) is relevant again ("The non-specificity of 'schizophrenic' symptoms brings into question all research that uses them as the primary method of diagnosis") because, if accurate, it directly invalidates the studies of schizophrenia cited as indicative of two diseases, and it indirectly questions the validity of schizophrenia as a disease separate from psychotic mood disorders therefore supporting unification to a single disease (Tables 1.1, 10.1, 11.1, and 11.2).

Although there is no definitive proof either way, certainly most authors and a preponderance of the data continue to support the Kraepelinian dichotomy implying that these are two different disorders (Lapensee 1992a, b; Lapierre 1994; Pearlson et al. 1997; Hirayasu et al. 1998; Altshuler et al. 2000; Fischer and Carpenter 2009).

However, in each study finding differences, the patients in the cohort with schizophrenia were diagnosed based on the presence of nonspecific psychotic symptoms and/or chronicity of course, common to psychotic bipolar disorders and therefore may have suffered from a psychotic mood disorder with only subtle unaddressed disturbances of mood (Pope and Lipinski 1978). For example, one review found support for two disorders based on the misconception that a disorder of thought is unique to schizophrenia. She concluded that there is

> "… no evidence to suggest a common pathophysiology for schizophrenia and bipolar disorder," since, according to the author's stated differentiating feature of schizophrenia, a "thought disorder is a … useful symptom in distinguishing schizophrenia [from bipolar] …"
>
> (Lapierre 1994).

As discussed in Chap. 13, psychotic mood disorders are disorders of thought, as well as of the emotions.

Even without pathophysiological proof, a growing international comparative literature across a wide array of disciplines reports similarities and overlap that invite now the conclusion that patients diagnosed with schizophrenia have no unique diagnostic symptom, prognosis, course, epidemiology, heritability, cognitive defect, or any other characteristic not accounted for by psychotic bipolar disorder (Table 11.3; Figs. 3.1, 3.2). Molecular pathophysiology suggests that bipolar disorder "… arises from abnormalities in synaptic and neuronal plasticity cascades, leading to aberrant information processing in critical synapses and circuits" (Schloesser et al. 2008). These abnormalities are thought to cause the disturbances in mood, changes in psychovegetative function, cognitive performance, psychosis, and general health, heretofore attributed to the disease that has been called schizophrenia (Post 2007; Schloesser et al. 2008). Neither a "disorder of thought" (Lapierre 1994) nor a "massive volume of research [on schizophrenia]" (Nasrallah 2006) can continue to distinguish schizophrenia or any other disease as a "bona fide" disorder. Ockham's razor is invoked.

Figures 3.2 and 11.2 depict the hypothesized diagnoses for psychotic patients over the past century and a half. The percent of psychotic patients diagnosed with schizophrenia has dramatically fallen while that of psychotic mood disorders has increased. The estimated percentages for the year 2001 are supported by the data of Pini et al. (2001) from one substantial academic medical center (Table 3.5). The extrapolation of these curves leads to the hypothesis that eventually the diagnoses of schizoaffective disorder and schizophrenia will be eliminated maybe from the DSM-6, if not from the DSM-5.

Of the major psychiatric disorders named in the nineteenth century or before, bipolar disorder has proved valid. Bleuler was unlucky; he chose to dedicate his life to the wrong disease, dementia praecox, instead of manic-depressive insanity. As previously stated, "Bleuler did not discover schizophrenia, he invented it." (Szasz 1976) Bleuler counted on future neuroscience finding a unique neuropathology as had been the case for syphilis and other infectious diseases, but this has not

11.8 Conclusions

happened leading to several appropriate conclusions (Table 11.2, Quotes 4, 17, 18, 26–29, and 33). Kraepelin's recantation, although ignored, appears to have been insightful and accurate (Table 11.13, Quote 1).

Weaknesses of these conclusions include the biased selection of quotes when the authors of the quoted papers may not have intended to be so definitive and may have also supported a dichotomy. However, several authors have been clear in their doubt of the validity of the dichotomy and/or of schizophrenia (Tables 1.1, 10.1, 11.2–11.9, and 11.13). No single publication proves the hypotheses presented herein; it is, rather, the strength of so many different studies across such a wide array of disciplines that report conclusions that contradict the established dogma of a dichotomy and of schizophrenia that encourages this proposal.

Chapter 12
The Subtypes and the Positive and Negative Diagnostic Symptoms of Schizophrenia Are Explained by Psychotic Mood Disorders

...many patients whose conditions are diagnosed as paranoid schizophrenia actually suffer from an affective illness...

(Abrams et al. 1974)

There are no known pathognomonic symptoms for schizophrenia, nor even any cluster of symptoms,... to be valid in diagnosing schizophrenia. The non-specificity of "schizophrenic" symptoms brings into question all research that uses them as the primary method of diagnosis.

(Pope and Lipinski 1978)

They [schizophrenia and mania] have a number of properties in common, including heritability, response to neuroleptics and the tendency to post-psychotic depression. In the area of psychotic phenomena such as delusions, hallucinations and passivity phenomena [the negative symptoms], the overlap is almost complete.

(Brockington et al. 1980b)

12.1 Introduction: The Subtypes Are the Same as the Diagnostic Criteria

The three core subtypes of schizophrenia, originally called dementia praecox, are hebephrenic, now called disorganized, catatonic, and paranoid (Tables 3.4, 6.3, 12.1). All date from the nineteenth century. Morel (1851) differentiated dementia praecox from manic-depressive insanity based on severity and chronicity. Hecker (1871) described hebephrenia, and Kahlbaum (1874) wrote about catatonia (Doran et al. 1986). Kraepelin in the 1880s added the paranoid subtype and grouped the three as comprising dementia praecox. Bleuler (1911) defined schizophrenia as "... The Group of Schizophrenias" meaning that his disease was made up of subtypes and did not exist as an entity separate from the subtypes. Bleuler (1911, p. 10) added a fourth

Table 12.1 Changes and lack thereof of the subtypes and the positive and negative diagnostic symptoms of schizophrenia from the DSM-IV-TR to the DSM-5 (proposed)

DSM-IV-TR (APA, DSM 2000)
Subtypes of schizophrenia
1. Catatonia[b]
2. Disorganized[c]
3. Paranoid[d]
4. Residual
5. Undifferentiated

Criterion A. Diagnostic criteria for schizophrenia in the DSM-IV-TR
A. Characteristic symptoms: Two or more during a 1-month period:
   Positive Symptoms[a]
   1. Delusions[d]
   2. Hallucinations[d]
   3. Disorganized speech (frequent derailment, incoherence)[c]
   4. Grossly disorganized or catatonic behavior[b,c]

   Negative Symptoms[a]
   5. Negative symptoms (affective flattening, alogia, or avolition)

Note: Only one symptom is required if delusions are bizarre or hallucinations are a voice commenting on one's behavior/thoughts, or two or more voices are conversing with each other. [These are Schneider's first-rank symptoms]

DSM-5 (APA, DSM 2011/2013)
Subtypes of schizophrenia:
NONE
All subtypes proposed for elimination

Criterion A. Diagnostic criteria for schizophrenia in the DSM-5 (proposed)
A. Characteristic symptoms: Two (or more) during a 1-month period. At least one of these should include 1–3.
   Positive symptoms[a]
   1. Delusions[d]
   2. Hallucinations[d]
   3. Disorganized speech[c]
   4. Catatonia[b]

   Negative symptoms[a]
   5. Negative symptoms, i.e., restricted affect or avolition/asociality

Note: The use of Schneider's first-rank symptoms is proposed for elimination.

---
[a]Headings are not part of the DSM
[b]Catatonia as a subtype to be eliminated in the DSM-5 but to be retained as a diagnostic symptom
[c]Disorganized as a subtype to be eliminated in the DSM-5 but to be retained as a diagnostic symptom
[d]Paranoid (hallucinations and delusions) as a subtype to be eliminated in the DSM-5 but hallucinations and delusions are to be retained as diagnostic symptoms

subtype, simple schizophrenia, but this subtype was dropped upon the publication of the DSM-III in 1980. The three core subtypes, disorganized, catatonic, and paranoid, have survived intact from the nineteenth century and apparently until 2013 when the DSM-5 is due to be published. Two other less specific subtypes, residual and undifferentiated, were added at least by 1968 with the publication of the DSM-II and, like the core three subtypes, have been retained through the current DSM-IV-TR. From the publications of Kraepelin and Bleuler through the present, a century, the

12.1 Introduction: The Subtypes Are the Same as the Diagnostic Criteria

validity of schizophrenia as a disease depended upon the validity of the three subtypes that double as diagnostic criteria. This has been a cornerstone of psychiatry of equal import to Kraepelin's dichotomy. The accuracy of this statement is based on the current widely accepted diagnostic manuals, the DSM-IV-TR and the ICD-10 as well as textbooks of psychiatry (Tables 2.5, 3.4, 9.3, 9.4, 12.1). That there is no schizophrenia without the subtypes may change in 2013. The proposed draft revision for the DSM-5 includes the statement regarding the subtypes of schizophrenia: "The workgroup is recommending that these subtypes not be included in the DSM-5" (APA, DSM-5 2013) (Bruijnzeel and Tandon 2011). This proposal is a critical change representing a justified lack of confidence in the validity of the subtypes but also raising an even more central problem.

At issue is that the three core subtypes slated for oblivion have served dual roles: (1) as subtypes of schizophrenia and (2) as the core diagnostic criteria for the diagnosis of schizophrenia (Tables 2.5, 3.4, 12.1). If these subtypes warrant elimination from the DSM-5, what about the synonymous diagnostic criteria? That the subtypes proposed for elimination as subtypes are being retained as symptoms diagnostic of schizophrenia raise doubt about the wisdom of retaining schizophrenia at all in this author's opinion (Table 12.1). This chapter demonstrates how these "diagnostic" symptoms of schizophrenia, the three core subtypes synonymous with the core diagnostic symptoms, also called "positive symptoms" and "negative symptoms," are readily explained by psychotic mood disorders (Tables 12.1–12.3). Case summaries are given to illustrate examples of the initial misdiagnosis of schizophrenia in psychotic mood-disordered patients.

The positive and negative symptoms of schizophrenia have been extensively discussed in the literature with regard to their diagnostic specificity. The positive symptoms, i.e., hallucinations and delusions date at least from the first century CE but were attributed to manic-depressive insanity or organic/secondary psychoses until the mid-1800s when dementia praecox (or schizophrenia) was initiated as a separate disease and defined by the positive symptoms (Table 12.1). The negative symptoms, that is, disturbed affect, avolition, alogia (DSM-IV-TR), and asociality (DSM-5) were initiated by Kraepelin and Bleuler (Foussias and Remington 2010). The positive and negative symptoms are found in the current DSM and the proposed DSM-5 under criterion A "characteristic symptoms" that define the diagnosis of schizophrenia. There are five "characteristic symptoms" (Tables 2.5, 12.1). The first four are the positive symptoms, and number five includes several negative symptoms (Table 12.1). Five editions of the DSM dating from the DSM-III (APA, DSM 1980) through the proposed DSM-5 (APA, DSM 2013) have been generally consistent in requiring one or two of these positive or negative symptoms along with a chronic deteriorating course for the diagnosis of schizophrenia. These three factors, the positive symptoms, the negative symptoms, and a chronic deteriorating course, have consistently defined schizophrenia since the publication of Bleuler's textbook in 1911 but have varied as to the weight each has been given toward making a diagnosis of schizophrenia (Fig. 12.1). Prior to 1860, these three criteria (positive and negative symptoms and a chronic course) were associated in the literature with psychotic mood disorders (Table 3.1).

Kraepelin (1919) emphasized a chronic deteriorating course, psychotic symptoms which were to become the positive symptoms, and avolition, one of the negative

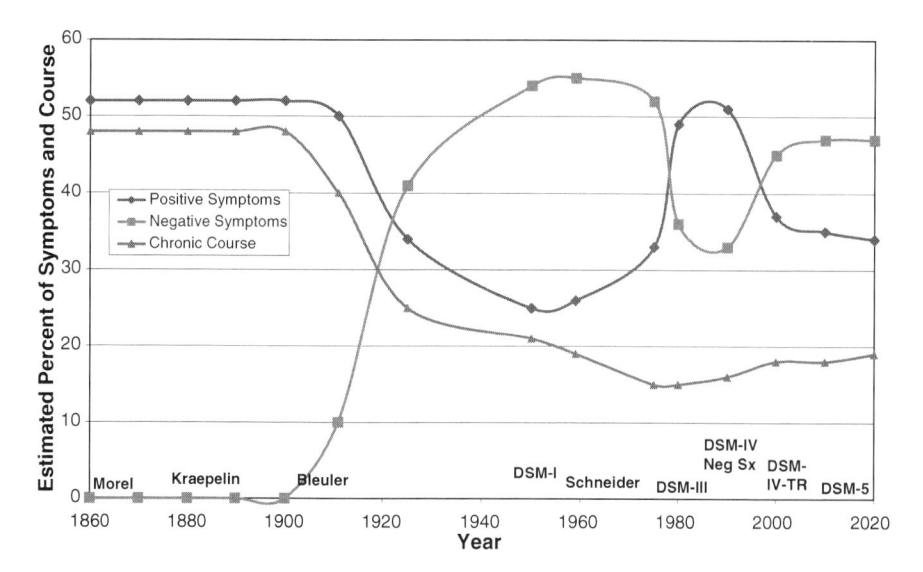

Fig. 12.1 Estimated diagnostic weight given to the positive and the negative symptoms and chronic course for the diagnosis of schizophrenia over time

Since the initiation of the concept of dementia praecox or schizophrenia in the 1850s by Morel, three factors have made varying contributions to the diagnosis of schizophrenia:

1. Positive symptoms such as hallucinations, delusions, disorganization, catatonia, and paranoia
2. Negative symptoms such as shallow, blunted, flat or inappropriate affect, mutism, alogia, apathy, indifference, avolition, loss of empathy, withdrawn or aggressive behavior, reduction in external attachments, and interests and asociality
3. Chronic course

Each of these three criteria has changed over time with respect to the weight given each of them toward arriving at a diagnosis of schizophrenia as estimated in the figure.

When Morel named dementia praecox as a disease separate from manic-depressive insanity, he emphasized the positive or psychotic symptoms and a chronic downhill course; he did not consider the negative symptoms. Kraepelin, in the late 1800s and early 1900s, also emphasized positive symptoms and a chronic course as differentiating dementia praecox/schizophrenia from manic-depressive insanity.

In 1911, Bleuler added a new subtype of schizophrenia, simple schizophrenia that did not require psychosis or chronicity but demonstrated his "fundamental symptoms of schizophrenia" that included what has become known as negative symptoms (Table 6.1). As shown in the figure, the value of negative symptoms rose with regard to its importance in diagnosing schizophrenia, while the importance of positive symptoms and chronicity fell. This trend continued through the 1940s and 1950s.

In 1959, Schneider introduced his first-rank symptoms (Chap. 8; Table 8.1) of schizophrenia emphasizing positive symptoms and de-emphasizing course chronicity. His focus on the positive symptoms may have decreased psychiatry's emphasis on the negative symptoms and on course chronicity.

The publication of the DSM-III in 1980 eliminated simple schizophrenia de-emphasizing the negative symptoms of Bleuler but did not totally eliminate them. As a result, the negative symptoms were reduced in diagnostic importance for a decade and the positive symptoms reinforced as diagnostic.

The negative symptoms were officially recognized in the DSM-IV (APA, DSM 1994) increasing their emphasis in making the diagnosis of schizophrenia. At the same time, there was increasing recognition that the positive symptoms and a chronic course were common to psychotic mood disorders so that the emphasis on the positive symptoms as diagnostic of schizophrenia may have declined. As a result, the negative symptoms were resurrected as was the concept of "nuclear schizophrenia" that gained popularity.

Although this figure is only a gross approximation by the author, it does emphasize substantial fluctuations in the concept of schizophrenia with wide variations of emphasis on the importance of various diagnostic criteria. Such variability raises questions as to the validity of schizophrenia as a scientifically based disease.

symptoms, as diagnostic of schizophrenia. There were no negative symptoms associated with schizophrenia until Kraepelin and especially Bleuler (1911) published his diagnostic criteria which included his fundamental symptoms or the "Four As of Schizophrenia" that morphed into some of the negative symptoms. His accessory or psychotic symptoms were similar to Kraepelin's and are the positive symptoms of schizophrenia (Tables 6.1, 12.1).

Bleuler (1911) de-emphasized the positive or psychotic symptoms and a chronic course as necessary diagnostic criteria and elevated the importance of his fundamental or the negative symptoms of schizophrenia as also diagnostic. This strategy enabled nonpsychotic and nonchronic individuals to receive a diagnosis of schizophrenia. Bleuler added the "simple" subtype of schizophrenia to the original three core subtypes to accommodate such nonpsychotic, nonchronic patients. This may have increased the pool of potential individuals subject to the diagnosis of schizophrenia by tenfold or more.

12.2 Catatonic Subtype

In another example of the shifting concept of the diagnosis of psychosis toward overlap between schizophrenia and psychotic mood disorders, the section on mood disorders in the DSM-IV-TR (pp. 417, 418, full text, APA, DSM 2000) lists catatonia as a potential feature for psychotic mood disorder patients (Tables 2.3, 2.4, 12.3). The description of catatonia is identical between the section on schizophrenia and that on mood disorders (compare Tables 2.4, 12.2 and 12.3) (pp. 417, 418 and 315, 316 from full text DSM-IV-TR). According to the DSM-IV-TR (pp. 417, 418, full text).

> Catatonic states have been found to occur in 5%-9% of inpatients. Among inpatients with catatonia, 25%-50% of cases occur in association with Mood Disorders, 10%-15% of cases occur in association with Schizophrenia, and the remainder occur in association with other mental disorders....

However, there has been no adjustment in the DSM section on schizophrenia to accommodate catatonia being added to the DSM mood disorders section. A minor adjustment to downgrade catatonia is proposed for the DSM-5 (see below). The literature finds that "catatonia is more frequently associated with mania, melancholia, and psychotic depression than it is with schizophrenia" (Fink and Taylor 2006). Abrams and Taylor (1976a, b) reviewed the literature and presented data discounting any meaningful relationship between catatonic symptoms and schizophrenia. They noted that Kraepelin in 1919 stated that,

> ... 47% of catatonic attacks begin with a depressive phase and that recovery occurred most frequently in just such patients. ... As a rule, catatonic symptoms mix with manic and the melancholic conditions, ... one can speak of a manic or a melancholic catatonia. ... A number of these patients are manifestly manic (with demonstrable flight of ideas); others are melancholic; ... or feel themselves persecuted.

Lang found symptoms of catatonia in about 25% of his manic-depressive patients, and Bonner and Kent (1936) also reported catatonic features in at least 34% of their manic-depressive patients (Abrams and Taylor 1976b). Swartz and Shorter (2007)

Table 12.2 Redundant descriptions of catatonia from the DSM-IV-TR chapters on schizophrenia versus the mood disorders

Catatonia in schizophrenia (see pp. 315–316, full text DSM-IV-TR or p. 156 abbreviated desk reference)

Diagnostic criteria for the catatonic subtype or the diagnostic criterion for schizophrenia

A type of schizophrenia in which the clinical picture is dominated by at least two of the following:

A. Motoric immobility as evidenced by catalepsy (including waxy flexibility) or stupor
B. Excessive motor activity (that is apparently purposeless and not influenced by external stimuli)
C. Extreme negativism (an apparently motiveless resistance to all instructions or maintenance of a rigid posture against attempts to be moved) or mutism
D. Peculiarities of voluntary movement as evidenced by posturing (voluntary assumption of inappropriate or bizarre postures), stereotyped movements, prominent mannerisms/grimacing
E. Echolalia or echopraxia

Catatonia in mood disorders (see pp. 417–418, full text DSM-IV-TR or p. 202 abbreviated desk reference)

Diagnostic criteria for catatonia in mood disorders (catatonic features specifier) with catatonic features (can be applied to the current or most recent major depressive episode, manic episode, or mixed episode in either major depressive disorder or bipolar I or II disorder)

The clinical picture is dominated by at least two of the following:

A. Motoric immobility as evidenced by catalepsy (including waxy flexibility) or stupor
B. Excessive motor activity (that is apparently purposeless and not influenced by external stimuli)
C. Extreme negativism (an apparently motiveless resistance to all instructions or maintenance of a rigid posture against attempts to be moved) or mutism
D. Peculiarities of voluntary movement as evidenced by posturing (voluntary assumption of inappropriate or bizarre postures), stereotyped movements, prominent mannerisms/grimacing
E. Echolalia or echopraxia

attribute symptoms of catatonia primarily to psychotic depression and consider "catatonic psychotic depression" as a major type of psychotic depression:

> A catatonic psychotic state is more frequently depression than Schizophrenia, …

They report the success of treating patients with catatonic symptoms with ECT, the treatment of choice for psychotic major depression, suggesting the association of catatonia with depression (Swartz and Shorter 2007) (Table 12.3).

The proposed DSM-5 demotes catatonia as a diagnostic symptom since it alone of the four positive symptoms cannot fulfill criteria with the negative symptoms (Table 12.1). Diagnostic characteristics 1, 2, and 3 are hallucinations, delusions, and disorganized speech, and any one of these plus number 5, negative symptoms, qualifies for the criterion A symptoms for the diagnosis of schizophrenia. Thus, catatonia is proposed as less significant in the symptoms of schizophrenia than hallucinations, delusions, and disorganized speech (Bruijnzeel and Tandon 2011).

This demotion does not go far enough since catatonia is disease nonspecific and diagnostically irrelevant. These data raise doubt about the validity of using catatonia to diagnose schizophrenia and, of more importance, question the validity of schizophrenia because catatonia is still being used as a diagnostic criterion.

12.2 Catatonic Subtype

Table 12.3 Selected quotes discounting the validity of catatonia as diagnostic or even characteristic of schizophrenia

Quote no.	Journal (year)	Author(s)	Field of study	Selected quotes of summary/conclusions	Results
1	*Dementia Praecox and Paraphrenia* (1919; pp. 133, 152, 211, 214)	Kraepelin	Book	"… 47% of catatonic attacks begin with a depressive phase and recovery occurred most frequently in just such patients. … As a rule, catatonic symptoms mix with manic and the melancholic conditions, … one can speak of a manic or a melancholic catatonia. … A number of these patients are manifestly manic (with demonstrable flight of ideas), others are melancholic, … or feel themselves persecuted."	Catatonic symptoms associated with mania and depression
2	*AGP* (1976b)	Abrams and Taylor	Catatonia	"We conclude that catatonic signs are nonspecific, homogenously distributed among a variety of clinical diagnostic entities, do not predict treatment response, and are seen most frequently in patients with diagnosable affective disorders, especially mania."	Catatonic symptoms nonspecific and associate with mania
3	*AJP* (2006)	Fink and Taylor	Catatonia	"Catatonia is more frequently associated with mania, melancholia and psychotic depression than it is with schizophrenia."	Catatonic symptoms indicate a Mood Disorder
4	*Psychotic Depression* (2007; pp. 6, 92)	Swartz and Shorter	Book	"In catatonic depression, the extreme form of which is stupor, movement and speech are slowed. … A catatonic psychotic state is more frequently depression than schizophrenia. …"	Catatonic symptoms associate with depression

12.3 Disorganized Subtype

Although disorganization/disorganized, like catatonia, is both a DSM diagnostic criterion and a subtype of schizophrenia, this symptom is a hallmark of moderate to severe mania (Tables 2.3, 2.4, 2.5, 3.4, 12.1). Distractibility, an established criterion of mania, readily leads to disorganization and psychosis (Sect. 12.5, Case numbers 7, 9, 10). Distractibility leading to disorganization in mania has been theorized on the basis of a defective selective attention mechanism (Chap. 13). Although disorganized is to be eliminated as a subtype in the DSM-5, it is being retained as a core diagnostic criterion of schizophrenia as though "disorganization" was disease specific.

12.4 Paranoid Subtype, i.e., Hallucinations and Delusions: Paranoia Hides the Grandiosity and Guilt of Psychotic Mood Disorders

Delusional paranoia has been associated with severe mental illness for some 2,000 years, and until the twentieth century, the mental illness was a mood disorder called manic-depressive insanity (Table 3.2). Kraepelin linked paranoia and mood when he used the term "paranoid depression" in the 1800s to describe an illness with a high rate of suicide, severe depression, paranoia, and auditory hallucinations. Kraepelin wrote a book titled *Manic Depressive Insanity and Paranoia* (Kraepelin 1921/1976). In 1905, Specht said that all psychoses were derived from mood abnormalities (Specht 1905). In addition, certain authors in the UK associated paranoia with depression and delusional guilt (Doran et al. 1986). According to Beck (1967, 1972), 46% of severely depressed patients believed themselves to be sinners or criminals deserving punishments such as torture or hanging which they feared surely awaited them. Some thought they were imprisoned as punishment, but they were actually in the hospital.

One group in the 1970s implied that about 95% of their sample of patients diagnosed with paranoid schizophrenia actually suffered from mania (Abrams et al. 1974). Despite these linkages of paranoia and psychosis with mood disorders, the concepts of Bleuler, Schneider, and even Kraepelin, who associated paranoia and all psychoses to schizophrenia, prevailed, and such cases typically have been diagnosed as paranoid schizophrenia or postschizophrenic depression, not as psychotic mood disorders (Abrams et al. 1974; Doran et al. 1986; Lake and Hurwitz 2006a, b; Lake 2008a, b). Paranoia continues to be associated with schizophrenia rather than with a mood disorder, both as the most common subtype and as a core diagnostic symptom incorporating delusions and hallucinations, as reflected in the current DSM-IV-TR (Tables 2.5, 12.1), the ICD, and major textbooks of psychiatry (APA, DSM 2000). However, when mood disorders are explored as a source of paranoia, a different causal relationship presents itself (Fig. 12.2).

12.4 Paranoid Subtype, i.e., Hallucinations and Delusions...

```
PSYCHOTIC DEPRESSION → DELUSIONAL GUILT OF PAST "SINS" → PUNISHMENT DESERVED AND IMMINENT ↘
PSYCHOTIC MANIA → DELUSIONAL GRANDIOSITY: POSSESSIONS OF WEALTH, KNOWLEDGE, FAME, STATUS, ETC → OTHERS WILLING TO KILL FOR THESE POSSESSIONS ↙
                  → PARANOID PSYCHOSIS FROM PSYCHOTIC MOOD DISORDERS
```

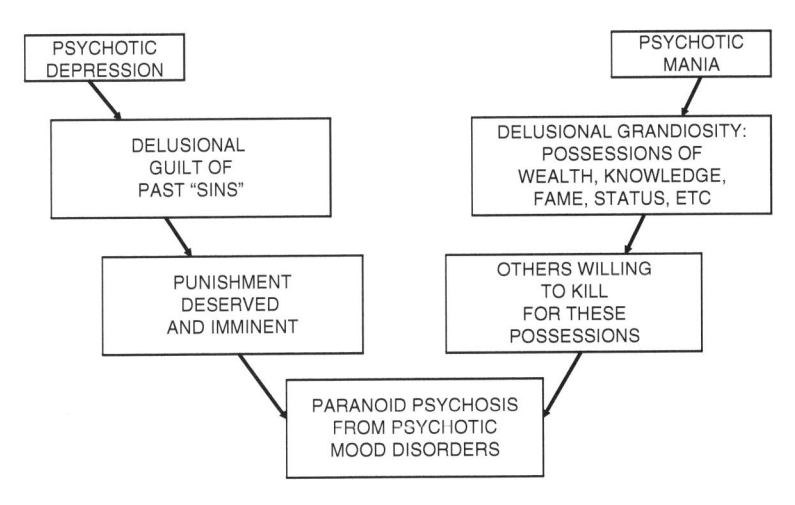

Fig. 12.2 Paranoia hides guilt and grandiosity: Psychotic mood disorders cause paranoid delusions

Psychotic depression can cause delusions of exaggerated severity of past "sins" leading to delusional guilt. Such guilt stimulates thoughts that punishment is deserved and imminent. The fear of punishment, torture, and/or execution defines the paranoid psychosis that consumes these patients' lives.

Similarly, psychotic mania can cause delusional grandiosity of ownership of valuable possessions. A logical result is the delusional belief that others want these possessions and are going to kill to get them, leading to paranoid psychosis. Since these patients present with complaints of fear for their lives, the core symptoms of the mood disorder may be overlooked, and a misdiagnosis of paranoid schizophrenia made

Two common mood-based symptoms, grandiosity and guilt, underlie the development of paranoia in certain psychotic patients. Mania explains paranoia when grandiose delusions involve beliefs that one's possessions or knowledge are so valuable that others are willing to kill for them. Similarly, depression explains paranoia when delusional guilt and sin convinces patients that they deserve punishment that is feared (Fig. 12.2) (Beck 1967, 1972; Lake 2008b). Patient and physician focus on paranoia rather than underlying mood symptoms can mislead the initial diagnostic process causing the misdiagnosis of paranoid schizophrenia (Lake 2008b). Since paranoid schizophrenia is by far the most common subtype, if psychotic mood disorders explain many paranoid presentations, as suspected over 30 years ago (Abrams et al. 1974; Doran et al. 1986), substantial questions are raised about the validity of any distinction between schizophrenia and psychotic mood disorders (Table 12.4; Fig. 12.2) (Abrams et al. 1974; Pope and Lipinski 1978; Schurhoff et al. 2003; Schulze et al. 2005; Lake and Hurwitz, 2006a, b, 2007a, b; Maier 2006; Maier et al. 2006; Lake 2008b, 2010a).

Recent molecular genetic studies show considerable overlap and similarities between schizophrenia and psychotic bipolar disorder (Sect. 11.3.6; Table 11.8) (Berrettini 2000, 2003a, b; Schurhoff et al. 2003; Hodgkinson et al. 2004; Schumacher et al. 2004; Craddock et al. 2005; Craddock and Owen 2005; Green et al. 2005;

Schulze et al. 2005; Fawcett 2005; Maziade et al. 2005; Maier et al. 2006; Williams et al. 2006). The symptom of paranoia, in particular, has been the focus of genetic studies. For example, familial aggregation data reveal that paranoid delusional proneness is an endophenotype common to patients diagnosed with "schizophrenia" and psychotic bipolar but not nonpsychotic bipolar (Schurhoff et al. 2003). Two years later, Schulze et al. (2005) extended this work by linking persecutory delusions (paranoia) to variance at a specific locus, the D-amino acid oxidase activator (DAOA/G30), located on chromosome 13q34, in patients diagnosed with "schizophrenia" and with psychotic bipolar disorder (Schulze et al. 2005). More recent results link this locus primarily to mood disorders "across the traditional bipolar and schizophrenia categories" (Williams et al. 2006). Such genotypic overlap, when considered with the phenotypic similarities, suggests the hypothesis that paranoid schizophrenia is a psychotic mood disorder and not a separate disorder.

The following cases of 12 patients, most initially diagnosed with schizophrenia, paranoid type, but subsequently revealed to suffer from a psychotic bipolar or unipolar disorder, serve to illustrate these ideas (Table 12.4).

12.5 Case Summaries of Psychotic Mood Disorders Misdiagnosed as Schizophrenia, Paranoid Subtype

The subjects whose cases are discussed gave their written informed consents to participate in this IRB-approved research.

Case 1

A 58-year-old Vietnamese veteran living in a suburban neighborhood presented to the emergency department (ED) in handcuffs accompanied by police. He reported to the interviewing psychiatrist that he had nailed shut his doors and windows except for small slits through which he "planned to fire on attacking CIA operatives." Having amassed numerous small arms weapons including an illegal, fully automatic machine gun, he brought attention to himself by placing multiple calls to CIA headquarters in Langley, VA, "to get them to lay off" and finally by spraying automatic gunfire through his attic because he thought "they had gotten into the attic."

The patient's resistance in the ED necessitated involuntary commitment. On the unit, he was agitated, fearful, avoiding eye contact, and communication. His fear was that "They are trying to eliminate me!," and his affect was appropriate to his persecutory delusions. He refused to cooperate with providing further history or taking anything by mouth because he feared he would be poisoned. He was diagnosed with schizophrenia, paranoid type. After 3 days of IM haloperidol (Haldol) 10 mg bid, he began to eat and drink as well as to reluctantly cooperate with the staff, providing further history.

12.5 Case Summaries of Psychotic Mood Disorders Misdiagnosed... 251

This individual said that he had led illegal US government operations in Cambodia during the Vietnam war and had become convinced that the CIA intended to eliminate him for fear he would publish his memoirs. He said that during the past 2 weeks, he had called the CIA over 300 times, frequently between midnight and 4 a.m. Further, he said he had not slept or eaten for fear of "getting overrun" and had lost over 15 lb. He admitted that his thoughts had been racing. The patient said a war buddy he had called told him to slow down and had finally hung up on him. He had stopped using his telephone for calls other than the CIA for fear of wiretaps.

His diagnosis was changed to bipolar disorder, type I, manic, severe with psychotic features. Lithium was rapidly titrated to a therapeutic blood level and effectively stabilized his mood over 2 weeks. In subsequent outpatient follow-up, the patient revealed that he had a paternal uncle who had previously been diagnosed with bipolar disorder, type I and was also taking lithium.

Case 2

Prior to the fall of the Soviet Union, a 48-year-old divorced senior aerospace engineer officer in the air force presented to military police (MP) afraid for his life and with his briefcase chained to his wrist. He was escorted by the MPs to the hospital ED where the intake psychiatrist found that his chief complaint was that the KGB and the NSA were following him and planned to "erase him." He tried to leave the ED when he became suspicious of the interviewing physician. He was restrained by the MPs and forcibly admitted to the locked unit. With affect of agitation and paranoia, he was prescribed an antipsychotic combined with a benzodiazepine. His physician contacted his military unit, learning of the patient's AWOL status for over 2 months, his rank as an officer, and his high-level security clearance. After 2 days on the unit, he admitted that he had "gone underground," had moved every 2–3 days, and had not reported for duty in order to escape assassination. He claimed to have received coded messages from the TV over the previous 3–4 weeks, telling him that he was in danger of attack by the KGB "who had conspired with the NSA to eliminate him." He was diagnosed with schizophrenia, paranoid type.

Subsequently, the patient said he had slept very little for the past 2 months because he had been working 20–24 h everyday and had developed a "Star Wars" ICBM interceptor system. A secret pocket of his briefcase contained several hundred pages of neatly drawn formulas, calculations, and scale drawings of his system. He believed the KGB was working with the NSA and planned to kill him and steal the plans. He had attempted to call the president, Ronald Reagan. He endorsed losing weight, racing thoughts, no need for sleep, and increased energy during the previous two and one-half months. He had suffered two episodes of major depression in the past and several hypomanic episodes when he became more productive. He was given carbamazepine (Tegretol) which was appropriately titrated, and his diagnosis was changed to bipolar disorder, type I, manic, severe with psychotic features.

Case 3

A 28-year-old Eastern European single male, working as a microbiology technician, was brought to the ED by his parents. He tried to leave the ED, became assaultive, was forcibly restrained, and was admitted involuntarily. On the unit, he was mute, fearful, and socially withdrawn. He paced the floors, refusing food, water, or medicine because of his fear of poison. His lab work and physical exam revealed marked dehydration. He suffered a major motor seizure, but subsequent neurologic work-up was negative, and the seizure was attributed to his electrolyte imbalance. He was given IM antipsychotic medication and was forced to take IV fluid. The patient was diagnosed with schizophrenia, paranoid type.

A medical student elicited the patient's history from his parents. They said that he had not slept for at least 2 weeks, had stopped going to work, and was working on his computer 24/7. They said he had appeared distracted, frightened, and suspicious but was noncommunicative about whatever was bothering him. After several days on the unit, the patient said he feared for his life because "God selected me as a prophet." He said Al-Qaeda operatives had found out about his "high Christian religious position" and intended to kill him on September 11, 2002. This delusion may have related to his having been in New York a year earlier. The patient believed that Al Qaeda intended to send him anthrax and that he would die and be blamed for the resultant holocaust. He admitted that he suspected that the staff on the inpatient unit had been infiltrated by Al-Qaeda operatives. It was learned that his maternal grandmother had suffered several "psychotic breakdowns." His diagnosis was changed to bipolar disorder, type I, manic, severe with psychotic features, and a mood-stabilizing medication was prescribed.

Case 4

A 29-year-old Hispanic single male musician, of Cuban descent, presented to the ED in police custody. Saying that he feared for his life, he became suspicious of ED staff and seemed to be attending to unobserved external stimuli. He was admitted involuntarily when he became aggressive because he was restrained from leaving the ED. He was diagnosed with schizophrenia, paranoid type and medicated with IM antipsychotics.

As his psychosis resolved, the patient began to cooperate, revealing that he believed he possessed the recording of a song he had composed and performed that was "worth millions of dollars." He believed the Cuban Mafia wanted the recording for the profit it would generate and was justifying their crime because his lyrics were anti-Castro in tone. Two weeks before his admission, he had begun staying up all night, vigilant to protect himself, and was getting signals from the television and radio warning him that the Cuban Mafia had located him. He had moved several times. The patient was apprehended after striking a passerby on the street who he believed was a Cuban agent about to kill him. As in the preceding cases, this patient's diagnosis and medications were appropriately changed with effective mood stabilization.

Case 5

A 48-year-old Columbian unemployed college graduate with a major in chemistry presented to the ED in a disheveled, unshaven, and unbathed state. He said he had been fleeing from Cali Cartel agents for over 6 months, and when he sought protection from the police, they had told him to come to the ED. He was disorganized and suspicious, appearing to address unseen external stimuli. He was admitted voluntarily and diagnosed with schizophrenia, paranoid type.

More careful interviews with him revealed that the reason behind his fears was his belief that he had developed a formula to cheaply produce a very potent narcotic. His synthetic drug would eliminate the need to grow opium or coca. He believed the Cali Cartel had discovered his invention and had sent agents to torture and kill him for the formula. He knew the names of the Cartel bosses and discussed them as if they were intimate acquaintances. He had not slept for days, fleeing the cartel's agents. Again, the diagnosis was changed.

Case 6

The police escorted a 56-year-old unemployed house painter to the ED, and he was voluntarily admitted to the psychiatric locked ward because "the devil is coming to take me away." A passerby called the police after seeing a man standing suspiciously on a bridge. Claiming that he deserved to die, he wanted to jump to his death before the devil got him. He was unshaven, unclean, and emaciated. On the unit, his affect remained terrified, tearful, and suspicious; he would not accept anything by mouth. He said he heard voices of the devil and God arguing over who should kill him. He said that he heard the devil say that he was "coming up the hospital stairs" and "had corrupted the nursing staff." He was diagnosed with schizophrenia, paranoid type, or postschizophrenic depression and forcibly treated with IM haloperidol (Haldol).

As he began to improve, he endorsed the symptoms of a major depressive episode that had escalated over the prior 8 months. He repeatedly said that he deserved to die for a past "sin." He asked for help to die in order to prevent "falling into the hands of the devil." Several days later, he revealed that his "sin" was stealing five dollars from the gas station where he worked when he was 15 years old. He said he had had "a first date with a girlfriend and no money," and he had never paid the five dollars back. His diagnosis was changed to major depressive disorder, severe with psychotic features, and he was given amitriptyline (Elavil) in addition to the haloperidol.

Nine months later, he was readmitted in handcuffs. His wife had called the sheriff after a dump truck entirely filled their front yard with 10,000 fresh oysters in the shell. The patient exhibited racing thoughts, pressed speech, irritability and said he had not slept "for weeks" while planning a party for the state legislature and governor. His diagnosis and medications were changed again. Lithium stabilized his mood. The implications of his misdiagnoses and inappropriate pharmacotherapy are discussed below.

Case 7

A 28-year-old single, never married male was escorted to the ED by law enforcement officers after neighbors reported his bizarre behavior. He had been kneeling motionless on his mother's front lawn and had remained in a stiff kneeling position (catatonic) when the police picked him up. He said the "hit men" hidden across the street had aimed "deadly ray guns all around me so that if I moved an inch, I was dead." He said the "hit men" had been after him for over a year but had recently picked up his trail, and his execution was imminent. He was college educated but worked menial jobs, had always lived with his mother, and described himself as a "loner." On the second night of his inpatient stay, the staff found him cowered in the far corner of his room, naked having smeared his feces in his hair, face, and mouth. He later said that he did this to get himself transferred to the state hospital because the staff at the academic medical center had been "infiltrated by the hit men." He was diagnosed as schizophrenic, paranoid type.

As his psychosis began to resolve, he volunteered for a student interview course where he revealed that 3 years prior to his admission he had suffered a major depressive episode followed by a hypomanic period when he began to think that ownership of a local bank was going to be transferred to him. Over the ensuing months, his delusional ownership of the bank became more concretized. He began to make plans about the use of his newfound wealth. He outlined several million dollars of purchases that included a specific mansion, a villa in France, and six cars. He said he had planned on running for governor of the state. Over the weeks before his admission, he said he could not sleep and had become terrified when he heard the voice of God warning him of danger from the hit men who were "closing in to kill me so that they could have the bank for themselves." His diagnosis and medications were changed.

Case 8

A 48-year-old female unemployed lawyer presented to the ED frightened for her life and unable to stop sobbing. She would not commit to safety saying that she deserved to die but was afraid. She had tried to escape punishment by not leaving her room for the past 2 weeks. She held a strong faith in God but believed He had told her that she would be punished and executed because she was a "worthless failure." She wanted to take her own life rather than continuing to suffer the knowledge that she would soon be tortured and killed. The patient said that over the past several months God had frequently kept up a running commentary on her activities, often threatening that her end was near. Because of her extensive auditory hallucinations, especially of God's voice "keeping up a running commentary"—one of Schneider's first-rank, pathognomonic symptoms of schizophrenia—she was diagnosed with schizophrenia, paranoid type.

As her condition improved, she said her father, also a lawyer, had named her after a famous lawyer and had influenced her to go to law school against her wishes. After graduation, she was fired from several law firms because of episodes of depression.

12.5 Case Summaries of Psychotic Mood Disorders Misdiagnosed... 255

She considered herself an overwhelming failure, having let God and her family down. Over the past 6 months, she began to believe that she had a special relationship with God to "save the world from evil" and to make up for her failures as a lawyer. As she became more and more involved in charity work, she lost her menial but paying job and believed that another failure mandated her death. Because of a history of hypomanic episodes, her diagnosis was changed to bipolar disorder, type II, depressed, severe with psychotic features. Lamotragine (Lamectal) was prescribed with stabilizing effects.

Case 9

This obese 54-year-old female artist from NYC was taken into custody in the Chicago airport by law enforcement officers after her loud warnings of the imminent assassination of President Reagan and herself. In the ED, she became aggressive and was admitted involuntarily. Upon admission, she was frightened for her life from "rogue CIA and Cuban agents" who she believed were plotting to kill her and the president. God had warned her in the airport that the CIA agents had followed her from New York. The patient believed that she received instructions through the TV and on one occasion had thrown a bucket of water over a new television set shorting it out to stop the voices coming from the TV. She was diagnosed with chronic paranoid schizophrenia since her records revealed over ten prior admissions with this diagnosis.

After several days, her fear was obscured by uncharacteristic irritability and anger. She did not sleep until medicated with antipsychotic drugs. She revealed her delusional involvement in an elaborate scheme that included the jewels of the Queen of Spain worth "millions of dollars," Fidel Castro, and President Reagan. Her delusions may have been seeded by the facts that she had visited Cuba and Spain as a small child and that a distant cousin held a low-level position at the CIA. The patient endorsed for the past 6 months a lack of need for sleep, racing thoughts, irritability, and increased activities. She had been similarly grandiose prior to past hospitalizations. She suffered with tardive dyskinesia, having been given IM injections of fluphenazine (Prolixin) monthly for over two decades. Again, her diagnosis and treatment were changed on the basis of her disease-specific grandiosity and other core diagnostic symptoms of mania.

Case 10

A 62-year-old widowed, unemployed female, found on the street inappropriately hiding behind a car and wearing a white sheet, was escorted to the ED by law enforcement. She appeared to be fearful and was carrying on an incomprehensible, running "conversation" with no obvious interlocutor. She was admitted involuntarily. Her daughter, an RN, said that her mother feared for her life from "anti-Jewish foreign agents" who she believed intended to assassinate her. She said that her mother moved frequently, sometimes weekly, and in the middle of the night and often slept on the street to get away from the agents. She learned when she was safe and when the agents had discovered her new residence by way of coded TV and radio messages. The patient's daughter said her mother had behaved in this manner for decades. She was diagnosed with schizophrenia, paranoid type.

Further history from the daughter revealed that the patient often did not sleep more than an hour or two per night over months to years because she "had to write critical letters" to her US government handlers. Saying that she held a US State Department undercover position as a "foreign affairs advisor" and was tasked for the "protection of the Jewish race," she had written hundreds if not thousands of multipage letters to the state department. Her daughter described her as never depressed but constantly vigilant, hyper, grandiose, and suspicious. The patient believed she had been involved in the J.F. Kennedy assassination. Her diagnosis, too, was changed to bipolar disorder, type I.

Case 11

This 36-year-old multiply divorced female nurse was brought by ambulance to the ED unconscious, having overdosed. After 3 days on a ventilator and 3 more days in the ICU, she was transferred to psychiatry. There, she said she wanted to die at her own hands rather than be executed by law enforcement. She believed her death was imminent. She had suddenly stopped going to work for fear of being apprehended and arrested. She had suffered multiple hospitalizations, all with the diagnosis of chronic paranoid schizophrenia, which was assigned at this admission as well. Postschizophrenic depression was also considered.

The patient said that once her incompetence was discovered by her hospital administration, she would be prosecuted and executed for murder. She felt she deserved to be punished but was afraid of her execution. Her "crime" involved the death of a 4-year-old child suffering from terminal leukemia and under her hospice care. Upon careful questioning, the patient admitted to past episodes of decreased need for sleep, increased activities, racing thoughts, the ability to work three jobs at once without fatigue, and poor decisions with potential for dangerous outcomes. These episodes lasted several months and were usually followed by severe depressions. Her diagnosis was changed to bipolar disorder, type I, depressed, severe with psychotic features.

Case 12

This 39-year-old Latino journalist presented to the ED saying he was going to be assassinated by the CIA or the FBI (Jaffee 2005). He said he had avoided mirrors because "they might be see-through" and that he received messages from both the TV and the radio that indicated his imminent execution. He had fled his home because he believed his wife was a CIA spy. Having recently read an article about the detrimental effects of toxic fumes on the brain, he avoided car washes and tire

Table 12.4 Case summaries of psychotic mood disorders misdiagnosed as schizophrenia

Case#	Age/sex, job	Emergency department presentation	Initial symptoms	Initial diagnosis	Subsequent symptoms	Specific causes of Paranoia	Actual patient experience ("thread of truth")	Final diagnosis
1	58/M, unemployed day laborer	Handcuffed, paranoid, fearful, agitated, resistant, involuntary	Feared elimination by CIA, poison	Paranoid schizophrenia	Decreased sleep with increased activities, grandiosity, lost 20 pounds due to "no time to eat," made over 300 phone calls to the CIA often between midnight and 4 a.m.	Believed he possessed critical knowledge about the Vietnam war that was embarrassing to the US government who had sent the CIA to eliminate him.	Had fought in Vietnam	BP-I manic, severe with[a]
2	48/M, military officer	Escorted by MPs, involuntary	Feared for his life from assassination by KGB and NSA, coded messages from TV	Paranoid schizophrenia	Decreased sleep with increased activities, grandiosity, called President Reagan.	Believed he had a "Star Wars" missile design that the KGB & NSA wanted.	Was a rocket engineer	BP-I manic, severe with[a]
3	28/M, microbiology technician	Restrained in E.D., involuntary	Feared his murder by Al-Qaeda was imminent, feared poison	Paranoid schizophrenia	Decreased sleep with increased activities, worked on his computer 24/7 for weeks, grandiosity, marked weight loss due to fear of poison.	Believed God had named him as a prophet and that Al-Qaeda would assassinate him with anthrax.	Was a microbiologist and in NY on 9/11/01	BP-I manic, severe with[a]
4	29/M, musician	Police escort, delusional, paranoia, violent, restrained, involuntary	Feared execution by Cuban Mafia, messages from TV and radio	Paranoid schizophrenia	Decreased sleep with increased activities, grandiose.	Believed he had a recording worth millions that the Cuban Mafia wanted.	Was a Cuban musician who supported the anti-Castro effort	BP-I manic, severe with[a]
5	48/M, biochemist	Voluntary, delusional, paranoia	Feared execution by Cali Cartel	Paranoid schizophrenia	Decreased sleep with increased activities, fleeing for his life, grandiose.	Believed he possessed a formula to make synthetic narcotics so the Cali Cartel wanted it and him dead.	Was from Columbia, SA and a chemistry major	BP-I manic, severe with[a]

(continued)

Table 12.4 (continued)

Case#	Age/sex, job	Emergency department presentation	Initial symptoms	Initial diagnosis	Subsequent symptoms	Specific causes of Paranoia	Actual patient experience ("thread of truth")	Final diagnosis
6	56/M, unemployed house painter	Delusional paranoia, suicidal, voluntary	Feared death at the hands of the devil and God, feared poison	Paranoid schizophrenia, postschizophrenic depression	Psychotic, suicidal depression followed by psychotic mania when he ordered 10,000 oysters in the shells for a party for the governor of the state of NC.	Believed he had sinned over 40 years before and deserved torture and death by God and the devil, believed he was friends with the governor.	Did steal $5 from his boss' gas station at 15 years of age	MDD, severe with[b], then BP-I, manic, severe with[a]
7	28/M, fast food restaurant worker	Handcuffs, catatonia, delusional paranoia	Feared his execution by "hit men," poison	Paranoid schizophrenia	Decreased sleep with increased activities, disorganization due to racing thoughts, grandiosity, premeditated coprophilia with a purpose to get transferred.	Believed he was to gain ownership of his bank but "hit men" were sent to kill him to get the bank for themselves.	Did make trips to the bank on a regular basis for his mom	BP-I manic, severe with[a]
8	48/F, unemployed lawyer	Delusional paranoia, voluntary	Auditory hallucinations keeping up a running commentary	Paranoid schizophrenia	Psychotic, suicidal depression, delusional guilt, persecutory delusions, history of hypomanic episodes.	Believed she was such a failure that she deserved torture and death, then feared her torture and death.	Lost several legal positions and then was fired from even menial jobs	BP-II, depressed, severe with[a]
9	54/F, artist	Police escort, delusional paranoia, involuntary	Feared "rogue CIA and Cuban agents" trying to kill her, messages from TV	Paranoid schizophrenia	Decreased sleep with increased activities, had flown from NY to Chicago at last minute, extensive grandiosity.	Complex grandiose delusional system incorporating the jewels of the Queen of Spain, Fidel Castro, and the assassination of President Reagan.	Had visited Spain and Cuba and had a distant relative with a low-level CIA position	BP-I, manic, severe with[a]

10	62/F, unemployed	Police escort, delusional paranoia, involuntary	Feared her imminent assassination by "anti-Jewish foreign agents"	Paranoid schizophrenia	Decreased sleep with extensive writing to the US Dept of State for 20–24 h a day for several weeks.	Believed she was an undercover "foreign affairs advisor" for the US State Dept tasked to protect the Jewish people.	Had held a low-level job in the US government	BP-I, manic, severe with[a]
11	36/F, nurse	Ambulance, unconscious due to overdose	Feared her capture by law-enforcement, sentencing to death and execution	Paranoid schizophrenia or postschizo- phrenic depression	Psychotic suicidal depression.	Believed she had "murdered" by neglect a terminal, 4-year-old patient under her care in hospice.	Had lost such a patient under her hospice care	BP-I, depressed, severe with[a]
12	39/M, journalist	Delusional paranoia, voluntary	Feared assassination by CIA or FBI, messages from TV and radio	Met criteria for paranoid schizophrenia	Mixed symptoms of psychotic, suicidal depression along with racing thoughts, decreased sleep with increased activities such as uncharacteristically walking 20 miles to escape harm.	Complex grandiose delusional system involving his assassination by the CIA and the FBI, messages from the TV and radio.	Was a journalist and expanded the subjects of some of his readings	BP-I, mixed, severe with[a]

[a]BP-I, manic, severe, with is bipolar type I, manic, severe with psychotic features
[b]MDD, severe, with is major depressive disorder, severe with psychotic features

dealerships to "avoid the chemical sprays" which he believed the perpetrators were designing to "destroy my memory." This presentation is consistent with the DSM criteria for schizophrenia, paranoid type. More detailed history revealed symptoms of both psychotic depression and mania with positive suicidal ideation and racing thoughts, a lack of need for sleep, increased energy, marked distractibility and excessive walking for miles to escape harm. He endorsed auditory hallucinations, and his delusional system was diverse. His diagnosis was most likely bipolar disorder, type I, mixed, severe with psychotic features.

12.6 Paranoid Schizophrenia Is a Psychotic Mood Disorder

These 12 cases clarify the idea that a core disturbance of mood is associated with delusional paranoia (Tables 12.4, 12.5). In contrast to the concept of Bleuler and Schneider, but as previously suggested (Specht 1905; Beck 1967, 1972; Doran et al. 1986; Lake 2008a,b), delusional guilt, usually due to severe depression, underlies the belief that punishment is deserved and imminent, but this is mixed with intense fear for survival (Fig. 12.2). Cases 6, 8, 11, and 12 are examples (Table 12.4).

Table 12.5 Symptoms indicating a psychotic mood disorder not schizophrenia in functionally psychotic patients

1. Paranoia (fear for one's life: punishment, poison, torture, execution)
2. Delusional grandiosity (valuable possessions)
3. Delusional guilt (past sins)
4. Persecution by high-profile groups (FBI, CIA, KGB, IRS, God, the devil, etc.)
5. Psychosis without organic cause (both mood-congruent and mood-incongruent hallucinations and/or delusions)
6. Atypical increase in goal-directed behavior/activities especially involving "spur of the moment" decisions: religious, legal, political, sexual activities, cleaning, phoning, writing, loud music, partying, travel
7. Atypical increase in emotion: anger, elation, irritability, intrusiveness, sadness, emotional flatness and withdrawal, crying, suicidality
8. Absence of pleasure and/or emotion (depression): anhedonia, flat affect, avolition, alogia
9. Behavior causing disturbance: police called, assaultive, loud, neighbor's complaints
10. History of major depression or mania/hypomania
11. Family history of bipolar or major depression
12. DSM criteria for bipolar, manic, depressed or mixed
13. Good premorbid or current social life: school officer, sports, gangs, dated, past long-term relationship, formally married, children

Table 12.6 Sources of paranoid delusional threats that suggest grandiosity of mania

FBI
CIA
NSA
IRS
KGB
Mafia
God
The devil
The police
The boss
The supervisor
The landlord
The government
The president
Politicians

Just as psychotic depression can lead to guilt-induced paranoia, manic grandiosity readily proceeds to paranoia and fear for one's life (Fig. 12.2). Cases 1–5, 7, 9, and 10 demonstrate that mania can lead to grandiose delusions of ownership of possessions of exaggerated value. The fear for survival, i.e., paranoid delusions, develops and escalates as patients begin to believe others are willing to inflict harm or kill them to gain their possessions or knowledge (Fig. 12.2). The significance of those imagined to be threatening, such as the FBI, CIA, IRS, KGB, the Mafia, God, or the devil, is an indication of grandiosity and of mania (Tables 12.4, 12.6).

Although these cases presented over a 40-year period, there are several commonalities. Each patient was admitted while experiencing an intense, delusional fear for his/her life. The majority were escorted to the ED by law enforcement, were handcuffed, or were involuntarily committed. Patient aggression and restraint were frequently due to a broadening paranoia that the ED or ward staff were part of the plot to kill them. At least four cases feared they would be poisoned. Case 7 engaged in coprophagia in order to get himself transferred to the state hospital to escape the "infiltrated" academic ward staff. Coprophilia and coprophagia, traditionally considered pathognomonic of schizophrenia, can occur in psychotic mood disorders as shown in case 7 and noted in the literature (Carlson and Goodwin 1973). At presentation, patient focus was on self-preservation, and these patients volunteered no mood symptoms, and questions about mood were apparently inadequate. The overwhelming paranoid psychoses consistently led to misdiagnoses of schizophrenia, paranoid type (Table 12.4). However, the acquisition of additional history by various means in each case revealed mood-based symptoms that led to the delusional paranoia and a change of diagnosis to one of a mood disorder, severe with psychotic features. Several "take-home messages" are given in Table 12.7.

Table 12.7 Take home messages for the diagnosis of psychotic patients

1. Depression causes paranoia through delusional guilt, feelings of deserved punishment, then fears of persecution, torture, and execution.
2. Manic grandiosity causes paranoia through delusions of ownership of a valuable possession followed by fears of persecution by others to gain the valued article.
3. Such patients complain only of their fears (paranoia), not their guilt or grandiosity.
4. For interviewing psychiatrists, explore for mood symptoms in psychotic patients, avoid focus on the "paranoia" and pursue symptoms of psychotic mood disorders.
5. A resultant misdiagnosis of paranoid schizophrenia in psychotic mood disorder patients results in inappropriate treatment putting patients and physicians at risk.
6. The functional psychoses, traditionally explained by three diseases, may be accounted for by only one, a psychotic mood disorder.

12.7 Undifferentiated Subtype

The history of the undifferentiated subtype of schizophrenia dates at least to the publication of the DSM-I (APA, DSM 1952) if not before. In the DSM-I, the undifferentiated subtype was further divided into an acute reaction versus a chronic reaction, and both were described as exhibiting "… a wide variety of schizophrenic symptomatology … a mixed symptomatology …" that did not fit into any of the other subtypes.

In the DSM-II (APA, DSM 1968), only the chronic undifferentiated subtype was retained and was described for patients showing "…mixed schizophrenic symptoms and who present definite schizophrenic thought, affect and behavior …" not better fitting another subtype.

In the DSM-III (APA, DSM 1980), specific diagnostic criteria were given that included "prominent delusions, hallucinations, incoherence, or grossly disorganized behavior… [that] does not meet the criteria for any of the previously listed types…"

There were no significant changes through the DSM-III-R (APA, DSM 1987), DSM-IV (APA, DSM 1994), or the DSM-IV-TR (APA, DSM 2000).

However, the DSM-5 proposal (APA, DSM 2013) intends to eliminate all subtypes to include this one.

12.8 The Positive and Negative Symptoms of Schizophrenia

Possibly as a response to the accumulating data showing the high prevalence of the positive symptoms of hallucinations, delusions, disorganization, and catatonia in psychotic mood disorders and their disease nonspecificity through the 1970s and 1980s (Chap. 10, 11; Tables 1.1, 10.1, 11.2), more recently investigators in schizophrenia seemed to reemphasize the diagnostic importance of the negative symptoms in schizophrenia (Fischer and Carpenter 2009) (Fig. 12.1). The DSM-IV (APA, DSM 1994) officially recognized the term "negative symptoms." This is reflected by an increasing number of PubMed cites of the negative symptoms of schizophrenia from the mid-1980s and continuing through the present (Fig. 12.3).

Carpenter and his co-workers have been proponents of differentiating schizophrenia based in part on the presence of the DSM's "negative symptoms" (Fischer and Carpenter 2009). They credit Kraepelin and Bleuler with initiating the concept of a negative symptom complex of schizophrenia. Kraepelin (1919/1971) considered two areas of psychopathology in patients with dementia praecox: (1) disorganization of thought and behavior that he called "dissociative pathology" and (2) avolition that he described as "…a weakening of the wellsprings of volition." Bleuler's fundamental features (1911/1950) included some of the current negative symptoms considered diagnostic of schizophrenia today. Fischer and Carpenter (2009) referred to "A long-term course [as] also discriminating [schizophrenia from bipolar disorder]." Fischer and Carpenter (2009), as had Kraepelin (1919), equate negative symptoms with "deficit" or "nuclear" schizophrenia as distinct from a psychotic mood disorder. Others have observed some once classic psychotic mood-disordered patients digress to this same chronic, persistent, treatment-resistant psychotic state (Carlson and Goodwin 1973; Goodwin 1989; Post 1992, 2010).

12.8.1 The Positive Symptoms

Academic psychiatry in the US interpreted Bleuler's teachings that his accessory or positive symptoms, i.e., hallucinations and/or delusions were not necessary for the diagnosis, although, if present, mandated the diagnosis of schizophrenia. His fundamental symptoms that encompassed some of the negative symptoms were broadly applied to the diagnosis of schizophrenia so that the positive symptoms received less diagnostic emphasis for decades following Bleuler's 1911 publication (Fig. 12.1). The positive symptoms regained prominence with the publication of the DSM-III in 1980 because simple schizophrenia was dropped, and delusions, hallucinations, incoherence, and catatonia or other grossly disorganized behavior became critical as symptoms diagnostic of schizophrenia. In fact, hallucinations and delusions became understood as synonymous with the diagnosis of schizophrenia and, when present, reduced or eliminated the consideration of mood disorders. Beginning in the 1970s and continuing through the present, an increasing number of authors recognized that these positive symptoms "of schizophrenia" were common to severe mood disorders, yet the positive symptoms have continued as the core diagnostic symptoms for the DSM diagnosis of schizophrenia largely unchanged through the proposed DSM-5. Possibly as a result of recognition of overlap in the positive symptoms between schizophrenia and psychotic mood disorders and in an effort to maintain separation between schizophrenia and mood disorders over the past two decades, the negative symptoms have regained prominence again in the diagnosis of schizophrenia (Fig. 12.1).

The positive symptoms are synonymous with the subtypes of schizophrenia that are discussed in detail above in this chapter and are scheduled for deletion from the DSM-5.

12.8.2 The Negative Symptoms

According to Makinen et al. (2008), the

> Negative symptoms refer to the weakening or lack of normal thoughts, emotions or behavior in schizophrenia patients. Their prevalence in first-episode psychosis is high, 50-90%, and 20-40% of schizophrenia patients have persisting negative symptoms. Severe negative symptoms during the early stages of treatment predict poor prognosis.

The first statement is striking in speaking of a "weakening... of normal thoughts..." as contributing to any diagnosis, especially one as ominous as schizophrenia. This terminology was used by Morel, Kraepelin, and Bleuler a century ago. Patients with psychotic depression suffer the "negative symptoms of schizophrenia" with a prevalence surely as high if not higher than the percentages noted above by Makinen et al. (2008). Psychotic mood-disordered patients have a striking "... weakening or lack of normal thoughts, emotions, and behavior." These prevalence figures suggest that a high percent of patients with psychotic depression are misdiagnosed as having schizophrenia (Swartz and Shorter 2007).

Before Bleuler (1911), there was little attention given to negative symptoms. Schizophrenia was defined by positive symptoms, i.e., psychosis, hallucinations, or delusions and a chronic course. Although Bleuler emphasized his fundamental symptoms as diagnostic of schizophrenia, with the publication of the DSM-III in 1980, his simple schizophrenia was dropped, and the diagnostic emphasis on his fundamental symptoms was reduced but not eliminated. One of his fundamental symptoms, a flat or restricted affect, has survived all editions of the DSM and at this point is scheduled to be included in the DSM-5 as a significant "negative" characteristic symptom of schizophrenia (Table 12.1). A second, loosening of associations continued at least until the publication of the DSM-IV in 1994. Thus, a disturbance of affect has survived as a diagnostic characteristic of schizophrenia, not mania or depression, for over 100 years. What is notable is that a disturbance in affect seems to relate to affect and mood without the need for any additional diagnosis.

The specific term "negative symptoms" has been used as a diagnostic criterion of schizophrenia in the DSM since the DSM-IV (APA, DSM 1994). With regard to the negative symptoms, there was no difference between the DSM-IV and the DSM-IV-TR (APA, DSM 2000) (Table 12.8). For the DSM-5, "restricted affect" is proposed to replace "affective flattening," "avolition" remains unchanged, and "asociality" is added. In the current DSM-IV-TR, alogia is given as one of the three negative symptoms (Table 12.1). Apparently, alogia has not been proposed for the DSM-5 and with good reason. As stated by Swartz and Shorter (2007),

> Patients with psychotic depression are typically severely behaviorally disturbed and ill. ... Some are incapable of expressing themselves accurately or coherently or even of saying anything at all.

This is alogia. Similarly avolition, asociality, and restricted or flattening of affect are also basic characteristics of moderate to severe major depression. Avolition means no motivation and an aversion to activities. Moderate to severely depressed patients typically sleep excessive hours or at least lay in bed or on the couch often

12.8 The Positive and Negative Symptoms of Schizophrenia

Table 12.8 A history of the negative symptoms of schizophrenia from Bleuler's accessory symptoms to the DSM-5

Quote #	Author	Publication (date)	Description of terms "diagnostic" of schizophrenia
1	Bleuler	Textbook (1911)	Ambivalence, affectivity[a], associations (loose), autistic thinking[b]
2	APA	DSM-I (1952)	Affective disturbances, emotional disharmony, regressive behavior, reduction in external attachments and interests[c], impoverishment of human relationships[c], apathy[d], indifference[d], shallow, inappropriate affect, stupor, mutism[e], negativism
3	APA	DSM-II (1968)	Ambivalent, constricted and inappropriate emotional responsiveness, loss of empathy with others, withdrawn or regressive behavior, a slow and insidious reduction of external attachments and interests[c], apathy and indifference leading to improvishment of interpersonal relations[c], shallow and inappropriate affect, stupor, mutism[e], negativism
4	APA	DSM-III (1980)	Loosening of associations, marked poverty of content of speech, blunted, flat or inappropriate affect
5	APA	DSM-III-R (1987)	Loosening of associations, flat or grossly inappropriate affect, marked social isolation or withdrawal[c], peculiar behavior, impairment in personal hygiene or grooming, blunted or inappropriate affect, poverty of speech or poverty of content of speech[e], odd beliefs, i.e., superstitiousness, "sixth sense," marked lack of initiative, interests or energy[d]
6	APA	DSM-IV[f] (1994)	Negative symptoms, i.e., affective flattening, alogia, avolition, inappropriate affect, extreme negativism or mutism, odd beliefs
7	APA	DSM-IV-TR (2000)	Negative symptoms, i.e., affective flattening, alogia, avolition, inappropriate affect, extreme negativism or mutism, odd beliefs
8	APA	DSM-5 (2013) (proposed revision published in 2010)	Negative symptoms, i.e., restricted affect or avolition/asociality (odd beliefs)

[a]Bleuler described the disappearance of affect, indifference, inappropriateness to content of thought, social isolation
[b]Akin to hallucinations and delusions
[c]Precursor to asociality
[d]Precursor to avolition
[e]Precursor to alogia
[f]First to use "negative symptoms"

unable to get work done or even read. They socially isolate. A loss or interest or pleasure called anhedonia has been a diagnostic criterion for major depression since the DSM-III (APA, DSM 1980) with "… markedly diminished interest or pleasure in all or almost all, activities most of the day nearly every day…" (APA, DSM 2000). Anhedonia readily leads to avolition as well as asociality. "Asociality," as associated with schizophrenia, dates from the publication of the DSM-I in 1952 when

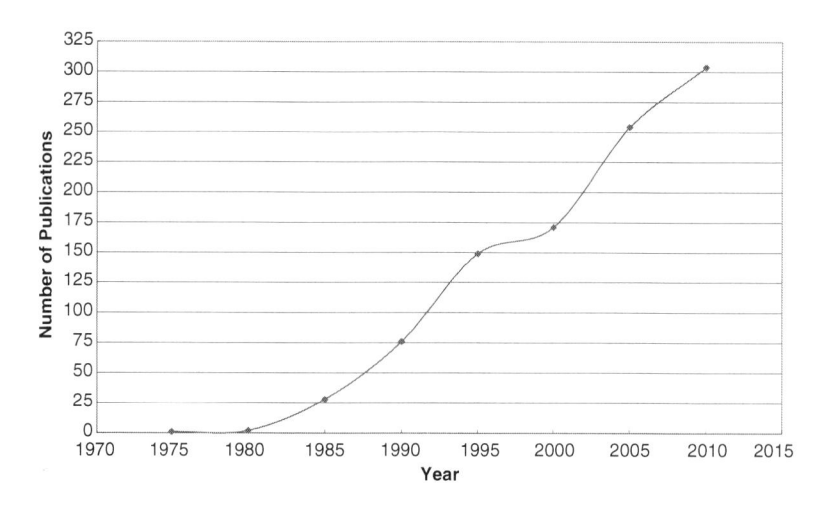

Fig. 12.3 PubMed cites of the negative symptoms of schizophrenia

Despite the elimination of simple schizophrenia in the DSM-III published in 1980 which should have de-emphasized the negative symptoms, as shown in Figure 12.1, the number of PubMed cites of negative symptoms of schizophrenia began a consistent increase from 25 cites in 1985 to over 300 cites in 2010. The negative symptoms were first officially introduced into the DSM in 1994 with the publication of the DSM-IV. This did not seem to increase the slope of increasing cites

symptom descriptions included "reduction in external attachments and impoverishment in human relationships" (Table 12.8). However, this description, misattributed to schizophrenia, is actually more logically explained by the social withdrawal and social isolation characteristic of major depression. Depressed patients are the ones who sometimes cover their windows with black construction paper or newspaper, turn off the lights, do not answer a ringing telephone, and do not leave their room sometimes even to go to the bathroom. "Asociality," as related to schizophrenia, seemed to be de-emphasized with the publication of the DSM-III (APA, DSM 1980) but is proposed for revival in the DSM-5. It is surprising to read that the DSM-5 intends to retain negative symptoms as having any influence whatsoever toward the diagnosis of any disease other than major depression. Also surprising is the observation that "odd beliefs," that have been given as a characteristic of schizophrenia since at least 1987 and the DSM-III-R, is also apparently proposed to be continued in the DSM-5.

One index of the increasing popularity from the 1980s of the concept of "negative symptoms" as diagnostic of schizophrenia is the number of PubMed cites of "negative symptoms of schizophrenia." A search found 4,054 cites initiating from 1975 and increasing steadily through the 1980s, 1990s, and 2000s (Fig. 12.3). As adequately documented, these negative symptoms are common to moderate through severe major depression whether bipolar or unipolar yet continue to be considered by some as diagnostic of schizophrenia.

12.9 Conclusions

The data are clear with regard to no diagnostic relevance of the symptom or subtype of catatonia. The rationale for eliminating catatonia as a subtype of schizophrenia in the DSM-5 but retaining catatonia, as well as hallucinations and delusions, as core diagnostic criteria for schizophrenia is puzzling (Tables 12.1, 12.2, 12.3, 12.9).

Distractibility, a source of disorganization, may reflect a primary defect in information processing in the manic brain involving selective attention (Chap. 13) (Oltmanns 1978; Carroll et al. 2005). This breakdown in mania can lead to gross disorganization of thought, speech, and behavior, including hallucinations, delusions, paranoia, and incoherence and seems to explain most, if not all, of the signs and symptoms of disturbed thought, behavior, and speech traditionally attributed to disorganized schizophrenia. Disorganization is a characteristic of a psychotic mood disorder and not any other functional disease. The rationale for eliminating disorganized as a subtype of schizophrenia in the DSM-5 but retaining disorganization of speech as core diagnostic criterion for schizophrenia is also puzzling (Tables 12.1, 12.9).

Misperceptions and exaggerations are common, predisposing mentally ill patients to grandiosity and then to paranoia. The extent of manic exaggeration and expansion from "a grain of truth" are highlighted by case 9's actual visits to Cuba and Spain and a CIA position held by a distant relative. The defective selective attention function in mania can also explain the loosely associated globalization of some delusional systems, such as case 9 when "rogue CIA agents," Cuban agents, the Queen of Spain, Ronald Reagan, and Fidel Castro were involved, or the loose,

Table 12.9 The subtypes of schizophrenia explained by mood disorders; are a prerequisite for schizophrenia's existence

Catatonic:
- In the DSM, identical definitions under schizophrenia and mood disorders chapters
- "Catatonia is more frequently associated with mania, melancholia, and psychotic depression than it is with schizophrenia" Fink and Taylor, AJP 2006
- "We found that a majority of patients admitted with one or more catatonic signs had diagnosable affective illness, most frequently mania" Abrams and Taylor, AGP 1976

Paranoid:
- Psychotic depression → Delusional guilt of past sins → Punishment deserved → Fear/paranoia
- Psychotic mania → Grandiose delusions of valuable possessions → Others want them → Fear/paranoia

Disorganized/hebephrenic:
- Manic defect in selective attention/prioritizer function → Distractibility → Disorganization/Psychosis

Undifferentiated and residual:
- Atypical or psychotic mood disorder without prominent disorganization, paranoia, or catatonia with persistent depression ("negative symptoms")

Note: Psychosis without obvious mood symptoms is most likely explained by (1) a psychotic mood disorder with obscured symptoms or (2) subtle organicity. Use psychosis, NOS only temporarily until etiology resolved

Table 12.10 Suggested initial screening questions for psychotic or paranoid patients (or their significant others)

For mania
1. How many hours of sleep per night have you averaged over the past days to weeks? Is this different from your baseline? Please explain further.
2. Describe your energy and activity levels during this time. What new activities have you begun?
3. Has your mind been going slower or faster than usual? Please explain.
4. Do you believe you possess special powers, connections, knowledge, or valuables? Please explain further.
5. Who (What) are you afraid of? Please explain.
6. Why are they after you? What do they want from you? Please explain further.
7. Have you been more irritable or more easily angered lately? How many physical or verbal altercations/fights have you been involved in lately? Is this typical for you? Give some examples.
8. What problems have you had with law enforcement?
9. Have you driven your car differently recently than is usual for you?
10. Has anyone asked you to slow down or shut up recently?

For depression
1. Describe how you have been feeling in your mood or spirits over the past days to weeks? Have you been more tearful or felt like crying recently? Have you felt sad or empty? Is this different from your baseline? Please explain further.
2. Describe your energy and activity levels during this time. What activities have you given up?
3. Have you been enjoying usually pleasurable activities as much as usual? Please explain further and give examples.
4. Have you had feelings of guilt most days? Please describe in detail.
5. Have you felt worthless and that you deserved punishment for transgressions or sins in the past? Please explain in detail.
6. Have you stayed at home or in your room or not answered you telephone or door? Is this unusual for you? Please give details.
7. Have you experienced difficulty concentrating or focusing on a task? Help me understand how this is different from the normal you.
8. Have you had thoughts that life was not worth living? How have you thought about hurting yourself? What plans have you made? What is the closest you have come to hurting yourself? How close have you come to killing yourself in the past?

disorganized delusions of case 12, diagnosed with bipolar-I, mixed. Paranoia is common to psychotic mania and depression (Fig. 12.2). Table 12.10 offers some initial screening questions for psychotic or paranoid patients or their significant others in order to reveal disturbances of mood. The rationale for eliminating paranoid as a subtype of schizophrenia in the DSM-5 while retaining hallucinations and delusions as core diagnostic criteria is questionable. That the paranoid subtype accounts for a very high percentage of all diagnoses of schizophrenia, possibly approaching 80% to 90%, leads to doubt about retaining schizophrenia itself.

Without the core diagnostic criteria of schizophrenia, there is no schizophrenia separate from a psychotic mood disorder. Table 12.7 summarizes some "take-home messages."

12.9 Conclusions

The observation of Barnes and McPhillips (1995) is appropriate:

> A major challenge in the clinical assessment of schizophrenia is the differentiation between depressive features, negative symptoms and neuroleptic side effects, including the adverse subjective experiences associated with this medication.

The caveat is that psychotic depression and antipsychotic drug side effects make the use of the diagnosis of schizophrenia redundant.

The positive symptoms of schizophrenia overlap with the subtypes of schizophrenia in the current DSM. The subtypes of schizophrenia are proposed for elimination in the DSM-5 for good reason. These symptoms or subtypes, paranoid (hallucinations, delusions), disorganization, and catatonia, occur in psychotic mood disorders, eliminating a need for a separate disease, schizophrenia. If the subtypes are proposed for elimination because of their nonspecificity, how are the synonymous positive symptoms still justified as diagnostic?

Possibly as a result of such findings of overlap of psychotic (positive) symptoms from the 1970s (Chaps. 10, 11), the negative symptoms of schizophrenia gained popularity in identifying schizophrenia (Makinen et al. 2008; Fischer and Carpenter 2009). The negative symptoms, whether from the DSM-IV-TR or the proposed DSM-5, are almost universally present in psychotic depression, thus eliminating their validity as specific diagnostic criteria for schizophrenia.

Psychotic depression lost favor as the diagnosis for psychotically depressed patients in the late 1800s and afterward with the influence of Kraepelin and Bleuler who taught that psychosis meant the new disease, schizophrenia. This was a major mistake and a substantial disservice to patients so misdiagnosed as they have not received proper treatment for their mood disturbance or organic/secondary causes for their psychoses. Such organic or secondary causes of psychoses, mania, and depression are discussed in Chap. 14.

Chapter 13
Psychotic Mood Disorders Are Disorders of Thought and of Mood

> *The data indicate that [1] most hospitalized manics are severely thought disordered; [2] hospitalized manics are as thought disordered as schizophrenics ... [5] even after the acute phase, some manics show severe thought pathology. ... [Upon two to four years post-hospitalization follow-up,] 30% of the manic patients showed severe positive thought disorder .... The results support formulations that thought disorder is not unique to schizophrenia. Some factors involved in manic and schizophrenic thought pathology are similar. There may be a general psychosis factor that cuts across psychotic diagnoses.*
>
> (Grossman et al. 1986)

> *The zone of rarity between schizophrenia and psychotic mood disorders is blurred because severe disorders of mood are also disorders of thought. This relationship calls into question the tenet that schizophrenia is a disease separate from psychotic mood disorders.*
>
> (Lake 2008b)

13.1 Introduction

Medical students and residents in psychiatry have been taught that schizophrenia is a disorder of thought, exclusive of disorders of mood. This dichotomy was imprinted upon academic psychiatry by the teachings of Kraepelin, Bleuler, and Schneider, despite almost 2,000 years of reports of cases of manic-depressive insanity whose behavior was described as psychotic suggesting disordered thought (Table 3.1). Only recently have serious questions been raised about this dichotomy despite these consistent observations of hallucinations and delusions in mood-disordered patients from the literature (Table 3.1) and also noted for 60 years in the DSMs (Tables 2.4, 9.3, 9.4, and 11.10). Psychotic thoughts, speech, and behavior that include hallucinations, delusions, and disorganization define a disorder of thought. Kraepelin's dichotomy between the disorders of thought, the schizophrenias, and the disorders

Table 13.1 Symptoms of disordered thought and speech traditionally indicative of schizophrenia or mania

Schizophrenia[a]	Mania
A disorder of thought	A disorder of mood
Delusions	Distractibility
Hallucinations	Racing thoughts
Paranoia	Flight of ideas
Tangentiality	Pressure of speech
Circumstantiality	Grandiosity
Loose associations	
Derailment	
Blocking	
Disorganized thought and speech	
Incoherence	
Echolalia	
Echopraxia	
Clanging	
Rhyming	
Punning	
Word salad	
Ideas of reference	
Ideas of influence	
Ideas of control	

[a] Note that no single symptom or combination of symptoms is disease specific for schizophrenia, and all are more likely explained by the core manic symptom of distractibility

of affect, mood disorders, was simple, seemed to have separation, and continues to be widely embraced forming the keystone of psychiatry's concept of the functional psychoses. Defective thought and speech garnered an extensive terminology that was sharply divided and mutually exclusive. Each term was indicative of either schizophrenia or bipolar disorder (Table 13.1). Most of these signs and symptoms were initially attributed to schizophrenia, not mania or depression. To explore such issues of disordered thoughts and speech, several investigators have studied the brain's selective attention mechanism and its dysfunction in severe psychiatric disorders of thought including schizophrenia, mania, and depression.

13.2 Selective Attention: The Brain's Filter-Prioritizer Mechanism

The human brain possesses the ability to selectively process incoming information. Attention is part of this processing and is a multidimensional construct. Selective attention refers to those mechanisms which lead consciousness to be dominated by one thing rather than another (Driver 2001). Partly under voluntary control, partly subconscious, and partly dependent on stimulus salience for each individual, some stimuli are blocked and some are processed more thoroughly than others. Experimental models, including

13.2 Selective Attention: The Brain's Filter-Prioritizer Mechanism

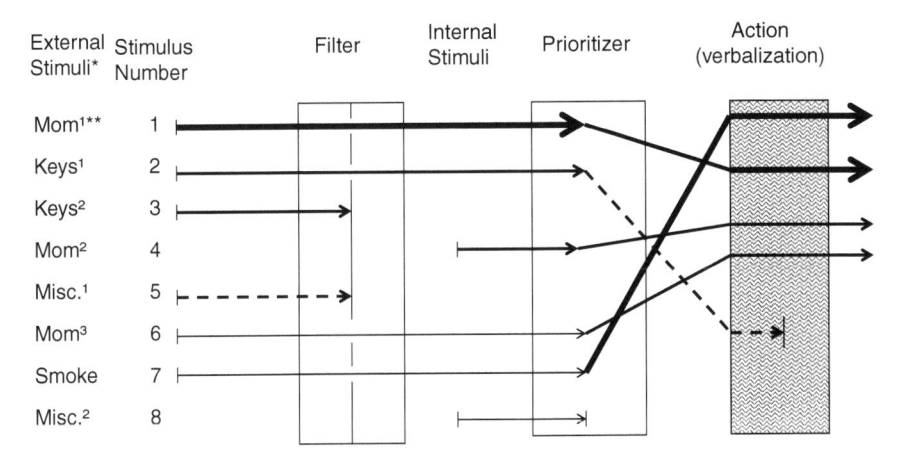

[Figure showing columns: External Stimuli*, Stimulus Number, Filter, Internal Stimuli, Prioritizer, Action (verbalization)]

External Stimuli*	Stimulus Number
Mom[1]**	1
Keys[1]	2
Keys[2]	3
Mom[2]	4
Misc.[1]	5
Mom[3]	6
Smoke	7
Misc.[2]	8

*The thicknesses of the stimuli lines indicate relative importance
**superscript number refers to the first or second stimulus to that subject

Fig. 13.1 Psychotic mood disorders are disorders of thought: euthymia

Three areas of CNS data processing are denoted by three boxes. Figs 13.1, 13.2, and 13.3 represent three states of mood. The examples of the stimuli used in the figure derive from an actual interview of a patient during a student case conference (see text). External stimuli appear to meet a filter that eliminates trivial data in euthymia, while most or all stimuli pass through the filter in mania. More stimuli may be stopped at the filter in depression. Internal stimuli are shown, but their filtration is not indicated in the figure. A second data-processing mechanism is represented by the *second box* and is likely a prioritizing function that can rearrange the importance of stimuli, diminishing or exaggerating attention to incoming data. The time elapsed during processing of the interview material differs between mood states. In euthymia, discussion of the eight stimuli take about 5 to 10 min; the 10 stimuli in mania, 2 min; and the five steps in depression, 10 min.

In euthymia, the psychiatrist's questions about "mom" are prioritized and are not overridden by the "keys" (neither "keys" stimuli 1 or 2) or by miscellaneous stimuli, 1 or 2. The first "keys (1)" stimulus is impactful enough to pass the filter but is shown as downgraded by the prioritizer function, and there is no action or verbalization. A second "keys (2)" stimulus when the professor picked up his keys does not pass filtration. Internal stimulus four ("mom 2") and external stimulus six ("mom 3" as in the form of another question from the interviewer) are appropriately prioritized and verbalized in continuing with the psychiatric interview. The dialogue about the topic of "mom" may last 5 to 10 min and is only overridden by a hypothetical stimulus, "smoke." The sight or smell of smoke (stimulus 7) readily passes the filter and is highly prioritized. Note increase in line thickness and elevation to the top of the "action" box, receiving immediate attention above the "mom" topic

Donald Broadbent's filter theory and various cognitive neuroscience techniques in psychiatric patients, have focused on selective attention and its malfunction (Oltmanns 1978; Posner and Petersen 1990; David 1993; Mialet and Pope 1996; Addington and Addington 1997; Driver 2001; Politis et al. 2004; Olincy and Martin 2005). Selective attention appears to govern an initial filtration process that is linked with a prioritization mechanism before stimuli reach consciousness (Fig. 13.1). Stimuli that reach consciousness are the basis of thoughts, verbalizations, and actions. This filter/prioritizer enables one to screen out and avoid attending to extraneous distractions during a conversation or other focused activity such as an initial diagnostic interview. Although there is wide individual variability in what is likely to attract or distract one's attention, stimuli indicating emergency or life-threatening situations are universally given priority in euthymic individuals. For example, the sudden smell of smoke appropriately overrides most conversations (Fig. 13.1). By contrast, at a ball game, depending on their individual interests, a home run or touchdown might appropriately distract only some from a serious discussion while others are appropriately oblivious to a score.

13.3 Defective Selective Attention Is Epitomized by Manic Distractibility

Distractibility is a recognized core diagnostic symptom of mania (Table 2.3) (APA, DSM-IV-TR 2000). In mania, the selective attention function apparently deteriorates, and the filter/prioritizer becomes more porous allowing inappropriate and irrelevant stimuli to gain attention and focus over important data which are lost (Fig. 13.2). This defect is observed clinically as manic distractibility, flight of ideas, racing thoughts, pressure of speech, circumstantiality, tangentiality, loose associations, and derailment that lead to paranoid delusions, hallucinations, disorganization, incoherence, dangerously poor judgment, and lack of insight. Most of these signs and symptoms have been associated with schizophrenia, not mania (Table 13.1). The level of distractibility and degree of the disturbance of thought and speech provide a clinical index reflecting the severity of the information-processing defect in manic patients (Oltmanns 1978; David 1993; Mialet and Pope 1996). Increasing damage to the filter/prioritizer in mania causes increasing distractibility leading to blocking, echolalia, clanging, punning, rhyming, word salad, speaking in tongues and disorganization of thought, speech, and behavior, increasing incoherence, and to psychosis. Although disorganization is still considered diagnostic of schizophrenia according to the DSM-IV-TR (APA, DSM 2000) (Table 2.5), it is a prominent characteristic of severe mania, likely exacerbated by failure of the selective attention function and increasing distractibility (Oltmanns 1978). Many of the symptoms of disordered thinking noted above are traditionally considered pathognomonic for schizophrenia not mania, such as tangentiality, derailment, loose associations, ideas of reference, influence, and control, blocking, rhyming, punning, echolalia, clanging, word salad, paranoia, disorganization, and incoherence (Table 13.1). How this set of symptoms derives instead from manic distractibility is considered below (Fig. 13.2).

In mild mania, the defect in the filter/prioritizer system is modest, allowing fairly appropriate evaluation of incoming data, but with reduced dampening so that there is an increase in the number of ideas and more activities than are usual for that individual. During this state, new ideas are triggered more readily, filtered less critically, and are expressed with less restriction and more confidence. Hypomanic patients typically become more productive in their areas of endeavor as well as in additional ventures. History demonstrates that some of the most famous and successful writers, composers, musicians, artists, generals, religious leaders, and politicians have suffered and benefited from mild bipolar mood disorders.

When the filter/prioritizer mechanism becomes less discriminating, however, rationality and the quality of productivity decrease. In moderately severe mania, multiple ventures may be undertaken with initial enthusiasm, but none completed due to inappropriate attention to the next new activity. Sequential stimuli demand attention even though they are tangential or seemingly unrelated to the subject of a conversation. For example, during an initial diagnostic interview to determine if hospitalization is warranted, a patient with moderate mania may attend to and comment on irrelevant stimuli from pictures on the wall, a clock, noises outside, the interviewer's keys, tie, jewelry or hair, and other inappropriate distractions rather than the interviewer's questions that govern disposition of the patient. Redirection of the patient may become difficult due to increasing distractibility and irritability.

In severe mania, the brain's filter/prioritizer is very porous to inappropriate distractions. The ability to distinguish and thus to discard trivial sensory input is lost, and the manic brain seems to attempt to process and vocalize myriad stimuli (Fig. 13.2). This defect results in the experience of racing thoughts, flight of ideas, and confusion, typically described by manic patients and observed by the interviewer as a pressure of speech extending to disorganization and incoherence. New ideas and thoughts come so fast that even speaking as rapidly as possible, a manic patient may be able to verbally express only a small percentage of them. Conversely, critical stimuli may be overlooked. Rational conversation becomes difficult because such patients are confused by sensory and thought overload, as demonstrated in the case conference below.

13.4 Student Case Conference: Schizophrenia Explained by Mania

The subjects whose cases are discussed gave their written informed consents to participate in this IRB-approved research.

The case of a 56-year-old married male, recently readmitted to the acute inpatient unit, was presented in a weekly student conference. He had carried the diagnosis of schizophrenia, disorganized type for decades. The student reported his presenting symptoms of derailment, loose associations, blocking, delusions, functional deterioration, and gross disorganization of thoughts, speech, and behavior for over 6 months (Table 2.5). He fulfilled DSM criteria for schizophrenia and demonstrated additional signs and symptoms usually associated with this diagnosis (Table 6.4). After the student's presentation, the patient was invited into the conference room for an interview with the attending professor. About 2 min into the interview, as the patient answered a question about his mother, with a normal rhythm but a modest pressure of speech, the professor "accidentally" knocked his heavy key chain off the table onto the floor. The patient stopped talking, remained silent for about 15 seconds, and then said, with appropriate emotion, "The pyramids are magnificent structures." After another unusual pause, the patient said, "May I have a glass of water?"

These appear to be textbook examples of "schizophrenic thought blocking," understood as the sudden obstruction in or loss of a thought during a flow of speech, and observed as an unusual silence followed by the emergence of a totally unrelated subject. There is no apparent association between "mother," "pyramids," and wanting water. This presentation appeared to meet all the DSM criteria for schizophrenia, but the rule out for psychotic mood disorder had been overlooked.

The patient was asked by the attending professor to try to focus his attention and explain how his thoughts had jumped from discussing his mother to pyramids to wanting water. With some redirection, he was able to maintain focus to say that the key chain stimulated the thought of "the key of life" leading to the idea that life began in Egypt's Nile River valley. "Egypt" brought him to pyramids and how "magnificent" they must be. This process of racing but linked thoughts apparently took about 15 seconds at which time he had time to say his "pyramids" statement. Egypt also stimulated the thought of a desert, of feeling hot and then thirsty, so he asked for a glass of water. This sequence of thoughts occurred in a matter of seconds. An analysis of what transpired in this interaction demonstrates distractibility, flight of ideas, and racing thoughts and may be explained by a defect in the selective attention function thought to be typical to mania (Fig. 13.2). The patient's filter/prioritizer failed to prevent his inappropriate distraction to and processing of "keys." Because he was unable to maintain appropriate focus on the interviewer's questions about his mom, this theme was lost. There were nine thoughts including the initial subject of "mom" and the extraneous stimulus of the attending professor's keys that led to a cascade of at least seven internally generated loosely associated ideas: (1) mom, (2) the professor's keys, (3) the key of life, (4) Egypt, (5) the magnificent pyramids, (6) the desert, (7) feeling hot, (8) being thirsty, and (9) wanting water. The patient's mind was racing to such an extent that he only had time to verbalize "pyramids are magnificent" and wanting water, items 5 and 9 (Fig. 13.2). Such a breakdown apparently allows so many thoughts to reach consciousness that there is no time to say them all. By the patient's report, there were connections to all his thoughts, but an observer is oblivious to the connections because only about 20% of this patient's thoughts are verbalized, and none have any relationship to the subject of "mom."

During euthymia, distraction to the keys falling to the floor would usually be blocked at the filter or given such low priority that the interview subject of "mom" would continue to hold focus appropriately and uninterrupted (Fig. 13.1). In depression, exclusion of stimuli may be increased (Fig. 13.3).

Bleuler and Schneider would interpret this interchange as thought blocking, loose associations, derailment, disorganization, and incoherence of thought and speech, leading to a diagnosis of schizophrenia, disorganized subtype (Bleuler 1911; Schneider 1959), but these signs are also compatible with manic distractibility. Upon additional inquiry, the patient under discussion endorsed the DSM, disease-specific symptoms diagnostic of a manic episode (Table 2.3) (APA, DSM-IV-TR 2000). The significant other of the patient confirmed his manic symptoms.

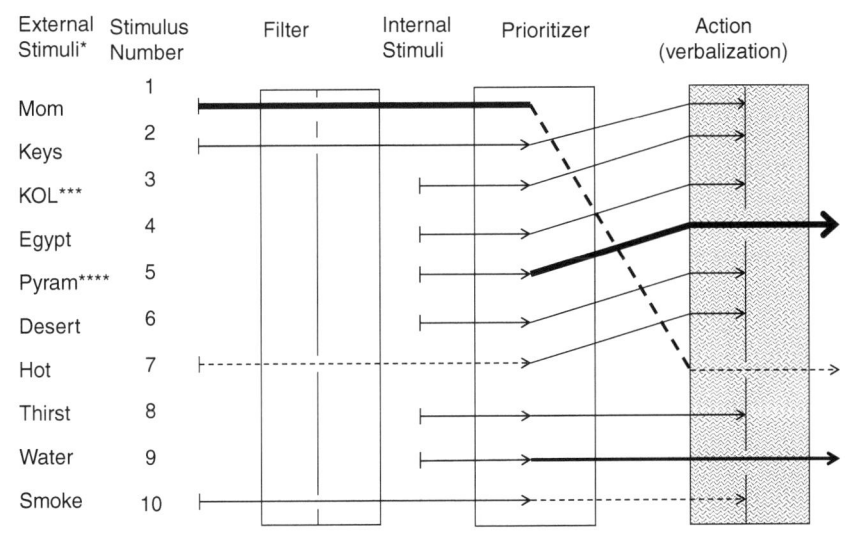

13.4 Student Case Conference: Schizophrenia Explained by Mania

External Stimuli*	Stimulus Number	Filter	Internal Stimuli	Prioritizer	Action (verbalization)
Mom	1				
Keys	2				
KOL***	3				
Egypt	4				
Pyram****	5				
Desert	6				
Hot	7				
Thirst	8				
Water	9				
Smoke	10				

*The thicknesses of the stimuli lines indicate relative importance
**superscript number refers to the first or second stimulus to that subject
***KEY OF LIFE
****PYRAMIDS

Fig. 13.2 Psychotic mood disorders are disorders of thought: mania

Three areas of CNS data processing are denoted by three boxes. Figs 13.1, 13.2, and 13.3 represent three states of mood. The examples of the stimuli used in the figure derive from an actual interview of a patient during a student case conference (see text). External stimuli appear to meet a filter that eliminates trivial data in euthymia, while most or all stimuli pass through the filter in mania. More stimuli may be stopped at the filter in depression. Internal stimuli are shown, but their filtration is not indicated in the figure. A second data-processing mechanism is represented by the second box and is likely a prioritizing function that can rearrange the importance of stimuli, diminishing or exaggerating attention to incoming data. The time elapsed during processing of the interview material differs between mood states. In euthymia, discussion of the eight stimuli take about 5 to 10 min; the 10 stimuli in mania, 2 min; and the five steps in depression, 10 min.

In mania, the subject of "mom" is inappropriately lost when stimulus 2, the "keys," is passed through the filter and prioritized, possibly due to its being the most recent stimulus. The "keys" idea is not verbalized because of a flurry of subsequent internal stimuli based initially on "keys" and then on subsequent stimuli (see text). This series of internal stimuli includes numbers 3–9. Stimulus 7 is shown as a dashed line of external input as the room may have been warm. Only 5 and 9 are verbalized. Although there are connections to each thought based on the patient's report, the failure to filter and prioritize causes stimuli to come so fast and demand attention (apparently based on most recent order) that there is not enough time to verbalize all of them. An observer hears only "mom," "pyramids," and wanting water, concluding there has been a "blockage of thought." The present explanation is predicated on the core manic symptoms of distractibility, flight of ideas, and racing thoughts. Manic thought is indeed disordered.

The potentially critical external stimulus of "smoke" (number 10) may pass the filter but may not be adequately prioritized in mania to receive action. "Smoke" may be quickly overridden by the next stimulus such as "cigarettes are expensive" or "Smokey the Bear is cute." The first nine stimuli are actual thoughts of the patient as discussed in the text; stimulus 10 is hypothesized. This exchange and series of thoughts might occur in as little as 2 min

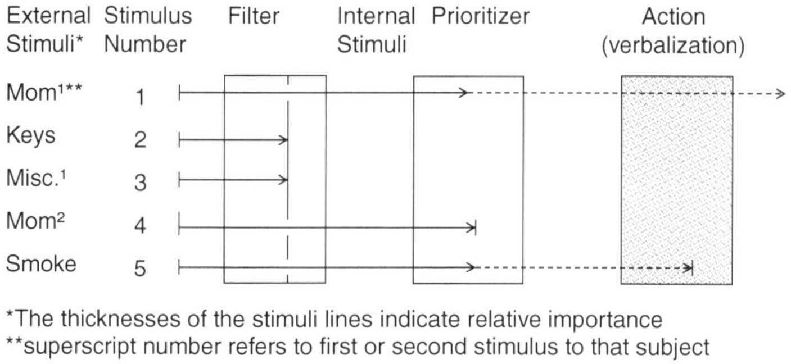

```
External  Stimulus    Filter     Internal  Prioritizer      Action
Stimuli*  Number                 Stimuli                (verbalization)

Mom¹**     1
Keys       2
Misc.¹     3
Mom²       4
Smoke      5
```

*The thicknesses of the stimuli lines indicate relative importance
**superscript number refers to first or second stimulus to that subject

Fig. 13.3 Psychotic mood disorders are disorders of thought: depression
Three areas of CNS data processing are denoted by three boxes. Figs 13.1, 13.2, and 13.3 represent three states of mood. The examples of the stimuli used in the figure derive from an actual interview of a patient during a student case conference (see text). External stimuli appear to meet a filter that eliminates trivial data in euthymia, while most or all stimuli pass through the filter in mania. More stimuli may be stopped at the filter in depression. Internal stimuli are shown, but their filtration is not indicated in the figure. A second data-processing mechanism is represented by the *second box* and is likely a prioritizing function that can rearrange the importance of stimuli, diminishing or exaggerating attention to incoming data. The time elapsed during processing of the interview material differs between mood states. In euthymia, discussion of the eight stimuli take about 5 to 10 min; the 10 stimuli in mania, 2 min; and the five steps in depression, 10 min.

In depression, all cognitive processes appear to be slowed. A patient may have difficulty maintaining focus on "mom" but because of his depression rather than because of subsequent interrupting stimuli. Other stimuli may be inappropriately filtered out or receive an unwarranted reduction in prioritization. Stimulus 5, "smoke," is shown as passing the filter but not receiving a high enough prioritization rank to produce an action. No internal stimuli are generated, in sharp contrast to the manic state where an excessive number of internal stimuli reach consciousness. In depression, only five stimuli may require as much as 10 min with less comprehension than the eight stimuli in euthymia in the same time

In severe psychotic mania with more extensive damage to the filter/prioritizer mechanism, patients may only focus on words or sounds that rhyme or may only be able to say words or make sounds with no apparent relationship to one another. These disorganized and incoherent patterns of speech, called rhyming, punning, clanging, echolalia, and word salad, are traditionally associated with schizophrenia and not mania (Table 13.1). An example of such manic incoherence comes from a recovered 25-year-old bipolar patient who said that, when manic, his mind raced so fast that he had been able to focus on the first letter of each word spoken by others and to "make entire [denovo] sentences beginning with each of those letters." His speech had been incoherent (word salad), and his behavior, disorganized, delusional, and psychotic, yet he said he had felt organized. He met disease-specific DSM criteria for mania (Table 2.3) (APA, DSM-IV-TR 2000).

Another extremely disorganized 45-year-old patient was brought to the Emergency Department (ED) by the police accompanied by his wife. He had been apprehended from the middle of a busy intersection gesturing frantically and speaking rapidly, nonstop in a "foreign language" or "in tongues" to any one or no one.

In the ED, he continued to speak rapidly without pause but with a rhythm that indicated a potential for meaning. No English words were discernable. His affect was of extreme excitement and agitation. His wife denied that he spoke a foreign language and said that he had been in this mental state for 2 days without sleep or food. In retrospect, his initial diagnosis of disorganized schizophrenia was likely incorrect because he probably suffered from excited mania, severe with psychotic features. Such a presentation can be understood as a severe disintegration in the manic filter/prioritizer function. A productive strategy in this case in the ED would have been to interview the significant other asking the questions given in Table 12.10 relevant to the diagnosis of mania. This case emphasizes the importance of considering a diagnosis of mania in disorganized, incoherent individuals observed to be "speaking in tongues" and inappropriately "preaching" on street corners.

13.5 Conclusions

The degree of distractibility is an index of the severity of a core defect in information processing in the manic brain involving selective attention (Oltmanns 1978). This breakdown in mania leads to gross disorganization of thought and behavior, hallucinations, delusions, and incoherence and seems to explain most, if not all, the signs and symptoms of disturbed thought, traditionally attributed to schizophrenia (Tables 2.3, 2.4, 2.5, 6.4, and 13.1). The cognitive deficits, including defects in selective attention, in schizophrenia and bipolar disorder share commonalities and overlap (Table 11.9) (Oltmanns 1978; Olincy and Martin 2005; Politis et al. 2004; Addington and Addington 1997; Mialet and Pope 1996; David 1993).

Psychotic mood disorders are disorders of thought as well as mood (Table 13.2) (Harrow et al. 1982; Grossman et al. 1986; Lake 2008b). Disorders of thought have been mistakenly considered the exclusive domain of the disorder called schizophrenia. That psychotic mood disorders are disorders of thought raises doubt about the validity of schizophrenia as a separate disorder. These data concur with prior conclusions that psychotic mood disorders are commonly misdiagnosed as schizophrenia (Pope and Lipinski 1978; Weiser et al. 2001; Angst 2002; Hafner et al. 2005; Lake and Hurwitz 2006a, b, 2007a,b; Maier et al. 2006; Lake 2008a, b).

Disordered thought and the functional psychoses can be accounted for by a single disorder, a psychotic mood disorder (Table 11.14; Figs. 3.1 and 11.3). A correct diagnosis is critical because psychotic bipolar or unipolar depressed patients misdiagnosed with schizophrenia or schizoaffective disorder do not receive standard of care treatment (Chap. 15).

Table 13.2 Psychotic mood disorders are:

DISORDERS OF MOOD

AND

DISORDERS OF THOUGHT

Chapter 14
Medical and Other Psychiatric Conditions Potentially Misdiagnosed as Schizophrenia

> *A wide variety of physical diseases masquerade as psychiatric disorders. The clinician must be alert to the possibility that organic disease may underlie overt psychiatric symptoms. ... approximately 30 percent of patients with underlying medical illnesses exhibit symptoms of functional psychoses [schizophrenia] ... No where in the practice of medicine is an accurate and detailed history more important than with patients whose organic disease is hidden by a façade of psychiatric symptoms.*
>
> (Martin 1983)

> *In a sample of 268 cases of first-episode schizophrenia, 15 patients [5.6%] were found to have organic disease which appeared relevant to the mental state. ... Physical illnesses for which appropriate treatments are available were present and apparently accounted for schizophrenia-like psychoses.*
>
> (Johnstone et al. 1987)

14.1 Introduction

Although psychotic mood disorders likely account for a large majority of misdiagnoses of schizophrenia, many medical disorders, medications, drugs, and some other psychiatric disorders can present with psychotic features that can also lead to misdiagnoses of schizophrenia or a mood disorder. Hall et al. (1978) reported an incidence of medical disorders in 9.1% of 658 consecutive psychiatric outpatients that they felt caused the patients' psychiatric symptoms. Such patients were most commonly misdiagnosed with schizophrenia and depression. A similarly designed study found 5.6% of first-episode patients diagnosed with schizophrenia had an unrecognized medical disorder that explained psychotic symptoms (Johnstone et al. 1987).

Such misdiagnoses of psychotic patients with no obvious mood symptoms can occur under several circumstances (Martin 1983). Most often, in psychotic mood-disordered patients, psychotic symptoms can obscure mood symptoms, and psychiatry's overemphasis on the diagnostic import of psychotic symptoms and underemphasis on mood symptoms most often leads to misdiagnoses of schizophrenia (Carlson and Goodwin 1973; Pope and Lipinski 1978; Pope 1983; Goodwin 1989). In addition, misdiagnoses of schizophrenia also occur in organically caused psychosis when the typical symptoms of the medical condition have yet to develop or go unrecognized (Johnstone et al. 1987). Similarly, some prescription and illegal drugs can cause a chronic psychotic state without continued use or abuse so that admission drug screens are negative. Tardive or supersensitivity psychosis reportedly caused by antipsychotic/antischizophrenia medications is a potential source for the continued misdiagnosis of schizophrenia. Since several medical diseases and substance usages can present with symptoms of mania or depression, misdiagnoses of mood disorders are also likely without adequate medical and drug screens. Conversely, mania and depression can present with overwhelming confusion and cognitive deficits, superficially suggesting a toxic cause (Caton et al. 2005).

This chapter discusses such organic conditions and tests useful to differentiate them from schizophrenia and psychotic mood disorders. Such differentiation of the etiology of psychosis between primary psychiatric (previously referred to as functional) and secondary (organic) is critical to the effective treatment of such psychotic patients. To misdiagnose a mood disorder or schizophrenia when a psychotic patient actually suffers from a medical condition is as egregious as misdiagnosing a psychotic patient with a medical condition when they suffer from a psychotic mood disorder. Much of the data in this chapter derived from several excellent reviews (Martin 1983; Freudenreich et al. 2007; Freudenreich 2010).

14.2 Medical and Surgical Causes of Psychosis (Table 14.1)

14.2.1 Autoimmune Disorders

Systemic lupus erythematosus is a multisystem autoimmune disease that can present with psychosis and/or seizures. Eleven percent of patients suffered from psychosis due to brain involvement. In addition, appropriate treatment with corticosteroids caused psychosis in about 5% of these patients. Hashimoto's encephalopathy is associated with autoimmune thyroiditis and episodes of psychosis (Freudenreich 2010). Corticosteroid treatment is very effective but can cause psychotic, manic, or depressive symptoms. Paraneoplastic limbic encephalitis, due to autoantibodies directed to neuronal antigens, can present with psychosis. This condition is associated with several tumor types, most commonly small-cell lung cancer. The progressive muscular weakness, easy fatiguability, listlessness, and irritability of myasthenia gravis can be misdiagnosed as a major depressive disorder.

14.2.2 Chromosomal Abnormalities

See Table 14.1 for rare disorders that can exhibit psychotic symptoms.

Table 14.1 Medical disorders with potential psychotic presentations (adapted from Freudenreich et al. 2007)

1. Autoimmune
   Systemic lupus erythematosus
   Hashimoto encephalopathy
   Paraneoplastic syndrome
   Rheumatic fever
   Myasthenia gravis
2. Chromosomal abnormalities
   Sex chromosomes (Klinefelter's syndrome, XXX syndrome)
   Fragile X syndrome
   Velocardiofacial syndrome
3. Chronic traumatic encephalopathy (History of head trauma)
4. Dementias and delirium
   Alzheimer's disease
   Pick's disease
   Lewy body disease
5. Demyelinating diseases
   Multiple sclerosis
   Leukodystrophies
   Schilder's disease
6. Electrolyte and fluid imbalance
   Hypernatremia
   Hypokalemia
   Hypercalcemia
   Hypomagnesemia
7. Endocrinopathies
   Hypoglycemia
   Insulinoma
   Addison's disease
   Cushing's syndrome
   Hyper- and -hypothyroidism
   Hyper- and hypoparathyroidism
   Hypopituitarism
   Pheochromocytoma
8. Epilepsy
9. Hydrocephalus
10. Infections
    Viral encephalitis (e.g., herpes simplex, measles [including subacute sclerosing panencephalitis], cytomegalovirus, rubella, Epstein-Barr, varicella)
    Neurosyphilis
    Neuroborreliosis (Lyme disease)
    HIV infection or AIDS
    CNS-invasive parasitic infections (e.g., cerebral malaria, toxoplasmosis, neurocysticerosis)
    Tuberculosis
    Sarcoidosis
    Cryptococcus infection
    Prion diseases (e.g., Creutzfeldt-Jakob disease)

(continued)

Table 14.1 (continued)

11. Metabolic diseases (partial list)
    Amino acid metabolism (Hartnup disease, homocystinuria, phenylketonuria)
    Porphyrias (acute intermittent porphyria, porphyria variegate, hereditary coproporphyria)
    GM-2 gangliosidosis
    Fabry's disease
    Niemann-Pick type C disease
    Gaucher's disease, adult type
    Tay-Sachs disease
12. Narcolepsy
13. Neuropsychiatric diseases
    Huntington's disease
    Wilson's disease
    Parkinson's disease
    Fahr's disease (Familial basal ganglia calcification)
    Friedreich's ataxia
    Spinocerebellar ataxia 2
14. Nutritional deficiencies
    Magnesium deficiency
    Vitamin A deficiency
    Vitamin D deficiency
    Zinc deficiency
    Niacin deficiency (pellagra)
    Vitamin B_{12} deficiency (pernicious anemia)
15. Space-occupying lesions and structural brain abnormalities
    Primary brain tumors
    Secondary brain metastases
    Brain abscesses and cysts
    Tuberous sclerosis
    Midline abnormalities (e.g., corpus callosum agenesis, cavum septi pellucidi)
    Cerebrovascular malformations (e.g., involving the temporal lobe)
    Pancreatic carcinoma
    Chronic subdural hematoma
16. Stroke

14.2.3 Chronic Traumatic Encephalopathy (History of Head Trauma)

Chronic traumatic head injury has received considerable and appropriate attention in athletes after repeated sports-related concussions. Concussion, especially repeated, "… is a risk factor for the development of a chronic psychotic syndrome that can be clinically indistinguishable from Schizophrenia. Head injury-related psychosis is typically a mostly paranoid-hallucinatory syndrome…" (Freudenreich 2010). Such patients with chronic traumatic encephalopathy are usually unaware of the relationship between their current psychotic state and repeated concussions often suffered years before when they were active athletes. Asking about past athletic activities such as boxing, mixed martial arts, soccer, hockey, diving, and football is critical.

14.2.4 Dementias and Delirium

Alzheimer's disease and other dementias are subject to misdiagnoses when referred to psychiatry for evaluation of psychotic, manic, or depressive symptoms. Psychosis is present in about 40% of Alzheimer's patients. Delirium has also been misdiagnosed as schizophrenia when the psychotic features overshadow the typical cognitive deficits (Freudenreich 2010).

14.2.5 Demyelinating Diseases

Multiple sclerosis is the most common demyelinating disease and is associated with the occurrence of psychosis and symptoms of mania and depression. Metachromatic leukodystrophy and adrenoleukodystrophy are rare inherited disorders associated with as high as a 50% rate of psychosis. An abnormal MRI, progressive cognitive decline, seizures, a neuropathy, or adrenal insufficiency with the usual onset in childhood usually distinguish these disorders, but they can have an adult onset.

14.2.6 Electrolyte and Fluid Imbalance

Depression may accompany hypernatremia, hypokalemia, hypercalcemia, and hypomagnesemia. A misdiagnosis and ineffective treatment of an electrolyte imbalance can occasionally cause an irreversible organic brain syndrome (Martin 1983).

14.2.7 Endocrinopathies

Endocrine diseases, although systemic, typically affect the brain and can present with psychotic, manic, or depressive symptoms. Thyroid disease has certainly been misdiagnosed as mania or unipolar depression as well as schizophrenia. Steroid-producing tumors such as Cushing's disease or syndrome (from small-cell lung cancer) can initially present with psychotic features. Insulinomas and pheochromocytomas are rare but occasionally present with psychosis. Severe repeated episodes of hypoglycemia caused by a rare insulin-secreting adenoma may result in brain damage, personality changes, dementia, and a psychotic state potentially misdiagnosed as depression or schizophrenia. Addison's disease usually develops gradually and is associated with progressive weakness, weight loss, and hyperpigmentation, but a severe depression of psychotic proportions can lead to the misdiagnosis of psychotic depression or schizophrenia (Martin 1983).

14.2.8 Epilepsy

Temporal lobe epilepsy has been linked with schizophrenia presumably because psychotic symptoms produced by an epileptic focus resulted in misdiagnoses of schizophrenia. There are reports of such patients misdiagnosed and mistreated with antipsychotic/antischizophrenia medications for years before the accurate diagnoses of a seizure disorder was made (Swartz 2001). Psychotic symptoms can occur during the ictal, postictal, or interictal phases. Postictal psychosis reportedly can last several days or weeks or can become chronic (Adachi et al. 2007). Such postictal psychosis can be treated but only if correctly diagnosed (Devinsky 2008). Serial EEGs and optimal lead placement such as pharyngeal leads improve the chances of correctly diagnosing epilepsy. Frontal lobe seizures can be particularly difficult to diagnose (Freudenreich 2010).

Arzy et al. (2006) described the repeated iatrogenic production of delusions as "a first-rank Schneiderian symptom of schizophrenia" in a patient undergoing presurgical deep brain stimulation for ablation of an epileptic focus. The electrode placement was in the left temporoparietal junction, and the sensation was described as the presence of "… somebody is nearby and no one is actually present…." Others have described inducing "out-of-body experiences" in normal controls consistent with schizophrenia using "… conflicting visual-somatosensory input in virtual reality to disrupt the special unity between the self and the body" (Ehrrson 2007; Lenggenhager et al. 2007).

14.2.9 Hydrocephalus

Normal pressure hydrocephalus is characterized by progressive cognitive decline similar to the course of senile dementia, but psychosis has been reported as well, with a potential for misdiagnosis of psychosis due to a psychiatric disorder (Freudenreich 2010).

14.2.10 Infections

CNS HIV infection and neurosyphilis can present with psychosis as can the other diseases listed under "Infections" in Table 14.1. General paresis of the insane or CNS syphilis was erroneously considered a functional psychotic disorder for decades. CNS parasitic infections are rare in the USA, and a history of travel or immigration can raise a suspicion. Herpes simplex encephalitis is important to consider in psychotic presentations since the administration of acyclovir greatly improves prognosis (Freudenreich 2010).

14.2.11 Metabolic Diseases

Acute intermittent porphyria is sufficiently common to be routinely considered in psychotic presentations especially if there are gastrointestinal complaints and a peripheral motor neuropathy. This is an autosomal dominant disease of heme synthesis caused by defective porphobilinogen deaminase resulting in an accumulation of porphobilinogen and aminolevulinic acid. Fasting, alcohol, and several porphobilinogenic medications can trigger episodes. A misdiagnosis of schizophrenia in such psychotic patients is a disservice.

Psychotic symptoms are possible in Tay-Sach's and Niemann-Pick's diseases.

14.2.12 Narcolepsy

Narcolepsy is generally characterized by excessive daytime sleepiness, cataplexy, sleep paralysis, and hypnagogic hallucinations, but the full tetrad is only present in 10% of patients. However, in some patients "… prominent psychosis-like experiences occur throughout the day and overshadow other symptoms of narcolepsy that can lead to a mistaken diagnosis of schizophrenia." One study found 7% of patients that were diagnosed with schizophrenia actually had narcolepsy (Douglas 2003).

14.2.13 Neuropsychiatric Diseases

Rare, inherited disorders of the basal ganglia that are associated with psychosis include Huntington's, Wilson's, and Fahr's diseases. The psychotic symptoms of Wilson's disease "… frequently resembles schizophrenia" (Martin 1983). Wilson's disease is a disorder of copper metabolism causing copper deposits in the liver and the lenticular nucleus of the brain, thus called hepatolenticular degeneration. Early diagnosis can prevent permanent end-organ damage so that a misdiagnosis of a psychiatric disorder can have permanent effects. Twenty-four-hour urinary copper screenings, serum ceruloplasmin levels, liver abnormalities, and Kayser-Fleischer rings of the cornea as detected by slit-lamp examination are diagnostic.

Huntington's disease is an autosomal dominant disorder in which psychotic features can precede the motor symptoms, but a positive family history of Huntington's should be diagnostic. Genetic testing can confirm a diagnosis. Since there is no effective treatment, a misdiagnosis has less negative impact.

Fahr's disease or familial basal ganglia calcification can produce psychosis.

Parkinson's disease can also present with hallucinations, grandiosity, or depression and can be misdiagnosed as schizophrenia, bipolar disorder, or major depression.

Spinocerebellar ataxia 2 has been misdiagnosed as schizophrenia, and the diagnosis missed for a decade (Rottnek et al. 2008).

14.2.14 Nutritional Deficiencies

Deficiencies of vitamin B_{12}, thiamin, and niacin (pellagra) are associated with psychotic symptoms. Vitamin B_{12} and thiamine deficiencies are readily correctable with an accurate diagnosis. Niacin deficiency is rare in the USA and typically recognizable by the presence of diarrhea, dermatitis, stomatitis, and glossitis.

14.2.15 Space-Occupying Lesions and Structural Brain Abnormalities

Primary or secondary brain tumors can cause psychosis as their first and, occasionally, the only manifestation and are particularly important to consider in the elderly. The location of the tumor and the rate of tumor growth influence the types of symptoms. Temporal lobe tumors increase the chances of psychosis. Occipital lobe lesions associate with visual hallucinations. Frontal lobe tumors frequently cause personality change, flatness of affect, and superficial euphoria. Parietal lobe tumors sometimes cause sensory or agnostic disturbances as well as a lack of awareness mistaken as denial. Rapidly growing tumors usually produce physical signs and symptoms indicative of brain impairment, while slow-growing tumors more often present with depression.

Pancreatic carcinoma frequently manifests as a severe depression. The incidence of depression is higher in pancreatic carcinoma than it is in any other tumor type. The reason is unknown. Clinicians are encouraged to consider pancreatic carcinoma when examining a middle-aged male suffering from severe depression. Hints of a cancer etiology to the depression are the absence of guilt and a negative premorbid psychiatric history (Martin 1983).

14.2.16 Stroke

Psychosis is rarely the presenting symptom of a stroke, but severe depression is common. Complex visual hallucinations of sudden onset mandate ruling out peduncular hallucinosis caused by focal midbrain (peduncular) lesions and the Charles Bonnet syndrome following occipital infarction. Causes of both conditions other than a stroke are possible. For example, the Charles Bonnet syndrome, first described in 1760, is thought to be caused by progressive visual impairment and manifests as complex visual hallucinations with preservation of cognition and insight (Mahgoub and Serby 2007).

14.3 Substances That Can Cause Psychosis

It is important to inquire about all drugs, medications, herbal remedies, and occupational and hobby exposures. Many toxins, drugs, and medications can cause psychosis without delirium. These include drugs bought over the Internet, over the counter, prescribed, nonprescribed, illegal, herbal preparations, as well as occupational exposure and hobbies such as gardening (Table 14.2).

Mood and psychotic symptoms are associated with recreational anabolic steroid use (Pope and Katz 1988). Use and abuse of alcohol, sedative-hypnotics, and illegal drugs are common causes of psychosis. Alcohol and sedative-hypnotic dependence can cause psychosis rarely during intoxication but more often during withdrawal such as delirium tremens. Persistent psychosis such as alcoholic hallucinosis occurs with chronic alcohol abuse. Stimulant drugs (methylphenidate, methamphetamine, dextroamphetamine, cocaine, crack, and less often caffeine) and psychotomimetics (LSD, hallucinogenic mushrooms, phencyclidine, "bath salts") can cause psychosis and symptoms of mania or severe depression (Gardner et al. 2011).

These classes of drugs, especially phencyclidine; the amphetamines, especially methamphetamine; crack cocaine; and, more recently, "bath salts" can cause permanent neuronal death resulting in permanent psychotic states. Bath salts contain man-made chemicals like mephedrone and methylenedioxypyrovalerone and are sold

Table 14.2 Substances that can cause psychoses (adapted from Freudenreich 2010)

Anesthetics
[a]Anabolic steroids
Antibiotics (ciprofloxacin)
[b]Anticholinergics
Anticonvulsants (high doses)
Antimalarial drugs (mefloquine)
Antineoplastics (especially ifosfamide)
[b]Antipsychotic drugs (especially typicals)
Antituberculosis drugs (D-cycloserine, ethambutol, isoniazid)
Antivirals: HIV medications (e.g., efavirenz at high plasma levels), acyclovir
Cardiovascular drugs (antiarrhythmics, digitalis)
[a, b]Corticosteroids
[a, b]Dopaminergic drugs (e.g., L-dopa, amantadine, ropinirole)
[a, b]Interferon
Miscellaneous (baclofen, caffeine, disulfiram, cyclosporine)
Pain medications (opioids especially meperidine, pentazocine, indomethacin)
[a, b]Stimulants
[a]Sympathomimetics (including over-the-counter preparations and ephedra-containing diet supplements)
[b]Bath salts (mephedrone and methylenedioxypyrovalerone; sold under the names of Aura, Ivory Wave, Loco-Motion, and Vanilla Sky)

[a]Substances particularly likely to cause mood symptoms
[b]Substances particularly likely to cause psychosis

under the names of Aura, Ivory Wave, Loco-Motion, and Vanilla Sky. If the drug use was in the past, the urine drug screen is negative, and the patient denies past illegal drug use, a misdiagnosis of schizophrenia is quite possible.

Dopamine agonists such as L-dopa and ropinirole used to treat Parkinson's disease and restless leg syndrome can cause psychosis (Perea et al. 2006).

The typical antipsychotic/antischizophrenia medications and other dopamine antagonist drugs may cause a syndrome called tardive psychosis as discussed in more detail below.

14.4 Tardive Psychosis Possibly Caused by Antipsychotic/ "Antischizophrenia" Medications and Misdiagnosed as Schizophrenia

Tardive psychosis is analogous to tardive dyskinesia as both are thought to be caused by antipsychotic/antischizophrenia medication induced dopamine supersensitivity. Dopamine supersensitivity is thought to be caused by long-term, that is, for months to years, administration of dopamine receptor blocking drugs, primarily the antipsychotic/antischizophrenia medications. The long-term blockade of dopamine receptors seems to cause either an increase in presynaptic cellular production of dopamine, a postsynaptic increase in cellular production of dopamine receptors, and/or an increased sensitivity of postsynaptic dopamine receptors.

Two Canadian researchers at McGill University, Montreal, Chouinard and Jones (1980) concluded that,

> Neuroleptics [antipsychotic/antischizophrenia medications] can produce a dopamine supersensitivity that leads to both dyskinetic and psychotic symptoms. An implication is that the tendency toward psychotic relapse in a patient who has developed such a supersensitivity is determined by more than just the normal course of the illness … the need for continued neuroleptic treatment may itself be drug induced.

Weinberger et al. (1981) considered the possibility of tardive psychosis as have several investigators since (Swartz 1995, 2004). In 2002, Lu et al. reported the onset of hallucinations and delusions in two patients after discontinuing treatment with the dopamine receptor blocking drug, metoclopramide, given for nausea, vomiting, and migraine headaches. Neither patient had a history of previous psychiatric symptoms. As stated by Swartz (2004), "This is tardive psychosis." Downs et al. (1993) described breakthrough tardive psychosis in treatment resistant nonpsychotic manic patients who had been treated for years with antipsychotic medications. Three additional reports described first onset of psychotic symptoms in patients who had received years of high-dose antipsychotic/antischizophrenia medications for Tourette's syndrome (Swartz 2004). The psychotic symptoms in these cases did not occur until the antipsychotic medication dose was decreased or stopped. Tardive psychosis was considered the accurate diagnosis in four patients apparently misdiagnosed with schizophrenia and treated with antipsychotic/antischizophrenia medications continuously for between 3 and 23 years (Swartz 1995).

The idea that antipsychotic/antischizophrenia medications can cause the very symptoms that are diagnostic of schizophrenia according to the DSM should have a major impact upon the use of such drugs. As Swartz (2004) noted however, the awareness of tardive psychosis among clinicians is low as judged by the absence of mention of tardive psychosis in the Physician Desk Reference (PDR). Antipsychotic medications are not the only group of drugs that can cause the symptoms for which they are used to treat. Antiarrhythmic drugs can cause deadly arrhythmias and after several months, benzodiazepines can cause rebound anxiety.

More potent dopamine receptor blocking drugs, such as the typical antipsychotics, risperidone, and metoclopramide, appear more likely to cause tardive psychosis (Swartz 2004). The prevalence of tardive psychosis is estimated to be similar to that for tardive dyskinesia, about 50%. The implications that long-term use of dopamine-blocking antipsychotic medications can cause tardive psychosis just as often as they cause tardive dyskinesia in patients diagnosed with schizophrenia are substantial. That about 33% of patients treated with chronic antipsychotic medications become "drug resistant" may be because of the induction of tardive psychosis. As with tardive dyskinesia, increasing the dose of the antipsychotic medication stops the symptoms but further breakthrough should be expected. It is now considered malpractice in cases of tardive dyskinesia to increase the dose of the offending antipsychotic/antischizophrenia medication in order to temporarily alleviate the movement disorder. In fact, standard of care mandates tapering and discontinuing the drug. Since tardive psychosis is underrecognized, the logical clinical approach to an increase in psychotic symptoms is to raise the dose of the antipsychotic medication. The worsening of psychotic symptoms upon reducing or discontinuing an antipsychotic medication is interpreted as an absolute requirement for antipsychotic medication compliance. The temporary alleviation of psychotic symptoms by reinstituting or raising the dose is more positive reinforcement for further increases in the drug and confirmation of the diagnosis of schizophrenia. Using antipsychotic/antischizophrenia medications long term to treat temporary or episodic psychotic or nonpsychotic conditions such as mood, anxiety, sleep, pervasive developmental, attention deficit, disruptive behavior, or mental retardation disorders places such patients at risk for developing persistent psychosis. This will be especially tragic if tardive psychosis is subsequently shown to occur in children and adolescents treated with long-term antipsychotic drugs.

Iatrogenic chronic tardive psychosis is a serious and debilitating condition because it is likely to be made worse by an increase in the offending drug. Tardive psychosis should be preventable by an increased awareness, by avoidance of the more potent dopamine receptor blocking antipsychotic medications, by minimizing the dose, by limiting use to a few weeks rather than years, and by very gradually tapering doses when discontinuing them (Swartz 2004).

The antipsychotic/antischizophrenia medications can cause apparent psychotic symptoms acutely in the form of delirium. Neuroleptic malignant and serotonin syndromes, potentially caused by antipsychotic medications, can include delirium sometimes mistaken as a worsening of schizophrenia.

14.5 Obsessive-Compulsive Disorder and "Hallucinations and/or Delusions" in Normals Can Be Misdiagnosed as Schizophrenia

Obsessive-compulsive disorder (OCD) has been reported to occur with some frequency in patients primarily diagnosed with schizophrenia. The obsessions and global dysfunctionality of OCD may have been misinterpreted as auditory hallucinations and dysfunctionality of schizophrenia (Doran et al. 1986; Poyurovsky et al. 1999; Tibbo et al. 2000; Hwang et al. 2005; Byerly et al. 2005; Bottas et al. 2005). As noted by Doran et al. (1986),

> Obsessional thoughts can border on schizophrenia, and some believe that obsessions can later develop into schizophrenia. It is not difficult to see why this boundary can easily be lost. ... Usually, the confusion centers around the distinction between an obsession and a delusion.

OCD can also be difficult to differentiate from major depressive disorder.

About 10% of nonpsychiatric subjects from the general population have reported experiencing hallucinations and/or delusions, far more frequently than might be expected (Verdoux and van Os 2002; Bentall 1990, 2006). Sources of misdiagnoses of psychosis can result from respondent misunderstandings, drug-induced states, schizotypal traits, antisocial personality disorder, and culturally sanctioned magical or religious beliefs (Kendler et al. 1996). Standard questions such as "Have you ever seen or heard things that others could not see or hear?" can be misunderstood and normal experiences such as illusions or patients' own thoughts or obsessions can be reported and considered psychotic. The overemphasis on finding psychoses in the forms of paranoia, hallucinations, delusions, and dysfunctionality can lead to the misdiagnosis of schizophrenia in cases of severe OCD as well as in eccentric but nonpsychotic, functioning individuals (Doran et al. 1986; Bentall et al. 1988; Bentall 1990, 2004, 2006; Honig et al. 1998; Poyurovsky et al. 1999; Tibbo et al. 2000; van Os et al. 2000; Moynihan et al. 2002; Verdoux and van Os 2002; Hwang et al. 2005; Byerly et al. 2005; Bottas et al. 2005; Moore et al. 2006; Bentall and Fernyhough 2008). Because of the traditional concept that "a touch of schizophrenia [hallucinations and/or delusions] is schizophrenia," once a patient is deemed psychotic, the diagnosis of schizophrenia may be made, and questions about OCD may be overlooked.

Patients do not recognize the diagnostic and pharmacological consequences of their endorsing "ideas of influence or reference," "paranoid thoughts," "voices," "seeing things," or other symptoms potentially interpreted as hallucinations, delusions, or other psychotic behavior. The misidentification of hallucinations and/or delusions and a diagnosis of schizophrenia have a substantial negative impact on treatment of the actual disorder, if any, as well as on outcome (Chap. 15).

OCD and schizophrenia have been associated in the literature as two separate disorders occurring together more often than expected (Doran et al. 1986; Poyurovsky et al. 1999; Tibbo et al. 2000; Hwang et al. 2005; Byerly et al. 2005;

14.5 Obsessive-Compulsive Disorder and "Hallucinations and/or Delusions"... 293

Bottas et al. 2005). However, this observation may depend, in some cases, on the misinterpretation by OCD patients and the evaluating physicians of obsessions as auditory hallucinations and the OCD patient's dysfunctionality as schizophrenia as demonstrated by the case summaries given below. The subjects whose cases are discussed gave their written informed consents to participate in this IRB-approved research.

Case 1

Obsessions were misinterpreted as "voices" during a routine annual exam of a healthy 22-year-old, single female who reported to her primary care physician (PCP) that she heard a "voice keeping up a running commentary" on her behavior. The PCP referred her to psychiatry with the question of ruling out schizophrenia. She again answered the psychiatrist's question affirmatively that the "voice kept up a running commentary on my behavior" and had persisted "on and off" for over a year. She was misdiagnosed with schizophrenia since this answer alone satisfies DSM core criteria for the diagnosis of schizophrenia (Table 2.5) and represents a key "first-rank system" of Schneider from 1959 (Table 8.1). She was prescribed haloperidol (Haldol). Upon further consultation a year later, while still taking haloperidol, she said her "voice" continued to speak to her, keeping her organized by telling her, for example, a list of products to buy in the grocery store and chores to do for the day. She admitted to several checking compulsions that "her voices" insisted she perform and that "her voices" could be her own thoughts. She functioned well in her work and social life. Her diagnosis was changed, haloperidol was tapered and discontinued, and her OCD responded positively to clomipramine (Anafranil).

Case 2

Severe OCD can also be misdiagnosed as schizophrenia because of the persistent and often chronic course with marked dysfunction. For example, a 36-year-old, never married male was so dysfunctional that he could not hold a job and was socially isolated and withdrawn, staying in his room in his parents' house. He had been an inpatient at the state mental hospital on several occasions for months at a time. His hospital summaries noted that he "... talked to the television and to a tree in his yard." He was diagnosed with schizophrenia and had been medicated with large dosages of antipsychotic/antischizophrenia medications for years. He had mild tardive dyskinesia but was considered so severely psychotic that the antipsychotic/antischizophrenia medications were continued. He had not been given a trial off his medications "for fear he would get worse." This decision was supported by his parents. He said his "voices were a little better" when he took these drugs, but he was oversedated and was still dysfunctional. During a "second opinion" interview at the hospital, his statement that he was worse in the late spring and summer stimulated the elucidating question to which he answered that he was worse then because the leaves came out on the large oak tree in his yard in the spring, and when he tried to go out of his house, he saw the tree and had to count each leaf before he could move. He "spoke to the TV" when he saw a number such as the channel number and then had to say that number, round to an even number, count by that number to 1,000, in a "perfect voice," which took hours. When he counted, he formed the numbers with his mouth and was thus thought to be talking to the TV and the tree. He endorsed more than enough DSM symptoms to fulfill criteria for severe OCD. His diagnosis was changed, his medications were discontinued, his TD worsened, and a high dose of a tricyclic antidepressant, coupled with psychotherapy, improved his daily function.

Case 3

A 44-year-old, never married male presented for the first time to an academic outpatient clinic "because his insurance had changed and his former psychiatrist was no longer on his provider list." His chief complaint was only that he needed psychiatric follow-up for his medications for his "major depressive disorder and schizophrenia, paranoid subtype." When questioned why he was diagnosed with schizophrenia, he said he told his psychiatrist some 5 years before that he was "paranoid" and "heard voices in his head." He was prescribed olanzapine (Zyprexa) for his continuing "psychosis." During his more recent intake interview, he was questioned about his "paranoia." He said that sometimes, when he saw the president of his firm talking to his direct supervisor, he believed that he was being discussed negatively and that "such thoughts kept going around and around in my head." This had been interpreted as "ideas of reference" commonly associated with the diagnosis of schizophrenia. He also stated that other "paranoid" thoughts occurred at church or at work when he said he felt "suspicions" that some people might be thinking that his new eyeglasses "looked stupid." He said he had difficulty getting these thoughts out of his mind and equated this with the "intrusive voices in his head." Further questions revealed that he also obsessed about his forgetting to turn off his electric stovetop burners. To try to avoid this conflict, he began having breakfast at restaurants to avoid ever turning his stove on, but he admitted that on several occasions before this, he had had to drive back to his house, over 10 miles, several times a day to check the burners. He scored high on the Yale-Brown OCD scales. Overall, he functioned marginally in his life and at work that did not require interpersonal interactions. This patient had not developed tardive dyskinesia but his glucose was elevated and he had gained over 35 pounds, possibly related to 5 years of daily atypical neuroleptic therapy that was unwarranted, ineffective, and detrimental. Fluoxetine (Prozac) improved his OCD symptoms.

For all of these patients it is most fortunate that none apparently developed tardive psychosis.

14.6 Conclusions

Psychotic patients presenting or brought to the Emergency Department or Acute Care Center can certainly present a diagnostic dilemma. The first diagnostic task in approaching a psychotic patient, once the patient and medical personnel are safe, is to determine whether the cause of the psychosis is primary/functional or secondary/organic. A secondary or organic etiology to the psychosis is suggested as the first consideration. Secondary or organic causes include dementia, delirium, and myriad medical illnesses and substances (Tables 14.1, 14.2). Of the secondary causes, intoxication with one or more substances is at the top of the rule out list. All patients presenting with a new-onset psychosis warrant a thorough medical and laboratory evaluation that excludes medical and toxic causes of the psychosis (Table 14.3). Neurologic and cognitive evaluations along with a comprehensive laboratory and possibly brain imaging are basic. Repeated serial cognitive testing may reveal a delirium or toxic psychosis. Consideration of the overall clinical and epidemiological circumstances is important to narrow the differential diagnosis of psychosis. As Freudenreich (2010) states, "If a disease is unlikely (low prior probability), a positive test result is probably a false positive, which argues against indiscriminate screening." He recommends selecting the most sensitive test available so that a negative result removes that disease from the differential. For example, a treponemal-specific test to rule out neurosyphilis is recommended. A positive finding on physical

Table 14.3 Suggested medical work-up for the rule out of secondary/organic psychoses (adapted from Freudenreich 2010)

Screen broadly
  CBC, glucose, full chemistry, LFTs, ESR, ANA, UA, UDS
  Consider brain imaging with CT or MRI[a]
Exclude specifically
  Abnormal levels of TSH, vitamin B12 and folate, ceruloplasmin, HIV, FTA-Abs
Investigate further as clinically indicated[b]
  Electroencephalogram
  Chest radiography, lumbar puncture, blood and urine cultures, arterial blood gases
  Serum cortisol levels
  Toxin search
  Drug levels
  Genetic testing

CBC complete blood count; *LFTs* liver function test; *ESR* erythrocyte sedimentation rate; *ANA* antinuclear antibodies; *UA* urinalysis; *UDS* urine drug screen; *TSR* thyroid-stimulating hormone; *FTA-Abs* fluorescent treponemal antibody absorbed

[a]There is no consensus of whether brain imaging should be part of a routine workup for patients with first-episode psychosis. The yield of brain imagines is low in a patient with first-episode psychosis who presents with typical psychopathological features and illness course, and no red flags by history (e.g., history of head injury), and without positive findings on a neurological examination

[b]A broader search is indicated if a delirium is present or suspected. The extent of the workup is guided by epidemiological considerations, the clinical situation, and the immune status

examination or laboratory testing alone does not establish causality. Although there is no consensus regarding routine brain imaging in first-episode psychosis, a CT or MRI is warranted for patients with an atypical presentation, positive neurological findings, or a treatment-refractory course. The Canadian Psychiatric Association recommends routine genetic screening in patients with psychosis to rule out velocardiofacial syndrome if it is clinically suspected.

Once reasonably confident that the psychosis is primary or functional, the initial priority is a detailed screen for mood symptoms especially since data indicate over 80% of functionally psychotic patients suffer from a mood disorder, not schizophrenia (Pini et al. 2001). There will certainly be a finite number of psychotic patients with no obvious mood symptoms or signs of an organic etiology at any time. Psychotic symptoms can obscure mood symptoms, and overemphasis on the psychosis and underemphasis on mood symptoms during the initial diagnostic interview may explain some of these cases (Kendell and Gourlay 1970a, b; Lake 2008c, d). Some organic causes may be difficult to identify such as past illegal drug use, like phencyclidine, that can cause a chronic psychotic state even without continued use so that current drug screens are negative. Unrecognized tardive or supersensitivity psychosis (Weinberger et al. 1981; Steiner et al. 1990; Swartz 1995, 2004; Viguera et al. 1997; Lu et al. 2002), subtle seizure disorders (Swartz 2001), subtle congenital or subsequent brain damage, Huntington's, Parkinson's, and Wilson's diseases, and other neurological disorders can account for some of these psychotic patients without mood symptoms who are misdiagnosed with schizophrenia (Johnstone et al. 1987).

A diagnosis of schizoaffective disorder is discouraged since this diagnosis actually translates to a psychotic mood disorder. If unsure about the correct diagnosis, consider a temporary diagnosis of Psychotic Disorder Not Otherwise Specified (DSM-IV-TR #298.9) while organic causes and subtle mood symptoms are explored further.

Severe OCD and nonpsychiatrically impaired individuals have been misdiagnosed with schizophrenia. In the case of severe OCD, a global dysfunctionality and/or obsessions misinterpreted as auditory hallucinations can lead to a misdiagnosis. In normal individuals, a misattribution of one's own thoughts as "voices," eccentricities, and a suspicious nature can cause a misdiagnosis of schizophrenia.

Chapter 15
The Negative Impact of the Misdiagnosis of Schizophrenia upon Patients, Their Families, and Their Caretakers

> *We raise the possibility that antipsychotic medication may make some schizophrenic patients more vulnerable to future relapse than would be the case in the natural course of the illness [without antipsychotic medications].*
>
> (Carpenter et al. 1977)
>
> *To misdiagnose schizophrenia as bipolar disorder rarely does harm; to misdiagnose bipolar disorder as schizophrenia may adversely affect a patient's entire future.*
>
> (Pope 1983)
>
> *This formulation highlights the critical importance of early intervention in the illness [Bipolar Disorder] in order to prevent malignant transformation to rapid cycling, spontaneous episodes, and refractoriness to drug treatment [possibly leading to a misdiagnosis of Schizophrenia].*
>
> (Post 1992)
>
> *[Antipsychotic medications] ... worsen long-term outcomes, ... and ... 40% or more of all ... patients would fare better if they were not so medicated ...The preponderance of evidence shows that the current standard of care ... continual medication therapy [with antipsychotic medications] for all [psychotic] patients ... does more harm than good.*
>
> (Whitaker 2004)

15.1 Introduction

Functionally psychotic patients misdiagnosed with schizophrenia or schizoaffective disorder are most likely to suffer from an undiagnosed psychotic mood disorder or, in a few percent, an unrecognized organic psychosis (Chap. 14; Tables 14.1 and 14.2). In either situation, such patients receive substandard care with increased morbidity

Table 15.1 Department of Justice National Crime Victimization Survey for 1993-1999; Annual rate for nonfatal violet crime

Occupation	Rate of violent crime per 1,000 workers
All workers	12.6
Physicians	16.2
Nurses	21.9
Psychiatrists and other mental health professionals[b]	68.2
Mental health custodial workers[b]	69

Rosack (2006)

[b]Violence upon workers in the mental health fields are assumed by current author to be perpetrated by psychiatric patients primarily suffering from acute psychotic mania or psychosis from drug intoxication (stimulants such as cocaine, crack and methamphetamine, or hallucinogens such as PCP or "bath salts") or organic brain syndromes

and mortality. Without a correct diagnosis of a mood disorder, patients are unlikely to receive first-line mood-stabilizing medications, i.e., lithium, valproic acid (Depakote), carbamazepine (Tegretol), and lamotrigine (Lamictal). Without one or more of these, recurrent mood disorders tend to cycle faster (Sect. 15.2; Fig. 4.1) (Goodwin 1989). Increased cycles mean an increased risk for treatment resistance, chronicity, suicide, and rarely homicide (Casey 1988; Post 1992; Calabrese et al. 2001; Whitaker 2004). Friends, family, mental health professionals, and caretakers are at increased risk of violence (Table 15.1). Mental health workers including psychiatrists are over five times as likely to sustain nonfatal criminal assaults as the average worker and four times as likely as physicians in general according to the Department of Justice Crime Victimization Survey between 1993 and 1999 (Tables 15.1 and 15.7) (Rosack 2006).

When there is an unrecognized organic cause of psychosis misdiagnosed as schizophrenia, no effective treatment is given for the physical disease. In addition, the antipsychotic/antischizophrenia medications may be prescribed long term and have substantial and unacceptable side effects (Sect. 15.3). Although antipsychotic medications may be appropriate for most psychoses regardless of the cause, with some clear exceptions such as elderly demented patients, if the diagnosis of schizophrenia is made, these drugs are typically given for much longer periods of time such as years to life and in larger dosages than for psychotic mood-disordered patients (Casey 1988; Whitaker 2004). Such overuse of the antipsychotic/antischizophrenia medications also occurs in patients with psychotic mood disorders since 95% of hospitalized psychotic mood-disordered patients prescribed antipsychotic medications while inpatients, are also discharged on these drugs and their "… ongoing neuroleptic exposure remained substantial" (Sernyak et al. 1994).

Schizophrenia has been considered a lifelong, incurable, incapacitating disease since Bleuler (1911) said that there was "no restituto ad integrum [no return to baseline]" in schizophrenia. Such patients carrying the diagnosis of schizophrenia tend to give up, become dependent upon Medicaid and SSI disability, and are heavily stigmatized. Jobs, cars, houses, friends, families, and physical health can be lost, possibly not because of schizophrenia but rather due to an underrecognized and undertreated psychotic mood disorder. This is not to say that appropriately diagnosed and treated psychotic mood-disordered patients never regress to a noncycling, treatment resistant, permanent state of psychosis, but the prognosis should improve if the correct diagnosis and treatments are given early in the course of the disease (Post 1992). Regrettably, the average time between onset of symptoms and the correct diagnosis and treatment of bipolar disorders is measured in years to decades (Chap. 18) (Post 2007). The goal should be to diagnose accurately, treat appropriately, and aggressively in order to give the best chance to prevent or postpone the next episode, suicide, and homicide.

Caretakers have difficult challenges because amotivation, avolition, irritability, aggression, abuse, and possible violence are not rare in acute or chronic, psychotic mood-disordered patients (Tables 15.1, 15.7, 15.8). Physicians who misdiagnose schizophrenia in patients with psychotic mood disorders may put themselves, other caretakers, and patients' families and friends at risk for violence and homicide from acutely psychotic manic or depressed patients and may be liable for malpractice.

15.2 The Absence of Mood-Stabilizing Medications due to Misdiagnoses of Schizophrenia Allows Recurrent Mood Disorders to Worsen

Psychotic patients diagnosed with schizophrenia generally are not given lithium or any other first-line mood-stabilizing drug (Table 15.2). For mood disorders, without mood-stabilizing medications, on average, the cycle length decreases (Fig. 4.1), the risk of dementia seems to increase with the number of episodes (Kessing and Anderson 2004), and there can be a "... malignant transformation to rapid cycling, spontaneous episodes, and a refractoriness to drug treatment" (Post 1992, 2007, 2010). Dozens of studies document that lithium, at oral dosages that provide a therapeutic blood level of between approximately 0.6 and 1.4 mEg/L, substantially reduces cycling and postpones manic and depressive relapses (Gershon and Yuwiler 1960; Schou 1967, 1968, 1979; Angst et al. 1970; Shopsin et al. 1971; Wehr and Goodwin 1987; Goodwin 1989; Goodwin and Jamison 1990, 2007). Schou (1979) concluded that,

On lithium therapy alone, relapse rates for patients of either polarity [bipolar or unipolar] decreased dramatically, and there was no bipolar-unipolar difference in response to lithium.

The other three first-line mood stabilizers are also documented to reduce cycling in bipolar patients (Post 1992; Calabrese et al. 2001; Goodwin and Jamison 2007).

Lithium and the three antiepileptic mood stabilizers have significant adverse effects (Table 15.3). The therapeutic index for lithium is low at about three, meaning that its toxic level is not much greater than its therapeutic level. At the therapeutic

Table 15.2 First-line mood-stabilizing medications

Generic name	Trade name
Lithium carbonate	Eskalith, Lithobid, Lithane
Lithium citrate	Cibalith-S
Valproic acid (divalproex sodium)	Depakote
Carbamazepine	Tegretol
Lamotrigine	Lamictal

Table 15.3 Adverse effects of the first-line mood-stabilizing medications

Medication name	Common, mild to moderate side effects	Rare, severe to life-threatening side effects	Comments
Lithium	Fine tremor in the hands; dehydration; mild nausea; headache; thirst; frequent urination; weight gain; symptoms of hypothyroidism; metallic taste.	Renal diabetes insipidus due to renal impairment; coarse tremor; irregular heartbeat; visual changes; rash; swelling of the eyes, face, lips, tongue, throat, hands, feet, ankles or lower legs; ataxia; dysarthria; nystagmus; confusion; seizures; coma; death.	Lithium inhibits antidiuretic hormone, thereby inhibiting the ability of the kidney to reabsorb water from the urine, i.e., an inability to concentrate urine leading to loss of body water and thirst. Thiazide diuretics are contraindicated with lithium. Must monitor plasma lithium levels and thyroid and kidney function on a regular basis. Lithium is a teratogen causing birth defects. Lithium inhibits thyroid hormone causing symptoms of hypothyroidism.
Antiseizure mood-stabilizing medications (carbamazepine, valproic acid, lamotrigine)	Dizziness; decreased coordination; nausea; sedation; headaches; double vision; insomnia; anxiety; vivid dreams; missed or painful menstrual periods; cough; dry mouth; constipation; diarrhea; weight gain; hair loss (valproic acid).	Cardiac arrhythmias; aplastic anemia; agranulocytosis; syndrome of inappropriate antidiuretic hormone (carbamazepine); cognitive anomalies; Stevens-Johnson syndrome and toxic epidermal necrolysis (especially lamotrigine); vomiting; fever; dark urine; jaundice; liver damage; blood in the urine; hallucinations; drug eruptions; DRESS syndrome (especially lamotrigine); seizures, coma, and death possible in overdose.	Carbamazepine (Tegretol) is a CYP450 inducer increasing clearance (decreasing blood level and effectiveness) of warfarin (Coumadin), phenytoin (Dilantin), theophylline, and valproic acid (Depakote). Drugs increasing the level of carbamazepine include erythromycin, cimetidine (Tagamet), propoxyphene (Darvon), and calcium channel blockers. Valproic acid inhibits the catabolism of carbamazepine and increases its activity. Lamotrigine (Lamictal) has relatively few side effects and does not require blood monitoring; valproic acid and carbamazepine do require blood level and liver function monitoring.

level, lithium may be associated with thirst, polydipsia, a fine tremor typically observed in the hands and fingers, a metallic taste, weight gain, anorexia, and nausea. At toxic levels, most of the above worsen, and confusion, seizures, coma, and death are possible (Table 15.3). After overdose and toxic levels are reached, treatment is available since lithium is dialyzable. Lithium is excreted by the kidney and must be used with care in patients with impaired renal function and those taking diuretics. Long-term use can adversely affect kidney and thyroid function (Table 15.3).

The list of adverse reactions of the antiseizure mood stabilizers is long. Lethal side effects are rare. All are metabolized in the liver, have drug-drug interactions, and must be used with care in patients with impaired liver function. Lamotragine can cause a fatal rash called Stevens-Johnson syndrome in about 1% of recipients. The rash usually occurs when titrating up the dose. All these drugs can suppress bone marrow production of blood cells leading to aplastic anemia and especially agranulocytosis, a reduction in white blood cells, that predisposes to infections and possible death. At toxic levels, seizures, coma, and death are possible. Nonlethal adverse effects include sedation (or occasional activation with lamotragine), hair loss, weight gain, nausea, dizziness, and headache (Table 15.3).

An asset of lithium, valproic acid, and carbamazepine is that the therapeutic plasma range for each is established and levels can be measured from routine venipuncture. Clinical experience with the mood-stabilizing drugs is extensive over the past 35 years with the exception of lamotrigine (Lamictal) that has been in use for over a decade.

Given the potential for a life-devastating course from recurrent or persistent psychotic mood disorders, the benefit-to-risk ratio for these drugs is considered large. A missed diagnosis usually eliminates chances for such benefit. Regular psychiatric follow-up, weekly to every other week, is recommended to maximize the chances of patient acceptance of their disease, medication compliance, and for recognizing early indications of the onset of an episode, enabling medication adjustment before a full-blown episode develops. The goal is prevention of episodes rather than the usual "catch-up" treatment after a full relapse has occurred.

15.3 Higher Dosages of Antipsychotic/"Antischizophrenia" Medications Are Given to Patients Diagnosed with Schizophrenia and for Longer Periods of Time

The antipsychotic/antischizophrenia medications are prescribed in larger, usually escalating dosages over the lifetime of patients diagnosed with schizophrenia (Table 15.4) (Whitaker 2004). One reason is the universal idea that schizophrenia is a lifelong disease, and that the antipsychotic medications are necessary to prevent relapse. With compliance, the antipsychotic medications do acutely reduce hallucinations and delusions, but,

> ... they have not enhanced functional recovery (for example, employment) for people [diagnosed] with schizophrenia.
>
> (Insel 2010)

Table 15.4 Antipsychotic/antischizophrenia medications; typical vs atypical

Typical		Atypical	
Generic name	Trade name	Generic name	Trade name
Chlorpromazine	Thorazine	Aripiprazole	Abilify
Chlorprothixene	Taractan	Clozapine	Clozaril
Fluphenazine	Permitil, Prolixin	Iloperidone	Fanapt
Haloperidol	Haldol	Lurasidone	Latuda
Loxapine	Loxitane	Olanzapine	Zyprexa
Mesoridazine	Serentil	Paliperidone	Invega
Molindone	Lidone, Moban	Quetiapine	Seroquel
Perphenazine	Trilafon	Risperidone	Risperdal
Pimozide (for Tourette's)	Orap	Ziprasidone	Geodon
Thioridazine	Mellaril		
Thiothixene	Navane		
Trifluoperazine	Stelazine		
Trifluopromazine	Vesprin		

Across Europe, less than 20% of patients diagnosed with schizophrenia were employed. Sustained recovery of only about 15% has been recorded by two groups; one within 5 years of a psychotic episode and a second group, after a 25-year follow-up. Relapse rates in patients diagnosed with schizophrenia approached 80% despite (or because of some would say) antipsychotic/antischizophrenia medications, and despite psychosocial treatment (that is very important in preventing relapse of any chronic mental illness). Other studies reported nearly 20% of such patients were homeless at 1-year follow-up and had a high rate of incarceration (Insel 2010).

If these data derive from mood-disordered patients misdiagnosed with schizophrenia, it is possible that these dismal statistics might improve with the correct diagnosis and the addition of mood-stabilizing medications long term and only temporary use of the antipsychotic medications. The psychotic episodes are so destructive to patients' lives, their families, and friends that psychiatrists have believed that larger lifetime dosages of antipsychotic medications even with substantial adverse effects were justified to try to delay or prevent these relapses. This practice continues even in some academic departments. This may be a terribly detrimental misconception.

Data reviewed by Whitaker (2004) suggest that the antipsychotic/antischizophrenia medications,

> ... worsen long-term outcomes, ... and that 40% or more of all schizophrenia patients would fair better if they were not so medicated. ... The preponderance of evidence shows that the current standard of care ... continual medication therapy [with antipsychotic/antischizophrenia medications] for all patients so diagnosed [with schizophrenia] ... does more harm than good. ... A small number [of researchers] ... have used MRIs ... to study the effects of neuroleptics on the brain. These investigators have found that the [antischizophrenia] drugs cause atrophy of the cerebral cortex and an enlargement of the basal ganglia. ...the drug-induced enlargement of the basal ganglia is "associated with greater severity of both negative and positive symptoms." In other words, they found that the drugs cause changes in the brain associated with a worsening of the very symptoms the drugs are supposed to alleviate. In 1977, Carpenter reported that only 35% of the non-medicated patients in his study relapsed within a year after discharge, compared to 45% of those treated with

neuroleptics [antipsychotic/antischizophrenia medications]. The non-medicated patients also suffered less from depression, blunted emotions and retarded movements. ... Thus, the literature suggests that relapse rates fall into three groups: lowest for those not placed on neuroleptics in the first place, higher for those who take [antischizophrenia] drugs continuously, and highest of all for those withdrawn from the drugs. ... The real-world first-year relapse rate for patients maintained on neuroleptics is understood to be 40%.

Carpenter et al. (1977) stated that,

> There is no question that, once patients are placed on medication, they are less vulnerable to relapse if maintained on neuroleptics. But what if these patients had never been treated with drugs to begin with? ... We raise the possibility that antipsychotic medication may make some schizophrenic patients more vulnerable to future relapse than would be the case in the natural course of the illness.

The antipsychotic medications given chronically have negative effects in patients diagnosed with schizophrenia as well as in patients diagnosed with psychotic mood disorders. For example, manic patients maintained on antipsychotic/antischizophrenia medications,

> ... were more likely to have a shorter time to depressive relapse, discontinue the study, and have increased rates of dysphoria, depressive symptoms and extrapyramidal symptoms. ... There were no short-term benefits with the continued use of a typical anti-psychotic [drug] after achieving remission from an episode of acute mania. In fact, its [antipsychotic/antischizophrenia medication] continued use was associated with detrimental effects.
>
> (Zarate and Tohen 2004)

In normal subjects, single doses of antipsychotic medications produced negative symptoms and drowsiness to severe sedation that may be important confounding factors in the assessment of negative symptoms in trials of antipsychotic drugs in patients diagnosed with schizophrenia (Artaloytia et al. 2006).

According to Casey (1988), psychotic mood-disordered patients, especially those in depression, are at increased risk for tardive dyskinesia when treated with antipsychotic medications. If tardive psychosis proves to be a valid entity, analogous to tardive dyskinesia, the antipsychotic/antischizophrenia medications may be responsible for many misdiagnoses of schizophrenia and the worsening and prolongation, if not the initiation, of psychotic symptoms. He continued,

> In the short term, neuroleptic drugs should be limited to managing acute psychotic symptoms in patients with mood disorders. In the long term, neuroleptics should be reserved for manic or depressive symptoms that do not respond to standard therapy. The overall goal is to use the lowest effective neuroleptic dose for the shortest period of time....
>
> (Casey 1988)

Adverse effects of the antipsychotic medications are common and involve disfiguring movement disorders as well as other life-threatening reactions (Tables 15.5 and 15.6). The mild-to-moderate adverse effects of the antipsychotic medications typically have been addressed by prescribing additional medications to attempt to counter the adverse effects of the original antipsychotic medications rather than reducing or discontinuing them for fear of another psychotic relapse. According to some, the antipsychotic/antischizophrenia medications themselves prevent full remissions or may cause relapses into psychotic episodes based on the concept of tardive psychosis

Table 15.5 Adverse effects of antipsychotic/antischizophrenia medications

Medication name	Common, mild to moderate side effects	Rare, severe to life-threatening side effects	Comments
Atypicals	Akathisia (restlessness); dry mouth; dizziness; irritability; sedation; insomnia; constipation; urinary retention; fatigue; orthostatic hypotension; increased appetite and weight gain (ziprasidone (Geodon) may cause less weight gain); missed periods; apathy; lack of emotion; hyperprolactinemia with breast enlargement and lactation, hyperglycemia and diabetes mellitus; brain zaps; dental problems and discoloration of teeth; impaired erectile function; increased salivation; lowered seizure threshold; stuffy nose; movement disorders but at a lower rate than with the typicals (Table 15.6).	Tardive dyskinesia; neuroleptic malignant syndrome; metabolic syndrome with substantial weight gain and diabetes mellitus; risk of death in elderly patients with dementia-related psychosis; torsades de pointes and other arrhythmias; acute dystonia; severe Parkinson syndrome; stroke; allergic reaction with swelling in the mouth and throat, itching, and rash; liver damage; inflammation of the pancreas; tardive psychosis; body temperature dysregulation; aplastic anemia; agranulocytosis; cognitive and motor impairment; in overdose, seizures, coma, and death.	Quetiapine (Seroquel) had annual worldwide sales of $5.7 billion and $2.9 billion in the USA. Eli Lilly (maker of olanzapine (Zyprexa)) agreed to pay up to $1.2 billion to settle lawsuits from people who claim they developed diabetes or other injuries. About 20 million people worldwide have taken olanzapine. Pfizer (ziprasidone (Geodon)) pleaded guilty to misbranding "with the intent to [commit] fraud or mislead," agreeing to pay $2.3 billion in settlement for promotion of its drug for use in conditions that have not been approved by the FDA. Several of these atypical antipsychotic/antischizophrenia medications have received FDA approval for use in psychotic mood disorders.
Typicals	Sedation; slurred speech; dry mouth; constipation; diarrhea; urinary retention; lowered seizure threshold; weight gain; glucose intolerance; rash; skin pigmentations especially in regions exposed to sunlight; hyperprolactinemia leading to breast swelling or discharge and amenorrhea, ovarian cycle dysfunction, loss of libido, hirsutism, false-positive pregnancy tests, risk for osteoporosis in women, in men, impotence and loss of libido; contact dermatitis; akathisia (restlessness); decreased night vision, tunnel vision, increased sensitivity to light; stuffy nose; increased salivation; movement disorders (Table 15.6).	Priapism; acute dystonic reaction; tardive dyskinesia; neuroleptic malignant syndrome; Parkinson syndrome; aplastic anemia; agranulocytosis; ocular tissue deposits; blindness; cardiac arrhythmias such as torsades de pointes and sudden death; tardive psychosis; seizures; coma; death; increased risk for stroke and death in demented elderly.	The typical antipsychotic/antischizophrenia medications, especially the more potent such as haloperidol (Haldol) and fluphenazine (Prolixin) may cause the movement disorder adverse effects more often than the atypicals (Table 15.6). Their use has decreased with the development and marketing of the atypicals.

15.3 Higher Dosages of Antipsychotic/"Antischizophrenia" Medications... 305

Table 15.6 Movement disorders caused by the antipsychotic/antischizophrenia medications

Movement disorder	Time to onset of symptoms[a]	Symptoms of movement disorder	Treatment	Side effects of the treatment
Akathisia	Hours to days	Restlessness; inability to sit still; agitation	Benzodiazepines	Sedation; tolerance; subject to abuse; difficult withdrawal
Acute dystonic reaction	Minutes to days; 50% within 2 days; 90% within 5 days	Sudden onset of frightening, painful muscle cramps; dramatic presentation sometimes confused with a seizure or stroke; muscles affected are neck, face, and eyes; torticollis with neck twisted or head drawn back and fixed to one side; oculogyric crisis causes the eyes to be turned upward and/or to one side.	Discontinue antipsychotic/antischizophrenia medication(s); stat IV push of diphenhydramine (Benadryl), 25–50 mg or benztropine mesylate (Cogentin) 1–2 mg PO/IM/IV; prophylactic anticholinergic agent such as benztropine mesylate (Cogentin) recommended for first five days (Boyer et al. 1987).	Additional anticholinergic side effects
Parkinson's syndrome	Days to a few weeks	Rigidity; instability; resting tremor; shuffling gait; masked facies; urinary retention; depression	Anticholinergic and/or dopaminergic agents	Additional anticholinergic side effects
Tardive dyskinesia	Months to years	Bucco-facial-lingual syndrome with repetitive lip pursing, grimacing, and tongue protrusions	None	Must discontinue antipsychotic/antischizophrenia medications typically resulting in a worsening of symptoms.

[a]From starting a course of an antipsychotic/antischizophrenia medication

(Sect. 14.4) (Swartz 1995; Whitaker 2004). The occurrence of tardive psychosis, theorized as antipsychotic medication induced psychosis after chronic use and especially exacerbated by missing several doses or a prescribed lowering of dose, usually leads to physician ordered increases of dosage with temporary improvement in the psychotic symptoms. Such improvement is mistaken as confirmation of schizophrenia and the need for lifelong antipsychotic/antischizophrenia medications at greater dosages after each breakthrough of dopamine supersensitivity over dopamine receptor blockade. Parallel with the established antipsychotic medications induced movement disorder, tardive dyskinesia, tardive psychosis is also thought to be caused by antipsychotic/antischizophrenia medication induced supersensitivity of brain dopamine receptors. When the dopamine receptor supersensitivity overrides the dopamine receptor blocking effects of the antipsychotic medication, tardive dyskinesia or tardive psychosis is thought to occur, depending upon the brain area most affected. As indicated by "tardive," its onset occurs months to years after taking an antipsychotic medication. The movements do not stop and tend to get worse with the discontinuation of the causative antipsychotic medication (Table 15.6).

In the case of tardive dyskinesia, continuation of the offending antipsychotic medication is considered malpractice despite the recognition that increasing the dose does usually lead to a temporary decrease in the abnormal movements based on increased dopamine receptor blockade temporarily overcoming the dopamine receptor supersensitivity. Tardive dyskinesia is untreatable except by increasing the dose of dopamine-blocking antipsychotic medications which is prohibited by standard of care. Symptoms can last for years to decades, are highly disfiguring, and life altering often leading to the loss of employment and dysfunction. Dozens of medications have been tried for treatment but with little success. Another name for tardive dyskinesia is the bucco-facial-lingual syndrome because the abnormal movements involve repetitive lip pursing, facial grimacing, and tongue protrusions on a fairly constant waking basis, worsened by anxiety (Table 15.6).

The other antipsychotic medication induced movement disorders are also disfiguring, disturbing, and life altering (Table 15.6). Akathisia can begin within hours to days of starting an antipsychotic/antischizophrenia medication. This movement disorder is described as an uncomfortable sensation of an inability to sit still or relax. Patients are driven into nongoal-directed movement and agitation. At least one patient described the sensation as having "ants in my pants." The benzodiazepine class of antianxiety drugs such as alprazolam (Xanax) and clonazepam (Klonopin) can give some relief but produce tolerance and sedation themselves. When tolerance develops, higher dosages are needed for continued relief, and these drugs are difficult to taper and discontinue after a few months of high dosages because of patient reluctance to taper due to withdrawal effects. Because of the fear of a psychotic relapse, these additional drugs are prescribed to try to counter the adverse effects of the antipsychotic medication rather than discontinue it. Akathisia usually goes away within days to a week or two after discontinuing the antipsychotic medication.

Acute dystonic reactions are acute in onset, dramatic, painful, and frightening. These symptoms occur due to muscle contractures typically in muscles of the neck and eyes called torticollis and oculogyric crisis. Onset typically occurs within minutes to a few days of beginning a course of an antipsychotic medication. A schizophrenia drug induced acute dystonic reaction is considered a psychiatric emergency and warrants a stat IV push of diphenhydramine (Benadryl), 25–50 mg. Prophylactic anticholinergic drugs (for example, benztropine, (Cogentin)) have been recommended in parallel with starting one of the potent typical antipsychotic/antischizophrenia medications especially in younger, muscular male patients (Boyer et al. 1987). The addition of such drugs adds to the side-effect profile of the treatment of schizophrenia.

Antipsychotic medication induced Parkinson's movements can begin within days to weeks of starting the drug (Table 15.6). These abnormal and disfiguring movements are basically the same as those seen in idiopathic Parkinson's disease. They include imbalance, a shuffling gate, limb rigidity, masked facies or flat affect (an inability to show emotions in the facial muscles), and a resting tremor. Depression is possible if not likely. These side effects usually resolve within weeks of discontinuing the antipsychotic medication, but as with akathisia, other drugs, in this case, the anticholinergic drugs are added to try to counter these Parkinson's side effects in order to continue the antipsychotic medication. These added anticholinergic drugs have adverse effects of their own (Table 15.6). In some cases, the drug induced Parkinson's syndrome does not resolve after discontinuing the offending antipsychotic medications (Jimenez-Jimenez et al. 1997).

Other adverse effects of the antipsychotic/antischizophrenia medications are considered by severity and frequency and by class of drugs: the typical antipsychotic medications versus the atypical antipsychotic medications (Table 15.5). The first typical antipsychotic medication was chlorpromazine (Thorazine), developed in the 1950s (Chap. 9). The typical antipsychotic medications have a substantial adverse-effect profile (Table 15.5) in addition to the drug induced movement side effects (Table 15.6). Life threatening but rare effects include sudden cardiac death, bone marrow suppression with aplastic anemia or agranulocytosis, neuroleptic malignant syndrome, and serotonin syndrome. Common but generally nonlife-threatening adverse effects are sedation, often severe; weight gain, often substantial; nausea; constipation or diarrhea; dizziness upon standing; blurred vision; rapid heartbeat; sensitivity to the sun; and others (Table 15.5).

One of the first atypical antipsychotic/antischizophrenia medications was olanzapine (Zyprexa) released in 1996, followed by quetiapine (Seroquel) and many others (Table 15.4). More are under development or in clinical trials, spurred by a $1 billion dollar a year market for this class of drugs. As is usual with the release and marketing of most new drugs, the atypicals were presented as a major advance in the treatment of schizophrenia because of the early belief of a substantial reduction of side effects compared to the typicals. They were not more effective in the treatment of hallucinations and delusions with the possible exception of clozapine (Clozaril). The atypicals seem to have a lower incidence of movement disorder side effects that were common to the typical antipsychotic medications (Tables 15.5 and 15.6). The atypicals also followed the usual course of other new classes of drugs; with time, substantial adverse effects were found (Table 15.5).

The atypicals may increase the risk of stroke and death in elderly patients with dementia. Abnormal shifts in sleep patterns with extreme fatigue and weakness were noted. The fatigue can cause avolition, amotivation, dysfunctionality, and an almost stuporous state. These adverse effects overlap with the "negative symptoms" of schizophrenia that are criteria for the diagnosis and are target symptoms for which these drugs are given. Cardiovascular disease and sudden death are possible adverse effects of the atypicals. Sexual side effects include a reduction in sexual interest, impaired sexual performance with failure to ejaculate in males, and abnormal menstrual cycles and infertility in females. Both sexes are subject to breast enlargement and lactation. Since 2003, the FDA has required all manufacturers of the atypicals to include a warning about the risks of hyperglycemia, hyperlipidemia, and diabetes. This group of side effects including substantial weight gain and diabetes has been called the neuroleptic metabolic syndrome. Hypertension is not unusual. One reference cited the prevalence of the metabolic syndrome in patients diagnosed with schizophrenia and treated with the atypical antipsychotic medications to be about 40% (McEvoy et al. 2005).

The term "atypical antipsychotics" has been criticized, and any substantial differences from the typicals has been questioned. It was said that,

> ... the second-generation drugs [atypicals] have no special atypical characteristics that separate them from the typical, or first-generation, antipsychotics. As a group they are no more efficacious, do not improve specific symptoms, have no clearly different side-effect profiles than the first-generation antipsychotics, and are less cost effective. The spurious invention of the atypicals can now be regarded as invention only, cleverly manipulated by the drug industry for marketing purposes and only now being exposed.
>
> (Tyler and Kendell 2009)

The misconception that the atypicals had a substantially improved benefit to risk ratio over the typicals served to increase the diagnosis and the perceived validity of schizophrenia.

15.4 The Stigma of Schizophrenia

The disease called schizophrenia is understood as a life-long, disabling disease with a downhill course mandating the taking of antipsychotic/antischizophrenia medications for life. The diagnosis of schizophrenia essentially eliminates chances for most employment including service in the military. Society's expectations of those diagnosed with schizophrenia are low, and with each psychotic relapse, patients' self-confidence and self-esteem fall further. Schizophrenia and bipolar disorder receive government disability status allowing survival at a poverty level. Once disability status is received, it is rarely given up and adds to amotivation and avolition. These patients can become homeless, living on the streets, and physically ill.

Society in general does not fully understand mental illness. Some believe willpower should be able to overcome the inertia, avolition, and absence of productivity of chronic or recurrent psychotic mental illness especially depression. Some attribute such dysfunctionality to laziness.

In addition to the stigma caused by the disease and the dysfunctionality, the antipsychotic/antischizophrenia medications given chronically to treat schizophrenia cause a host of adverse effects that are disfiguring and subject patients to further family and public ridicule. These side effects such as the movement disorders, sedation, and gross weight gain are sometimes considered willful. Tom Insel summarized the stigma of schizophrenia in his 2010 perspective article in *Nature*:

> In contrast to many other medical disorders, schizophrenia today too often defines a person rather than describing the illness. Our fear of psychosis or disruptive behaviour may keep us from seeing the heroic struggle that people with this disorder face just to survive amidst the internal chaos and panic that is part of this chronic illness. Our expectations of these citizens are low: they should stay out of jail, on their medications and not distress their families, friends and fellow citizens. They deserve better. As a vision for 2030, people who suffer from any stage of schizophrenia will be considered to be educable, employable and capable of living in intimate relationships with others.

This description of schizophrenia by Insel readily applies to the psychotic mood disorders, but the stigma is markedly less for mood disorders than for those with the diagnosis of schizophrenia. Since the mood disorders have been considered more treatable and likely to remit, such patients are more hopeful than patients diagnosed with schizophrenia. Such hope can improve prognosis. Stigma and hope are again addressed in a New York Times front page article about schizophrenia (Carey 2011):

> Moreover the enduring stigma of mental illness [schizophrenia] teaches people with such a diagnosis to think of themselves as victims, snuffing out the one thing that can motivate them to find treatment: hope.

Another factor that increases the stigma of the diagnosis of schizophrenia is the high rate of incarceration among psychotic psychiatric patients. Over the past 50 years, the psychiatric inpatient population decreased by about 75%, but during this time in the USA, there has been a marked increase in the prison population, as high as six-fold between 1970 and 2002 (Harcourt 2007). A majority of violent psychiatric patients, most diagnosed with schizophrenia, are now incarcerated in jails and prisons instead of in psychiatric facilities (Table 15.7) (Harcourt 2007; Mandal 2002). Patients diagnosed with schizophrenia are, "... nearly 20 times more likely to have committed murder than people in the general population, ... one in 300 people with schizophrenia has killed someone..." (Fazel et al. 2009, editors summary). For patients diagnosed with schizophrenia and who drink alcohol or abuse illegal drugs, especially stimulants, the risk factor for violence and prison is much greater (Fazel et al. 2009). As expected, these patients diagnosed with schizophrenia and with bipolar disorder have a rate of incarceration and homelessness as high as 20 times the rate of nonbipolar or nonschizophrenic individuals. By 2020, it has been estimated that 60% of patients diagnosed with schizophrenia will have a criminal record. With a diagnosis of schizophrenia, a criminal record, and homelessness, they are stigmatized and discriminated against even more. With a correct diagnosis of a mood disorder versus schizophrenia, and treatment with mood-stabilizing drugs, it is certainly possible that these statistics would improve.

15.5 Risk for Violence, Suicide, Homicide, and Filicide Is Increased in Psychotic Mood Disorders Misdiagnosed with Schizophrenia

The risk for suicide in major mood disorders in general has been estimated at 10–15%, that for bipolar disorders is as high as 20–25%. Suicide occurs predominantly in depressed patients with a few exceptions such as end-of-life decisions. The suicide rate in patients diagnosed with schizophrenia has also been reported as substantial at 7% (Insel 2010), but if these suicidal patients are misdiagnosed and have a psychotic mood disorder instead, then accurate diagnosis and treatment might lower the 7% rate of suicide in those cases attributed to patients diagnosed with schizophrenia. The most productive strategy for preventing suicide is a high rate of recognition of depression, a high index of suspicion in depressed patients, an effective risk assessment strategy, and intense follow-up or hospitalization with preventative care by a physician or psychiatrist (Chap. 18) (Lake 2008c, d; Lake and Baumer 2010). Other acts of violence are perpetrated by psychotic mood-disordered patients, putting their significant others at risk (Table 15.8).

Psychiatrists and other mental health workers are at risk of violence, injury, and murder by their psychotic patients.

> According to the Department of Justice National Crime Victimization Survey for 1993 to 1999, the annual rate for nonfatal violent crime for all occupations was 12.6 per 1,000 workers. For physicians, the rate was 16.2, and for nurses it was 21.9. But for psychiatrists and mental health professionals, the rate was 68.2, and for mental health custodial workers, 69. (Rosack 2006) (Table 15.1)

Friends, families, caretakers, counselors, and physicians of psychotic mood-disordered patients are at risk for injury and murder particularly from psychotic manic or depressed patients and especially when they are un- or misdiagnosed and not controlled with mood-stabilizing drugs (Tables 15.1 and 15.7). This risk increases for bipolar patients misdiagnosed with schizophrenia, unipolar depression, or postpartum depression. It is psychotic mania that associates with racing thoughts, uncharacteristic spur of the moment decisions, extremely poor judgment, abuse of alcohol, irritability, paranoia, intrusiveness, anger, aggression, psychosis, violence, and sometimes homicide (Sects. 12.4–12.6). However, in high-profile murder cases by mentally ill killers, the diagnosis in the media is typically paranoid schizophrenia. A Yahoo search crossing murder and severe mental illness from media sources revealed 33 cases that are reviewed here (Tables 15.7, 15.8). For example, the *Vancouver Sun*, Vancouver Canada on October 7, 2002, reported the occurrence of:

> … more than 130 murders and murder-suicides across Canada since 1997 in which mental illness played a prominent role … particularly schizophrenia, … Psychiatric patients are assaulting and murdering their loved ones at an alarming rate, with family members the victims in three out of four killings committed by the mentally ill, …

In the 108 killings between 1997 and 2002 in Canada that were unequivocally attributed to psychotic mental illness, over 95% of the victims were either related to their killers by blood or marriage, or were friends, neighbors, employers, employees, roommates, or fellow residents of an apartment or rooming house. Twenty-seven of the victims were parents or grandparents. The majority of the 130 Canadian diagnoses of the perpetrators in these cases was schizophrenia. Ten of these Canadian cases are summarized in Table 15.7 along with 23 cases of murder, suicide, or assault by psychotic patients that occurred in the USA for a total of 33 cases. At least 1 victim was murdered in 28 of the 33 cases.

One hundred percent of the perpetrators were male in the 32 of 33 cases in which there were murders or injuries. The one case with no injury involved an 18-year-old female perpetrator diagnosed with schizophrenia who had a vivid fantasy and made threats to murder her family by stabbing them to death in their sleep (Table 15.7, case #20). In 30 of the 33 cases, the victims were known to the perpetrator. Five victims were the patients' therapists, psychiatrists, or counselors (Table 15.7, cases #3, 7–9, 12). Eleven were parents, uncles, or children (cases #1, 10, 17–19, 21, 22, 26, 29, 30, 32). In seven events, the victims were spouses, fiancées, friends, roommates, or fellow students (cases #10, 11, 14, 16, 23, 28, 31). Of the three cases in which the victims were unknown, two were in China (cases #5, 15) with several seemingly random murders in each case including children in both. In the random US case (#24), Mr. Goldstein pushed his victim in front of the N train in the 23rd Street station, in an apparent spur-of-the-moment act. These three killers were diagnosed with schizophrenia.

All of the 33 perpetrators were psychotic and had a history of past psychotic behaviors (Tables 15.7 and 15.8). Several circumstances in many of the cases, such as no mention of a positive drug test or event-related drug use, positive past episodes of major depression, close family ties, a family history of a bipolar disorder, and some successes in their lives, at least suggest that illegal or prescription drugs were not the primary cause of the fatal actions. Thirty-one (94%) of the 33 cases of mentally ill murderers or attempted murderers from Tables 15.7 to 15.8 carried diagnoses of schizophrenia; three of these also were diagnosed with bipolar disorder, and one had diagnoses of schizophrenia and major depressive disorder. The remaining two had bipolar disorder diagnoses, only (6%). In two of the 33 cases, there were only threats (#20) or a sexual assault and kidnapping (#13). Two perpetrators were shot dead at the scene after their attacks. Five committed murders and then killed or attempted to kill themselves (cases #1, 8 (attempted suicide), 11, 18, 21).

There were relevant descriptions of some of the killers diagnosed with schizophrenia when they were apparently euthymic:

> ... [they] often led deceptively routine lives – honor-roll students, gifted athletes, kids who paddled canoes and peddled newspapers. ... He was cheerful, witty, unassuming, ... He was so tender and gentle and full of self-doubt that he didn't realize what a terrific person he was.

This description highlights the fact that cycling mood-disordered patients can have euthymic episodes in between episodes of mania and depression in which they can function normally or excel at least in the early stages of the disorder. Some bipolar patients throughout history have been successful in every endeavor of life (case #28). During relapse behavior is far from normal.

Table 15.7 Violence, homicide, and suicide committed by patients misdiagnosed with schizophrenia

Case no.	Year; location; reference	Patient/murderer age; diagnosis	Description of crime	Victim name(s)/ relationship to patient
1	Mar. 2011; New Orleans, LA; Urbaszewski, nola.com Mar. 6, 2011 Braxton; Fox 8 TV, Mar. 7, 2011	John Reynolds, 22; *schizophrenia*	Leon (9 years old) and Dawania (10 years old) Reynolds were shot in the heads by their uncle who also shot himself at about 3 a.m.	Leon Reynolds, 9; Dawania Reynolds, 10; *nephew* and *niece*; killer *suicided*
2	Jan. 2011; Tucson, AZ Johnson et al., *New York Times*, Jan. 10, 2011 Becker et al., *New York Times*, Jan. 11, 2011 and Jan. 16, 2011 Gardner et al., *Washington Post*, Jan. 13, 2011 Sulzberger & Carey, *New York Times*, Jan. 19, 2011 Wikipedia (2011)	Jared L. Loughner, 22; *paranoid schizophrenia*	Apparently the night before the shooting, Mr. Loughner got little or no sleep posting an incoherent note on MySpace at 4:12 a.m. MST that discussed the literacy rate, wanting to make it out alive, the longest war in the history of the United States, the current currency, and job employment. He signed "Thank you. PS—plead the fifth!" At 7:04 a.m. MST, Loughner went out to buy ammunition, was stopped for running a red light but not detained. Upon returning home, he had an argument in the front yard with his father who had told a neighbor the 22-year-old was "out of control." Mr. Loughner ran away and took a cab to the murder site. "… Jared L Loughner, 22, wearing a black hooded sweatshirt, blue jeans and sunglasses,…" asked an aid for "… time with his Congresswoman." He was told to stand at the end of the line of about 20 people, and at first, he complied but then came back, "… walking swiftly… eyes steeled, heading for the table where Ms. Giffords was speaking. He raised his arm and opened fire…. <u>Mr. Loughner kept up his fatal barrage, dancing up and down excitedly</u>, turning from Ms. Giffords before firing, apparently indiscriminately, at her constituents, staff and the random passers-by."	*Six dead and 13 wounded including Rep. Gabrielle Giffords, D-AZ.* Among the dead were Judge John M. Roll; Christina Taylor Green, 9 years old; Gabriel Zimmerman, an aid to Ms. Giffords

Symptoms	Comments
According to a NOPD spokesperson, "… the man [perp] was staying temporarily at the residence and suffered from schizophrenia. He had stopped taking his medication and had been awake for several days." He abused alcohol.	This double murder and suicide occurred at about 3 a.m. after the murderer "… had not slept for several days and had been drinking shortly before the shooting…." Such insomnia coupled with activity and drinking suggests a psychotic manic episode. Although there was likely a paranoid delusion, no information was found about such. The perpetrator was said to have had a history of severe mental illness and domestic violence.
"He played… marathon games of monopoly with his buddies. He went with friends on family vacations…. He had a girlfriend. He laughed and he loved and he knew things-about jazz, cars, fantasy games. And then Jared Loughner slipped into a world of fantasy that was no online game." Police were called at least twice to Mr. Loughner's high school…. During his late high school years and thereafter, Loughner moved through a blur of entry-level jobs at chain stores and restaurants"…. In the past year or so the crumbling of what was once Loughner was clear to anyone who bothered to look. Teachers, fellow students,… suspected mental illness…. A student in Loughner's math class at Pima Community College usually sat near the classroom door for fear that he might turn violent,…" Loughner was *inappropriate and disruptive* in a remedial Algebra class, was "Asked to quiet down,… sent… to see a school counselor,… [and] told… to stop disrupting class,… on his first quiz, Loughner doodled in the margins, drew cartoon figures and wrote nonsensical equations such as 'Eat + Sleep + Brush Teeth = Math' and words 'MAYHEM FEST'… Students and teachers had reported his odd comments and inappropriate behavior. [One of his teachers] described a pattern of behavior by Mr. Loughner, marked by hysterical laughter, bizarre non sequiturs and aggressive outbursts,… [One teacher] asked police to send an officer to his class every day [that Loughner attended]… 'I was afraid he was going to pull out a weapon.' From Feb to Sept 2010 Loughner had five contacts with Pima Community College police for classroom and library disruptions. On Sept 29, 2010 college police discovered a UTube video shot by Loughner… stating that the college was illegal according to the United States Constitution. [This resulted in] a campus police officer visiting Loughner at home and reading him a letter of immediate suspension…. Loughner… told the officer, 'I realize now that this is all a scam'… On one [web] site, Above Top Secret, Loughner left dozens of posts with bizarre theories about U.S. currency, the Constitution and grammar…. [A friend said] 'He would call me at 2 am and ask, are you hanging out in front of my house, stalking me?' He started to get really paranoid and said he did not want to see us anymore and did not trust us… 'He thought we were plotting to kill him or steal his car.'" "…. some members of extended family may have had mental illness. 'There is a history in the family of what they used to call manic depression, which I guess they now call bipolar disorder'" Loughner apparently abused marijuana and alcohol but stopped using both in 2008.	Some important symptoms that might have conclusively given a diagnosis of psychotic mania were not found in the material reviewed. Still there are behaviors described that are convincing indications that Mr. Loughner was in an excited, psychotic, manic state and may not have slept the night before the shootings as well as other nights. His erratic, loud, inappropriate and intrusive disruptions documented in some of his classes caused the police to be called on at least five occasions. Grandiosity is indicated by his focus on a U.S. Congresswoman. Grandiosity, paranoia, inappropriate, loud, intrusive disruptions, psychosis and violence are compatible with psychotic mania.

(continued)

Table 15.7 (continued)

Case no.	Year; location; reference	Patient/murderer age; diagnosis	Description of crime	Victim name(s)/ relationship to patient
3	Jan. 2011; Revere, MA Manganis, SalemNews.com, Jan. 22, 2011 Sontag, *New York Times*, June 17, 2011	Deshawn James Chappel, 27; *schizophrenia, head trauma*	Ms. Moulton was working her solo shift as counselor at the group home. The other residents had left the house to attend programs while she had been scheduled to accompany Mr. Chappel to a therapy session. "He [Chappel] believed she [Moulton] was sending his information to President Obama.… Mr. Chappel beat her, stabbed her repeatedly and then dumped her partially nude body in a church parking lot,… [There were] 'multiple, deep penetrating stab wounds to her neck,… blunt impact injuries to her head, torso and upper extremities,' the pants and underwear 'dangling from one ankle'… After depositing her body in the parking lot, Mr. Chappel abandoned the car and stole clothes to replace his bloody ones,… He then called his grandmother."	Stephanie Moulton, Resident Counselor, 25; *patient's counselor*
4	Sept. 2010; Kansas City, MO Vendel and Williams, *Kansas City Star*, Sept. 16, 2006	Casey Brezik, 22; *paranoid schizophrenia*	Mr. Brezik learned that Governor Nixon was to speak at the community college that he had been attending in KC, MO and wore a bullet-resistant vest to class that day. He apparently mistakenly stabbed Al Dimmit Jr. the Dean of Instruction in the hallway outside the computer lab where a lectern had been set up for Nixon's speech. Nixon had not arrived yet.	Intended victim was *Missouri Governor* Jay Nixon, but he, Brezik, mistakenly stabbed Al Dimmit Jr., a Metropolitan Community College-Penn Valley *Dean*

Symptoms	Comments
Mr. Chappel was the oldest of five children in an intact family. He was "… a running back on his high school football team and went to work … after graduation. He had been an outgoing, church going boy, and his mother thought he would grow up to be a minister.… 'He took a girl with a prosthetic leg and arm to her senior prom because nobody else would… That was the kind of stuff he'd do before he changed.'… [He was] a snappy dresser but began neglecting his appearance… stopped talking about God and started talking about <u>the devil</u>… 'He would say <u>the devil was telling him to do things</u>,… He would talk about curses and hexes and a lot of things that didn't make sense.'… By the time he turned 21,… the <u>voices in</u> his head <u>prevented him from sleeping</u>… He said <u>he felt so angry that he feared he would hurt himself or someone else</u>, and he asked her [his mom] to take him to the hospital,…. [He] was admitted to Massachusetts General Hospital for a couple of weeks. That is when schizophrenia was diagnosed and he was prescribed anti-psychotic medication… Over the next couple of years,… <u>he was hospitalized… at least four more times</u> [and] he was also <u>arrested several more times on assault charges</u>… In 2007 [he seemed to be doing better.] 'This was the son I raised,' [his mother said]. 'He talked about going back to school and getting a college degree.' [However,]… he mostly stayed in his room and did not participate in day programs. He got anti-psychotic injections every other week. [By Thanksgiving (2010)] 'He was talking intensely about <u>people watching him</u>,… He felt too uneasy to leave the house.' [By Christmas]… He began phoning relatives and 'making delusional statements.'…" He believed Ms. Moulton was *sending his information to President Obama*. "The psychologist [who examined him] cited non sequiturs that Mr. Chappel had spouted in a private session.… Mr. Chappel…told him variously that he <u>hailed from Texas and rooted for the Washington Redskins and that he wanted 'a lawyer from UCLA with a 3.5 grade-point average</u>.'"	Assuming Mr. Chappell's head trauma did not have a role in his psychosis and the murder, his belief of "his information" being sent to President Obama and his demand for "… a lawyer from UCLA with a 3.5 grade-point average," indicates a level of grandiosity compatible with psychotic mania. He said he couldn't sleep due to the voices in his head that were likely his racing thoughts. His paranoia, episodes of depression and violence are compatible with psychotic bipolar disorder.
Reportedly, "Brezik did not have a particular beef with Nixon, the sources said, but wanted to harm him because he was <u>a top government official.… in Jackson County Circuit Court</u> …, onlookers could see an anarchist symbol tattooed on his right hand and a star, hammer and sickle on his left hand.… His… father… said Brezik talked about '<u>big brother watching</u>' and harbored anti-government views'… Brezik had a history of 'lack of personal hygiene, delusional thoughts, drug abuse, erratic behavior and homelessness.'"	Assuming illegal drugs are not a source of his psychotic behavior, his paranoia, grandiosity, symptoms of major depression, and violence are consistent with a diagnosis of psychotic bipolar disorder (Chap. 12; Fig. 12.2).

(continued)

Table 15.7 (continued)

Case no.	Year; location; reference	Patient/murderer age; diagnosis	Description of crime	Victim name(s)/ relationship to patient
5	Apr. 2010, Xizhen, China LaFraniere, *New York Times*, Nov. 11, 2010	Yang Jiaqin, 40; *schizophrenia*	"On a warm, sunny afternoon in April, Mr. Yang burst from his home in this rural village near the Vietnamese border, carrying a kitchen cleaver. He encountered three youngsters headed home from school … he hacked two primary schoolers, badly wounding both, and slit a second grader's throat, leaving him dying on the ground. Then he moved on…. Running from house to house, Mr. Yang killed a 70-year old woman who was making firecrackers, and a man who was watching a television drama on his sofa. He slashed the man's wife and a girl drawing well water."	Three primary school children, a 70-year-old woman and a man watching television, the man's wife, and a girl drawing water. He *killed a total of three people and injured four*. All were apparently *unknown* to Mr. Yang.
6	Mar. 2010; Washington DC, at the Pentagon Klein et al., *The Washington Post*, Friday, Mar. 5, 2010	John Patrick Bedell, 36; paranoid *schizophrenia*, according to his father	Mr. Bedell "… walked up to an entrance to the Pentagon … approached two police officers, calmly pulled a gun from his coat pocket and opened fire, wounding the officers before they shot and seriously wounded him."	Two Pentagon *police officers*

15.5 Risk for Violence, Suicide, Homicide, and Filicide Is Increased in Psychotic... 317

Symptoms	Comments
Five years prior to the murders, Mr. Yang's wife said, "… that her husband … needed [psychiatric] treatment. Always excitable and easily frightened, she said, he became obsessed with the notion that <u>people were after him</u>. One night that autumn, he fled his house during a raging storm. Relatives found him the next day pacing near a pond, covered with scratches, shaking violently,… 'It was very scary' he told her. <u>'People were chasing me all night.</u>'… Relatives ferried Mr. Yang to the Hepu County Psychiatric Hospital,… Still, his episodes grew more severe. In 2007, she said, Mr. Yang <u>leaped from a third-floor window to escape imaginary pursuers</u>, breaking his leg. In 2008,… he called the police from a <u>Shanghai television tower, threatening suicide</u>.… By last spring, Mr. Yang, was afraid to leave his dim mud-clay house. <u>'All he did was stay home and cry,</u>'… Last April 9, the demons inside him took control. That evening, Mr. Yang smashed through the wooden door of his 63-year old neighbor,… and struck him in the head with an axe."	Stages of success interspersed with psychotic episodes that include depression, delusional paranoia, and violence are compatible with a bipolar disorder.
Mr. Bedell apparently lived in California. Before the shooting, "… <u>he had crises-crossed the country in a frenetic and sometimes in a doped-up state</u> that had his parents so worried they alerted the police that he might be armed.…[he] had been slipping into increasingly disturbed thinking for years but whose <u>behavior became uncharacteristically erratic only in recent months</u>.… In early January, <u>a Texas highway patrol officer stopped Bedell… for speeding</u>. Bedell's car was in 'disarray.'" His parents, "… had filed a missing persons' report… according to police, [Bedell] said he was heading to the East Coast but instead drove home.. [about 1,500 miles the opposite direction back to California].. He wouldn't stay long. On February 1, Bedell hit the road again and was stopped by an officer in Reno.… He was charged with possession of marijuana… In an audio address posted on the internet, he suggested that <u>after the 1963 assassination of President John F Kennedy the United States had been infiltrated by a cabal of gangsters he called the 'coup regime.'</u>" In another internet posting, he discussed, "… his <u>invention of a stock market-like information exchange</u>.…[According to his parents,] Bedell 'had gone off the deep end right before he left,…'" At 24, "… his skepticism began to turn to deep rooted suspicion. And soon it became paranoia, his brother said.… He believed <u>songs he heard on the radio were meant as warnings</u> [and that] <u>'they' were watching him</u>.… his father, [a former California Deputy Attorney General said,] 'there were symptoms of a mental disorder, approaching <u>paranoid schizophrenia</u>,…'" It was said that Bedell, "… <u>moved to Austin [TX] to live with a woman he met at a bookstore</u> at the University of California at Davis.… [his thoughts were] laden with <u>conspiracy theories</u>,… He was interested in <u>developing a different currency</u>,…"	His erratic, spur-of-the-moment decisions, frantic state, multiple trips, speeding, grandiosity, and paranoia are compatible with psychotic mania and a bipolar disorder.

(continued)

Table 15.7 (continued)

Case no.	Year; location; reference	Patient/murderer age; diagnosis	Description of crime	Victim name(s)/ relationship to patient
7	2009; Boston, MA Ward, Boston.com/news; Oct. 27, 2009	Jay Carciero, 37; *likely bipolar since event happened in the bipolar clinic*	During a therapy session in the bipolar clinic near the Massachusetts General Hospital, Mr. Carciero, a patient, stabbed his psychiatrist, Dr. Astrid Desrosiers, an MGH psychiatrist. Mr. Carciero was shot dead by an off-duty security guard and Dr. Desrosiers survived.	Dr. Astrid Desrosiers was the *patient's psychiatrist*.
8	Feb. 2008; North Andover, MA *Eagle Tribune*, Feb. 7, 2008 *North Andover Citizen*, Feb. 8, 2008	Thomas Balenger, 18; *severe bipolar disorder*; *head trauma*	Ms. Mattian, a counselor and social worker, made a house call to Mr. Balenger's house where she was fatally stabbed in the back after she allegedly failed to persuade him to give up a knife. He then slit his own throat, but survived.	Diruhi Mattian, MSW, 53; patient's *psychotherapist*; killer *attempted suicide*, but failed.
9	Feb. 2008; Upper East Side, New York City, NY *New York Times*, May 21, 2008 and Oct. 15, 2008	David Tarloff, 39; *paranoid schizophrenia*	Mr. Tarloff went to his psychiatrist's suite of offices. He intended to rob Dr. Shinbach and, with the money, take his incapacitated mother out of her nursing home to Hawaii. Seeing Dr. Faughey alone in her office, he murdered her with a meat cleaver. Dr Shinbach, hearing her screaming, came to her office and was himself attacked, robbed, and cut badly.	Kathryn Faughey, Ph.D., 56, officed in the suite with Mr. Tarloff's *psychiatrist*, Dr. Kent Shinbach, M.D. Dr. Shinbach was severely injured.

Symptoms	Comments
No symptoms or diagnoses were given in the article.	The patient was being seen in the bipolar clinic and demonstrates the danger of psychotic bipolar patients.
Four years earlier, "… Thomas Balenger, then 14, was involved in an episode that led to multiple charges of assault with a knife and a fire extinguisher, as well as assault on a public official." A neighbor said he watched football games with Mr. Balenger, whom he described as a "… lonely, gentle kid."	The diagnosis of bipolar disorder is likely accurate based on the assumptions that he was not intoxicated with psychoactive drugs, that his head trauma was not a factor and that he had had episodes of violent behavior and a long history of mental illness with remissions. His neighbor described him as a "gentle kid" emphasizing the contrast between baseline euthymia and psychotic mania.
Mr. Tarloff had been diagnosed with paranoid schizophrenia at 22 years of age by Dr. Shinbach. He was enrolled at Syracuse University but when he came home, "… he was changed,… he was moody… 'All of a sudden, he became catatonic,… He couldn't talk.' … [and he] would see things and believe that people were looking at him and were against him. He could not hold a job for longer than a day; he also attended St. John's University and the University of Miami, but left both times before one semester was through.… he had obsessions. 'There were times when he would take showers 15 or 20 times in a day,… He would walk the streets picking up cigarette butts,… He'd call back 20 times or more to say it [the compulsion] right so that it [the compulsion] would go away.'" He was *committed more than a dozen times and treated with lithium, Depakote*, Haldol, Seroquel, and Zyprexa. "He'd feel better and then say to himself, 'I feel good. There's nothing wrong,' and stop taking his medications." He may have made *a spur-of-the-moment decision* to travel to Baltimore to see his brother and "He called me [his father] and says he's on Staten Island and in a taxi and the cab driver can't find me." Mr. Tarloff believed his plan was, "… sanctioned by God … [and] that he believed he was on a mission from God--to rescue his mother from a nursing home …"	The description of Mr. Tarloff's early psychotic break of "catatonic [and] He couldn't talk" is compatible with psychotic depression, and his paranoia is consistent with a psychotic mood disorder (Chap. 12; Fig. 12.2). His delusion of God is grandiose and indicative of psychotic mania. His activity and plan to take his mother to Hawaii as well as his violence are compatible with acute psychotic mania. His past prescriptions of lithium and Depakote suggest at least one physician thought he suffered from bipolar disorder. He also had symptoms of OCD.

(continued)

Table 15.7 (continued)

Case no.	Year; location; reference	Patient/murderer age; diagnosis	Description of crime	Victim name(s)/ relationship to patient
10	July 2007; Augusta, MA Kim Fletcher, *The Lincoln County News*, Augusta, MA; Dec. 17, 2008	John A Okie, 22; *schizophrenia*	Okie believed that his girlfriend, "… was part of an evil group and that she could read his mind because it 'was exposed to her.' In killing Mills July 10, Okie believed the world would thank him. Okie killed his father … six days later … [because] Okie developed the belief that his father had actually been the reason he couldn't use his mind and was part of the 'evil group.'"	Elexandra Leigh Mills, patient's former *girlfriend* and John S. Okie, patient's *father*
11	Apr. 2007, Virginia Polytechnic Institute and State University (Virginia Tech) in Blacksburg, VA Wikipedia (2011)	Seung-Hui Cho, 23; *schizophrenia, major depressive disorder*, and a severe anxiety disorder called selective mutism	"Around 7:15 am EDT … on April 16, 2007, Cho killed two students, … [in their] dormitory [rooms].… Cho returned to his room to re-arm himself and mailed a package to NBC News that contained pictures, digital video files and documents. At approximately 9:45 am EDT…, Cho then crossed the campus to Norris Hall, a classroom building on the campus where, in a span of nine minutes, Cho shot dozens of people, killing 30 of them. As police breached the area of the building… Cho committed suicide in Norris 211 with a gunshot wound to his temple.… Cho… had left a note in his dormitory which contains a rant referencing Christianity.… He stated that 'Thanks to you I died like Jesus Christ, to inspire generations of weak and defenseless people.'"	Emily Hilscher and Ryan Clark, were "friends" and the first two of the *32 killed*, and in addition, *25 students and teachers* were wounded at Virginia Tech. Mr. Cho *suicided*.

15.5 Risk for Violence, Suicide, Homicide, and Filicide Is Increased in Psychotic…

Symptoms	Comments
"[His sister] described Okie as distant, distracted, and often unresponsive in conversations.… We called him The Sloth. He was always tired.… Okie told his sister he was convinced he had to use cocaine to prevent cancer. He also *insisted his mother was raping him* in the night, and injecting heroine into his feet to kill him. He reasoned to protect himself, he would have to kill her to save himself." Therefore, he was hospitalized in 2004 and described as "… quiet, depressed, and distant, and very much different." In a "… 2005 incident Johnny 'took off' to New Hampshire and Massachusetts, and was locked in a woman's restroom. He was arrested but not charged due to his mental status." Another incident involved his *driving to visit his sister* "… in Boston following a tonsillectomy surgery, and arrived covered in blood.… In a hospital emergency room, Okie was admitted for blood loss."	At least two apparent spur-of-the-moment trips were described. The use of cocaine was implied and could explain the trips and the murders but for the hospitalization in 2004 that had similarities to the 2007 paranoid symptoms. His symptoms in the hospital in 2004 were that of depression, possibly explained by withdrawal from stimulants. His paranoid delusions can be explained by psychotic mania or psychotic depression (Chap. 12; Fig. 12.2).
Cho immigrated to America in about the second grade. He finished the 3-year elementary school program in a year and a half and was noted to be good at Mathematics and English and was pointed out by teachers as a good example for other students. In middle school, Cho was diagnosed with *major depressive disorder* and selective mutism. His inability or unwillingness to speak brought him ridicule in secondary and high school. He "… was transfixed by [the Columbine High School massacre]" that occurred when he was in the eighth grade. At Virginia Tech, some of his professors found him "menacing" and became concerned for their safety as did some of his fellow students. Cho told another student during a telephone call that he was "… vacationing with Vladimir Putin" in North Carolina. He sent another message with the words, "I might as well kill myself now." Campus authorities were contacted and police escorted Cho to the Virginia Mental Health Agency serving Blacksburg. There, he was found to be "… mentally ill and in need of hospitalization," and he was described as having "… a flat affect and depressed mood." Outpatient treatment was recommended. The package Cho *mailed to NBC News in New York contained 25 minutes of video, 43 photographs, 23 pages of written material, and 23 PDF files* that were last modified at 7:24 a.m. after the first shooting. In his writings sent to NBC, Cho "… made threatening messages to then-US President George W Bush, Vice-President Dick Chaney and Secretary of State Condoleezza Rice.… in another video, he compared himself to Jesus Christ,…"	Autopsy toxicology showed the absence of either psychiatric or any illegal drugs. A history of major depression, paranoia, grandiosity, i.e., President Vladimir Putin and President George Bush, violence upon others, and suicide are compatible with a psychotic mixed mania and bipolar disorder.

(continued)

Table 15.7 (continued)

Case no.	Year; location; reference	Patient/murderer age; diagnosis	Description of crime	Victim name(s)/ relationship to patient
12	Sept. 2006; Bethesda, MD Rosack, *Psychiatric News*, 2006	Vitali A. Davydov, 19; *schizophrenia and bipolar disorder*	Dr. Fenton, a psychiatrist, agreed to an emergency meeting with his 19-year-old patient and the patient's father on Sunday, Sept. 3, 2006, the day before Labor Day. Dr. Fenton had apparently seen the patient for the first time the day before and had made a follow-up appointment for the next week. "… the patient's father called Fenton, pleading with him to see his son again [sooner]." Fenton agreed to see them at 4 p.m. Sunday afternoon. "The patient's father brought his son to Fenton's office, then apparently left to do an errand while his son talked with Fenton." When he returned from errands the father waited for his son in the parking lot, and the patient beat Dr. Fenton to death with his fists saying, "… that he had killed Fenton in self-defense. <u>He was afraid that Fenton was about to sexually assault him.</u>"	Dr. Wayne Fenton, M.D., was the *patient's doctor* and was an Administrator at the National Institute of Mental Health (NIMH) and renowned world expert in the diagnosis and treatment of schizophrenia.
13	Oct. 2005, New York City, NY Hartocollis, *New York Times*, May 24, 2007	Peter Braunstein, 43; *paranoid schizophrenia*	"… Mr. Braunstein dressed as a firefighter, his face hidden behind a helmet and visor, and set off a smoke bomb to trick the woman, a former colleague, into letting him into her apartment … once inside, Mr. Braunstein knocked her out by putting a chloroform-soaked rag over her mouth, stripped her, tied her to her bed with a green parachute cord and sexually molested her [but apparently, did not rape her] over a period of 13 hours.… He told her… that he was an Aquarius, and left a message written in makeup on her bathroom mirror: 'Bye-Hope things turn around for U soon.'"	36-year-old female ex-colleague, former editor at W Magazine who had worked in the same newsroom as Mr. Braunstein; victim was sexually assaulted for 13 hours.

Symptoms	Comments
"In the nine months leading up to Fenton's murder, Davydov was spiraling deeper and deeper into psychosis, ... several different Psychiatrists who diagnosed him [Davydov] with schizophrenia and bipolar disorder had tried to treat him with medication. But,... Davydov was <u>afraid to take his medication</u> because he thought it would allow the Psychiatrists to control his mind.... Davydov was delusional, had auditory hallucinations, believed that he <u>received messages from the television</u> and had an obsessive belief that his fraternal twin <u>brother had been sexually abused</u> and was in danger." After their first visit on the day before the murder, "... Davydov believed that Fenton asked Davydov to kill him,... Davydov believed that 'Dr. Fenton asked [Davydov] to kill him because <u>he had been the victim of a rape</u> and wanted his soul to leave his body,... he thought if he killed Dr. Fenton, his real body would live on.'" The patient was "... reportedly suffering ongoing paranoid and complex delusions ... The patient reportedly was very agitated."	Mr. Davydov likely suffered from an acute psychotic manic episode because of his paranoid delusions especially of a sexual nature, defective judgment, and violence, but additional symptoms compatible with mania would have had to be assessed such as sleep, activity, energy, speech, and thoughts. However, like case #9 in Chap. 12.5, he believed that he received messages from the TV and was described as paranoid which is compatible with psychotic mania (Chap. 12; Fig. 12.2).
Mr. Braunstein was a *successful former fashion writer at Women's Wear Daily* from which position he was fired in 2002. At the trial, "... the testimony included his <u>readings of long, rambling passages from a diary</u>... in which he <u>compared himself to the victims of hurricane Katrina</u>, expressed admiration for serial killers, and threatened to kill Anna Wintour, the editor of Vogue. 'I'm going to kill Anna Wintour--because I feel like it,'... Just shooting would be too 'impersonal,'... he considered blowing up Ms. Wintour's townhouse, then dashing inside the ruins dressed as a firefighter and killing her. He also wrote that Ms. Wintour would be <u>'escorted by eunuchs to a place in hell run entirely by large rats.'</u>... a former girlfriend, Jane Larkworthy, the beauty editor for W Magazine... testified in detail about the violent unraveling of their relationship. Mr. Braunstein... taped her to a chair and menaced her with a knife,... She called the police, who took Mr. Braunstein to a psychiatric hospital." Mr. Braunstein also wrote that, "<u>In terms of my own criminal MO, that's hard to categorize.... It's like Munchausen by proxy via arson. It's kind of an 'all you can eat' buffet of crime, comprising as it does; arson, robbery, home invasion, rape, assault, unlawful imprisonment, murder and --oh yeah--impersonating a fireman.</u> If it doesn't constitute 'Criminal Anarchy,' well, I don't what does."	Stages of success interspersed with psychotic episodes of focused activity and grandiosity that include violence are compatible with a bipolar disorder.

(continued)

Table 15.7 (continued)

Case no.	Year; location; reference	Patient/murderer age; diagnosis	Description of crime	Victim name(s)/ relationship to patient
14	2004; San Francisco, CA Healthy Place.com staff writer *The Daily Review*, San Francisco Bay, CA, Nov. 19, 2004	Michael Diamond, 35; *schizophrenia* and *bipolar disorder*	Strangled his roommate, Dong Tran, with two rubber bicycle tire inner tubes tied together.	Dong Tran, 50, *roommate* in an independent living facility for people with psychiatric disabilities
15	2004; Beijing, China; *New York Times*, Aug. 5, 2004	Xu Heping, 51; *schizophrenia*	Mr. Xu, "A 51-year old security guard at a Beijing kindergarten slashed 15 children and three teachers with a kitchen knife, killing one of the children, …"	15 kindergarten children and 3 kindergarten teachers; one child died
16	2003; New York City, NY Albin, *New York Times*, July 29, 2003	Luis M. Perez, 21; *schizophrenia*	Mr. Perez, "… fatally stabbed his mother's girlfriend … suffering from the delusion that the victim, Juanita Hernandez, had sexually assaulted him,…"	Juanita Hernandez, *friend of the family*
17	May 2003; Brownsville, TX Ortiz, *The Brownsville Herald*, July 20, 2010	John Allen Rubio; 23; *paranoid schizophrenia*	"… allegedly strangled, stabbed and cut the heads off of [his and] his common-law wife's three children …"	*Children* of Mr. Rubio— Julissa Quesada, 3 years old; John Rubio, 14 months; Mary Jane Rubio, 2 months
18	Sept. 2002; Lorraine, Quebec, Canada Mandal, *Vancouver Sun*, Oct. 7, 2002	Andre Letellier, 30; *schizophrenia*	"… killed his parents and hanged himself."	Killed *parents* and committed *suicide*
19	Apr. 2002; Windsor, Canada Mandal, *Vancouver Sun*, Oct. 7, 2002	Thomas Demers, age unknown; *schizophrenia*	Mr. Demers murdered his father, heart specialist, Dr. Percy Demers.	Dr. Percy Demers, *father*
20	2001; Windsor, Ontario, Canada Mandal, *Vancouver Sun*, Oct. 7, 2002	Robbi-Lynn Jessop, 18; *schizophrenia*	"In 2000, she tried to set the family home on fire. Last year, she admitted to visions of stabbing her parents and two sisters, arranging their bodies like toppled dominoes in a pool of their own blood. … the Jessop's took the extraordinary step of barricading Robbi's bedroom each night and taking turns standing watch…. to prevent their daughter from killing them."	Potentially *parents* and *two sisters*

Symptoms	Comments
Chronic mental illness; "The once gregarious, smart and athletic boy suddenly became uncommunicative and withdrawn. … His weight began to drop, from about 130 to 93. … a psychiatrist gave [the] diagnosis: bipolar disorder and schizophrenia. … His father… 57… is bipolar."	Mr. Diamond likely suffers from psychotic bipolar disorder based on his positive family history, symptoms of a major depressive episode, and his diagnosis of bipolar disorder.
"… Mr Xu had been hospitalized for schizophrenia for five months in 1999…"	Psychosis and violence are associated with psychotic mood disorders.
Committed murder while psychotic, delusionally *believing that the victim, a family friend, had sexually assaulted him.*	Psychosis, paranoia of a sexual nature, and violence are associated with psychotic mood disorders.
"… Rubio believed that an ultimate battle between good and evil would take place and [he] was only thinking about what his delusions compelled him to do, regardless of the consequences,… Rubio believed he was killing demons when he committed the murders… he secluded himself with his family… during the three days in the house before the murders, [when] Rubio allegedly cleaned the place with bleach in an effort to keep evil away,… when Rubio's hamsters got agitated, Rubio took it as a sign of demonic possession and killed them with a hammer,…When he chocked the children and they gasped for air, Rubio interpreted that as a further sign of possession,… After the murders, Rubio told his wife that no one would understand their actions and persuaded her to have sex one last time,… His regular [illegal] drug use made the condition worse."	Acute intoxication with stimulant or hallucinogenic drugs could explain his actions but probably not a long-term diagnosis of paranoid schizophrenia. The delusional system has a flavor of grandiosity. Necessary information would be additional signs and symptoms of mania such as hours of sleep per night, racing thoughts, pressed speech, and increased energy and activities. Although he was evaluated by two psychiatrists, such symptoms were not noted in the newspaper article. Paranoia, psychosis, and violence are compatible with psychotic mixed mania.
"… neighbors said [he] had a history of schizophrenia and roamed the neighborhood singing and talking to himself…"	Inadequate descriptions of the patient's behavior were given to suggest a psychiatric diagnosis beyond a psychosis. Some data indicate that over 80% of functional psychoses are explained by psychotic mood disorders.
Thomas "… had stopped taking his medication, [and his father] was unable to get his mentally ill son… admitted to the hospital … earlier that day…"	Inadequate descriptions of the patient's behavior were given to suggest a psychiatric diagnosis beyond a psychosis. Some data indicate that over 80% of functional psychoses are explained by psychotic mood disorders.
Robbi had been described as a gifted student.	Inadequate descriptions of the patient's behavior were given to suggest a psychiatric diagnosis beyond a psychosis. Some data indicate that over 80% of functional psychoses are explained by psychotic mood disorders.

(continued)

Table 15.7 (continued)

Case no.	Year; location; reference	Patient/murderer age; diagnosis	Description of crime	Victim name(s)/ relationship to patient
21	May 2001; Montreal, Canada Mandal, *Vancouver Sun*, Oct. 7, 2002	Geoff Fertuck, 35; *schizophrenia*	Stabbed to death his parents before throwing himself in front of a freight train. *Suicided.*	Ed and Margaret Fertuck, *parents*; committed *suicide*
22	2000; Toronto, Canada Mandal, *Vancouver Sun*, Oct. 7, 2002	David Patten, 45; *schizophrenia*	Mr. Patten "… bludgeoned [to] death his parents… and a retired nurse, with whom Patten lived. He beat them in their driveway with a red-handled spade."	Manus Patten, 81, Clare Patten, 73—*parents*; and an unnamed retired nurse who was his *roommate* or *landlady*
23	2000; Fort Qu'Appelle, Sask., Canada Mandal, *Vancouver Sun*, Oct. 7, 2002	Brian Eugene Wessel, 30; *schizophrenia* likely	"…Mr. Wessel cleaved the pair [his wife and brother-in-law] in their sleep."	*Wife* and *brother-in-law*
24	Jan. 1999; in the subway in New York City, NY Barnes, *New York Times*, Mar. 24, 2000 Rohde, *New York Times*, Feb. 29, 2000	Andrew Goldstein, 30; *schizophrenia*	Mr. Goldstein and Ms Webdale did not know each other and had no connection except that they were waiting with others for the N train at the 23rd Street station. Mr. Goldstein said, "She was leaning against a pole with her back to me near the edge of the platform by the tracks, … I looked to see if the train was coming down the tracks. I saw that the subway train was coming into the station. When the train was almost in front of us, I placed my hands on the back of her shoulders and pushed her. My actions caused her to fall onto the tracks [where she was killed]."	Kendra Webdale, 32; *no relationship, random*
25	1998; New York City, NY *New York Times*, Oct. 14, 1999	Kevin Cerbelli, 30; *schizophrenia*	Mr. Cerbelli, "… walked into the 110th Precinct Station House in Queens … and stabbed a sergeant in the back. Police officers shot him to death after he refused to drop a screwdriver and a large kitchen knife."	New York City police officer
26	1998; Victoria, Canada Mandal, *Vancouver Sun*, Oct. 7, 2002	Aaron Millar, 24; *schizophrenia*	"One night, as Ruth [his mother] was doing the supper dishes, Aaron, tormented by voices which told him Ruth was going to harm the family, plucked a ceremonial sword off the wall and drove it through her heart."	Ruth Millar, 49; *mother*

15.5 Risk for Violence, Suicide, Homicide, and Filicide Is Increased in Psychotic... 327

Symptoms	Comments
"…Fertuck was found to be schizophrenic in August 2000 while he was being treated for depression. In January 2001, a psychiatrist told Fertuck's parents it would be dangerous to keep him at home." One family friend described Mr. Fertuck as, "… cheerful, witty, unassuming,… He was so tender and gentle and full of self-doubt that he didn't realize what a terrific person he was."	Ruling out intoxication on illegal drugs, his violence, posttreatment for depression, and suicide are compatible with psychotic mania or depression. The article noted that he had been treated for depression in the past (Chap. 12; Fig. 12.2).
"…he thought he was the 'leader [General] of the British Army' heading into the third World War and could advert the conflict by killing the devil possessing his parents,… 'He thought he was killing the devil inside his father and that his father was still alive and the devil was then transferred to his mother, so he killed her.'"	Grandiosity, paranoia, and violence suggest psychotic mania and a bipolar disorder.
Mr. Wessel said in court, "I lost my mind, and two people lost their lives,…"	Inadequate descriptions of the patient's behavior were given to suggest a psychiatric diagnosis beyond a psychosis. Some data indicate that over 80% of functional psychoses are explained by psychotic mood disorders.
Mr. Goldstein has been diagnosed with schizophrenia for 10 years prior to the murder. Before his arrest, he had "… a history of violent behavior and [made] requests for treatment." It was noted in the *New York Times* that he *suffered from depression* and "… made erratic requests to take his medication again,…"	In this case, there are very few symptoms available describing Mr. Goldstein's behavior before the murder. It is clear from the material reviewed that he was psychotic and there were no indications of any organic cause. If there was a delusional rationale Mr. Goldstein held in pushing Ms. Webdale, it was not given. According to at least some data, functional psychoses are predominately caused by psychotic mood disorders.
"… Mr. Cerbelli … suffered from schizophrenia and psychosis and had a history of violence.… He failed to keep [outpatient care] appointments."	Psychosis and violence are associated with psychotic mood disorders.
Paranoia, auditory hallucinations, and *violence*.	Inadequate descriptions of the patient's behavior were given to suggest a psychiatric diagnosis beyond a psychosis. Some data indicate that over 80% of functional psychoses that include paranoia, auditory hallucinations, and violence are explained by psychotic mood disorders.

(continued)

Table 15.7 (continued)

Case no.	Year; location; reference	Patient/murderer age; diagnosis	Description of crime	Victim name(s)/ relationship to patient
27	July 1998; United States Capitol, Washington DC Wikipedia Jones, projects.Idc.upenn.edu, June 26, 2000 ALombardi, *New York Times*, Aug.30, 1998 *New York Times*, Mar. 7, 2001	Russell E. Weston, 42; *paranoid schizophrenia*	At 3:40 p.m., armed with a .38 caliber Smith & Wesson handgun, Mr. Weston Jr., "… was accused of bursting into the [United States] Capitol and fatally shooting two [United States] Capitol guards and wounding a bystander."	Jacob Chestnut and John Gibson, *United States Capitol police officers*
28	June 1998; Hastings-on-Hudson, NY Berger and Gross, *New York Times*, June 19, 1998 Foderaro, *New York Times*, May 12, 2000 Fried, *New York Times*, May 26, 2002	Michael B. Laudor, 35; *schizophrenia or schizoaffective disorder*	Mr. Laudor stabbed his pregnant 37-year-old fiancée more than ten times in the back and neck in their kitchen of the apartment they shared on the banks of the Hudson River. He reportedly "…<u>thought Ms. Costello but a 'robot' or 'doll' acting on behalf of a conspiracy to kill him</u>." Mr. Laudor then drove to Binghampton, NY and took a bus to Ithaca, NY where at Cornell University, "… he flagged down a patrol car and told an officer that he had hurt his girlfriend and possibly killed her,… he was covered in blood, but he assured them 'he was not hurt, but the blood on his person was Carolyn's blood,'… he was alternately calm and agitated and, at one point, struck a Cornell police officer, who was treated at a local hospital. He had no prior record for violence." Subsequently while in confinement, Mr. Laudor had at least two additional assault charges, one against a corrections officer.	Carolyn Costello; *fiancée*

Symptoms	Comments
In 1983, after Mr. Weston's "80-something [year-old] landlady took her cane and struck him in the face,… [Mr. Weston] commenced a $2.5 million lawsuit against the woman… [that] was dismissed… He had delusions that someone was attempting to get him because he had top-secret knowledge of some kind…. In 1991, Weston wrote two threatening letters to then-Montana Gov. Stan Stephens." Six years before the shooting, he was diagnosed with paranoid schizophrenia in Montana after threatening a resident. He spent 53 days in a mental hospital. At one time, he "… thought a neighbor was using his television satellite dish to spy on his actions. He also believed that Navy SEALs were hiding in his cornfield…. Weston earlier had been investigated by the Secret Service after acquaintances reported hearing him make threats toward the government and President Clinton,… Weston had traveled to Washington [DC] before. He went to CIA headquarters and allegedly told officials that he was a clone and that President Clinton was a clone as well…. Two days prior to the capitol shooting, at his grandmother's insistence to do something about cats which were becoming a nuisance, Weston shot and killed 14 cats with a single barreled shotgun, leaving several in a bucket and burying the rest…. he explained that he stormed the capitol to prevent the United States from being annihilated by disease and legions of cannibals…. On March 6, 2008 Weston filed a motion requesting a hearing on his mental status." He apparently organized two witnesses, a psychologist, a vocational rehabilitation specialist, and his public defender to make the request for his release, but it was denied.	The numerous examples of delusional paranoia, grandiosity, travel, and violence that seemed to occur in cycles, all seem to suggest a psychotic bipolar disorder. To drive from Montana to Washington, DC in less than two days, just under 2,000 miles, Mr. Weston may have driven nonstop and exceeded the speed limit, both consistent with manic behaviors.
Mr. Laudor "… had graduated Summa Cum Laude from Yale University in three years and …," graduated from Yale Law School and "… signed a book and movie deal for his life story worth $2.1 million." Although Mr. Laudor's story did not get told, he may have inspired the writing of "A Beautiful Mind" about the math genius John Forbes Nash Jr. who was assumed to have schizophrenia. He was asked to join Yale Law School as an associate after his graduation. He was described by a friend as "…unbelievably charismatic, unbelievably bright, someone you'd never forget…. He is handsome, kind, spiritual, a wonderful conversationalist, a wonderful sense of humor and was destined for what everyone thought was greatness…. The golden boy. Over the last year he definitely deteriorated…. he was withdrawn and depressed… he'd complain that he couldn't get out of bed in the morning…. He complained that his friends phones were tapped." He believed Ms. Costello was *part of a plot to kill him.*	Some of the most successful and famous people in all fields of endeavor have suffered from bipolar disorder. These people are often brilliant, charismatic, and leaders. However, when mania worsens in such individuals, they are subject to increasing irritability, anger, fury, violence, and homicide (Table 3.11, quote #6). As is typical for bipolar patients, Mr. Laudor also seemed to suffer episodes of nonproductive, disabling depression alternating with sometimes lengthy periods of brilliant productivity. His depression was described in the *New York Times* as, "… he complained that he couldn't get out of bed in the morning" (Berger and Gross 1998).

(continued)

Table 15.7 (continued)

Case no.	Year; location; reference	Patient/murderer age; diagnosis	Description of crime	Victim name(s)/ relationship to patient
29	1997; Toronto, Canada Mandal, *Vancouver Sun*, Oct. 7, 2002	Gregory Workman, 44; *schizophrenia*	"… Workman … said he stabbed his mother Noel, 77, five times in the neck, chest and back because he believed he was a surgeon carrying out a medical procedure."	Noel Workman, 77; *mother*
30	June 1997; Toronto, Canada Mandal, *Vancouver Sun*, Oct. 7, 2002	Joseph Meehan, 43; *schizophrenia* or *bipolar disorder*	Mr. Meehan "… nearly dismembered his … [son] Michael, 8, … [after] falling under the delusion that his son was the devil." Kenny Meehan, the 11-year-old brother told the 911 operator "My dad's killing my brother, … He's got blood all over him … I'm gonna die … He was strangling him. Oh, my God … I think he's [brother] not alive."	Michael Meehan, 8; *son*
31	Jan. 1996, Philadelphia *New York Times*, Feb. 4, 1996 *New York Times*, Sept. 22, 1996 *New York Times*, Jan. 28, 1997 Longman, *New York Times*, Dec. 10, 2010 Wikipedia (2011)	John E. du Pont, 57; *paranoid schizophrenia*	Mr. Schultz, who lived on Mr. du Pont's estate in suburban Philadelphia was "… repairing his car radio, when Mr. du Pont drove up and shot him, without provocation. … Mr. Schultz's last words were, 'Hi, coach,' to which Mr. du Pont replied, 'You got a problem with me?' and shot him. … du Pont used hollow point bullets and fired the last shot into Schultz's back while Schultz was bleeding to death from a gunshot wound in his chest and crawling face down in the snow trying to get away.… Mr. Schultz was a long time friend of Mr. du Pont who had repeatedly tried to help him."	Mr. Schultz, 36, was an Olympic gold medal winner in wrestling and had been *an invited guest* living with the US Olympic wrestling team on Mr. du Pont's estate.

15.5 Risk for Violence, Suicide, Homicide, and Filicide Is Increased in Psychotic... 331

Symptoms	Comments
Mr. Workman *believed he was a surgeon and performing surgery.*	Grandiosity and violence are compatible with psychotic mania and a bipolar disorder.
Mr. Meehan believed "… that his [8-year-old] son was the devil."	Inadequate descriptions of the patient's behavior were given to suggest a psychiatric diagnosis beyond a psychosis. Some data indicate that over 80% of functional psychoses that include paranoia, auditory hallucinations, and violence are explained by psychotic mood disorders.
Mr. du Pont was described "… as a shy, gawky teen-ager who never had a girlfriend and avoided school dances. …" At his high school graduation party he was described as "… very, very happy." After high school, Mr. du Pont's life was characterized by cycles of "… throwing himself into a series of passions over which he at first would take total control, then would totally withdraw.…He earned a BS in Biology from the University of Miami, has two species of birds named after him because he first identified them, earned an MS at Villanova University, won the 1965 Australian National Pentathlon Championship, became an accomplished wrestler and housed the Olympic wrestling team on his estate." Forbes Magazine in 1987 estimated his worth at $200 million. Yet, he was described as an unhappy man. His cycles were described as occurring at four year intervals. Mr. du Pont "… believed Schultz was part of an international conspiracy to kill him.… he believed people would break into his house and kill him, the reason he put razor wire in his attic." Other episodes contained psychotic behavior that included "… pointing a machine gun at a wrestler, holding a gun to his wife's temple while suggesting she was a Russian spy, placing infrared 'ghost-finding' cameras in his house, believing the walls were moving and growing afraid that clocks on the treadmills were taking him back in time,… driving two Lincoln Continentals into his pond, loosing his temper and yelling, firing cooks and security guards as if he were George Steinbrenner firing baseball managers, starting to carry a gun, accusing people of betraying him, hiring a company to X-Ray his columns and walls fearing that people or spirits were tunneling into his house to attack him, believing that he was the Dalai Lama, the last Russian Czar, the target of international assassins or the CIA's top consultant [and firing his highly respected defense lawyers] when he accused them of conspiring against him with the Central Intelligence Agency." Such episodes	Although there were no notations of other symptoms of mania such as increased energy simultaneously with a decreased need for sleep, the grandiosity, paranoia, and violence, as well as cyclic episodes of depression are suggestive of a psychotic bipolar disorder. His father may have carried a diagnosis of manic depressive disorder. Alcohol abuse and dependence are also common in bipolar disorders.

(continued)

Table 15.7 (continued)

Case no.	Year; location; reference	Patient/murderer age; diagnosis	Description of crime	Victim name(s)/ relationship to patient
32	1993; Vancouver, Canada Mandal, *Vancouver Sun*, Oct. 7, 2002	Mark Andrew Bottomley, 24; *schizophrenia*	Mr. Bottomley murdered his 79-year-old aunt with whom he was living and left *her partially clad body* in the lane behind her basement suite early Christmas Day.	Kathleen O'Sullivan, 79; *aunt*
33	Mar. 1981; Washington DC Wikipedia, 2007	John Hinckley Jr., 25; paranoid schizophrenia and erotomania	At 2:27 p.m. ET, as Pres. Reagan walked out of the Washington Hilton Hotel to his waiting limousine, Hinckley opened fire getting off six shots in 1.7 seconds, missing the President with all six shots. The sixth bullet ricocheted off the armored side of the limousine and hit Reagan under his left arm lodging in his lung and stopping about an inch from his heart.	President Ronald Reagan-seriously injured with a bullet lodged in his lung; James Brady, White House Press Secretary was hit in the head, survived with neurologic deficits; Thomas Delahanty, a District of Columbia police officer was hit in the back of his neck, survived; Timothy McCarthy, a Secret Service Agent was hit in the abdomen, survived.

Symptoms	Comments
seemed to have been interspersed with episodes of loss of interest, "… plunging into tailspins that drained his enthusiasm and distracted his focus, leaving him impatient, self-destructive fearful and ultimately threatening to other people." Mr. du Pont abused alcohol, if not meeting criteria for alcohol dependence.	
No specific symptoms were given.	Inadequate descriptions of the patient's behavior were given to suggest a psychiatric diagnosis beyond a psychosis. Some data indicate that over 80% of functional psychoses are explained by psychotic mood disorders.
Hinckley was a well adjusted, privileged child. "… he played football, basketball, learned to play the guitar, and was elected president of his class twice. As a teenager he suffered episodes of withdrawal and became obsessed with public figures such as John Lennon. He attended Texas Tech University off and on from 1974 to 1980." "In 1976 Hinckley <u>left home for Hollywood hoping to become a famous songwriter</u>." He became infatuated with the actress Jodie Foster. During these years, "… he developed a pattern of living on his own for a while and then returning home poor." In the late 1970s and early 1980s, "… Hinckley began purchasing weapons… [and] also began taking <u>anti-depressants</u> and tranquilizers." Hinckley followed Foster around the country even enrolling in a course at Yale University in 1980 when he learned that she was a student there. He *wrote numerous letters and notes* to her in late 1980. He also called her on the telephone but she rejected him. Hinckley became convinced that by becoming a national figure he could impress Foster. He decided he could accomplish this by *assassinating the President of the United States. He trailed President Jimmy Carter* from state to state, was arrested in Nashville, TN on a firearms charge, went home again and received psychiatric treatment for depression. "… Hinckley wrote that the shooting was <u>'the greatest love offering in the history of the world</u>' and was upset that Foster did not reciprocate his love." In 2009, Hinckley was allowed to visit his mother for a dozen visits of ten days at a time and obtain a driver's license. "Recently, a forensic psychologist at the hospital [St. Elizabeth's Hospital for the criminally insane] testified that <u>'Hinckley has recovered to the point that he poses no imminent risk to himself or others.</u>'"	Although symptoms that might have been more indicative of a psychiatric diagnosis were not available from the literature reviewed, the public were led to believe that Mr. Hinckley suffered from schizophrenia. Mr. Hinckley's fascination with Jodie Foster earned him the diagnosis of erotomania, and there is some overlap between this disorder and the grandiosity characteristic of mania. There are other examples of grandiosity including his pursuit of the President of the United States and his trip to Los Angeles to become a famous songwriter. He was treated with antidepressant medications and apparently suffered episodes of depression. Over the past years, Mr. Hinckley has demonstrated the ability to organize and write numerous motions for permission for unsupervised visitation. Cycles in mood that include depressions and focused activities, grandiosity, and violence suggest a bipolar disorder.

Table 15.8 Epidemiology of psychotic murderers and their victims

Category	Number of cases	Case # on Table 15.7
Perpetrators	33	1–33
Mean age	32 years old	
Range	18–57 years	
Sex	32 Males; 1 Female	Female case #20 (fantasy)
Murder, suicides (4 suicides, 1 suicide attempt failed; 2 other perps. shot dead at scene)	5 (plus 2 perps. killed)	1, 8 (attempt), 11, 18, 21; (7, 25—perps. shot dead at scene)
Guns used	7	1, 2, 6, 11, 27, 31, 33
Knives used	16	3–5, 7–9, 15–17, 20 (fantasy), 21, 23, 26, 28, 29, 30
Miscellaneous weapon	6	12 (fists), 13 (sexual assault), 14 (bicycle tubing), 22 (spade), 24 (pushed under train), 25 (screwdriver and knife)
Unknown weapon	4	10, 18, 19, 32
Feared sexual abuse	3	10, 12, 16
Committed sexual abuse	3	3, 13, 32
Diagnoses		
Schizophrenia	31 (94%)	1–6, 9–33
Schizophrenia and bipolar disorder	3	12, 14, 30
Schizophrenia and major depressive disorder	1	11
Bipolar disorder	2 (6%)	7, 8
Victims		
Murders (victims and perps died) (total # of deaths: 80, including 4 perp suicides and 2 perps were killed)	26 (plus 2 perps. killed)	1–3, 5, 8–12, 14–19, 21–24, 26–32 (perp. suicided—1, 11, 18, 12; killed—7, 25)
Severe injuries (without victim deaths) (total # of injuries 71 including 1 perp. injury)	7	2, 4, 6(perp. shot but survived), 7(perp. shot to death), 13(sexual assault), 25(perp. shot to death), 33
Cases of single victim	17	3, 4, 7, 8, 12–14, 16, 19, 24, 26, 28–32
Cases of multiple victims (range of number of victims)	15 (2–57)	1, 2, 5, 6, 9–11, 15, 17, 18, 21–23, 27, 33
No victim, no injuries, only threats	1	20 (fantasy)
Mental health professionals	5	3, 7–9, 12
Parents or children	11	1 (niece and nephew), 10, 17–19, 21, 22, 26, 29, 30, 32
Spouse, fiancée, girlfriend	3	10, 23, 28
Roommates, friends, classmates	4	11, 14, 16, 31
Random victims	3	5, 15, 24
Suffered sexual abuse	3	3, 13, 32
Famous victims	6	2, 4, 6, 25, 27, 33
Delusions of perpetrators		
Grandiose delusions		
Presidents, governors, congresspersons, general, czar, CIA, Dalai Lama, Surgeon	9	2–4, 6, 11, 22, 27, 31, 33
U.S. Capitol, Pentagon, NYC police	3	6, 25, 27
Mission of God, UCLA lawyer (3.5 GPA)	2	3, 9
Fear of sexual abuse	3	10, 12, 16
Paranoid and grandiose delusions		
Devil	3	17, 22, 30
Conspiracy against	12	4, 5, 9, 10, 15, 17, 22, 26–28, 30, 31

Beyond psychosis, several descriptions of the killers' behaviors and symptoms were detailed enough, even in newspaper articles, to speculate on a diagnosis different than schizophrenia. Apparently, the diagnoses of schizophrenia were made based on the presence of psychosis, paranoid delusions, hallucinations, bizarre behavior, and in some cases, chronicity of course. As previously discussed, such symptoms are disease nonspecific and, according to some, explained by psychotic mood disorders over 80% of the time (Pini et al. 2001). Cycles of depression alternating with psychotic episodes of grandiosity, paranoia, spur-of-the-moment poor decisions, anger, aggression, violence, homicide, and/or suicide are suggestive of psychotic mood disorders (Chap. 12). Increased activities, decreased need for sleep, and racing thoughts were rarely more than suggested among the 33 cases, but grandiosity was apparent in at least 20 cases (Tables 15.7, 15.8—#2–6, 9–12, 15–17, 22, 25–28, 30, 31, 33). Grandiosity is assumed when patients' delusions involve famous individuals or institutions including political, religious, or media stars or involve evil plots and threats against the patients themselves (Chap. 12) (Tables 12.6, 15.7, 15.8, 15.9). Delusional grandiosity and paranoia in a violent, functionally psychotic mental patient implies mania and a bipolar disorder. In one case with the diagnosis of schizophrenia in 2011 (Table 15.7, #1), the killer "… had been awake for several days" despite drinking alcohol before he murdered his 9-year-old nephew and 10-year-old niece; then he suicided at around 3 a.m. (nola.com 2011). Activity, the lack of need for sleep and violence are indicators of mania. In addition, there were suggestions of past episodes of major depression in many of these 33 cases diagnosed with schizophrenia that rather suggest a psychotic mood disorder.

Ten of the cases involved grandiose delusions about political figures such as US or Russian Presidents (cases #3, 11, 27, 31, 33), members of Congress, governors, generals (cases #2, 4, 22, 27), or individuals representing government institutions such as the CIA, the Pentagon, the US Capitol, or the New York City Police (cases #6, 25, 27, 31). All of these involved famous victims except for case #22 where the perpetrator believed he was the "leading [General] of the British Army."

Specific examples include, Mr. David Patten, 45 (Table 15.7, #22) (Mandal 2002), who murdered his parents and a nurse in 2000 believing he (Mr. Patton) was the "leading [General] of the British Army" going into World War III and could abort the conflict only by killing the devil possessing his parents. Mr. Gregory Workman, 44 (Table 15.7, #29), according to the press, believed he was a famous surgeon operating on his mother who he murdered with multiple stabs to the neck, back, and chest in 1997 (Mandal 2002). Two fathers and one son developed the delusion that their children or parents were possessed by the devil or demons and killed them (Table 15.7, #17, 22, 30). Too little data were found in case #1, who murdered his 9- and 10-year-old niece and nephew to know what Mr. Reynolds' delusion was before he shot them in the heads (Braxton 2011). Speculation would include paranoid and grandiose delusions similar to those in cases #17, 22, and 30 (Table 15.7). Twelve other cases involved delusions that there was an evil conspiracy threatening the perpetrators or that they were on a mission of God (cases #4, 5, 9, 10, 15, 17, 22, 26–28, 30, 31). These include the two cases from China in which the perpetrators appeared to be terrified for their own lives from an apparent evil threat (#5, 15). Although the perpetrators were diagnosed with schizophrenia, these delusions of the devil, demons, or an evil conspiracy against them and being on a mission directed by God hint at grandiosity and are compatible with several of the cases discussed previously in Chap. 12 that were initially misdiagnosed with paranoid schizophrenia but, upon gathering additional history, were revealed to suffer from a bipolar disorder.

An example is Mr. John du Pont (case #31) who, at various times, believed that he was the Dalai Lama, the last Russian Czar, a target of international assassins, the CIA's top consultant, that his wife was a Russian spy, and that international conspirators would break into his house and kill him. He placed razor wire in his attic, "ghost-finding cameras" in his house, and had his houses' columns and walls x-rayed to prevent anyone tunneling into his house to attack him. In 1996, Mr. du Pont murdered his guest and long-time friend, the US Olympic wrestling coach. Despite this description of grandiosity and paranoia, his diagnosis was paranoid schizophrenia (Sect. 12.4) (Longman 2010; Wikipedia 2011).

Mr. Michael Laudor (case #28), a Summa Cum Laude, graduate of Yale University Undergraduate School and Yale Law School, a member of the Yale Law School faculty, holding a $2.1 million contract for his biography, was engaged to be married and living on the Hudson River in New York City murdered his fiancée in 1998 believing she was involved in a conspiracy to kill him. His diagnosis was schizophrenia although he was described as,

> … unbelievably charismatic, unbelievably bright, someone you'd never forget.… He is handsome, kind, spiritual, a wonderful conversationalist, a wonderful sense of humor and was destined for what everyone thought was greatness.… The golden boy.…

Such a description of brilliance and success is somewhat similar to that of John Nash, also diagnosed with schizophrenia but who displayed symptoms consistent with a bipolar disorder. Nash inspired *The Beautiful Mind* (Chap. 16). Laudor's charisma seems similar to that of some cult leaders such as Jim Jones who led and killed 909 Temple members in Jonestown, Guyana, South America in 1978. Some speculated in the press that Jones suffered from schizophrenia, but he was also known to abuse prescription and illegal drugs especially LSD. Such characteristics as charisma, leadership, brilliance, success, the ability to excel with only two or three hours of sleep a night coupled with psychotic episodes, and other episodes of major depression with reduced productivity suggest a bipolar disorder although additional signs and symptoms are necessary for a conclusive diagnosis (Berger and Gross 1998; Foderaro 2000).

Undiagnosed, misdiagnosed, and mismanaged psychotic bipolar patients, especially when manic, are a threat to doctors, therapists, counselors, and caretakers. Of the five murders involving mental health professionals, one of the most notable was the murder of Dr. Wayne Fenton by Vitali Davydov in Bethesda, MD (case #12). In 2006, Mr. Davydov was delusional, had been diagnosed with both schizophrenia and bipolar disorder, and at a Sunday afternoon emergency therapy session, beat Dr. Fenton to death with his fists. Such paranoia, intense aggression, and violence is in keeping with an acute manic episode and one of his diagnoses, a bipolar disorder (Chap. 12), but Dr. Fenton did not have the opportunity to diagnose and treat him with mood-stabilizing medications (Rosack 2006).

Another example is the case of Mr. Peter Braunstein, a fashion writer (case #13), who was diagnosed with paranoid schizophrenia but while psychotic in 2005 dressed as a firefighter, set off a smoke bomb to gain entry in to the apartment of a former female colleague, knocked her out with chloroform, stripped her, tied her to a bed, and sexually molested her for about 13 h. He said to her that he was an "Aquarius." He apparently wrote excessive and rambling passages in a diary (Hartocollis 2007). There were also signs of grandiosity in his thoughts. Such symptoms suggest mania and a bipolar disorder.

In 2007, Mr. Seung-Hui Cho (case #11) murdered 32 and wounded 25 students and teachers on his campus at Virginia Tech. He was diagnosed with paranoid schizophrenia and major depressive disorder, but said at one time that he was "… vacationing with Vladimir Putin," wrote "… threatening messages to then US President George W. Bush, Vice-President Dick Chaney, and Secretary of State Condoleezza Rice… [and] compared himself to Jesus Christ…" (Wikipedia 2011). The history and diagnosis of major depression, blatant grandiosity, paranoia, multiple homicides (necessitating considerable planning and activity), and suicide suggest a psychotic bipolar disorder.

In 2011, Jared L. Loughner (case #2) murdered 6 and wounded 13 in Tucson, AZ. His diagnosis in the media was paranoid schizophrenia. The focused anger on the government and a congresswoman suggest grandiosity. His multiple inappropriate, erratic, loud, intrusive, angry, and aggressive disruptions in his community college classes over several months that required calling campus security, coupled with an apparent lack of need for sleep and increased activities that include, "dancing up and down excitedly" as he murdered his victims also suggest mania and a bipolar disorder (Johnson et al. 2011; Becker et al. 2011).

Filicide is an especially tragic type of homicide also sometimes associated with suicide and psychosis. Some of the most likely causes for filicide are abuse, neglect, and revenge, but there are numerous cases when the perpetrator is psychotically ill, usually with a bipolar disorder, major depression, or postpartum depression. However, the perpetrators are often misdiagnosed with schizophrenia because of bizarre psychoses when sometimes subtle grandiosity is overlooked (Bourget et al. 2007; Anonymous 2006, http://myth-one.com/memorial.htm). In their review of filicide, Bourget et al. (2007) reported that 50–85% of perpetrators had histories of psychiatric diagnoses that included schizophrenia, major depressive disorder, and postpartum depression; bipolar disorders were not noted. A common scenario in such cases is that the killer is so psychotically depressed, manic, or mixed that he or she believes that the rest of the family including children and infants must be spared living in "this hell on earth." Killing friends and family is seen as a service and a duty in order to send them to a better place (Table 15.9) (Anonymous 2006). In such cases, the murderer often intends suicide but if the subsequent suicide fails, the killer is charged with murder. Typically, these psychotic patients are diagnosed with schizophrenia and thus have not received standard-of-care treatment for a psychotic mood disorder (Table 15.2). Even when such psychotic killers are misdiagnosed with major depressive disorder or postpartum depression/psychosis, if they really suffer from a bipolar depression instead, then they also do not receive mood-stabilizing drugs, and the antidepressants can worsen their bipolar disorder (Table 15.9).

One example of multiple filicide is the case of Andrea Yates who at 37, killed her five young children by drowning them one by one in the bathtub at home in Austin, TX on June 20, 2001, an hour after her husband left for work (Table 15.9, case #6). In high school, Ms. Yates was class valedictorian, captain of her swim team, and an officer in the National Honor Society. She then graduated in 1986 from the University of Texas School of Nursing in Houston and worked as an RN from 1986 to 1994 at the University of Texas M.D. Anderson Cancer Center. She was diagnosed with schizophrenia and postpartum depression with psychotic features after the birth of her first son in 1994 when,

> …she felt Satan's presence shortly after Noah's birth and "heard Satan's voice tell her to pick up the knife and stab the child." …The symptoms of schizophrenia didn't resurface until Yates' fourth son, Luke, was born in 1999.… Yates attempted suicide twice that year.
>
> (Anderson 2002)

She reportedly first spoke of suicide and suffered from depression at the age of 17 (Wikipedia 2011). She suffered numerous psychotic episodes most associated with diagnoses of schizophrenia, psychotic depression, and/or postpartum psychosis. After hospitalizations in 1999, she was medicated with "… a mixture of medications,…" Medications prescribed included Haldol (haloperidol), an antipsychotic/antischizophrenia medication; Cogentin (benztropine), an anticholinergic drug given prophylactically in an attempt to counter the side effects of Haldol (haloperidol); Effexor (venlafaxine); Wellbutrin (bupropion); and trazodone. No mood-stabilizing drugs were mentioned, and the several antidepressants might have worsened a bipolar disorder (Wehr and Goodwin 1987; Goodwin 1989):

> After being discharged [in late 1999 or early 2000], her condition worsened. "Staying in bed all day,… she experienced visions and voices. She would hear commands: Get a knife! Get a knife!."
>
> (Walsh 2002)

She seemed to recover, and in between episodes she apparently functioned fairly normally. Although warned against future pregnancies by a psychiatrist based on the fear of future psychotic postpartum episodes,

> The Yates' conceived their fifth and final child approximately seven weeks after her discharge [from a psychiatric inpatient stay and]. … gave birth to Mary Yates on November 30 of that year [2000]. She seemed to be coping until the death of her father on March 12, 2001.

Although she seemed to avoid a psychotic episode after the birth of Mary, her father's death and the miscarriage of her sixth pregnancy caused a further deterioration in her condition resulting in two additional hospitalizations in March and May of 2001. Ms. Yates

> … then stopped taking medication, mutilated herself and read the Bible feverishly. … believed that the children would be tormented and perish in the fires of hell unless they were killed.
>
> (Walsh 2002)

She believed her children would suffer in hell because the mark of the devil was hidden under her hair. She was evil; possessed by Satan. She had to kill her children before it was too late for them to get to heaven. (http://Karisable.com).

She murdered her children in June 2001.

While in prison, Ms. Yates continued to have psychotic episodes, at one time, refusing food and losing more than 20 lb. She has been placed on suicide watch at least four times in prison. She said that, "... she could not destroy Satan and that 'Gov. Bush would have to destroy Satan.'"

Ms. Yates was clearly psychotic and may have warranted the short-term prescription of an antipsychotic/antischizophrenia medication such as Haldol. The discontinuation of Haldol 4–6 weeks before the murders raises a question of tardive psychosis. Her episodic course, onset of a major depressive episode at 17, her episodes of postpartum depression/psychosis, her grandiosity marked by the delusion that she was possessed by Satan, and belief that Gov. Bush was involved in her life and could kill Satan as well as a reference to her "reading the Bible feverishly" raise a possibility of manic episodes and bipolar disorder. If accurate and bipolar disorder was diagnosed, a prescription of mood-stabilizing medications would have occurred with the possibility of better control of Ms. Yates' psychosis. See Chap. 17 for other differential diagnostic data to distinguish bipolar disorders from major depressive disorders and schizophrenia.

Another example of filicide by a psychotic mother is a woman who murdered, mutilated, and ate parts of her infant son in 2009 at 4:30 a.m. (Table 15.9, case #1). The autopsy showed that Ms. Sanchez must have spent a considerable amount of time mutilating her infant certainly consistent with a psychotic state. She seemed to have a healthy life until about five years prior to the murder when "... her behavior became erratic. She had trouble staying employed, bouncing from one low-paying job to another." Such a work history is typical of rapid-cycling bipolar disorders. The year before the murder, while psychotic, Sanchez may have made a spur-of-the-moment decision to travel to Austin, TX from San Antonio, TX (about 80 miles) with a friend. Ms. Sanchez was found in a CVS store after wandering around for seven hours, "... shopping for an imaginary trip to China." The Austin police took her to the State Mental Hospital where she spent the next 16 days, was diagnosed with paranoid schizophrenia, and was prescribed antipsychotic/antischizophrenia medication. She stopped this medication during her subsequent pregnancy, began taking it again after her delivery, but stopped it again nine days before the murder. She had paranoid delusions that other women were trying to breast-feed or take her baby away. She believed "... the devil made me do it" (Mann 2009, 2010). Such paranoia, grandiosity, violence, and hyperactivity are compatible with mania and a bipolar disorder.

A misdiagnosis of schizophrenia, major depressive disorder, or postpartum psychosis, in patients with a bipolar disorder, makes it unlikely these patients will have been prescribed first-line mood-stabilizing drugs (Table 15.2). Such an oversight heightens the risk of violence, suicide, homicide, filicide, and incarceration. Most of the killers described above were or had been under psychiatric or other mental health care. Appropriate diagnosis and follow-up might have changed some of these tragic outcomes.

Table 15.9 Risk for filicide is increased in psychotic bipolar disordered patients misdiagnosed

Case no.	Year/location/ reference	Patient/murderer age; diagnosis	Description of crime
1	July 2009; San Antonio, TX Mann, *Texas Observer*, 2009, 2010 *Fox News*, 2009.	Otty Sanchez, 33; paranoid schizophrenia, major depressive disorder, postpartum psychosis.	"Around 4:30 am, while the rest of the family slept, she attacked her infant son with a large kitchen knife.... Sanchez had decapitated her three-week-old son, mutilated his body and eaten some of the flesh.... mutilated [his] genitals, and flayed the skin. Authorities said Sanchez ate parts of her son, including the brain, and the medical examiners found apparent bite marks across the body. ... and [there were] missing fingers and toes."
2	July 2005; Dyer IN Anonymous, Children Murdered by Their Christian Parents Memorial Page, 2006.	Magdalena Lopez; bipolar disorder.	"Police reported that she beat her two sons to death with a ten-pound dumbbell because she thought they'd be better off in heaven.... 'They're in a much better place now.'"

15.5 Risk for Violence, Suicide, Homicide, and Filicide Is Increased in Psychotic... 341

with schizophrenia, major depressive disorder, or postpartum depression

Victim name(s)/ relationship to patient	Symptoms	Comments
Scott Wesley Buchholz-Sanchez; 3-week-old son.	Otty "… finished high school and began taking pharmacy-technician classes." At 27 years of age, "Her behavior became erratic. She had trouble staying employed, bouncing from one low-paying job to another.… In late May 2008, Sanchez went to Austin, TX with a friend. While her friend was getting an acupuncture treatment, Sanchez wandered off. She walked into a CVS and prowled the store for the next seven hours, 'shopping for an imaginary trip to China.'" "Austin, police arrived and took her to the State Mental Hospital where she stayed 16 days. She was prescribed anti-schizophrenia medication and diagnosed with paranoid schizophrenia. She stopped this medication during her pregnancy, was prescribed it after delivery, but stopped taking it again nine days before she murdered her child." She had paranoid delusions that "… other women were trying to breastfeed her baby. She was 'hearing voices which have informed her that others would like to take her baby away' … [and seeing] visual images of other children's faces transposed on her baby's face." She "… wailed about how the devil made her do it."	Ms. Sanchez was diagnosed with paranoid schizophrenia that is often a misdiagnosis when patients actually suffer from a psychotic mood disorder (Chap. 12). It was said that her mother, aunts, and cousins "… have all had similar mental illness [to Otty's]." "… family friends often described Otty as one of the most level-headed people in the family." Her saying "the devil made me do it" suggests a paranoid and grandiose delusion. That she committed the homicide at 4:30 a.m. and perpetrated the number of injuries revealed by the autopsy suggests possible lack of need for sleep and hyperactivity. Even if there were no other signs of mania, and the diagnosis is postpartum depression and major depressive disorder, severe with psychotic features, the diagnosis of schizophrenia is redundant because both depression diagnoses can encompass psychosis. That she stopped taking her medicine nine days before the murder, raises the question of tardive psychosis.
Antonio Lopez, son, 9; Erik Lopez, son, 2.	Was diagnosed with bipolar disorder.	Was diagnosed with bipolar disorder.

(continued)

Table 15.9 (continued)

Case no.	Year/location/ reference	Patient/murderer age; diagnosis	Description of crime
3	Nov. 2004; Plano, TX USA Today, Nov. 23, 2004 MSNBC, Nov. 23, 2004 CBSNews.com, Feb. 11, 2009 Wikipedia (2011).	Dena Schlosser, 35; postpartum depression/psychosis.	Ms. Schlosser "… 'euphorically' told a 911 operator she had cut off the baby's arms; police found Schlosser covered in blood and holding a knife while listening to a hymn." 911 had called Ms. Schlosser after day care workers had called 911 after talking to her and becoming concerned.
4	May 2003; New Chapel Hill, TX (Tyler, TX) Associated Press, 2004 Anonymous, Children Murdered by Their Christian Parents Memorial Page, 2006.	Deanna Laney, 39; postpartum depression.	A crime scene video showed her 8 and 6 year olds lying dead in the yard near garden signs that read "Mom's Love Grows Here" and "Thank God For Mothers. … the boys were found in their underwear with heavy rocks on their chests. The video also showed a large spot of blood in a baby bed, where Deanna Laney severely injured the couple's youngest son, Aaron, 14 months old at the time."

Victim name(s)/ relationship to patient	Symptoms	Comments
Margaret Schlosser, daughter, 10 months old.	Neighbors described her as "… a loving, attentive mother…. The children had always been healthy, happy and cared for…. In January, the [Child Protective] agency was called to the home after Schlosser was seen running down the street, with one of her daughters bicycling after her,… the child told them her mother had left her six-day-old sister alone in the apartment." She was hospitalized and diagnosed with postpartum depression. In a conversation with her mother the day before the slaying, Ms. Schlosser "… seemed oddly 'euphoric.'" Her mother said, "She was euphoric and it bothered me a little,… She wasn't herself." Her attack was described as a "religious frenzy."	Ms. Schlosser's mother described her as "… just a gentle soul." Neighbors seemed to agree. Ms. Schlosser had three children, all girls. The two older daughters were six and nine and were at school when the murder occurred. Ms. Schlosser had been previously diagnosed with postpartum depression or major depressive disorder. She had at least two psychotic episodes both involving substantial activities. Less than a year before the murder, she was found psychotic while running down the street. She had apparently "… taken a television news story about a boy being mauled by a lion as a sign of the apocalypse…. [and] … had heard God commanding her to remove her baby's arm and then her own. The attack was later described as a 'religious frenzy.'" Her mother described her as euphoric the day before the murder. A "religious frenzy," "euphoria," a delusion about the apocalypse, hearing God's voice commanding her, and violence are compatible with psychotic mania or a mixed state.
Joshua Keith, son, 8; Luke Allen, son 6; Aaron, son, 14 months (injured).	Ms. Laney was a stay-at-home mother who homeschooled her children and was deeply religious. She "… believed God ordered her to kill her children last Mother's Day weekend. 'She struggled over whether to obey God or to selfishly keep her children.' … she [believed she] saw Aaron with a spear, then throwing a rock, then squeezing a frog and believed God was suggesting she should either stab, stone or strangle her children. … She would read every day events or objects as messages from God. When her baby had abnormal bowel movements, … she thought it was a message from God that she was not properly 'digesting' God's word.	The delusions and auditory hallucinations communicating with God suggest grandiosity and a potential for mania and a bipolar disorder rather than major depressive disorder or postpartum depression. The risk for a postpartum depression potentially psychotic is common in bipolar disorders.

(continued)

Table 15.9 (continued)

Case no.	Year/location/ reference	Patient/murderer age; diagnosis	Description of crime
5	Mar. 2002; Austintown, OH Tristate A.M. Report, www.enquirer.com, 2002 Anonymous, Children Murdered by Their Christian Parents Memorial Page, 2006.	Sherry Marie Delker, 27; diagnosed with a mental illness.	"Mrs. Delker admitted to running her daughter down with her car outside a church. Police said she wanted to sent her daughter to a 'better place' because 'they were trying to take her baby away' and 'to stop the abuse.'"
6	June 2001, Houston, TX Walsh, wsw.org, 2002; CNN Justice, 2002 Anderson, Associated Press, 2002 CBSNews.com, 2011 Wikipedia (2011).	Andrea Yates, 37; schizophrenia, postpartum psychosis, major depressive disorder.	About an hour after her husband left for work, "She started with the youngest boys, and after drowning them in the bathtub, laid them in her bed. She then drowned Mary, who she left floating in the tub. Her oldest son, Noah, came in and asked what was wrong with Mary. Noah then ran, but Andrea soon caught up with him and drowned him. She then left him floating in the tub and laid Mary in the arms of her brothers. Afterwards, she called the police. Then, she called her husband saying and repeating only two words: 'It's time.'"

Victim name(s)/ relationship to patient	Symptoms	Comments
	..."A previous psychotic episode occurred several years earlier when she thought she smelled sulfur and believed this was God's warning that the devil was near."	
Samantha Mae Martin, daughter, 6.	Psychotic behavior	Data inadequate
Noah, son, 7; John, son, 5; Paul, son, 3; Luke, son, 2; Mary, daughter, 6 months.	After a healthy childhood, Ms. Yates suffered a major depressive episode with suicidal ideation at 17. After the birth of her first child, she suffered a psychotic episode, "… feeling the presence of Satan …" that was diagnosed as schizophrenia and postpartum psychosis. She had multiple subsequent psychotic episodes and the diagnoses of schizophrenia, major depressive disorder, and postpartum psychosis (when the psychotic episode followed a birth). Ms. Yates said, "I am Satan … It was the seventh deadly sin. My children weren't righteous. They stumbled because I was evil. The way I was raising them, they could never be saved. They were doomed to perish in the fires of hell.… She believed her children would suffer in hell because the mark of the devil was hidden under her hair. She was evil; possessed by Satan. She had to kill her children before it was too late for them to get to heaven." She also discussed Gov. George Bush being able to kill the devil. During one episode, she was said to "… read the Bible feverishly."	Ms. Yates certainly suffered from psychotic depression including postpartum psychosis. Still, there are hints of grandiosity that include delusions of Satan and the governor of Texas. At one point, she was said to have read the Bible feverishly. More symptoms of mania would be necessary to assure a diagnosis of bipolarity, such as a lack of need for sleep and increased activities such as reading the Bible, pressed speech, and racing thoughts, all occurring during one episode when she is also psychotic. The early episode of a major depression, multiple episodes, and psychosis add to the list suggestive of bipolarity versus unipolar depression. Since 50% of patients diagnosed with unipolar, turned out to be bipolar, addition of a mood-stabilizing medicine may have helped to minimize her violence.

(continued)

Table 15.9 (continued)

Case no.	Year/location/ reference	Patient/murderer age; diagnosis	Description of crime
7	Feb. 2000; Warrensburg, MO Tammeus, *Kansas City Star*, 2000 Samuels & Franey, *Kansas City Star*, Feb. 15, 2000 Simmons, http://larryrobison.org/pages/raymond_wood.htm.	Raymond Wood, 37; schizophrenia, schizoaffective disorder, bipolar type.	Mr. Wood shot and killed his pregnant wife and four of their six children wounding the other two with a rifle. "… Jared, 10, was found laying face down just outside the Woods' below-ground home. Joshua, 8, lay on a nearby hill. Inside, … 1 yr old Katlin [was found] toddling around in bloody clothes. On the floor lay her sisters Emily, 7 and Moriah, 3 … 5 year old Hannah … was found curled up underneath a bed, … their 31 year old mother, Tina Wood [was found] inside the family van, which had crashed into an embankment."
8	Mar. 1999; Naperville IL Hanna & Ferkenhoff, *Chicago Times*, 1999 Coen & Barnum, Chicagotribune.com, 2002 Anonymous, Children Murdered by Their Christian Parents Memorial Page, 2006.	Marilyn Lemak, 41; "seriously depressed".	"She murdered her 6 and 3 year olds in the afternoon when they arrived home from school and her oldest son, 7, when he arrived home around dusk after school activities. Mrs. Lemak fed the children peanut butter laced with antidepressants, aspirin and sedatives. She laid them down to sleep, then placed a hand over their mouths and pinched their nose until they suffocated. She then took a dose of the same concoction but when she woke the next morning, she called 911 and then … 'she slashed her arm at the spot where physicians and nurses take blood,' … doctors repaired a severed artery.'"

Victim name(s)/ relationship to patient	Symptoms	Comments
Tina Wood, wife, 31; Jared Wood, son, 10; Joshua, son, 8; Emily, daughter, 7; Hannah, daughter, 5; Moriah, daughter, 3—injured; Katlin, daughter, 18 months—injured.	"Growing up, Ray [Wood] was normal. He was an average student, an all-American boy. He participated in sports: cross-country … karate, swimming and wrestling. He played chess and was in a band." He was described by friends in Missouri "… as a kind, gentle man devoted to his family and his faith in God … '[He] was the nicest guy. He was really sweet. He was shy, but when you talked to him he would talk very calmly.'" His first break was in 1985 [at 22] when he was arrested for breaking into a home. He told police that he was God, and he was committed to the Psychiatric Institute. He had 13 psychotic episodes, some requiring hospitalization between the ages of 22 and 37. Some of these episodes were described as follows: "He was despondent, … He thought everybody was against him … he [believed he] talked to God and he was God … started talking about revelations he received from God, stopped sleeping, stopped eating,…".	The diagnoses of schizophrenia and schizoaffective disorder, bipolar type are typical misdiagnoses of a psychotic bipolar disorder. Mr. Wood's cycles from psychoses to relative euthymia during which times he fell in love and married his wife in 1987, fathered and cared for his children ("… he would always have that baby in is arms … He loved his family …"). When psychotic, he was both grandiose (talked to God; was God) and paranoid (thought everybody was against him), stopped sleeping, and stopped eating. During other episodes, he was described as despondent. These psychotic symptoms are entirely compatible with a psychotic bipolar disorder. What remains unclear are the details of his delusions that led him to kill his family.
Nicholas, son, 7; Emily, daughter, 6; Thomas, son 3; Ms. Lemak attempted suicide.	Ms. Lemak was "… described as seriously depressed" and was said to have "… lost her sanity as the marriage dissolved. She killed her children and attempted suicide believing they would be reunited in a better place,…".	Ms. Lemak was a registered nurse, and her husband was a doctor. They were in the midst of a divorce. She was "… described as seriously depressed" and said to have lost her sanity as the marriage dissolved. Her suicide attempt after murdering her children was a bona fide attempt, and she was said to believe that "… they would be reunited in a better place…. Prosecutors said that Ms. Lemak killed her children out of anger after her husband began dating."

(continued)

Table 15.9 (continued)

Case no.	Year/location/ reference	Patient/murderer age; diagnosis	Description of crime
9	Sept. 1998; St. Paul, MN Anonymous, Children Murdered by Their Christian Parents Memorial Page, 2006.	Khoua Her, 24; depression.	"… strangled her six children … She then hanged herself in a failed suicide attempt. … thought she would be reunited with the children in the afterlife."
10	Nov. 1997; Sherwood, AK Anonymous, Children Murdered by Their Christian Parents Memorial Page, 2006.	Christina Marie Riggs, 26; major depressive disorder.	"Christina Marie Riggs smothered her two children … with a pillow… She then attempted suicide by swallowing twenty-eight Elavil tablets and injecting enough potassium chloride to kill five people." She lived.
11	Mar. 1985 Anonymous, Children Murdered by Their Christian Parents Memorial Page, 2006 Huffpost Chicago, 2009 Amandolare, Finding Dulcinea, 2009.	Debra Lynn Gindorf, 20; postpartum psychosis, depression.	"[Ms.] Gindorf swallowed lethal doses of alcohol and sleeping pills but worried about her children when they woke up crying. So she … fed her twenty-three month old daughter Christina and three month old son Jason lethal doses of crushed sleeping pills in a cup of juice. She then unsuccessfully attempted suicide. She believed she and her babies would be reunited in heaven, where they would be safe and happy together for eternity."

15.6 The Negative Impact of the Misdiagnosis of Major Depressive Disorder or Postpartum Depression in Patients Who Have Bipolar Disorder, Depressed

Patients with bipolar, unipolar, or postpartum depression have the same neurovegetative symptoms, but distinguishing between the three is critical since patients with unipolar depression (major depressive disorder) or postpartum depression are generally prescribed antidepressants without mood stabilizers. The antidepressants given alone to bipolar-depressed patients can cause a switch to mania in about 10% and thus increase the rate of cycling making the condition worse (Fig. 4.1) (Carlson and Goodwin 1973; Wehr and Goodwin 1987; Goodwin 1989). This increases the

15.6 The Negative Impact of the Misdiagnosis of Major Depressive Disorder... 349

Victim name(s)/ relationship to patient	Symptoms	Comments
Kouaeai Hang, 11; Samson Hang, 9; Nali Hang, 8; Tang Lung Hang, 7; Aee Hang, 6; Tung Hang, 5; Ms. Her attempted suicide.	Described as melancholy and depressed.	Possibly major depressive disorder or bipolar depressed, severe with psychotic features.
Justin Thomas, son, 5; Shelby Alexis, son, 2; Ms. Riggs attempted suicide.	Ms. Riggs should not have survived her suicide attempt, but did and "… requested and … fought for her right to die [by lethal injection].… [She said,] 'I'll be with my children and with God. I'll be where there's no more pain. Maybe I'll find some piece.'" She was executed by lethal injection on May 3, 2000 in Pine Bluff, AK.	Her statements and her bona fide attempt suicide suggest major depression as a part of a psychotic mood disorder.
Christina, daughter, 23 months; Jason, son, 3 months; Ms. Gindorf attempted suicide.	Ms. Gindorf had suffered an episode of postpartum depression after the delivery of her first child and after delivery of the second, "… was hearing voices, not sleeping – since her son's birth [for three months] … started hearing voices and had crying spells." She was unemployed, had no car or phone.	Too little data are given to know if the severe postpartum depressions were a part of unipolar or bipolar disorders. More signs and symptoms would be required of Ms. Gindorf's thoughts and behaviors during the three months between the birth of her son and the murders. One statement in the newspaper said that she had been "hearing voices, not sleeping- since her son's birth [3 months].…", suggestive of mixed mania.

risk for violence, homicide, filicide, and suicide. Since data suggest that as many as 50% of patients initially diagnosed with major depressive disorder actually have a bipolar disorder, some recommend using lithium for patients with unipolar depression. Some data suggest lithium is as effective in unipolar as in bipolar disorders (Carlson and Goodwin 1973; Wehr and Goodwin 1987; Schou 1979; Goodwin 1989, 1990, 2007; Calabrese et al. 2001). To emphasize the utility of lithium and the liability of antidepressants in recurrent mood disorders, even unipolar depression, Fred Goodwin said that,

> … the one year relapse rate among the recurrent unipolar patients [major depressive disorder] treated with tricyclics [antidepressants] was 50% higher than among those treated with lithium (35% vs 22%).

> [Prien et al. (1972, 1973, 1984) found that] …antidepressant-treated bipolar patients experienced more than twice the rate of manic episodes than did bipolar patients who were treated with either placebo or the combination of lithium and imipramine.
>
> (Goodwin 1989)

Further,

> In a methodologically rigorous, longitudinal prospective comparison of lithium versus lithium plus imipramine in bipolar I patients, Quitkin et al. (1981) found a 50% higher rate of relapse in the combined treatment group, an increase accounted for by the two-and-a-half fold increase in manic episodes; these relapses occurred particularly among mania-prone patients. Shapiro et al. (1989) subsequently confirmed the vulnerability to relapse of bipolar patients admitted for treatment for a manic episode who were administered combined lithium and imipramine. That is, even with the protection of lithium, use of tricyclic medications can heighten the rate of cycle-induction among certain bipolar patients.
>
> (Wehr and Goodwin 1987)

Goodwin concluded that the antidepressant medications may cause an acceleration of cycle rate even in recurrent major depressive disorders (Carlson and Goodwin 1973; Wehr and Goodwin 1978).

These data support the potential for an increased risk for violence, filicide, homicide, and suicide when there is a misdiagnosis of major depressive disorder (unipolar depression) or postpartum depression that results in treatment with antidepressants in patients who actually have bipolar depression. Table 15.9 summarizes 11 cases of filicide. Three were diagnosed with schizophrenia (cases #1, 6, 7), one with bipolar disorder (case #2), eight with major depressive disorder and/or postpartum psychosis (cases #1, 3, 4, 6, 8–11), and in one case, no specific diagnosis was given (case #5). Some patients had multiple diagnoses. A bipolar disorder diagnosis was given to only one patient (case #2) despite suggestions of bipolarity in several others (cases #1, 3–7). Too little data were available in cases 8–11 but, in each, a bona fide effort was made at suicide suggesting major depression. One in four patients with bipolar disorder suicide during an depressive episode, and the risk is exacerbated during the postpartum period when the infant and other children are also at increased risk for death by filicide. In ten of the cases, the murderers were mothers, in one, a husband/father (case #7).

Table 15.7 also lists three cases of filicide (cases #1, 17, 30). Two of the murderers were fathers, one an uncle, and in two cases (#17, 30), the fathers believed their child was the devil or a demon. In case #1, no data about the delusion were given, and the uncle killed himself. All were diagnosed with schizophrenia.

An example from Table 15.9 is the case of Ms. Schlosser (case #3) who cut the arms off her ten-month-old daughter while listening to a hymn in 2004. Ms. Schlosser had been diagnosed with postpartum depression and postpartum psychosis. Neighbors had described her as a loving and attentive mother, but ten months prior to the murder, Ms. Schlosser was hospitalized after being observed "running down the street [in a psychotic state], with one of her [older] daughters bicycling after her." The day before the murder, Ms. Schlosser's mother said, "She was euphoric and it bothered me a little, … She wasn't herself." Ms. Schlosser had interpreted a television news story about a boy being mauled by a lion as a sign of the apocalypse and heard God commanding her to remove the baby's arms. The attack by Ms. Schlosser was described in the media as a "religious frenzy" (Wikipedia

2011). Such euphoria, grandiosity, religious frenzy, hyperactivity, violence, and psychosis are compatible with mania and bipolar depression or a mixed state rather than unipolar or postpartum depression. The treatment of postpartum depression or major depressive disorder consists of antidepressant medications that have the potential to make a bipolar condition worse. If Ms. Schlosser did suffer from a bipolar disorder, the appropriate use of mood-stabilizing medications would have been warranted and might have better regulated her psychotic behavior (Table 15.9, case #3).

15.7 Conclusions

As quoted at the beginning of this chapter, according to Pope (1983), "To misdiagnose schizophrenia as bipolar disorder rarely does harm; to misdiagnose bipolar disorder as schizophrenia may adversely affect a patient's entire future." This is certainly still true today, and the harm done can include violence, suicide, and murder.

Patients with psychotic mood disorders are terribly misserved when misdiagnosed with schizophrenia. The result often is that such psychotic bipolar manic, depressed, or mixed patients do not receive mood-stabilizing drugs and psychotic unipolar-depressed patients may not receive an antidepressant, lithium, or potentially life-saving ECT. Further, a bipolar-depressed patient misdiagnosed with major depressive disorder or postpartum depression may receive an antidepressant without a mood stabilizer and thus get worse. An accurate diagnosis is the key to effective treatment.

The antipsychotic/antischizophrenia medications, typicals and atypicals, are first-line antipsychotic drugs designed to treat schizophrenia but are not first-line (or even third- or fourth-line in this author's opinion) mood-stabilizing drugs and carry a substantial adverse effects profile (Tables 15.5 and 15.6). They can be life saving in acute psychoses but ideally are to be used in psychotic mood-disordered patients sparingly, only on a temporary basis for days to a few weeks because of their substantial adverse effects. Several of the antipsychotic/antischizophrenia medication side effects can be permanent (Casey 1988). A few authors discourage any use of the antipsychotic/antischizophrenia medications in psychotic patients because of the severity of possible adverse effects such as tardive psychosis (Whitaker 2004).

The stigma of the diagnosis of schizophrenia is substantial. The movement disorders and other adverse effects such as obesity add to this stigma. An increasing rate of incarceration of psychotic patients, most diagnosed with schizophrenia, adds more stigma. The misdiagnosis of psychotic mood disorders as schizophrenia and their treatment as schizophrenia can increase the chances for violence, injury, and homicide of friends, family, therapists, and psychiatrists as well as patient suicide (Tables 15.7, 15.8, 15.9). Likewise, the misdiagnosis of bipolar depression as unipolar or postpartum depression increases the risk of violence, filicide, homicide, and patient suicide. The misdiagnosis and mismanagement may constitute malpractice. Appropriate diagnoses and treatment with mood-stabilizing medications offer the best chance of diminishing if not avoiding such outcomes.

Chapter 16
How Has Schizophrenia Survived?

> *One possible reason for this lack of progress [in discovering the etiology of schizophrenia] is that schizophrenia is not a valid object of scientific enquiry. Data from published research (mainly carried out by distinguished psychiatrists) are reviewed casting doubt on: (i) the reliability, (ii) the construct validity, (iii) the predictive validity, and (iv) the aetiological specificity of the schizophrenia diagnosis.*
>
> (Bentall et al. 1988)

16.1 Introduction

In the last half of the nineteenth century, a new psychiatric disorder overcame 2,000 years of knowledge that manic-depressive insanity could encompass psychosis and chronicity (Table 3.1) (Bruijnzeel and Tandon 2011). Some influential psychiatrists believed that a new diagnosis was needed for the most severely psychotic and most chronically mentally ill patients that they felt could not be explained by manic-depressive insanity. Scientists gain esteem by naming and describing new species or diseases. According to these investigators, the new disease, dementia praecox or schizophrenia separated itself from manic-depressive insanity. The diagnoses of dementia praecox and schizophrenia captured only the most severely psychotic, bizarre, chronic, dysfunctional, and challenging cases until 1911.

Eugene Bleuler (1911) was a prolific writer and an influential teacher, and he dedicated his efforts to promoting his disease, schizophrenia. Although the original concept of schizophrenia was defined by chronicity and psychosis, in 1911 Bleuler eliminated these as necessary criteria for the diagnosis, enlarging the potential population subject to the diagnosis many fold (Chap 6). Academic psychiatry embraced Bleuler's concept of schizophrenia and the Kraepelinian dichotomy. This broad concept of schizophrenia flourished for 70 years, bolstered by a second prolific and influential psychiatrist, Kurt Schneider who published his book in 1959 (Chap 8). The publication of the DSM-III (APA, DSM 1980) eliminated "on paper" Bleuler's subtype of simple schizophrenia. This substantial change served to more narrowly focus the disease concept of schizophrenia back to psychosis and chronicity and to further enhance confidence in its validity.

Today there are thought to be around two million patients with the diagnosis of schizophrenia in the USA (Goodman 1999). Inhibiting the consideration of eliminating the diagnosis of schizophrenia, besides the large population with the diagnosis, is that some of these two million patients do not want to give up or lose their diagnosis of schizophrenia and the disability support that accompanies it (Pierre et al. 2003; Pierre 2009). As noted by Pierre (2009),

> When I made the mistake of suggesting that a patient might not have schizophrenia, the reaction was often one of outrage. ... A diagnosis of schizophrenia is one of the best ways to gain access to a disability income and other social services ... So, despite my best intentions, my patients were far from relieved when I "took away" their schizophrenia diagnosis or an anti-psychotic medication. On the contrary, their very existence was threatened.

Nor do legal guardians of patients diagnosed with schizophrenia usually want to consider any other diagnosis. Such a large population of patients with a diagnosis of schizophrenia, some insistent on keeping the diagnosis, supports its validity (Goodman 1999).

Hundreds of millions if not billions of federal dollars over five decades have funded basic and clinical research on the schizophrenias. Like numbers of dollars, if not more, from the pharmaceutical industry have supported research on schizophrenia that included the design, development, clinical trials, and marketing of new antipsychotic/antischizophrenia medications. This encouraged the diagnosis of schizophrenia and solidified it as a bona fide disease.

The cost to taxpayers for government support of patients disabled with "schizophrenia" is substantial. These factors have further stimulated research that generates thousands of manuscripts, conferences, seminars, and lectures annually (Table 16.1; Fig. 16.1). There are at least three psychiatric journals dedicated to schizophrenia. The June 2011 issue of Psychiatric Annals was dedicated to schizophrenia (Janicak 2011). The number of publications about schizophrenia has continued to increase from an estimated 1,500 publications in 1990 to 2,500 in 2000 to almost 4,500 in

Table 16.1 Factors prolonging the recognition of schizophrenia as valid

Academic psychiatry endorses schizophrenia as valid
Schizophrenia is recognized in all textbooks and diagnostic manuals of psychiatry
Students and residents in psychiatry are taught and tested on schizophrenia
The ABPN[a] includes questions about schizophrenia
Complex condition, poor prognosis thus low expectations, challenging diagnosis, increased esteem for its management
Disability common and expensive
2,000,000 patients may be diagnosed with schizophrenia
Schizophrenia is widely accepted by the public and media
Broad NIMH sponsored research extends support for schizophrenia
Large profit potential for antipsychotic/antischizophrenia medications
Massive pharmaceutical investment in antipsychotic/antischizophrenia medication development, clinical trials, and marketing, leading to increasing diagnoses of schizophrenia
Massive volume of published research implies schizophrenia is valid

[a]ABPN—American Board of Psychiatry and Neurology

16.1 Introduction

```
                    ┌─────────────────────────┐
                    │  Academic Psychiatry    │
                    │  embraces the validity of│
                    │  schizophrenia          │
                    └─────────────────────────┘
                              ↓↑
                    ┌─────────────────────────┐
                    │ Broad recognition and   │
                    │ attention to schizophrenia│
                    │ by mental health, the   │
                    │ public, media,          │
                    │ government, pharma      │
                    └─────────────────────────┘
```

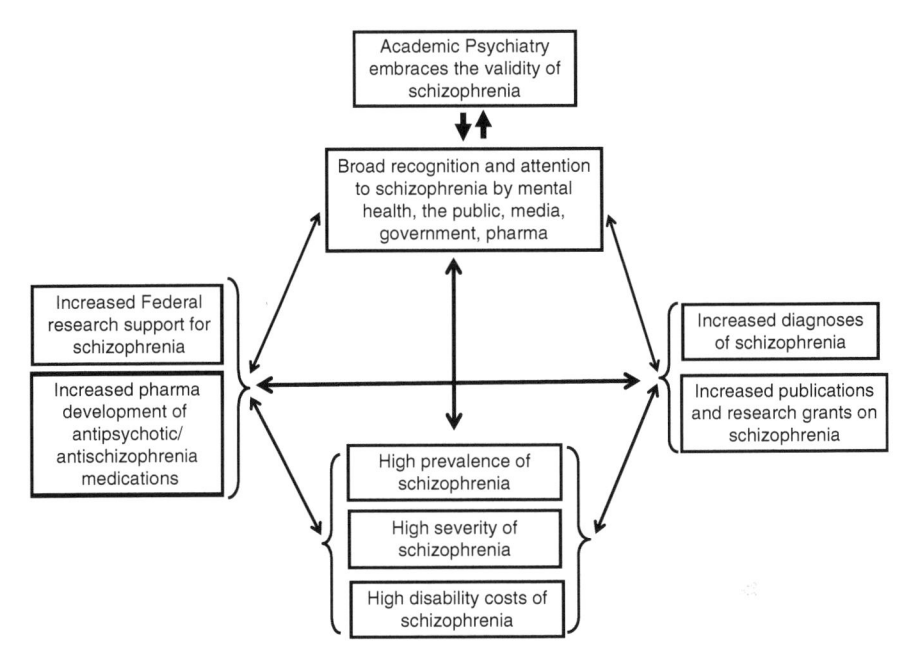

Fig. 16.1 Feedback loop enhancing the promotion of the concept of schizophrenia

Academic psychiatry, especially in the USA, embraced the validity of schizophrenia. By teaching medical students and residents in psychiatry, schizophrenia became widely recognized by all mental health professionals, the public, the media, government-granting agencies, and the pharmaceutical industry.

Such recognition led to increased diagnoses of schizophrenia as well as increased publications and research grants to study schizophrenia. These factors led to the concept of schizophrenia as common, severe in causing disability, and costly.

All these factors led to increased federal research support to study schizophrenia and increased investment by the pharmaceutical companies in developing drugs to treat schizophrenia.

These factors increased the recognition and attention to schizophrenia by academic psychiatry in a continuous positive feedback loop

2007 (Table 9.2; Fig. 9.1). The validity of schizophrenia has been justified by some based on this massive volume of research data published (Nasrallah 2006). This is despite the statement that,

> Although schizophrenia has been studied as a specific disease entity for the past century, its precise nature (core definition, precise boundaries, causes and pathogenesis) remains undefined. Since its demarcation as dementia praecox by Kraepelin and schizophrenia by Eugen Bleuler, its definitions have varied and its boundaries expanded and receded in the past century.
>
> (Tandon et al. 2011)

Consistent with the statement by Bentall et al. (1988) at the beginning of this chapter, and that of Kendell and Jablensky (2003) at the beginning of Chap. 1, this statement should raise doubt as to the validity of schizophrenia. With regard to the justification of schizophrenia as valid based on the "massive volume" of research data published on schizophrenia, Pope and Lipinski (1978) said:

> The non-specificity of "schizophrenic" symptoms brings into question all research that uses them as the primary method of diagnosis.

Of course all research on patients diagnosed with schizophrenia used the "schizophrenia" symptoms from the diagnostic manuals (the DSM and the ICD) "as the primary method of diagnosis." There is no laboratory test or pathophysiology to definitively rule in or rule out schizophrenia, inhibiting questions about the validity of such a long-standing disease. The basis for considering schizophrenia as separate from a psychotic mood disorder is governed by the Kraepelinian dichotomy, a concept that originated almost a century ago. The Kraepelinian dichotomy has been a cornerstone of psychiatry. It is a simple concept and

> … allows psychiatrists to demonstrate diagnostic expertise by exercising judgment over an often complex clinical picture and reach a clear diagnosis.
>
> (Craddock and Owen 2005)

Based on overlap and similarities between patients diagnosed with schizophrenia and psychotic mood disorders, the Kraepelinian dichotomy is approaching tombstone status (Craddock and Owen 2005, 2010a, b).

Schizophrenia is widely accepted as a "bona fide" disorder by the general medical and scientific communities, the media and the public. "Schizophrenic" is misused daily as an adjective. The power base and influence of researchers, academics, editors, reviewers, and administrators invested in the longevity of the disease called schizophrenia has been substantial and influential in the regulation of publications including the DSM and the funding of research grants on schizophrenia. Schizophrenia has received media attention both in the news and in film and has been evoked as the explanation for numerous high-profile murders by psychotic individuals (Sect. 15.5; Tables 15.7, 15.8, 16.3). For reasons such as these, schizophrenia has maintained its place as the most widely known mental disorder in the world (Table 16.1). Such broad acceptance along with the massive accumulation of research data seems to place the concept of schizophrenia as a disease beyond question.

16.2 The Overemphasis on Hallucinations and Delusions by Academic Psychiatry

Academic psychiatry regulates the global concepts of mental illnesses. No other group has such a powerful influence over tens of thousands of students, residents, and seminar and conference attendees every year. What professors teach is generally taken as accurate. Regarding the functional psychoses, academic psychiatry dictates its concepts to students and residents as well as to psychologists, psychiatric nurses, social workers, the media, and the public. Academic psychiatrists, especially in the USA, embraced and disbursed certain core beliefs of Kraepelin, Bleuler, and Schneider to their students and residents throughout the twentieth century.

16.2 The Overemphasis on Hallucinations and Delusions by Academic Psychiatry

Table 16.2 Core beliefs of E. Kraepelin, E. Bleuler, and K. Schneider promoted schizophrenia

Author	Core beliefs remembered for
Emil Kraepelin (1856–1926)	Schizophrenia defined by psychosis and chronicity
	The dichotomy: schizophrenia separate from bipolar disorders
Eugene Bleuler (1857–1939)	Greatly broadened the concept of schizophrenia with his fundamental symptoms and simple subtype
	Although unnecessary for the diagnosis, his accessory symptoms, hallucinations and delusions mandated the diagnosis of schizophrenia and have been embraced by academic psychiatry
	Concurred with dichotomy that schizophrenia different from bipolar
Kurt Schneider (1887–1967)	First-rank symptoms of special auditory hallucinations, pathognomonic of schizophrenia
	Second-rank symptoms of schizophrenia supported Bleuler's very broad concept
	Concurred with dichotomy that schizophrenia different from bipolar

This could amount to around 1.5 million doctors. The original beliefs of these "fathers of psychiatry" were condensed and simplified by subsequent authors to just a few basic concepts (Table 16.2). The two core keystones have been (1) the importance of chronicity, hallucinations, and delusions in defining schizophrenia and (2) the existence of schizophrenia as different from mood disorders. Schizophrenia became equated with hallucinations and delusions, i.e., the functional psychoses and more. The "more" were Bleuler's fundamental symptoms that allowed an explosion of the population diagnosed with schizophrenia. Schneider cemented the equation of hallucinations and delusions with the diagnosis of schizophrenia, and his second-rank symptoms of schizophrenia (Table 8.1) perpetuated Bleuler's broad concept. The increased population of patients diagnosed with schizophrenia solidified its acceptance among mental health professionals, the public, the media, and government-funding agencies. Even the publication of the DSM-III (APM, DSM 1980) did not entirely eliminate Bleuler's broad concept of schizophrenia (Sect. 10.10).

There have been a few doubters as to the validity of schizophrenia such as Kendell and Gourlay (1970a, b), Szasz (1976), Pope and Lipinski (1978), Bentall et al. (1988), Brockington (1992), and Kendell and Jablensky (2003), but it is unlikely their departmental chairpersons and directors of student and resident education assigned them the student and resident lectures on schizophrenia.

Every specialty and subspecialty of medicine has its most dreaded, widest known, and most severe diseases. For a century, psychiatry's most important disease has been schizophrenia, although it is really major depression, bipolar, or unipolar (Chap. 18). There is more emphasis on such important diseases in the core lectures, on wards, and in clinics so that most students, during their psychiatry clerkships, have been encouraged to recognize schizophrenia based on the elicitation of hallucinations and delusions. In the initial diagnostic interview, solicitation of hallucinations, delusions, and disorganization has taken priority over inquiring about mood symptoms (Sect. 16.3). Once confident of the presence or history of hallucinations and delusions, the diagnosis of schizophrenia could be justified. The diagnosis of schizophrenia has been self-serving for another reason, its prognosis. Patient improvement brought accolades because a worsening of symptoms and deterioration was expected.

That hallucinations and delusions define schizophrenia has been a consistent theme in a majority if not all of departments of psychiatry in the USA and in diagnostic manuals and has influenced the understanding of schizophrenia by physicians, by the public, and the media (Sect. 16.3). Psychosis is not rare, and it has typically received the diagnosis of schizophrenia reinforcing the validity of schizophrenia, especially in cases warranting media coverage.

16.3 Media Examples of the Endorsement of Schizophrenia

There have been several high-profile murder cases in which the killer has received the diagnosis of schizophrenia and that have garnered considerable press exposure. Examples are John Hinckley's assassination attempt on President Reagan in 1981 (Table 15.7, case #23); Theodore John "Ted" Kaczynski, the Unabomber, who terrorized the nation between 1978 and 1995 (Table 16.3, case #9); John du Pont who murdered the Olympic gold medal winner in wrestling while he was a guest on du Pont's estate (Table 15.7, case #31); Seung-Hui Cho who murdered 32 and wounded 25 classmates and teachers at Virginia Tech (Table 15.7, case #11); and most recently, Jared L. Loughner who murdered six and wounded 13 including Representative Giffords, D-AZ (Table 15.7, case #2). See Tables 15.7 and 15.8 for 33 cases that were described in newspapers from North America of murders by psychotic perpetrators, the majority diagnosed with schizophrenia. Since these infamous killers were diagnosed in the press as having schizophrenia, such publicity adds to the stigma and the acceptance of the diagnosis of schizophrenia as valid. Table 15.9 reviews 11 cases of filicide from the media where the parent who killed his or her children was often diagnosed with schizophrenia. There are several other media examples of attention to schizophrenia.

Goodman's (1999) New York Times article titled, *TELEVISION REVIEW; A New Role for the Family in Cases of Schizophrenia* is another example of schizophrenia in the press. He said, "… schizophrenia produces headlines when a tormented mind produces an act of violence that is often described as senseless or random." This article discussed cases said to be of schizophrenia including that of

> … a Long Island man who had a breakdown while an art student. He tells of believing he was King Tut, throwing bottles and phones through windows and spending time in jails and mental wards.

This description of "believing he was King Tut" associated with violence, time in jails, and mental wards suggests grandiosity and behavior compatible with mania and a bipolar disorder but the presentation emphasized schizophrenia. Also reviewed was the prime-time television A&E documentary titled, *INVESTIGATIVE REPORTS: The Shattered Mind*. The NBC special first aired on May 27, 1996, and then again on December 17, 1999. The plot involved a young wife and mother named Suzy who was diagnosed with schizophrenia and "… suddenly develops several alternate personalities …" Despite the misrepresentation of the concept of schizophrenia, such exposure in newspapers and prime-time television about schizophrenia increases the acceptance of the disease as valid.

16.3 Media Examples of the Endorsement of Schizophrenia

Table 16.3 summarizes nine cases of stories from the press over the past 20 years that feature schizophrenia. The front page of the Sunday Business Section of the New York Times on February 24, 2008, featured a half-page article and picture titled, *Daring to Think Differently About Schizophrenia* (Berenson 2008) (Table 16.3, case #4). This article continued on page 10 and consumed the page. The article discussed the development, marketing, and sales by the pharmaceutical industry of drugs used to treat schizophrenia, showing a sharply rising demand for the atypical antipsychotic/antischizophrenia medications (Table 15.4). The article stated that the overall sales of such drugs "… have doubled in the past five years" to over a billion dollars annually. Spending a billion dollars a year on a class of drugs designed to treat schizophrenia certainly promotes its validity.

Within one week, in June 2011, there were two front-page New York Times articles focused on schizophrenia (Sontag 2011; Carey 2011). The first (June 17, 2011) featured a large color photograph at the top of the page about a "schizophrenic" patient who murdered his counselor. A back-page follow-up consumed two pages with six color photographs (Table 15.7, case #3). The second article (June 23, 2011) also began on the first page of the New York Times and continued to take 75% of a back page with two black and white photographs (Table 16.3, case #1). This article titled, *Expert on Mental Illness Reveals Her Own Fight*, described Dr. Marsha M. Linehan, Professor of Psychology at the University of Washington, Seattle, WA. At 68 years old, she

> … told her story in public for the first time last week before an audience of friends, family and doctors at the Institute of Living, The Hartford Clinic where she was first treated … at age 17.

There she was diagnosed with schizophrenia and treated with Thorazine and electroshock therapy. Subsequently, Dr. Linehan earned her Ph.D. at Loyola of Chicago in 1971 and completed a postdoc program at Stony Brook, Long Island, NY. She

> … climbed the academic ladder, moving from Catholic University of America [Washington, DC] to the University of Washington in 1977, …

There she used dialectical behavior therapy to successfully treat a very difficult patient population, i.e., self-injurious, suicidal borderline personality disorders. In addition to her ability to succeed in academia, other symptoms revealed in the article at least suggest consideration of a bipolar disorder, not schizophrenia. Episodes of depression were suggested by descriptions of her

> … trying to kill herself so many times … while weathering gusts of dark emotions or delusions that would quickly overwhelm almost anyone.

She also described an event that occurred while kneeling in her church when

> … the whole place became gold … It was this shimmering experience, and I just ran back to my room and said, "I love myself." … "I felt transformed" … The high lasted about a year, before the feelings of devastation returned …

These quotes describe what appear to be multiple episodes of depression alternating with other episodes of productivity and success and at least one episode of mania or hypomania that lasted a year before a return to depression. If accurate, this defines a bipolar disorder, yet schizophrenia was given as her diagnosis in the press.

Mr. Zacarias Moussaoui, accused of participating in the planning of the September 11, 2001, bombings of the World Trade Towers in New York City, may or may not have any psychotic illness, but a diagnosis of paranoid schizophrenia was noted in the New York Times (Lewis 2006) (Table 16.3, case #6). Mr. Hosam Maher Husein Smadi, 20 years old, was drawn into an FBI undercover sting and drove a truck he believed carried explosives into a garage under the 60-story Fountain Place Building in Dallas, TX. He was arrested, and in his New York Times write-up on October 20, 2010, the diagnosis of schizophrenia was noted. Mr. Smadi may or may not have had any psychiatric condition, but the diagnosis of schizophrenia in the media promotes acceptance of schizophrenia (Table 16.3, case #2). Another example is Mr. Isaac Brown, 40 years old, who was chosen as a poster advertisement for successful treatment of mentally ill individuals. In his write-up in the New York Times, November 7, 1999, as well as on his New York City Public Transport poster, the diagnosis of paranoid schizophrenia was given. This was despite Mr. Brown's belief that Jesus Christ and Jim Morrison had been talking to him (Jim Morrison was a nationally known law-enforcement officer and district attorney from New Orleans who promoted a conspiracy theory about the assassination of President John F. Kennedy.). Further, Mr. Brown said that,

> What kept on happening to me is I'd have these episodes and walk the street all hours of the night. (Table 16.3, case #7)

Such symptoms at least hint at bipolarity due to grandiosity, episodes of a lack of need for sleep with increased activity, and psychosis.

In addition to wide exposure in the news and television, schizophrenia has been the diagnosis of the star characters in books and movies such as *A Beautiful Mind*. This was a 2001 American film based on the life of Dr. John Nash, a Nobel Laureate in Economics, inspired by a best-selling, Pulitzer Prize–nominated 1998 book of the same name by Sylvia Nasar. The movie grossed over $313 million worldwide and won four Academy Awards including Best Picture and Best Director. Dr. Nash was diagnosed with paranoid schizophrenia but was the recipient of the prestigious Carnegie Prize for Mathematics along with his Ph.D. at Princeton University. He then accepted an appointment at the Massachusetts Institute of Technology (MIT). Nash married, had at least two children (one possibly out of wedlock), divorced, and then remarried his first wife. The brilliance of his work was rewarded with the Nobel Memorial Prize in Economics in 1994. His psychosis, that must have been episodic given his successes, included auditory hallucinations, grandiose, and paranoid delusions that involved the United States Department of Defense, the Pentagon, a Soviet plot, and Soviet agents. Another scene described distractibility when Nash left his infant son in the bathtub. Such success, grandiose and paranoid delusions suggest a bipolar disorder.

It is unknown by the current author whether the diagnosis of schizophrenia was ever changed. If Dr. Nash suffered from episodes of depression as well as episodes of a lack of need for sleep, increased activities, and racing thoughts along with grandiose and paranoid delusions, the bipolar diagnosis would seem even more likely. Regardless, the diagnosis of schizophrenia was understood as valid by tens if not hundreds of thousands of moviegoers and readers of the book and the press.

Table 16.3 Media emphasis on schizophrenia

Case no.	Year/location/ reference	Patient/age/diagnosis	Description of event/crime	Victim name(s)/ relationship to patient	Symptoms	Comments
1	June 2011; Hartford CT; Carey, *New York Times*, June 23, 2011.	Dr. Marsha M. Linehan, 68; *schizophrenia*.	Very successful academic career despite many episodes of suicidal feelings and "... gusts of dark emotions or delusions ...."	None.	Long-term success in the stressful field of academics. Episodic "... gusts of dark emotions or delusions ... " apparently associated with suicidal thoughts and depression. One episode was described that might have indicated a manic episode and it was stated that "The high lasted for about a year, before the feelings of devastation returned ...."	Suicidal ideations are associated with depression. Dr Linehan "weathered gusts of dark emotions or delusions" likely coordinated with episodes of depression and suicidality. One episode was described that might have indicated a manic episode and it was stated that "The high lasted for about a year, before the feelings of devastation returned ...." The diagnosis of schizophrenia, however, promotes the acceptance of schizophrenia.
2	Sept. 2009; Dallas, TX McKinley, Jr. *New York Times*, Oct. 20, 2010.	Hosam Maher Husein Smadi, 20; *schizophrenia*.	"... undercover FBI agents drew Mr. Smadi into a fake plot to blow up the 60-story Fountain Place building. Mr. Smadi drove a truck that he believed carried an explosive into a garage under the building and activated the false bomb. ... Mr. Smadi agreed to plead guilty to attempted use of a weapon of mass destruction in exchange for a reduced sentence."	Intended victims were thousands of employees in the 60-story Fountain Place building in Dallas, TX.	Mr. Smadi "... married an American woman and began dabbling in radical Islamic politics. ... Defense lawyers had argued that he suffered from depression and had received a diagnosis of Schizophrenia."	Mr. Smadi may not have been psychotic but only a radical. However, the diagnosis of schizophrenia in the media endorses schizophrenia as a valid disease.
3	Nov. 2008; Indianapolis, IN ESPN.com, December 1, 2008.	Leonard Taylor, Jr. 32, *paranoid schizophrenia*.	"... faces one felony stalking count and one misdemeanor count of telephone harassment." Over 2 days, Nov 24, 25, 2008, Mr. Taylor left 29 voice mails on Mr. Barry Alvarez's, (University of Wisconsin Athletic Director), office phone, "... leaving six to seven disturbing messages each night since the beginning of football season." In one of these, Mr. Taylor said, "Barry, you heard that [expletive] message, [expletive] it. I hate that [expletive] Maria Sharapova.... I just want to look at you one [expletive] last time before I pull the, [expletive] trigger, Barry...." No physical violence was perpetrated.	Barry Alvarez, University of Wisconsin *Athletic Director*; (Mr. Taylor was a former Wisconsin football player); Maria Sharapova, has been #1 in the world in *Women's Professional Tennis*.	Mr. Taylor made excessive and focused phone calls and threats of violence toward famous individuals and their families. The messages left were described as "bizarre." "He [Taylor] said he wanted to marry her [Sharapova] and kill her [Sharapova] and her family." Mr. Taylor has been prescribed medication, apparently antipsychotic/antischizophrenia medications, but had not taken them for 3 months.	In the context of major mental illness, excessive activities such as multiple phone calls, threats, and delusional and grandiose attention to famous people such as Sharapova indicate mania. In a nonpsychotic, milder but still excessive form of attention to a famous person, a diagnosis of erotomania might be appropriate. The overlap in symptoms is indicated by the "mania" in erotomania. His diagnosis of schizophrenia in the media promotes the validity of schizophrenia.

(continued)

Table 16.3 (continued)

Case no.	Year/location/reference	Patient/age/diagnosis	Description of event/crime	Victim name(s)/relationship to patient	Symptoms	Comments
4	Feb. 2008; North Wales, PA Berenson, *New York Times*, Feb. 24, 2008 (Sunday Business).	Dr. Darryle D. Schoepp: *no diagnosis*.	Dr. Schoepp has helped develop new drugs for treating schizophrenia.	No victim(s).	This article titled, *Daring to Think Differently About Schizophrenia* took the top half of the first page of the Sunday Business Section of the New York Times and a full back page. "Overall sales of drugs treating Schizophrenia have doubled in the past five years" totaling over $1 billion in 2008.	The press exposure dedicated to drugs used to treat schizophrenia promotes the acceptance of schizophrenia as a valid disease. How could the USA spend over $1 billion dollars a year for a misdiagnosis?
5	2002; New York City, NY Bernstein, *New York Times*, August 9, 2002.	Jason Eric Wilson, 16; *schizophrenia*.	Mr. Wilson took an overdose of medication and died at a shelter for homeless people in New York.	Suicide.	Suicide.	Suicide is associated with psychotic depression, but the diagnosis of schizophrenia in the press promotes schizophrenia as a valid disease.
6	Sept. 2001; Trade Centers, New York City, NY Pentagon, Alexandra, VA Lewis, *The New York Times*, April 19, 2006.	Zacarias Moussaoui; *paranoid schizophrenia*.	The bombings of the World Trade Towers in New York City and the Pentagon in Alexandra, VA.	Thousands were killed and injured.	"A defense psychologist … told the jury that … [Moussaoui] is a paranoid schizophrenic … [because he] holds firmly to the delusions that President Bush will soon set him free and that his court-appointed lawyers are engaged in a plot to kill him. … another delusion was that the FBI had planted a bug in an electric fan …."	Mr. Moussaoui may not suffer from any DSM, Axis I diagnosis, but the media on several occasions published schizophrenia as his diagnosis, promoting the validity of schizophrenia.
7	1996; New York City, NY Lee, *New York Times*, November 7, 1999.	Isaac Brown, 40; *paranoid schizophrenia*.	Mr. Brown, "… was picked up by a city ambulance after he got down on his knees somewhere in the Bronx and started talking to a military statue."	No victim(s).	"… Mr. Brown was in his 20s when mental illness threatened to define his life. He started having auditory and visual hallucinations in 1982 while serving in the Israeli Army. He thought Jesus Christ and Jim Morrison were talking to him." Jim Morrison was in law enforcement in New Orleans, LA and wrote a book and promoted a conspiracy theory about the assassination of President Kennedy. [Mr. Brown was diagnosed with *paranoid schizophrenia*, "… lost his wife, his job, his friends and his home. He was hospitalized seven times…. 'What kept on happening to me is I'd have these episodes and walk the street all hours of the night.'" He began working effectively, received a series of promotions, and became the executive director of the Brooklyn Peer Advocacy Center; he remarried and has had at least one child. His picture was featured on a subway poster that read, "For People With Mental Illness Treatment Is Working."	Although Mr. Brown was not involved in a violent act, he and his diagnosis of schizophrenia were the subject of a New York Times article on November 7, 1999 and featured on a subway poster. His delusions of talking to Jesus Christ and Jim Morrison, a high-profile media person at that time, are grandiose and suggest mania. His history of "episodes" when he would "walk the streets all hours of the night" also suggests manic hyperactivity and the lack of need for sleep. His subsequent success is also compatible with a bipolar disorder.

8	May 1996; Salt Lake City, UT *New York Times*, September 15, 2001.	Ryan Tate Eslinger, 19; *paranoid schizophrenia*.	Mr. Eslinger bought a shotgun at a Kmart and killed himself on May 23, 1996.	Suicide.	No symptoms except for the suicide were given in the article.	Suicide is associated with depression, usually psychotic depression either bipolar or unipolar, but his diagnosis of schizophrenia in the press promotes schizophrenia.
9	1978–1995; There were three fatalities: Dec. 11, 1985, Dec. 10, 1994, and April 24, 1995. There were at least eight other serious injuries; multiple locations Wikipedia (2011).	Theodore John "Ted" Kaczynski (the Unabomber), was between 36 and 53 when he sent the bombs; *paranoid schizophrenia*.	Between 1978 and 1995, Mr. Kaczynski mailed 16 bombs which injured 23 people and killed three. One bomb failed to explode on an American Airlines Boeing 727 flying from Chicago to Washington, DC.	23 injured and three killed. Victims were selected based on Mr. Kaczynski's research into those individuals that he felt were ignoring and destroying nature and the wilderness. Some were university professors, others were industry leaders. He placed a bomb on a commercial jet that failed to explode.	Mr. Kaczynski was a child prodigy, accepted into Harvard University at 16. After graduation he earned a Ph.D. in Mathematics from the University of Michigan and became an assistant professor at UC Berkley at age 25, but he resigned 2 years later after receiving negative feedback from his students concerning his teaching ability. In 1971, he moved to a remote cabin without electricity or running water in Lincoln, MT where he lived as a recluse and decided to begin a bombing campaign after seeing the wilderness around his cabin being destroyed by development. His IQ was 167. He wrote a 50+ page, 35,000-word manifesto titled *Industrial Society and Its Future*. He demanded it be published or he would continue his bombings. It was published by the New York Times and The Washington Post on September 19, 1995. The content of the manifesto indicates at least eccentricity if not psychosis. He was arrested on April 3, 1996 in his cabin. *40,000 handwritten journal pages were found*. A court-appointed psychiatrist diagnosed him as suffering from paranoid schizophrenia. Two prison psychologists who saw him almost everyday for 4 years said, "… that they saw no indication that he suffered from [schizophrenia]…and that the diagnosis of his being paranoid schizophrenia was 'ridiculous' and a 'political diagnosis.'" On Jan. 7, 1998, Kaczynski *attempted to hang himself. In prison, he has been an active writer corresponding with over 400 people. He is involved in a Federal Court action in Northern California over the auction of his journals.	It is unclear based on the information available whether any psychiatric diagnosis is warranted for Mr. Kaczynski. What is important here is that his fame as the Unabomber was associated with the diagnosis of schizophrenia, promoting the concept that schizophrenia is a valid disease.

16.4 The Neuroses Became Obsolete in 1980 with the DSM-III: Why Not Schizophrenia?

Reflecting the multiple, idiosyncratic subtypes of the neuroses and the schizophrenias, the DSM, second edition (DSM-II) (APA, DSM 1968), listed at least ten neurotic disorder subtypes and at least 12 schizophrenia subtypes (Table 9.4). For some diagnoses more than others, beginning with the DSM-III (APA, DSM 1980), there was an attempt to replace subjective observations and opinions with available scientific data as the basis for subtypes and diagnostic criteria. This led to cataclysmic changes in the DSM-III (APA, DSM 1980) regarding the neuroses and a bit less drastic changes for the schizophrenias. Recognizing that the diagnosis of neurosis was confusing, misunderstood, socially stigmatizing, and lacked a scientific basis, the DSM-III (APA, DSM 1980) eliminated the term "neurosis" and all its subtypes from the official nomenclature. Its subtypes were either dropped or reorganized, renamed, and integrated into other diagnostic categories such as the anxiety disorders.

In contrast, for the schizophrenias, only one subtype, simple schizophrenia, was eliminated. Simple schizophrenia was the newest of the four core subtypes and was originated by E. Bleuler in 1911. The significance of dropping it from the DSM-III is substantial because the diagnosis of simple schizophrenia may have accounted for as many patients diagnosed with schizophrenia as all the other subtypes together between 1911 and 1980. Despite such a major concession by schizophrenophiles in 1980, the concept of schizophrenia overall was not eliminated as were the neuroses. In fact, the concept of schizophrenia was solidified because it was narrowed back to psychosis and chronicity that were easier to substantiate than Bleuler's vague fundamental symptoms that defined simple schizophrenia. Although the population of individuals with a potential for the diagnosis of schizophrenia shrunk considerably, academic psychiatry was substantially assured of the validity of this new, narrowed concept of schizophrenia. Other than the changes from the elimination of simple schizophrenia, the diagnostic criteria for the schizophrenias remained the same, and there were no changes for the core three subtypes dating from the 1800s (Tables 3.14, 12.9).

The concept of schizophrenia as "insanity" focused the diagnosis mostly on psychotic patients with high morbidity and chronicity usually requiring hospitalization. The costs for patients diagnosed with schizophrenia on government disability status have garnered considerable attention from government, taxpayers, and society in general. The neuroses, which may have been as common but were usually managed in outpatient clinics at lower costs, received less attention and rarely had disability status. As a result, hundreds of millions of federal dollars have funded research on the schizophrenias, while relatively few dollars supported research into the neuroses. Far greater numbers of pharmaceutical dollars supported the development and clinical trials of new antipsychotic/antischizophrenia medications, encouraging the diagnosis of schizophrenia and substantiating it as a disease. A small fraction of such pharmaceutical expenditures have been invested in the benzodiazepines to treat the neuroses and anxiety disorders. The power base of researchers, academics, editors, and administrators invested in the schizophrenias has been greater and more influential than that of those studying the neuroses. Schizophrenia has received more media attention than the neuroses both in the news and in film and has been evoked as the explanation for numerous high-profile murders (Sects. 15.5 and 16.2). Evidence for the media and the public acceptance of schizophrenia is demonstrated by their misuse of the term "schizophrenic" as an adjective to signify "flip-flops" in behaviors, statements, or policies. For reasons such as these, schizophrenia has maintained its place as the most widely known mental disorder in the world, and the neuroses are history.

16.5 The DSM and the ICD Perpetuate Schizophrenia and the Dichotomy

The diagnostic manuals and textbooks are held as authoritative in defining the psychiatric disorders and the diagnostic criteria for every relevant profession such as medicine, law, and government. They are used in the determination of injury, damages, legal responsibility, competency, disability, and compensation. Schizophrenia has maintained a prominent place in all such manuals and psychiatry textbooks. Hallucinations and delusions have been consistently given as diagnostic criteria for schizophrenia throughout the history of the DSM from 1952. Chapters on schizophrenia in the major textbooks on psychiatry often contain as many or more pages than on any other group of disorders. For example, *Kaplan & Sadock's Comprehensive Textbook of Psychiatry*, eighth edition 2005, dedicates 230 pages to the chapter on *Schizophrenia and Other Psychotic Disorders* while giving 159 pages to *The Mood Disorders*. Based on the proposed drafts of the next editions of the manuals, the ICD-11 and the DSM-5, schizophrenia and schizoaffective disorder will be retained (Bruijnzeel and Tandon 2011). Such consistency supports the validity of schizophrenia without the scientific support of disease-specific diagnostic criteria (Table 11.11). In a relatively minor concession, the subtypes of schizophrenia are scheduled for elimination in the DSM-5, but this step hardly addresses the implications of the considerable overlap in signs and symptoms between patients diagnosed with schizophrenia versus those with psychotic mood disorders (Tables 1.1, 4.3, 10.1, 11.1, 11.2, 11.10, 11.11, and 12.4). No Kraepelinian dichotomy suggests one disease, a mood disorder, to explain the functional psychoses.

16.6 The Pharmaceutical Profit Motive Promotes Schizophrenia

The antipsychotic/antischizophrenia medications have been formulated to treat schizophrenia since the 1950s because there were ample patients and prescriptions written for patients with schizophrenia. By 1964, some 50 million people had taken chlorpromazine (Thorazine). The typical antipsychotic/antischizophrenia medications have been credited with enabling the emptying of the state mental hospitals from over 0.5 million in 1955 to about 100,000 by the 1990s. The majority of these inpatients had diagnoses of schizophrenia, and instead of hospital inpatient beds, many now are incarcerated in jails and prisons or are on the street. The perceived effectiveness of the antipsychotic medications promoted the diagnosis of schizophrenia since doctors tend to diagnose disorders for which they believe effective treatment is available.

The antipsychotic/antischizophrenia medications are expensive to design, develop, test, and market. This is especially true for the atypical and the newer glutamate class of antipsychotic medications. Such front-end expenses necessitate sales. Marketing of some of the atypicals has been aggressive, to include television advertisements during prime time. The sales of drugs designed for treating schizophrenia doubled between 2003 and 2008 to an estimated $1.0 billion in 2008 (Berenson 2008). Such a profit from the antischizophrenia class of drugs is motivation to reinvest more effort and money in developing new antipsychotic medications such as the glutamate drugs. In 2008, Pfizer and Merck each invested over $20 million to gain the right to develop new glutamate antipsychotic medications (Berenson 2008). New antipsychotic/antischizophrenia medications and even drug development spur more diagnoses of schizophrenia through recruitment of patients for clinical trials and aggressive marketing by pharmaceutical representatives in doctors' offices. Even assuming only 50% of patients with a diagnosis of schizophrenia are taking antipsychotic medications, this would amount to one million patients treated yearly. All of these data uphold the validity of schizophrenia without a scientific basis.

Until the 1980s there was a large enough population of patients diagnosed with schizophrenia for pharmaceutical companies to make significant profit from such patients. However, the decline in the number of new patients diagnosed with schizophrenia that began in the 1980s may have contributed to a new strategy for maintaining such profits from the antipsychotic medications (Fig 3.2) (Sect 9.6). For example, in 1981, Mahendra published an article titled, "Where Have All the Catatonics [Schizophrenics] Gone?" In 1990, Der et al. published their article in *The Lancet* titled, "Is Schizophrenia Disappearing?" It was not that there were fewer severely mentally ill patients, but apparently, it was that fewer were being diagnosed with schizophrenia (Fig. 3.2). There was a parallel increase in the use of mood disorder diagnoses (Stoll et al. 1993; Kramer et al. 1969; Cooper et al. 1972). One study in 2001 at a major academic medical center indicated that only about 10% of functionally psychotic patients were diagnosed with schizophrenia, while about 80% received diagnoses of psychotic mood disorders (Table 3.5) (Pini et al. 2001). Despite this, the number of publications on schizophrenia continued to increase (Table 9.2; Fig. 9.1). The contrast of decreasing numbers of new diagnoses of schizophrenia with increasing publications about schizophrenia and increasing profit from sales of antipsychotic/antischizophrenia medications reflects the influence of researchers, academia, and the pharmaceutical industry versus clinicians in perpetuating the concept of schizophrenia.

This apparent decrease in the number of patients diagnosed with schizophrenia may have resulted in some concern in the boardrooms of the major pharmaceutical companies that owned the rights to an antipsychotic/antischizophrenia medication. One strategy appears to have been a broadening of the targeted patient population to embrace disorders in addition to schizophrenia, both psychotic and nonpsychotic. One example was revealed by a federal government audit, requested by Senator Charles E. Grassley, Republican of Iowa, of nursing home prescriptions for antipsychotic/antischizophrenia medications (Harris 2011). The article indicated that about 15% of the 2.1 million elderly nursing home patients, many with dementia, "had at least one Medicare claim for an antipsychotic medication" during the first 6 months of 2007 and that over half were inappropriate based on nonapproved usage, excessive dosages, or duration of use. Daniel R. Levinson, inspector general of the Department of Health and Human Services was quoted as saying in response to the audit results that the atypical antipsychotic medications,

> "... are 'potentially lethal' to many of the patients getting them and that some drug manufacturers illegally marketed their medicines for these uses, 'putting profits before safety.'" Also, "In response to the audit, the Centers for Medicare and Medicaid Services said that some of the inappropriate use of antipsychotics in elderly nursing home patients is a result of drug makers' paying kickbacks to nursing homes to increase prescriptions for the medicines. Omnicare Inc, a pharmacy chain for nursing homes, paid $98 million in November 2009 to settle the accusations that it received kickbacks from Johnson & Johnson and other drug makers for antipsychotic prescriptions."
>
> (Harris 2011)

In addition to patients diagnosed with schizophrenia and the elderly nursing home residents, other patient populations and conditions have been solicited by pharmaceutical companies for sales of antipsychotic/antischizophrenia medications. These include bipolar disorders, depression, anxiety, and sleep disorders, as well as several disorders of childhood. The continuing profitability of around one billion dollars gross annual income from the atypical antipsychotic medications, for patients diagnosed with schizophrenia or other disorders, continues to give credence to the diagnosis of schizophrenia.

16.7 Conclusions

There were several similarities between the neuroses and the schizophrenias, but the neuroses were essentially eliminated from the psychiatric nomenclature, while the concept of schizophrenia was strengthened in 1980 with the publication of the DSM-III. The schizophrenias, like the neuroses, (1) were described in the nineteenth century, (2) have diagnostic symptoms based on observation and opinion, (3) have no disease-specific signs or symptoms, (4) convey considerable social stigma, and (5) are confusing and misunderstood by many including the public and the media.

Despite these similarities, schizophrenia has remained as the most widely known and feared mental health condition. Schizophrenia has survived as a diagnosis and

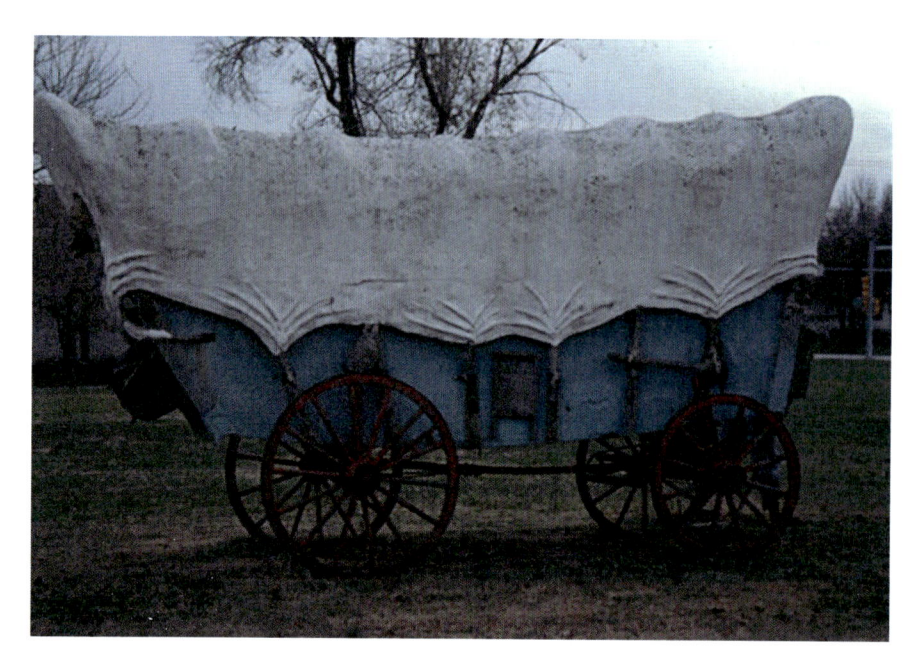

Fig. 16.2 Schizophrenia: a covered wagon
Like the neuroses, it is anticipated that the concept of schizophrenia has become obsolete with the fall of the Kraepelinian dichotomy and substantial overlap and similarities between patients diagnosed with schizophrenia and psychotic mood disorders. A goal in science is to simplify as suggested by Ockham's razor and as The Nobel Laureate Dr. Julie Axelrod constantly reminded his research associates

thrived in the literature for several reasons (Table 16.1; Fig. 16.1). Most basic to the continuing acceptance of schizophrenia is that there is no specific pathophysiology to rule it out despite enormous expenditures of research time and money for over a half century. Bentall et al. (1988) have addressed this issue saying,

> One possible reason for this lack of progress [in discovering the etiology of schizophrenia] is that schizophrenia is not a valid object of scientific enquiry. Data from published research (mainly carried out by distinguished psychiatrists) are reviewed casting doubt on: (1) the reliability, (2) the construct validity, (3) the predictive validity, and (4) the aetiological specificity of the schizophrenia diagnosis.

The influence of the originators of the concept of the Kraepelinian dichotomy and schizophrenia as psychosis has been large and pervasive especially among academic psychiatrists. However, as Craddock and Owen (2005) said,

> Now molecular genetic studies are beginning to challenge and will soon, we predict, overturn the traditional dichotomous view [that schizophrenia and bipolar are separate].

16.7 Conclusions

Despite the growing volume of data questioning the validity of schizophrenia as separate from psychotic mood disorders, the data are indirect and have not led to significant changes from the original concepts, at least since 1980. Academic psychiatry has dictated the concept of schizophrenia throughout the mental health and medical communities. As a result, the public and the media accept schizophrenia as valid. Media portrayals of schizophrenia broaden the public's knowledge about schizophrenia as a psychotic, potentially violent, common, dysfunctional, deteriorating, and costly disease that requires government support.

The severity and expense of schizophrenia generated the interest of psychiatrists, basic science researchers, federal-granting agencies such as the NIMH and the pharmaceutical industry. Increased research and the discovery of the apparent effectiveness of chlorpromazine (Thorazine) in schizophrenia led to increased diagnoses of schizophrenia, more money for research, the development and marketing of dozens of additional and profitable antipsychotic/antischizophrenia medications, and research foundation and laboratory focus on schizophrenia. The volume of research on schizophrenia is massive which for many seems to support its validity (Fig. 9.1). The DSM, the ICD, and textbooks continue to promote schizophrenia as a diagnosis.

Despite the above, this author believes the broad overlap from comparative neuroscience and clinical studies between patients diagnosed with schizophrenia and psychotic mood disorders, now documented from myriad sources, warrant the idea that, like the neuroses, the diagnosis of schizophrenia is as relevant as a covered wagon (Fig. 16.2).

# Chapter 17
What to Do if You, a Family Member, or Friend Is Diagnosed with Schizophrenia or Suffers with Psychotic Symptoms

> *Yet psychotic bipolar disorders can explain every sign, symptom, course, and other characteristics traditionally assumed to indicate schizophrenia. The literature, ... marshals a persuasive argument that patients diagnosed with schizophrenia usually suffer from a [psychotic] bipolar disorder.*
>
> (Lake and Hurwitz 2006a)

17.1 Introduction

If you or a significant other believe you might suffer from a psychotic mental illness or already have a diagnosis of schizophrenia, work with a trusted family member, friend, or caretaker to get the most effective treatment possible. The first step is the determination of whether or not there is a major psychiatric illness present (Table 17.1). This step can usually be accomplished by an appointment with an experienced psychiatrist for an initial diagnostic interview. Such an interview should take at least 50 min, but preparation before such an appointment is important and requires some research conducted by patients and their significant others.

Psychotic symptoms can be caused by street drugs and abuse of prescription medications, but when these are eliminated as the primary cause, the most common psychiatric disorders that can cause psychotic thoughts and behaviors include severe mania and depression.

Once drugs are ruled out as causative, a next step is to research the correct diagnosis because only with the correct diagnosis will the treatment plan be most effective. A new psychiatrist will not know much about you, so a concise outline of one page or less describing a recent psychotic episode can be very helpful. Begin by listing your or the patient's symptoms, behaviors, thoughts, and feelings that are considered abnormal or to have changed from baseline behavior. Include the most outrageous, striking actions atypical of normal behavior. Also record dates of historical episodes with similar symptoms you have experienced or observed. With the

Table 17.1 Outline of what to do if you or a significant other has a diagnosis of schizophrenia

Steps to take

1. Voice and discuss significant concerns about the presence of a severe mental illness
2. Accept responsibility for having a lifelong illness requiring your attention; listen to input of significant others
3. List your or the designated patient's signs, symptoms, behaviors, thoughts, speech, and feelings considered abnormal for that person or for the average person. Document the most atypical thoughts, behaviors, and actions; the most risky behaviors that led to trouble with authority figures are important
   - Record symptoms, dates of past episodes, and medicines prescribed
   - Document history of substance use/abuse
   - Record diagnoses, symptoms, and medications of family members with mental illness
4. Journal on a daily or twice daily basis (5–10 min a day) on daily flow sheet (Fig. 17.2)
   - Hours of sleep
   - Mood estimate on a 1–100 scale, once or twice daily; give examples
   - Rate of speech on a 1–100 scale, once or twice daily, give examples
   - Irritability level on a 1–100 scale, once or twice daily, give examples
   - Activity level on a 1–100 scale, once or twice daily, give examples
   - Grandiosity level on a 1–100 scale, once or twice daily, give examples
   - Fear/paranoia/suspiciousness level on a 1–100 scale, once or twice daily, give examples
   - Crying spells: the number per day, record once daily
   - Sociability/isolation level on a 1–100 scale, once or twice daily, give examples
   - Enjoyment/pleasure level on a 1–100 scale, once or twice daily, give examples
5. Research correct diagnosis from Tables in this book, DSM-IV-TR, Wikipedia, and Google
6. Research insurance
7. Research psychiatrist
8. Make an appointment with an experienced psychiatrist for an initial diagnostic interview
   - 50 min
   - $200–400
9. Clarify psychiatrist's impressions: the diagnoses with DSM codes, the treatment plan including frequency and length of future visits, medications, dosages, and psychotherapy
10. The goal of treatment is prevention of a next episode; must have correct diagnosis to get optimum treatment

availability of so much information through the internet, considerable research can be accomplished by a patient and his or her family and/or significant others by matching the symptoms exhibited by the patient with the symptoms diagnostic of some psychotic disorders from Tables 2.1, 2.2, 2.3, 2.4, 2.6, and 3.1. Search the internet via Google or Wikipedia for the DSM-IV-TR and contrast these diagnostic descriptions with the actual symptoms displayed by the patient. Research the family history including all blood relationships for any mental health contacts such as hospitalizations. Try to find what symptoms were exhibited by the relative just before hospitalization. Research what treatments were used, what medications.

A characteristic of manic thought and behavior is the use of denial and rationalization. Manic patients usually are not aware that they are acting abnormally even when

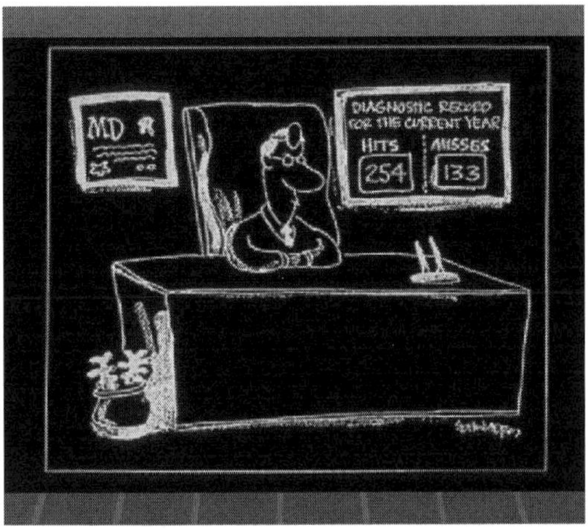

17.1 Introduction

Fig. 17.1 Get the diagnosis right

As emphasized in this cartoon, arriving at the correct diagnosis as quickly as possible is critical to effective treatment. Hopefully, this doctor is inexperienced since he does not have a very impressive "hits" to "misses" ratio

they are psychotic and are frightening friends and family. If you are a significant other and the patient does not recognize a problem or take responsibility, make the list of symptoms yourself enlisting help from others who have observed the individual's aberrant behavior and speech. The list becomes a daily journal of recorded abnormal behaviors, speech, and thoughts. Rather than trying to convince a manic (or hypomanic) or severely depressed patient that they are out of control, document the words and actions for presentation later when the patient has returned to baseline and is euthymic and more receptive. Hospital commitment may be necessary but even that may not be convincing evidence of a problem especially for a manic patient. Still, his or her psychiatric inpatient records are helpful as evidence to support the presence of a problem, and the patient has a right to obtain such records. Critical for the identified patient is to recognize and take responsibility for having a lifelong disease analogous to diabetes and hypertension in that daily attention is necessary even when feeling just fine. If you are the patient, accept observations and input from your significant others. Own having the diagnosis but get the right one (Fig. 17.1); get over the stigma.

Make an appointment with a psychiatrist for an initial diagnostic interview. Bring your list of your or the patient's symptoms and if possible, descriptions of other mentally ill family members' signs and symptoms. List family members who drink too much alcohol. If the psychiatrist confirms that there is a major psychotic disorder, document the specific diagnosis with the DSM code number. If the psychiatrist says you or the identified patient has schizophrenia, a second opinion is advised. If a psychotic mood disorder, bipolar or unipolar, is diagnosed, record the psychiatrist's treatment plan and medications. Expect frequent follow-up and the prescription of several drugs at the same time depending upon the severity of the condition. Treatment plans including medications recommended by the current author are given below (Figs. 17.3 and 17.4).

17.2 How Do You Tell If There Is a Severe Psychiatric Problem?

Answer the following questions honestly. How has your life been going over the past years to decades? Have you lost several jobs, friends or family or failed courses in school after doing well earlier in your life? Would you describe your life over the months and years as steady or up and down? Consider how up and how down and if these heights and depths are substantial and beyond the average. Have there been episodes for days or weeks when you may have lost touch with reality or when you were so down that you felt life was not worth living or when you were "high as a kite, on top of the world" and did not have time to sleep? Is it possible that a psychiatric disorder could be responsible for some of your failures and dysfunctionality? Ask significant others and listen to their input. Recognize that denial and rationalization, that is blaming others or other circumstances for your failures, are a symptom of some psychiatric disorders like mania in bipolar disorder. To effect any change, you or the identified patient must take responsibility for having a psychiatric disorder. Psychiatric disorders are treatable, but only after they are identified and a correct diagnosis is made (Fig. 17.1). You can take steps to help insure a correct diagnosis.

The influence of illegal or prescription drug use/abuse on the abnormal behavior must be distinguished. The most likely offending drugs that can mimic the signs and symptoms noted below are from the stimulant and hallucinogenic classes of illegal drugs and include such drugs as speed, cocaine, crack, amphetamine, and methamphetamine as well as LSD, PCP, psilocybin, khat, and bath salts containing man-made chemicals like mephedrone and methylenedioxypyrovalerone (sold under the names of Aura, Ivory Wave, Loco-Motion, and Vanilla Sky). If drugs can be eliminated as the primary cause of the psychotic symptoms, focus on episodes of depression and seek to identify one or more episodes of mania or hypomania from the past or in the present. A definitive answer can be determined by an appointment with a psychiatrist, but some preparation before the meeting can be productive. To gain confidence of a diagnosis, chart past and current mood swings on a form like the one in Fig. 17.2.

17.3 Journal Daily Symptoms, Dates, History, and Family History

Estimate the date of the first episode, the lifetime total number of episodes, how often they occur, how long they last and whether the episodes are generally the same or whether one or more have been strikingly different. How are they different? Record the level of dysfunctionality caused by the episodes. Going forward, journal on a daily basis such signs and symptoms. There are convenient forms already

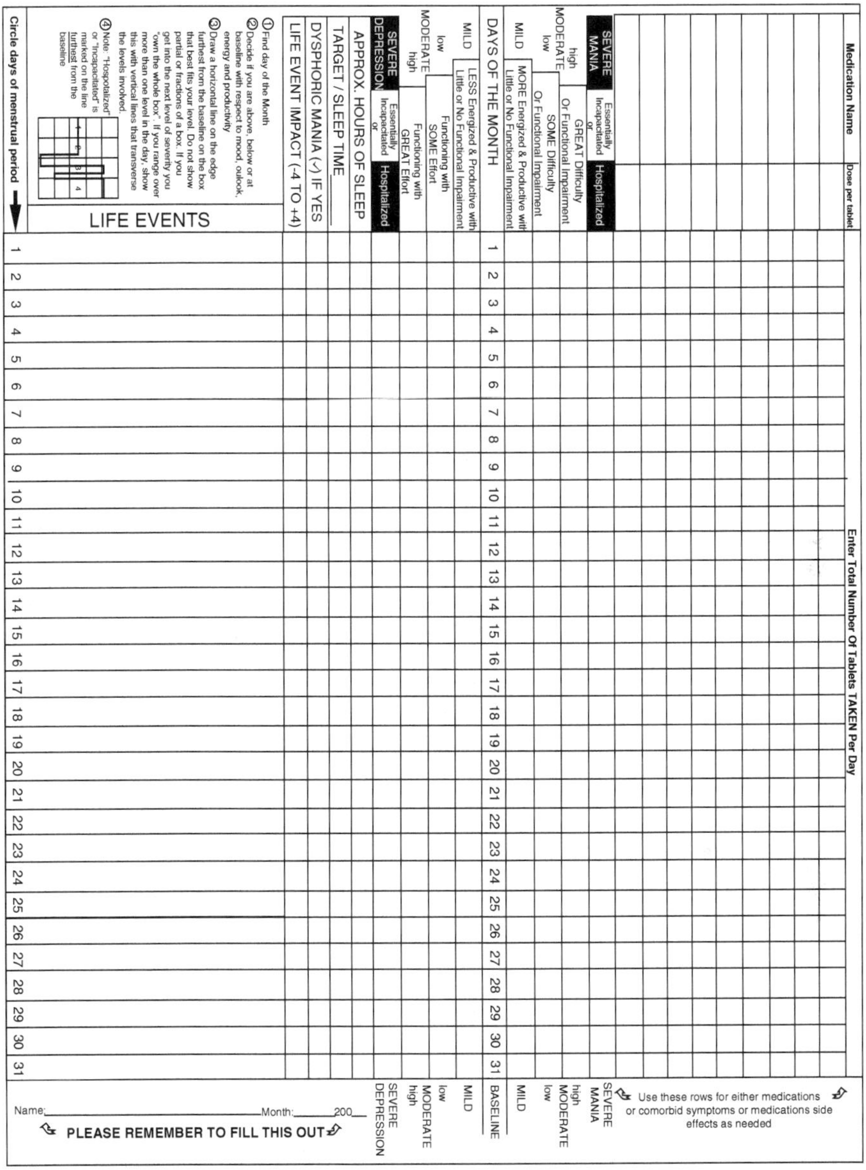

17.3 Journal Daily Symptoms, Dates, History, and Family History

Fig. 17.2 Daily mood, energy level, and sleep flow sheet for recurrent mood-disordered patients

This form is to be used daily by patients with recurrent mood disorders, either bipolar or unipolar. Begin each month by printing your name, the month, and the year on the new sheet at the bottom right of the form. Next, add the names of your medications and the number of milligrams in each tablet at the top of the form. See instructions, bottom left, for rating daily mood. Try to rate at approximately the same time every day. Abbreviate life events at the bottom of the form and rate the impact of each between a −4 and +4 depending upon negative or positive impact upon one's mood. Note the hours of sleep on the morning after. Women circle days of menstrual period at the very bottom of the form. Medication side effects can be noted under life events or in one of the rows available for medications at the top of the form. Target sleep time is one's average hours of sleep per night when euthymic.

Bring this form with you to your appointments with your psychiatrist.

established for this (Fig. 17.2). Ask or rate the mood and energy level once or twice every day on a 100-point scale with 0–10 signifying severe depression/no energy, 90–100, mania/super energy, and 40–60 as baseline mood/energy. Record the number of hours of sleep, medication taken, appetite, level of enjoyment of day-to-day activities that are usually enjoyable, rate of speech, activity level, crying spells, and sociability/isolation level. Several of these can also be evaluated on a 0–100 scale. Also record delusional thoughts, typically involving grandiosity, guilt, suspiciousness, paranoia, and fear of harm (Chap. 12). Grandiosity would include atypical ideas of the possession of very valuable powers, knowledge, wealth, or abilities. Often involved in delusional systems are figures of authority such as nationally or internationally known politicians, media, performing arts, sports, military, or religious figures that include the president, congresspersons, senators, governors, God, the devil, CIA, FBI, secret service, drug gangs, mafia, etc. On a different flow sheet record dates and symptoms of past episodes. The symptoms must occur together in time in an episode of 4 days to several months or more and be clearly uncharacteristic of the patient's baseline behavior. Document history of substance use/abuse. Journal on a daily basis on the form until your doctor tells you to stop. This effort will take less than 5 min a day and, over months and years, forms an invaluable database that can yield a pattern of episodes that is critical to ideal treatment and can give the best chance for the prevention of rapid cycling and treatment resistance.

17.4 Learn About the Disorders: Study Diagnostic Symptoms and Compare to Your Symptoms

The correct diagnosis is critical to optimal treatment. Substantial effort is warranted to accomplish this step. Read and take notes on as much data about bipolar and unipolar disorders as is reasonably possible. Begin with Tables 2.1, 2.2, 2.3, 2.4, 2.6, and 3.1, the DSM-IV-TR, and other sources such as textbooks, Wikipedia, and Google. The most comprehensive book about bipolar disorder is by Goodwin and Jamison (2007). The DSM-IV-TR is the best for the strict diagnostic criteria for mania and depression which are summarized below. Even a single episode of mania or hypomania distinguishes a bipolar from a unipolar disorder.

Compare the diagnostic symptoms from the tables in this book noted above and the DSM to the patient's recorded behavior, speech, and sleep at the peaks of the highs and depths of the lows. Symptoms of mania and depression typically, but not always, occur in distinct and separate episodes. Symptoms of mania must occur over a period of time lasting between several days and several months with an average of 3 months. The symptoms and behaviors must be clearly different from the patient's baseline behavior. Some of the important criteria of mania from the DSM-IV-TR are:

17.4 Learn About the Disorders: Study Diagnostic Symptoms...

... a distinct period of abnormally and persistently elevated, expansive or irritable mood, lasting at least 1 week (or any duration if hospitalization is necessary). During this period ... three or more of the following ... have persisted ... and [are] present to a significant degree: ... inflated self-esteem or grandiosity, a decreased need for sleep [coupled with an] increase in goal-directed activity, ... [that includes] excessive involvement in pleasurable activities that have a high potential for painful consequences [poor judgment], more talkative ... or pressure [of speech], flight of ideas ... thoughts racing, distractibility. (DSM-IV-TR, APA, DSM 2000)

Delusions, hallucinations, gross disorganization, and incomprehensibility are typical of psychotic mania or depression. These conditions can stop cycling and become persistent and chronic.

Symptoms of a major depressive episode from the DSM-IV-TR include:

... the presence of five or more of the following symptoms present during the same 2 week period or more that represent a clear change from previous functioning and that cause clinically significant distress or impairment of function. At least one of the symptoms must be:

1. Depressed mood [OR]
2. Loss of interest or pleasure in the usually pleasurable activities of life

   [The others are]
3. Weight loss or gain of at least 5% in a month
4. Insomnia or hypersomnia
5. Psychomotor agitation or retardation
6. Fatigue and loss of energy
7. Feelings of worthlessness or delusional guilt
8. Decreased ability to think and concentrate
9. Thoughts of death, recurrent suicidal ideation, or a suicide plan or attempt (APA, DSM-IV-TR 2000)

More than one major depressive episode, without a hint of mania or hypomania ever, defines a major depressive disorder, recurrent, also referred to as unipolar depression. A patient with major depression can exhibit psychotic behavior including hallucinations, delusions, catatonia, avolition, amotivation, a flat affect, and a deterioration to a chronic nonepisodic course. An episode of major depression in bipolar disorder has symptoms identical to those in a major depressive episode in unipolar depression. Bipolar disorders have episodes of both mania or hypomania and, usually but not always, depression; unipolar disorders have only episodes of depression that are indistinguishable from bipolar depression.

A bipolar disorder is important to distinguish from a major depressive disorder as well as from a diagnosis of schizophrenia. Table 17.2 distinguishes a bipolar depression from a unipolar depression. Table 17.3 lists signs and symptoms indicative of a bipolar disorder rather than a diagnosis of schizophrenia in a psychotic patient.

Table 17.2 Differentiating a bipolar disorder in a depression from a major depressive disorder[a]

Likely bipolar disorder, depressed, not major depressive disorder, if there has been:
1. A past manic or hypomanic episode
2. Prescription in the past of a mood stabilizing medication (Table 15.2)
3. A positive family history of bipolar disorder
4. Recurrent (more than three) major depressive episodes that begin before 25 years old
5. Postpartum onset
6. A typical but brief course (less than 3 months)
7. Psychotic features, hallucinations, delusions, disorganization in past depressive episodes
8. Resistance to antidepressants (more than three)
9. Antidepressant-induced mania or hypomania

[a]Absence of any or all does not rule out a bipolar disorder

Table 17.3 Differentiating a bipolar disorder from the diagnosis of schizophrenia[a]

Likely bipolar disorder, not schizophrenia, if there has been:
1. A past manic, hypomanic, or major depressive episode
2. Prescription in the past of a mood-stabilizing medication (Table 15.2)
3. A positive family history of bipolar disorder or a psychotic major depressive disorder
4. Any excessive, atypical emotion: irritability, grandiosity, elation, anger, verbal or physical conflict, sadness, tearfulness, hopelessness, guilt, suicidal ideations
5. Excessive, atypical and/or risky goal-directed behavior/activities: religious, legal, political, sexual, criminal, cleaning, phoning, writing, traveling, loud music, neighbor's complaints, police involved
6. Good premorbid social adjustment: school officer, sports, gangs, dated, "hung out with" buddies, past long-term relationship, formally married, children
7. Current social support: empathetic spouse, family, best friend
8. Psychosis, that is, hallucinations/delusions that are mood congruent: grandiose, guilt laden, paranoid, persecutory, conspiratorial OR mood incongruent hallucinations/delusions

[a]Absence of any or all does not rule out a bipolar disorder

17.5 Preparation for Seeing a Doctor/Psychiatrist

Even if confident of your or your significant other's diagnosis, an appointment with a psychiatrist is necessary for confirmation of the diagnosis and for formulation and implementation of a treatment plan. Research those psychiatrists included in your insurance plan, or go out of network if necessary for a more qualified and experienced psychiatrist. If available within 100 miles, see a psychiatrist rather than a nonpsychiatrist. Google available psychiatrists in your area. You must see a doctor with an M.D. or D.O. degree and ideally who has completed a Psychiatry Residency Program in the USA. The better the ranking of the residency program in general, but certainly not always, the better the training. The psychiatrist should be boarded in psychiatry by the American Board of Psychiatry and Neurology (ABPN). Certification in psychopharmacology is an asset as well. Other relevant questions include: What have they published? Do they teach at a medical school? What disorders do they teach? Select one who writes and teaches about bipolar disorders and depression.

The information you bring into your appointment must be a brief summary, preferably typed on less than one page double spaced. List the most outrageous, risky behaviors and hours of sleep during an episode. A past or family member's inpatient mental hospital stay with a diagnosis of schizophrenia indicates psychotic and/or chronic symptoms and is likely explained by a psychotic mood disorder, not schizophrenia. Look at your list of past symptoms and the mentally ill family member's symptoms, and you should be able to gain some idea of the diagnosis for you or your significant other.

Once at the appointment, share your data and clarify how long the psychiatrist plans to see you for the initial evaluation. If less than 45–60 min, consider another psychiatrist after stating that you understood that an initial diagnostic interview required that amount of time. If 45 min or more is okay, ask for 10 min at the end to ask questions and have them ready. Always include at the top of the list of questions the confirmation of the psychiatrist's diagnostic impressions with DSM code numbers and a description of the treatment plan including medications, dosages, and psychotherapy, individual and/or group therapy. If the diagnosis of schizophrenia or schizoaffective disorder is considered and an antipsychotic/antischizophrenia medication alone is recommended (Tables 15.4 and 15.6), consider a second opinion.

17.6 Treatment Plans for Major Mood Disorders

Different psychiatrists have different ideas about which symptoms are most important in making a diagnosis and about which medicines are better than others. For a century, psychiatrists have been taught that hallucinations and delusions mean schizophrenia, but this is not the case. The correct diagnosis matters; it is critical because the diagnosis narrows the treatment plan. Treating symptoms rather than the diagnosis does not meet standard of care. For example, a patient who has a past history of one or more manic episodes now presents in a florid psychotic state with minimal or no obvious mood symptoms. Treating the psychotic symptoms with an antipsychotic/antischizophrenia medication alone is malpractice because the patient suffers from a psychotic bipolar disorder and deserves one or more mood-stabilizing drugs in addition to the antipsychotic medication (that should only be given temporarily for days to weeks).

Different psychiatrists' treatment plans for the same diagnosis can also vary substantially. The mood-stabilizing drugs have been on the market for so long that they are available in generic form. This means they should be relatively inexpensive to purchase and not be a major income source for the manufacturers. This reduces or eliminates motivation by the pharmaceutical companies to invest in having their sales representatives market these drugs to doctors or directly to the public in media advertisements. Several of the newer atypical antipsychotic medications are not yet available generically, are expensive to purchase, are a potential source for large profit, and are heavily marketed by pharmaceutical sales representatives. Samples are given to doctors to pass on to their patients along with drug company generated data about the advantages of their drugs. Some psychiatrists are not critical enough of the bias of the drug representatives' pitches. This has been highlighted by FDA regulatory fines for the marketing of the antipsychotic/antischizophrenia medications for other non-FDA-approved disorders, some nonpsychotic. As stated above, the advertisement of any atypical antipsychotic medication as a first-line backup to an initial antidepressant drug to treat nonpsychotic depression is a substantial disservice in this author's opinion.

17.6.1 Major Depressive Disorder

Examine Table 17.2 carefully to rule out any hints of a bipolar disorder. Lithium would be prescribed first by several psychopharmacologists even if all nine of the points in Table 17.2 are negative and the diagnosis is a major depressive disorder (Schou 1967, 1968, 1979; Wehr and Goodwin 1987; Goodwin 1989; Calabrese et al. 2001). If one or more of the items in Table 17.2 are positive, the choice of lithium as the first medication is supported. Lithium is inexpensive but does have the potential for severe, life-threatening side effects (Table 15.3). Other psychopharmacologists would recommend one of the selective serotonin reuptake inhibitor (SSRI) or serotonin norepinephrine reuptake inhibitor (SNRI) antidepressants as the first drug (Table 17.4; Fig. 17.3).

If there are psychotic symptoms, expect a prescription for an atypical antipsychotic drug (Table 15.4) in addition to lithium, an SSRI, or an SNRI. If the patient is agitated, addition of a short-term course of a longer-acting benzodiazepine is appropriate. See below for recommendations of how to use these antipsychotic/antischizophrenia medications in psychotic mood disorders (Fig. 17.3).

If lithium is prescribed, it is reasonable to begin with 300 mg twice a day and to titrate this dosage up by 300 mg as tolerated over several days to as much as 600 mg twice a day. At this time, it is appropriate to have blood drawn to measure the level of lithium in the blood and establish baseline renal function. One should not have taken a dose of lithium within 8 h of having their blood drawn. Mild side effects are to be expected such as some tremor in the hands, thirst, and increased urination (Table 15.3). Depending on the individual patient's metabolism, between 600 mg per day and 2,100 mg/day can be tolerated to yield a therapeutic plasma level of between 0.6 and 1.4 meq/L. Note that if the person who achieves a therapeutic plasma level on 600 mg/day takes more than triple this amount, they are likely to become toxic and possibly die.

If an antidepressant was prescribed first and there has been no response, the first step is to raise the dose of that antidepressant as rapidly as tolerated per doctor's recommendations to the recommended maximum dose (Fig. 17.3). If the risk for suicide is deemed low, the patient can expect to be followed weekly or every other week as an outpatient. If there is no improvement after a week on the maximum dose tolerated or recommended of the initial antidepressant drug, a second step is to add a mood stabilizer such as lithium and titrate to a therapeutic blood level as described above. If still there is no improvement after a week with the lithium level in the therapeutic range in addition to the first antidepressant, a third drug can be

17.6 Treatment Plans for Major Mood Disorders

Table 17.4 Second-generation antidepressive medications

SSRI	
Trade name	Generic name
Celexa	Citalopram
Lexapro	Escitalopram
Luvox	Fluvoxamine
Prozac	Fluoxetine
Sarafem	Fluoxetine
Zoloft	Sertraline

SNRI	
Trade name	Generic name
Cymbalta	Duloxatine
Effexor	Venlafaxine
Pristiq	Desvenlafaxine
Paxil	Paroxetine
Pexeva	Paroxetine

Miscellaneous antidepressants	
Trade name	Generic name
Wellbutrin (dopaminergic)	Bupropion

Stimulants	
Trade name	Generic name
Adderall	Amphetamine
Concerta	Methylphenidate
Dexedrine	Dextroamphetamine
Ritalin	Methylphenidate
Strattera	Atomoxetine
Vyvanse	Lisdexamfetamine

SSRI selective serotonin reuptake inhibitor, *SNRI* serotonin norepinephrine reuptake inhibitor

added, either a second antidepressant (Table 17.4) or a second mood stabilizer (Table 15.2; Fig. 17.3). If the first antidepressant was an SSRI and the decision is made to choose a second antidepressant, some would recommend adding an SNRI or bupropion (Wellbutrin) (Table 17.4). Similarly, the dose of either the second mood stabilizer or the second antidepressant should be titrated up as rapidly as tolerated to the maximum recommended or tolerated dose. If there is no improvement in mood a week after reaching the maximum recommended or tolerated dose of the third medication, either a fourth medication can be added (an antidepressant if drug three was a second mood stabilizer or a mood stabilizer if drug three was an antidepressant), or ECT can be considered. The order depends on the condition of the patient. If deteriorating, ECT is used sooner. The benefit-to-risk ratio for ECT in the treatment of severe major depression is superior to that for an antipsychotic/antischizophrenia medication according to Swartz and Shorter (2007). If ECT is not chosen and the addition of a fourth drug does not begin to improve the depression,

OPTION A

STEP #1 — LITHIUM ± ATYP (if psychotic) / ± BZD (if agitated depression)

STEP #2 — + 1st SSRI or bupropion

STEP #3 — + 1st SNRI or bupropion | + CBZ or VPA

STEP #4 — + CBZ or VPA | + 1st SNRI or bupropion

STEPS #5-9 — +ATYP | +STIM | +LAM | +VPA or CBZ | +ECT | +VPA or CBZ | +LAM | +STIM | +ATYP

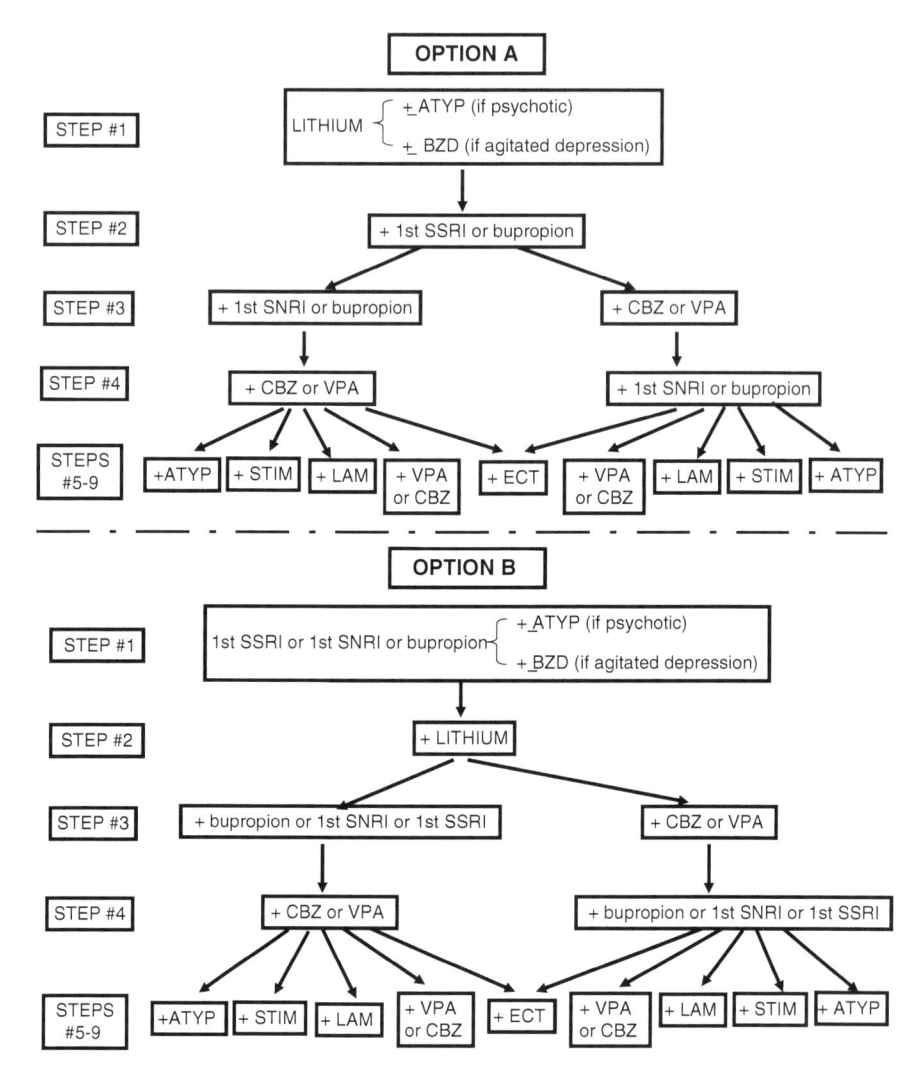

OPTION B

STEP #1 — 1st SSRI or 1st SNRI or bupropion { +ATYP (if psychotic) / +BZD (if agitated depression) }

STEP #2 — + LITHIUM

STEP #3 — + bupropion or 1st SNRI or 1st SSRI | + CBZ or VPA

STEP #4 — + CBZ or VPA | + bupropion or 1st SNRI or 1st SSRI

STEPS #5-9 — +ATYP | +STIM | +LAM | +VPA or CBZ | +ECT | +VPA or CBZ | +LAM | +STIM | +ATYP

Fig. 17.3 Medication treatment plan for unipolar depression (major depressive disorder, MDD)

Two options are presented for the medication treatment of unipolar depression. The differences between option A and option B only involve whether lithium or an antidepressant is given first or second. Under both options, an atypical antipsychotic drug and/or a benzodiazepine can be given initially if the patient is psychotic and/or agitated. Both are used sparingly as needed and titrated down and discontinued when psychosis and agitation resolve. In moderate to severe unipolar depression, because of substantial morbidity and mortality, the first drug prescribed (lithium in option A, an antidepressant in option B) is started at the recommended starting dose and titrated up as rapidly as tolerated until an improvement in symptoms occurs, adverse effects appear or a maximum recommended dose is reached. In inpatients, the rate of titration can be increased. There is flexibility regarding "maximum recommended dose" depending upon physician familiarity with use of larger doses. If there is no improvement, add the second medication (an antidepressant in a fifth drug or ECT are the choices. The fifth drug can be another antidepressant, another mood-stabilizing drug, a stimulant (Table 17.4), or an atypical antipsychotic medication (Table 15.4) unless the patient is already taking one of the antipsychotic/antischizophrenia medications because they presented in a psychotic state.

Aripiprazole (Abilify) is an example of an atypical antipsychotic/antischizophrenia medication that is FDA approved for depression and is advertized on prime-time television. In the TV ad, aripiprazole is said to be doctor recommended as a first-line backup choice to be added to an initial antidepressant to treat what is advertised as unresponsive depression. No mention is made of increasing the dosage of the antidepressant medication to a maximum recommended or tolerated amount. The cartoon ad implies that the addition of aripiprazole causes the patient's depression to go away. This is misleading, in the current author's opinion, and is an example of attempts by the pharmaceutical industry to influence clinical decisions by encouraging patients to ask for aripiprazole. In the current author's view, adding an atypical antipsychotic/antischizophrenia medication might be an appropriate fifth or sixth backup step in the treatment of a nonpsychotic, four or five drug-resistant depression as discussed above (Chap. 15).

Although some of the antipsychotic/antischizophrenia medications have won FDA approval for treating mania and depression, they are not first- or even second-line choices, in this author's opinion. These drugs are designed and developed to treat psychotic symptoms, not mood symptoms. They do appear to be effective in acutely psychotic mania and depression, but their long-term mood-stabilizing effects are not adequately tested when compared to the long-term trials conducted over multidecades of use of the first-line mood stabilizers, especially lithium, valproic acid, and carbamazepine.

Although controversial if antipsychotic/antischizophrenia medications should ever be given, even to psychotic patients, when given, dosages of an antipsychotic/antischizophrenia medication should be minimized (Calabrese et al. 2001; Whitaker 2004). Dosages should be titrated up as tolerated in inpatients and tapered down and discontinued when the psychosis has resolved, ideally before discharge, and as soon as the appropriate medicines such as mood stabilizers for long-term stabilization of the core disorder are at therapeutic levels. The most sedative mood stabilizers such as carbamazepine and valproate can be given in larger dosages to sedate dangerous, manic patients in addition to a short-term course of a long-acting benzodiazepine. The benzodiazepines can be used safely in sedating dosages.

Fig. 17.3 (continued) option A and lithium in option B) and titrate up as described above. Steps 3–9 are similar between option A and option B. Step 3 involves the addition of a second antidepressant but typically of a different class than the first or the addition of a second mood-stabilizing medicine. The fourth medication suggested if there is no improvement is either another antidepressant or another mood stabilizer. Steps 5–9 include choices of ECT, an atypical antipsychotic/antischizophrenia medication, a stimulant, lamotragine, or other first-line mood stabilizer.

Abbreviations: *Li* lithium, *SSRI* selective serotonin reuptake inhibitor (Table 17.4), *SNRI* serotonin norepinephrine reuptake inhibitor (Table 17.4), *CBZ* carbamazepine (Tegretol), *VPA* valproic acid (Depakote), *LAM* lamotragine (Lamectal), *STIM* stimulants (Table 17.4), *ECT* electroconvulsive therapy, *BZD* benzodiazepine, *ATYP* atypical antipsychotic/antischizophrenia medications

In cases of chronic, persistent psychosis, the smallest effective dose of an antipsychotic/antischizophrenia medication is recommended by some psychiatrists over time with regular weekly to monthly follow-up to assure some effectiveness of the drug and to monitor for tardive dyskinesia and tardive psychosis. When used for months at a time, drug holidays can be revealing of detrimental antipsychotic medication side effects related to dopamine receptor supersensitivity. The current author now errs on the side of minimizing use and dosages of the antipsychotic/antischizophrenia medications. If movement disorder side effects occur, some now recommend discontinuing the antipsychotic medication rather than adding other drugs to try to counter the side effects. This is especially encouraged by the data that suggest that the antipsychotic medications can worsen or cause psychosis (Swartz 1995; Whitaker 2004).

17.6.2 Bipolar Disorders

A bipolar disorder can present in a depression or in a mania, and the management with medication can be surprisingly similar in light of the marked differences in mood and behavior. Presentations in depression are more common and not infrequently occur postpartum. In psychotic bipolar depression, short-term use of an atypical antipsychotic/antischizophrenia medication may be appropriate (Table 15.4; Fig. 17.4), and its administration is similar to that given above for a psychotic unipolar depression. One of the first-line mood-stabilizing medications would be started simultaneously (Table 15.2). If lithium is chosen, its dose would be titrated up as described above. Lamotragine (Lamectal) is not a good first-drug choice because its titration is more gradual than the other mood stabilizers because of the risk of a fatal rash that usually occurs during the upward titration, especially if rapid. Valproic acid (Depakote) and carbamazepine (Tegretol) are good choices because of their sedative side of effects in agitated or mixed manic depressions. If there is no or only minimal response within a week after arriving at a therapeutic blood level of the first mood-stabilizing medication prescribed, a second mood stabilizer is appropriate, also to be titrated up as rapidly as tolerated. If still no response, a third mood stabilizer such as lamotragine is a good choice. If still depressed, some psychiatrists

Fig. 17.4 (continued) CBZ before LAM since LAM requires a slower upward titration rate. If necessary, both options recommend implementing all four of the first-line mood-stabilizing medications (Table 15.2). If the patient has not responded with therapeutic plasma levels of three of the mood-stabilizing medications and a daily dosage of LAM between 200 and 400 mg per day, consider adding an atypical antipsychotic, or if depressed, an antidepressant or ECT.

Abbreviations: *Li* lithium, *LAM* lamotragine (Lamectal), *SSRI* selective serotonin reuptake inhibitor (Table 17.4), *STIM* stimulants (Table 17.4), *SNRI* serotonin norepinephrine reuptake inhibitor (Table 17.4), *ECT* electroconvulsive therapy, *CBZ* carbamazepine (Tegretol), *BZD* benzodiazepine, *VPA* valproic acid (Depakote), *ATYP* atypical antipsychotic/antischizophrenia medications (Table 15.4)

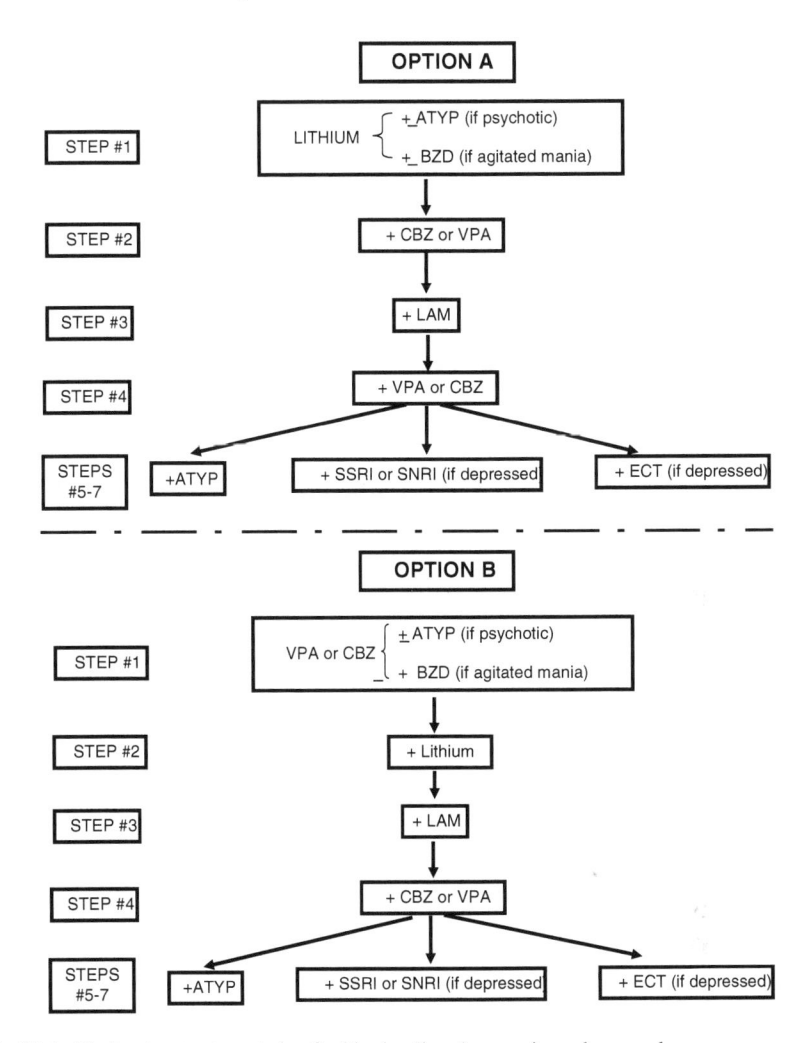

17.6 Treatment Plans for Major Mood Disorders 385

OPTION A

- STEP #1: LITHIUM { ± ATYP (if psychotic); ± BZD (if agitated mania) }
- STEP #2: + CBZ or VPA
- STEP #3: + LAM
- STEP #4: + VPA or CBZ
- STEPS #5-7: +ATYP | + SSRI or SNRI (if depressed) | + ECT (if depressed)

OPTION B

- STEP #1: VPA or CBZ { ± ATYP (if psychotic); + BZD (if agitated mania) }
- STEP #2: + Lithium
- STEP #3: + LAM
- STEP #4: + CBZ or VPA
- STEPS #5-7: +ATYP | + SSRI or SNRI (if depressed) | + ECT (if depressed)

Fig. 17.4 Medication treatment plan for bipolar disorder, manic or depressed

Two options are presented for the medication treatment for bipolar disorders. The differences between option A and option B only involve whether lithium or an antiseizure mood stabilizer is given first or second. Under both options, an atypical antipsychotic drug and/or a benzodiazepine can be given initially if the patient is psychotic and/or agitated. Both are used sparingly as needed and titrated down and discontinued when psychosis and agitation resolve. The schedules, options A and B, are applicable to bipolar mania or depression. Because of substantial morbidity and mortality, the first drug prescribed (lithium in option A, VPA or CBZ in option B) is started at the recommended starting dose and titrated up as rapidly as tolerated until an improvement in symptoms occurs, adverse effects appear or a dose that yields a therapeutic blood level is reached. In inpatients, the titration rate can be increased. If an inpatient, manic and potentially dangerous, VPA or CBZ may be a better first choice than lithium because of their sedative effects. Step 2, if inadequate improvement, is the addition of CBZ or VPA to lithium in option A and the addition of lithium to VPA or CBZ in option B. Steps 3 and 4 may be interchangeable when there is an inadequate response after step 2. If the patient still has anger control issues after step 2, consider adding VPA or might consider an antidepressant, given there are three mood-stabilizing medications on board at therapeutic levels. If still no response in the severely depressed bipolar patient, ECT becomes a choice as does a stimulant, a fourth mood-stabilizing medication, a second antidepressant, or a low dose of an antipsychotic medication. Once psychotic symptoms resolve, titration down and discontinuation of any antipsychotic medication is recommended by some (Calabrese et al. 2001; Whitaker 2004).

In case of psychotic manic presentations, an antipsychotic/antischizophrenia medication plus a mood-stabilizing drug are recommended by most psychopharmacologists. A benzodiazepine can also be useful. One of the more sedative mood stabilizers such as carbamazepine or valproate can lower the necessary dose of the antipsychotic medication. Next steps involve use of all four mood-stabilizing drugs titrated up to maximum tolerated or recommended dosages followed by addition of a second antipsychotic/antischizophrenia medication (Fig. 17.4, option B).

Patients are encouraged to participate in their titration schedules under doctor guidelines if they are able. This gives patients the ability to hold a given dose if there are mild adverse effects. They are encouraged to avoid stopping a drug altogether unless side effects are moderate to severe, rather, it is recommended that they take the dose down one step to see if adverse effects diminish or go away. Then one can titrate backup at a more gradual rate. Patients should recognize that there are a limited number of drugs in each class such as the mood stabilizers (Table 15.2). It is self-defeating to declare a drug unacceptable based on only mild, discomforting side effects. First try a smaller starting dose and going up more gradually.

17.6.3 Psychotherapy

Psychotherapy is a valuable therapeutic modality to combine with pharmacotherapy. Individual psychotherapy requires more than the 15-min medication checks that managed-care and insurance companies encourage psychiatrists to practice. For ideal patient care, both pharmacotherapy and psychotherapy are administered by the same doctor. Psychotic mood disorders are typically episodic early in their course, lifelong and can be markedly debilitating. Such conditions warrant major patient and significant other involvement in their care when capable. The goal is to prevent these episodic disorders from becoming rapid cycling, chronic, persistent, and treatment-resistant disasters. Full 45–50-min psychotherapy sessions weekly or every other week are recommended with the psychiatrist. Patients are expected to bring to each appointment their updated mood and sleep charts (Fig. 17.2). Therapy sessions must be a top priority in one's life and seen as a lifeline to sanity and functionality. If a priority overrides, reschedule the same week or twice the next week.

Weekly or twice a week group psychotherapy is also a very valuable experience. Group members, suffering with bipolar or unipolar disorders, learn from one another and monitor each other for early symptoms that can herald the onset of another episode. Group therapy is cost-effective, usually no more than $100 per session. Many insurance policies cover group therapy.

17.7 Conclusions

Once it is determined that there is a major psychiatric illness present and responsibility is accepted, the next step is to find the correct diagnosis. The overriding goal is to institute the most effective treatment plan, and this necessitates an accurate diagnosis. There are several impediments to this task. Some patients diagnosed with schizophrenia and their families or caretakers may be opposed to the conclusions of this book that a diagnosis of schizophrenia usually means a psychotic mood disorder because they have accepted and are comfortable with their diagnosis or believe their disability income might be jeopardized if their diagnosis were changed. Since psychotic mood disorders also warrant government disability, income issues should not be a major concern but changes in diagnosis and medications often meet resistance. Mental health professionals, including psychiatrists, are still likely to diagnose schizophrenia in cases of severe psychotic presentations because of the curriculum in Academic Psychiatry that continues in some cases to perpetuate the outdated concepts of Kraepelin, Bleuler, and Schneider (Table 16.2). They believed that psychotic symptoms trumped mood symptoms mandating the diagnosis of schizophrenia. Another substantial problem for patients with diagnoses of schizophrenia and long-term treatment with antipsychotic/antischizophrenia medications is the possibility of tardive psychosis, that is, psychotic symptoms, developing or worsening when the diagnosis is changed and the antipsychotic medication is titrated down. The onset or worsening of psychotic symptoms when antipsychotic medication dosages are reduced is likely to be misinterpreted as confirming the diagnosis of schizophrenia, the need for higher doses, and no further attempts to reduce dosages of antipsychotic medications.

An initial diagnostic interview and follow-up with a psychiatrist is mandatory. With so much information available online, patients and their families can facilitate arriving at the correct diagnosis and treatment plan. This is accomplished by journaling episodes of abnormal signs, symptoms, behaviors, actions, thoughts, and feelings. Journal on a daily basis. Then compare the patient's symptoms to the diagnostic criteria given in this book, the DSM-IV-TR, and from online data. Bring your journal of symptoms and ideas to the psychiatrist. Be prepared to ask his or her diagnostic impressions and to discuss the treatment plan options. In today's world of medicine, the patients and their families are their own best advocates.

Chapter 18
Vision for the Future: Conclusions and Solutions

> *There is, in short, no such thing as schizophrenia.*
>
> (Szasz 1976)
>
> *It is important to loosen the grip which the concept of "schizophrenia" has on the minds of psychiatrists. Schizophrenia is an idea whose very essence is equivocal, a nosological category without natural boundaries, a barren hypothesis.*
>
> (Brockington 1992)
>
> *Future research should focus on factors that may reveal overlap between schizophrenia and affective disorder ....*
>
> (Taylor 1992)
>
> *Dr. Wolfgang Gaebel, MD [Dusseldorf, Germany] suggested that the diagnostic concept of schizophrenia be abandoned ....*
>
> (First 2006)

18.1 Introduction

The focus of this book has been the position that schizophrenia is not a valid disorder different from psychotic mood disorders. This chapter assesses responsibility for the perpetuation of the concept of the validity and separateness of schizophrenia and addresses critical negative spin-off phenomena that detrimentally impact graduating MDs not entering psychiatry and their mentally ill patients. The negative spin-off phenomena from academic psychiatry's focus on schizophrenia include the underrecognition and undertreatment of depression and the risk for suicide by nonpsychiatric physicians. For 25 years, academic psychiatry and primary care have known that only 10–50% of depressed patients are adequately treated primarily because of the failure by their doctors to recognize depression. There are substantial negative consequences to the failure to recognize including death by suicide. Suicide occurs during depression, so the recognition of depression is the critical first step to preventing suicide.

Every medical doctor graduating from medical school in the USA has some exposure to psychiatry. Recently noted is that one barrier to recognition in nonpsychiatric medical settings is academic psychiatry's traditional attempt at comprehensive coverage of the field of psychiatry including schizophrenia and the thorough psychiatric interview that may actually reduce recognition because it takes too much time. Any screening psychiatric inquiry requiring more than a few minutes is impractical in primary care settings.

Medical student exposure to psychiatry is limited, and only a small minority enter psychiatry residencies, yet a large majority of patients with psychiatric problems first present to nonpsychiatric physicians (Lake et al. 1984). Given these somewhat unique circumstances, it has been suggested that academic psychiatry focus its limited time with medical students on only the most critical of psychiatric disorders and prepare its students both to recognize these disorders under time-limited circumstances and to know their referral and treatment options. The most critical disorders in any specialty of medicine are usually determined by four criteria: (1) the highest rates of mortality and morbidity, (2) high prevalence rates, (3) high response rates to treatments, and (4) substantial scientific data supporting them as actual disorders. Mood disorders, the disorders that primary care physicians underrecognize and undertreat, stand out in all four categories. These deserve sufficient emphasis to maintain students' knowledge throughout nonpsychiatric residencies and into practice even at the cost of several traditional topics in psychiatry taught for most of a century to medical students such as schizophrenia, schizoaffective disorder, and the comprehensive 50-min initial diagnostic interview.

Suggestions are given for changes in the DSM to eliminate schizophrenia and schizoaffective disorder that are already encompassed by the psychotic mood disorders.

18.2 The Failure to Recognize Depression and the Risk for Suicide in Nonpsychiatric Clinical Settings

Depression is a very common illness; nearly 19 million American adults have depression (Zung and King 1983; Prestidge and Lake 1987; Regier et al. 1993; Simon and VonKorff 1995; Hirschfeld et al. 1997; Lieberman 2002; Pignone et al. 2002; U.S. Preventive Services Task Force 2002; Vedantam 2002). The 6-month prevalence of major depression in the general population in the USA is about 6.6%, and for any mood disorder, 13.5–17% (Zung and King 1983; Prestidge and Lake 1987; Regier et al. 1993; Simon and VonKorff 1995; Kessler et al. 1996; Hirschfeld et al. 1997; Lieberman 2002; Pignone et al. 2002; U.S. Preventive Services Task Force 2002; Vedantam 2002). Depression has a high comorbidity in medically ill patients (Follette and Cummings 1967; Jacobs et al. 1968; Goldberg et al. 1970; Rodin and Voshart 1987; Culpepper 2002; Goodwin and Jamison 2007). Among outpatient primary care high utilizers, about 50% are depressed, whereas nonpsychiatric inpatients have an even higher rate (Zung and King 1983; Prestidge and Lake 1987; Regier et al. 1993;

Simon and VonKorff 1995; Kessler et al. 1996; Hirschfeld et al. 1997; Lieberman 2002). Despite being so common, depression is substantially underrecognized and undertreated (Zung and King 1983; Lake et al. 1984; Prestidge and Lake 1987; Regier et al. 1993; Simon and VonKorff 1995; Kessler et al. 1996; Hirschfeld et al. 1997; Arbabzadeh-Bouchez et al. 2002; Lieberman 2002; Pignone et al. 2002; Vedantam 2002; van't Veer-Tazelaar et al. 2009).

Primary care physicians too often fail to recognize and adequately treat mood disorders and suicidality (Robins et al. 1959; Prestidge and Lake 1987; Blumenthal 1988; Lonnqvist et al. 1995; Hirschfeld et al. 1997; Pirkis and Burgess 1998; Henriksson et al. 2001; Goldman et al. 2002; Luoma et al. 2002; Coyle et al. 2003; Gaynes et al. 2004; Mann et al. 2005). In their "consensus statement," Hirschfeld et al. (Hirschfeld et al. 1997) stated that,

> ... there is overwhelming evidence that the vast majority of patients with chronic major depression are misdiagnosed, receive inappropriate treatment, or, are given no treatment at all.

The Epidemiologic Catchment Area study found that only about one in ten depressed patients (10%) receives adequate treatment (Regier et al. 1993). Of depressed primary care high utilizers, less than 50% are treated for depression and only about 10% receive adequate antidepressants (Katon et al. 1992). Failure to recognize and treat has critical consequences.

Depression is the fourth highest cause of disability resulting in pain and suffering to patients and their families in the USA and around the world (Zung and King 1983; Prestidge and Lake 1987; Pignone et al. 2002; Vedantam 2002; Arbabzadeh-Bouchez et al. 2002). The morbidity is significant even in the milder forms of depression called dysthymia, subsyndromal depression, and minor depression (Shelton et al. 1997; APA, DSM-IV-TR 2000; Lyness et al. 2007). Although these dysthymic patients respond well to antidepressant medication, dysthymia and subsyndromal depression are typically not recognized (Shelton et al. 1997). Mortality is substantial in major depression.

Suicide is the most tragic consequence of severe depression (Guze and Robins 1970; Barraclough et al. 1974; Murphy 1975; Coombs et al. 1992; Hendin et al. 2001; Luoma et al. 2002; Goodwin et al. 2003; Dalton et al. 2003; Leverich et al. 2003). It is the eighth leading cause of death in the USA and is unchanged in rate since 1900 (Luoma et al. 2002; Dalton et al. 2003; Mays 2004). About 32,000 deaths per year result from suicide in the USA, of which over 14% occur in people over 65 (Conwell and Thompson 2008). Lifetime mortality from suicide for recurrent major mood disorders (both major depressive disorder and bipolar disorder) is about 15%, and for bipolar depression, 20–25% (Guze and Robins 1970; Barraclough et al. 1974; Prestidge and Lake 1987; Regier et al. 1993; Hirschfeld et al. 1997; Arbabzadeh-Bouchez et al. 2002; Lieberman 2002; Dalton et al. 2003; Goodwin et al. 2003; Leverich et al. 2003; Simon and VonKorff 1995). Among older adults, a far higher percentage of suicidal acts are fatal than among those younger than 65 (Conwell and Thompson 2008). Use of alcohol and both prescription and illegal drugs increases the risk of suicide to about 40% in bipolar-depressed patients (Guze and Robins 1970; Barraclough et al. 1974; Dalton et al. 2003; Mays 2004). Evaluation of the risk for suicide is important in any patient with major depression, especially when there is a comorbid substance abuse problem (Raue et al. 2006). At least 90% of patients who commit suicide have a psychiatric disorder (predominately depression), and more than 80% are untreated at the time of death (Lonnqvist et al. 1995; Henriksson et al. 2001; Mann et al. 2005). Suicidal ideations are present in 1–10% of primary care patients (Schulberg et al. 2005), with rates up to 54% in primary care patients suffering from depression (Wells et al. 1999). Suicide is a tragedy in terms of loss of life and is estimated to cost approximately $11.8 billion in lost income (Goldsmith et al. 2002; Mann et al. 2005).

More than twice as many patients who commit suicide see a primary care physician instead of a psychiatrist (Luoma et al. 2002). About 33% of suicide decedents see a mental health professional prior to their death, whereas 75–83% see a primary care physician within a year of their death (Luoma et al. 2002). Approximately 45–66% of patients who commit suicide have had contact with a primary care physician within 1 month of killing themselves; 10–40% see their primary care physician in the week before committing suicide (Robins et al. 1959; Blumenthal 1988; Pirkis and Burgess 1998; Luoma et al. 2002; Gaynes et al. 2004; Mann et al. 2005; Nutting et al. 2005). Thus, primary care physicians have a critical role in detecting patients with depression who are at a high risk for suicide and for whom effective interventions are readily available (Nutting et al. 2005). The failure to recognize the risk of suicide has been called a crisis because of the severity of the negative consequences, the prevalence of mood disorders, and patients' responsiveness to appropriate treatment (Fawcett 2004). Encouraging primary care physicians attention to this issue are the data showing that suicide is a common cause for legal action against the treating physician (Goodwin 1989).

Mania and/or hypomania, which define the diagnoses of cyclothymia, bipolar disorder type II, and bipolar disorder type I, are also underrecognized, misdiagnosed, and inadequately treated. Academic psychiatry may have some responsibility for more effective education of their medical students so that, as future nonpsychiatrists, they will better recognize depression, other mood disorders, and a risk for suicide among their patients.

18.3 The Responsibility of Academic Psychiatry for Improving the Recognition of Mood Disorders in Nonpsychiatric Clinical Settings

In the interest of mood-disordered patients who present to nonpsychiatric clinics, the sources of the failure to recognize must be identified and the changes necessary to reverse them must be established. Academic psychiatry certainly shares responsibility for making these changes because the traditional curriculum does not appear to resonate with the 90–95% of medical students who choose nonpsychiatric residencies. This, and the finding that 80% of patients with psychiatric disorders first present to nonpsychiatric physicians, is important when trying to understand the causes of the failure to recognize mood disorders and suicidal ideations, and the curriculum changes needed to address these problems (Prestidge and Lake 1987).

Students' limited exposure to psychiatry requires curriculum restriction to priority disorders to meet the needs of future nonpsychiatrists who will first see the vast majority of patients with mood disorders. Although mania, depression, and suicide are addressed in every psychiatry student clerkship, current levels of under-recognition in primary care lead to the assumption that psychiatry's emphasis on depression, suicidal ideation, and other mood disorders is inadequate, ineffective, and inefficient.

The previous discussion suggests that academic psychiatry must consider changing to a curriculum more focused on preparing future physicians for nonpsychiatric practices by making sure medical students thoroughly understand the most critical psychiatric disorders typically underrecognized in time-pressured, nonpsychiatric clinics. This means intense focus on the most critical psychiatric disorders; the broad spectrum of psychiatric disorders and a more thorough diagnostic interview can be addressed in residency training. Suggestions have been made as to some curriculum changes that could improve the poor recognition and treatment statistics for mood-disordered patients (Lake 2008d).

18.4 Simplify and Consolidate the Functional Psychoses for DSM-5 and/or DSM-6

The lessons from multiple sclerosis and syphilis establish a basic tenet in medicine (i.e., Ockham's razor: when one disease can explain a variety of symptoms, there is likely only one disease, not several.). The wide spectrum of severity and course of manic-depressive insanity prevented continued recognition of only a single disease to account for the whole spectrum of severe mental illness past the mid-nineteenth century when schizophrenia was introduced as separate from bipolar disorder, taking the most psychotic and chronic cases previously diagnosed with manic-depressive insanity. More recently, patients diagnosed with schizophrenia or schizoaffective disorder are again recognized to suffer from a severe, psychotic mood disorder and not different disorders (Kendell and Gourlay 1970b; Pope and Lipinski 1978; Post 1992).

As previously reported, the degree and breadth of commonality among the three psychotic psychiatric disorders reviewed herein are provocative and appear to justify this next step in the changing concept about choosing a diagnosis for functionally psychotic patients. The hypothesis that a mood disorder accounts for all three psychotic disorders eliminates many of the inconsistencies in comparative research results when differences are recognized to occur between psychotic and nonpsychotic mood disorders. Recognizing again that mood disorders can include psychosis and chronicity makes schizophrenia and schizoaffective disorder redundant and allows a consolidation of diagnoses that meets the criteria of Ockham's razor and the teachings of J. Axelrod (1976, personal communication) to simplify concepts.

Table 18.1 Suggested changes for the DSM-5 and/or the DSM-6

Traditional	Proposed
• Schizophrenia, nonchronic/chronic, catatonic, paranoid, undifferentiated or disorganized type	• BP I, manic, depressed or mixed, severe, **without/with mood cong/incong**[a] psychotic features, **non-chronic**/chronic; catatonic, **paranoid, undifferentiated or disorganized type**
• SA D/O, mainly schizophrenia, nonchronic/chronic	• BP II, depressed, severe, **without/with** mood cong/incong psychotic features, **nonchronic**/chronic
• SA D/O, BP/mainly affective, depressed with cong/incong psychotic features, nonchronic/chronic	• MDD, recurrent, severe, **without/with** mood cong/incong psychotic features, **nonchronic**/chronic
• SA D/O, BP/mainly affective, manic with cong/incong psychotic features, nonchronic/ chronic	• MDD, single episode, severe, **without/with mood cong/incong** psychotic features, **nonchronic**/chronic
• BP I, manic, depressed or mixed, severe, without/with mood cong/incong psychotic features, nonchronic/chronic	• BP II, hypomanic, **nonchronic**/chronic
• BP II, depressed, severe, without/with mood cong/ incong psychotic features, nonchronic/chronic	• Cyclothymia
• MDD, recurrent, severe, without/with mood cong/incong psychotic features, nonchronic/chronic	• Dysthymia
• MDD, single episode, severe, without/with mood cong/incong psychotic features, nonchronic/chronic	• Euthymia
• BP II, hypomanic, nonchronic/chronic	
• Cyclothymia	

(Severity ↑)

Abbreviations: *SA D/O* schizoaffective disorder, *BP* bipolar disorder, *MDD* major depressive disorder, *Cong/incong* congruent/incongruent
[a] Proposed changes in bold font

This chapter proposes a consolidation of diagnoses for the DSM-5 or the DSM-6 with a simplified hierarchy of diseases for psychotic patients that uses only mood disorders rather than using all three of the traditional psychotic disorder diagnoses. (Table 18.1). Bipolar-I, bipolar-II, depressed and major depressive disorders, severe with mood incongruent psychotic features, chronic, and with or without treatment resistance replace the various schizophrenia and schizoaffective disorder diagnoses. Expansion of the "specifiers" for mood disorders may be prognostically useful (Table 18.2). Mood incongruent versus mood congruent psychoses, chronic versus nonchronic, and "with" versus "without treatment resistance" seem to predict more severe prognoses (Lake and Hurwitz 2006a, b). Congruency is already included in the DSM-IV-TR but is not assigned a fifth digit code. Assigning ".x4" as "severe with mood congruent psychotic features," ".x5" as "severe with mood incongruent psychotic features" and increasing the fifth digit by one for "in partial remission" to .x6 and "in full" to .x7 would emphasize congruency to accommodate the transition from schizophrenia and schizoaffective disorder to severe mood disorders. "Nonchronic" might be a productive addition to "chronic," which is already present

18.5 Potential Judicial Sources for Change to Psychiatric Diagnostics

Table 18.2 Proposed additions to the DSM specifiers for mood disorders

Severity—mild (.x1); moderate (.x2); severe, without psychotic features (.x3); severe **with mood congruent (.x4)/incongruent psychotic features (.x5)**[a]; partial (.x6); full remission (.x7)

Course—**nonchronic/chronic** (symptoms >2 years); seasonal affective disorder; rapid cycling; postpartum onset, with/without full interepisode recovery

Features—catatonic; **paranoid/grandiose**; **disorganized**; **undifferentiated**; melancholic; atypical

[a] Proposed additions (shown in bold font)

in the DSM-IV-TR with the goal of adding focus to "course." Catatonia has been given as a potential "feature" for mood disorders for more than 10 years. If desired for further historical continuity, the other conventional subtypes of schizophrenia, more likely accounted for by psychotic mood disorders, might be added to the "features" subsection of "specifiers" for additional descriptors for very severe psychotic mood disorders when disorganization, paranoia/grandiosity, or none of these (undifferentiated) predominate diagnoses (Table 18.2). These suggestions now seem unlikely since the DSM-5 apparently eliminates the subtypes of schizophrenia but not schizophrenia or schizoaffective disorder (Bruijnzeel and Tandon 2011).

18.5 Potential Judicial Sources for Change to Psychiatric Diagnostics

The judicial system can have substantial impact upon psychiatric diagnoses. For example, in the early 1990s some psychotherapists began to "uncover" repressed memories of childhood sexual abuse that allegedly occurred one or more decades earlier. Patients were usually adult females, and their alleged abusers were often fathers or uncles. Several of the alleged abusers were charged, tried, and sent to prison. Families were wrecked and "memory recovery" increased in popularity among therapists. Memory research revealed that "memories" can be influenced during therapy, and memory terminology expanded to include the recovery of "false memories." There was not a question that memories of actual childhood sexual abuse could be repressed, but the persistence of some therapists to "uncover" such memories led to many unfounded cases. The identification of memories of repressed childhood sexual abuse stopped abruptly when accused fathers and uncles sued and won cases against the "recovered memory" therapists.

The diagnosis of schizophrenia may be similarly impacted by successful pursuit of malpractice claims against psychiatrists who misdiagnose schizophrenia in patients who actually suffer from documentable psychotic mood disorders. The size of a potential class action is considerable given an estimate of two million patients with the diagnosis of schizophrenia. Damages could be substantial due to years to decades of treatment with antipsychotic/antischizophrenia medications alone with their attendant long-term side effects as well as the absence of appropriate mood stabilization medications that would be argued to have improved functionality if they had been prescribed.

18.6 Conclusions

Although two participants in the DSM-5 planning meeting titled "deconstructing psychosis" in February 2006 stated either that the concept of schizophrenia should be abandoned or could not be distinguished from bipolar disorder (First 2006), schizophrenia continues to be the most recognized mental illness in the world and is scheduled for continuation in the DSM-5. Although the massive volume of data on "schizophrenia" inhibit doubt of its credibility, all research on schizophrenia has been questioned based on the overlap of diagnostic symptoms with psychotic bipolar disorders (Pope and Lipinski 1978). This massive volume of literature is not a sound scientific basis for the continuing recognition of schizophrenia. The current data support the suggestion of eliminating not only the subtypes of schizophrenia (paranoid, disorganized, catatonic, and undifferentiated) but eliminating schizophrenia and schizoaffective disorder as well from the DSM-6, if not the DSM-5 diagnoses (Table 18.1). Substitution of "psychosis" for "schizophrenia" is warranted. The continuum, dimensional, or spectrum approach to severity of symptoms and chronicity of course in the functional psychoses is appropriate, but the entire spectrum can be accounted for by the mood disorders only. Schizophrenia and schizoaffective disorder are redundant with psychotic mood disorders.

Any change must originate from academic psychiatry that has been deeply invested in schizophrenia. Impetus for change may result from two arenas: (1) basic science confirming even more overlap and similarities between patients diagnosed with schizophrenia versus a psychotic mood disorder and/or (2) a successful law suit against a psychiatrist who misdiagnosed schizophrenia in a patient suffering with a psychotic mood disorder. The patient could have suicided; developed tardive dyskinesia, obesity, and diabetes; and/or died during a neuroleptic malignant syndrome (Chap. 15).

The failure to recognize mood disorders and suicidal tendencies has persisted for more than four decades, with substantial ill effects for patients such as death by suicide, and the resulting impact upon their primary care physicians (Zung et al. 1983; Prestidge and Lake 1987). Blame has fallen on the educational system in psychiatry (Davis 2002) because suicide prevention begins with recognition and adequate treatment of depression. Under the traditional curriculum in academic departments of psychiatry, most graduating medical students who do not enter psychiatry do not adequately learn and retain information about mood disorders, which is critical for their future patients with depression and those at risk for suicide. Academic psychiatry faces the difficult choice to either maintain the traditional curriculum that likely will not improve recognition, or to eliminate some topics heretofore considered cornerstones of psychiatry such as schizophrenia, schizoaffective disorder, and the 50-min diagnostic interview, to dedicate more time to teaching disorders of mood and suicide prevention. A curriculum change to emphasize greater understanding of mood disorders and suicidal ideation should increase future primary care physician retention, which will, in turn, promote recognition and improved treatment or referral and will thus benefit primary care physicians, their patients, and psychiatry as well.

References

Abrams, R., & Taylor, M. A. (1976a). Mania and schizoaffective disorder, manic type: A comparison. *American Journal of Psychiatry, 133*, 1445–1447.

Abrams, R., & Taylor, M. A. (1976b). Catatonia, a prospective clinical study. *Archives of General Psychiatry, 33*, 579–581.

Abrams, R., Taylor, M. A., & Gaztanaga, P. (1974). Manic-depressive illness and paranoid schizophrenia. *Archives of General Psychiatry, 31*, 640–642.

Adachi, N., Ito, M., Kanemoto, K., Akanuma, N., Okazak,i M., Ishida, S., Sekimoto, M., Kato, M., Kawasaki, J., Tadokoro, Y., Oshima, T., Onuma, T. (2007). Duration of postictal psychotic episodes. *Epilepsia, 48*, 1531–1537.

Addington, J., & Addington, D. (1997). Attentional vulnerability indicators in schizophrenia and bipolar disorder. *Schizophrenia Research, 23*, 197–204.

Aires, D. J., & Hurwitz, N. G. (2010). Schizophrenia and schizoaffective are psychotic mood disorders. *Psychiatric Annals, 40*, 98–102.

Albin, S., & Ramirez, A. (2003, July 29). Metro Briefing/New York: Queens: Mentally ill man sentenced to prison. *The New York Times*.

Altshuler, L. L., Bartzokis, G., Grieder, T., Curran, J., Jimenez, T., Leight, K., Wilkins, J., Gerner, R., & Mintz, J. (2000). An MRI study of temporal lobe structures in men with bipolar disorder or schizophrenia. *Biological Psychiatry, 15*, 147–162.

al-Mousawi, A. H., Evans, N., Ebmeier, K. P., Roeda, D., Chaloner, F., Ashcroft, G. W. (1996). Limbic dysfunction in schizophrenia and mania. A study using 18F-labelled fluorodeoxyglucose and positron emission tomography. *British Journal of Psychiatry. 169*, 509–516.

Amandolare, S. (2009, May 6). Gindorf case could ease stigma of postpartum depression and psychosis. www.findingdulcinea.com.

American Psychiatric Association. (1952). *Diagnostic and statistical manual of mental disorders* (1st ed.). Washington, DC: American Psychiatric Press, Inc.

American Psychiatric Association. (1968). *Diagnostic and statistical manual of mental disorders* (2nd ed.). Washington, DC: American Psychiatric Press, Inc.

American Psychiatric Association. (1980). *Diagnostic and statistical manual of mental disorders* (3rd ed.). Washington, DC: American Psychiatric Press, Inc.

American Psychiatric Association. (1987). *Diagnostic and statistical manual of mental disorders* (3rd ed.-R.). Washington, DC: American Psychiatric Press, Inc.

American Psychiatric Association. (1994). *Diagnostic and statistical manual of mental disorders* (4th ed.). Washington, DC: American Psychiatric Press, Inc.

American Psychiatric Association. (2000). *Diagnostic and statistical manual of mental disorders* (4th ed.-TR.). Washington, DC: American Psychiatric Press, Inc.

American Psychiatric Association. *Diagnostic and statistical manual of mental disorders* (5th ed.). Washington, DC: American Psychiatric Press, Inc. Proposed release date 2013. http://www.dsm5.org.
Anderson, J. (2002, February 26). *Witness testifies Yates was insane.* Associated Press. www.beliefnet.com/news/2002/03/Witness-Testifies-Yates-Was-Insane.aspx.
Angst, J. (2002). Historical aspects of the dichotomy between manic-depressive disorders and schizophrenia. *Schizophrenia Research, 57,* 5–13.
Angst, J., Weis, P., Grof, P., Baastrup, P. C., & Shou, M. (1970). Lithium prophylaxis in recurrent affective disorders. *The British Journal of Psychiatry, 116,* 604–614.
Angst, J., Felder, W., & Lohmeyer, B. (1979). Schizoaffective disorders. Results of a genetic investigation: I. *Journal of Affective Disorders, 1,* 139–153.
Angst, J., Scharfetter, C., & Stassen, H. H. (1983). Classification of schizoaffective patients by multidimensional scaling and cluster analysis. *Psychiatry Clinics, 16,* 254–264.
Anonymous. (2006). *Children murdered by their christian parents memorial page.* http://myth-one.com/memorial.htm.
Applegate, S. (2009, February 8). Another murder in North Andover. *North Andover Citizen.*
Arbabzadeh-Bouchez, S., Tylee, A., & Lepine, J. P. (2002). A European perspective on depression on the community: The DEPRESS study. *CNS Spectrums, 7,* 120–126.
Artaloytia, J. F., Arango, C., Lahti, A., Sanz, J., Pascual, A., Cubero, P., Prieto, D., & Palomo, T. (2006). Negative signs and symptoms secondary to antipsychotics: A double-blind, randomized trial of a single dose of placebo, haloperidol, and risperidone in healthy volunteers. *The American Journal of Psychiatry, 163,* 488–493.
Arzy, S., Seeck, M., Ortigue, S., Spinelli, L., & Blanke, O. (2006). Induction of an illusory shadow person. *Nature, 443,* 287.
Asherson, P., Mant, R., Williams, N., Cardno, A., Jones, L., Murphy, K., Collier, D. A., Nanko, S., Craddock, N., Morris, S., Muir, W., Blackwood, B., McGuffin, P., & Owen, M. J. (1998). A study of chromosome 4p markers and dopamine D5 receptor gene in schizophrenia and bipolar disorder. *Molecular Psychiatry, 3,* 310–320.
Astrup, C., Fossum, A., & Holmboe, R. (1959). A follow-up study of 270 patients with acute affective psychoses. *Acta Psychiatrica et Neurologica Scandinavica, 34*(Suppl 135), 1–65.
Atre-Vaidya, N., & Taylor, M. A. (1989). Effectiveness of lithium in schizophrenia: Do we really have an answer? *The Journal of Clinical Psychiatry, 50,* 170–173.
Averill, P. M., Reas, D. L., Shack, A., Shah, N. N., Cowan, K., Krajewski, K., Kopecky, C., & Guynn, R. W. (2004). Is schizoaffective disorder a stable diagnostic category? A retrospective examination. *Psychiatric Quarterly, 75,* 215–227.
Azorin, J. M., Kaladjian, A., & Fakra, E. (2005). Current issues on schizoaffective disorder. *Encephale, 31,* 359–365.
Baastrup, P. C. (1964). The use of lithium in manic-depressive psychosis. *Comprehensive Psychiatry, 5,* 396–408.
Badner, J. A., & Gershon, E. S. (2002). Meta-analysis of whole-genome linkage scans of bipolar disorder and schizophrenia. *Molecular Psychiatry, 7,* 405–411.
Bailer, U., Leisch, F., Meszaros, K., Lenzinger, E., Willinger, U., Strobl, R., Heiden, A., Gebhardt, C., Doge, E., Fuchs, K., Sieghart, W., Kasper, S., Hornik, K., Aschauer, H. N. (2002). Genome scan for susceptibility loci for schizophrenia and bipolar disorder. *Biological Psychiatry, 52,* 40–52.
Barnes, J. E. (2000, March 24). Subway killer to be treated in cell or in hospital, or both. *The New York Times.*
Barnes, T. R., & McPhillips, M. A. (1995). How to distinguish between the neuroleptic-induced deficit syndrome, depression and disease-related negative symptoms in schizophrenia. *International Clinical Psychopharmacology, 10,* 115–121.
Barraclough, B., Bunch, J., Nelson, B., & Sainsbury, P. (1974). A hundred cases of suicide: Clinical aspects. *The British Journal of Psychiatry, 25,* 355–373.
Bearden, C. E., Hoffman, K. M., Cannon, T. D. (2001). The neuropsychology and neuroanatomy of bipolar affective disorder: a critical review. *Bipolar Disorder, 3,* 106–150.
Beck, A. T. (1972). *Depression: Causes and treatment.* Philadelphia: University of Pennsylvania Press.

Beck, AT. (1967). *Depression: clinical, experimental and theoretical aspects.* New York: Hoeber Press.

Becker, J., Johnson, K., & Kovaleski, S. F. (2011, January 11). Police say they visited Tucson suspect's home even before rampage. *The New York Times.*

Becker, J., Kovaleski, S. F., Lou, M., & Barry, D. (2011, January 16). Jigsaw picture of an accused killer. *The New York Times.*

Belmaker, R. H. (2004). Bipolar disorder. *The New England Journal of Medicine, 351,* 476–486.

Benabarre, A., Vieta, E., Colom, F., Martinez-Aran, A., Reinares, M., & Gasto, C. (2001). Bipolar disorder, schizoaffective disorder and schizophrenia: Epidemiologic, clinical and prognostic differences. *European Psychiatry, 16,* 167–172.

Bentall, R. P. (1990). The illusion of reality: A review and integration of psychological research on hallucinations. *Psychological Bulletin, 107,* 82–95.

Bentall, R. (2004, March 20–23). Roll over Kraepelin, *Mental Health Today.*

Bentall, R. (2006). Madness explained: Why we must reject the Kraepelinian paradigm and replace it with a 'complaint-oriented' approach to understanding mental illness. *Medical Hypotheses, 66,* 220–233.

Bentall, R. P., & Fernyhough, C. (2008). Social predictors of psychotic experiences: Specificity and psychological mechanisms. *Schizophrenia Bulletin, 34,* 1012–1020.

Bentall, R. P., Jackson, H. F., & Pilgrim, D. (1988). Abandoning the concept of 'schizophrenia': Some implications of validity arguments for psychological research into psychotic phenomena. *The British Journal of Clinical Psychology, 27,* 303–324.

Berenson, A. (2008, February 24). Daring to think differently about schizophrenia. *The New York Times.*

Berger, J., & Gross, J. (1998, June 19). From mental illness to Yale to murder charge. *The New York Times.*

Bernstein, N. (2002, August 9). Mayro wants investigation into homeless boy's death. *The New York Times.*

Berrettini, W. H. (2000). Are schizophrenic and bipolar disorders related? A review of family and molecular studies. *Biological Psychiatry, 48,* 531–558.

Berrettini, W. H. (2001). Molecular linkage studies of bipolar disorders. *Bipolar Disorders, 3,* 276–283.

Berrettini, W. (2003a). Evidence for shared susceptibility in bipolar disorder and schizophrenia. *American Journal of Medical Genetics, 123,* 59–64.

Berrettini, W. (2003b). Bipolar disorder and schizophrenia: Not so distant relatives? *World Psychiatry, 2,* 68–72.

Berrettini, W. (2004). Bipolar disorder and schizophrenia. *Neuromolecular Medicine, 5,* 109–117.

Berrettini, W. H. (2005). Genetic bases for endophenotypes in psychiatric disorders. *Diologues in Clinical Neurosciences, 7,* 95–101.

Berrios, G. E., & Beer, D. (1994). The notion of unitary psychosis: A conceptual history. *History of Psychiatry, 5,* 13–36.

Bertelsen, A., Harvald, B., & Hauge, M. (1977). A Danish twin study of manic-depressive illness. *The British Journal of Psychiatry, 130,* 330–351.

Bilder, R. M., Wu, H., Bogerts, B., Ashtari, M., Robinson, D., Woerner, M., Lieverman, J. A., Degreef, G. (1999). Cerebral volume asymmetries in schizophrenia and mood disorders: a quantitative magnetic resonance imaging study. *International Journal of Psychophysiology, 34,* 197–205.

Blackwood, D. H., Fordyce, A., Walker, M. T., St Clair, D. M., Porteous, D. J., & Muir, W. J. (2001). Schizophrenia and affective disorders – Cosegregation with a translocation of chromosome 1q42 that directly disrupts brain-expressed genes: Clinical and P300 findings in a family. *American Journal of Human Genetics, 69,* 428–433.

Bleuler, E. (1911/1950). *Dementia praecox or the group of schizophrenias.* New York: International Universities Press.

Blumenthal, S. J. (1988). Suicide: A guide to risk factors, assessment and treatment of suicidal patients. *Medical Clinics of North America, 72,* 937–971.

Bonner, C. A., & Kent, G. H. (1936). Overlapping symptoms in catatonic excitement and manic excitement. *The American Journal of Psychiatry, 92*, 1311–1322.

Borkowska, A., & Rybakowski, J. K. (2001). Neuropsychological frontal lobe tests indicate that bipolar depressed patients are more impaired than unipolar. *Bipolar Disorder, 3*, 88–94.

Bottas, A., Cooke, R. G., & Richter, M. A. (2005). Comorbidity and pathophysiology of obsessive-compulsive disorder in schizophrenia: Is there evidence for a schizo-obsessive subtype of schizophrenia? *Journal of Psychiatry & Neuroscience, 30*, 187–193.

Bourget, D., Grace, J., & Whitehurst, L. (2007). A review of maternal and paternal filicide. *Journal of American Academic Psychiatry Law, 35*, 74–82.

Boyer, W. F., Bakalar, N. H., & Lake, C. R. (1987). Anticholinergic prophylaxis of acute haloperidol-induced acute dystonic reactions. *Journal of Clinical Psychopharmacology, 7*, 164–166.

Braxton, A. (2011, March 7). *Murder/Suicide shocks seventh ward neighborhood*. Fox 8 TV, New Orleans.

Brockington, I. F. (1992). Schizophrenia: Yesterday's concept. *European Psychiatry, 7*, 203–207.

Brockington, I. F., & Leff, J. P. (1979). Schizoaffective psychosis: Definition and incidence. *Psychological Medicine, 9*, 91–99.

Brockington, I. F., Kendell, R. E., Wainwright, S., Hillier, V. F., & Walker, J. (1979). The distinction between the affective psychoses and schizophrenia. *The British Journal of Psychiatry, 135*, 243–248.

Brockington, I. F., Wainwright, S., & Kendell, R. E. (1980a). Manic patients with schizophrenic or paranoid symptoms. *Psychological Medicine, 10*, 73–83.

Brockington, I. F., Kendell, R. E., & Wainwright, S. (1980b). Depressed patients with schizophrenic or paranoid symptoms. *Psychological Medicine, 10*, 665–675.

Brown, S., Barraclough, B., & Inskip, H. (2000). Causes of the excess mortality of schizophrenia. *British Journal of Psychiatry, 177*, 212–217.

Bruijnzeel, D., & Tandon, R. (2011). The concept of schizophrenia: From the 1850s to the DSM-5. *Psychiatric Annals, 41*, 289–298.

Byerly, M., Goodman, W., Acholonu, W., Bungo, R., & Rush, A. J. (2005). Obsessive-compulsive symptoms in schizophrenia: Frequency and clinical features. *Schizophrenia Research, 76*, 309–316.

Cade, J. F. J. (1949). Lithium salts in the treatment of psychotic excitement. *Medical Journal of Australia, 36*, 349–352.

Calabrese, J. R., Shelton, M. D., Bowden, C. L., Rapport, D. J., Suppes, T., Shirley, E. R., Kimmel, S. E., & Caban, S. J. (2001). Bipolar rapid cycling: Focus on depression as its hallmark. *The Journal of Clinical Psychiatry, 62*(Suppl 14), 34–41.

Cardno, A. G., Marshall, E. J., Coid, B., Macdonald, A. M., Ribchester, T. R., Davies, N. J., Venturi, P., Jones, L. A., Lewis, S. W., Sham, P. C., Gottesman, I. I., Farmer, A. E., McGuffin, P., Reveley, A. M., & Murray, R. M. (1999). Heritability estimates for psychotic disorders: The Maudsley twin psychosis series. *Archives of General Psychiatry, 56*, 162–168.

Cardno, A. G., Rysdijk, F. V., Sham, P. C., Murray, R. M., & McGuffin, P. (2002). A twin study of genetic relationships between psychotic symptoms. *The American Journal of Psychiatry, 159*, 539–545.

Carey, B. (2011, June 31). Expert on mental illness reveals her own fight. *The New York Times*.

Carlson, G. A., & Goodwin, F. K. (1973). The stages of mania. A longitudinal analysis of the manic episode. *Archives of General Psychiatry, 28*, 221–228.

Carpenter, W. T., Strauss, J. S., & Muleh, S. (1973). Are there pathognomonic symptoms in schizophrenia? An empiric investigation of Schneider's first-rank symptoms. *Archives of General Psychiatry, 28*, 847–852.

Carpenter, W., McGlashan, T., & Strauss, J. (1977). The treatment of acute schizophrenia without drugs: An investigation of some current assumptions. *The American Journal of Psychiatry, 134*, 14–20.

Carroll, B. T., Thomas, C., Jayanti, K., Hawkins, J. M., & Burbage, C. (2005). Treating persistent catatonia when benzodiazepines fail. *Current Psychiatry, 4*, 56–64.

Casey, D. E. (1988). Affective disorders and tardive dyskinesia. *L'Encéphale, XIV*, 221–226.

Casey, D. E., Daniel, D. G., Wassef, A. A., Tracy, K. A., Wozniak, P., & Sommerville, K. W. (2003). Effect of divalproex combined with olanzapine or risperidone in patients with an acute exacerbation of schizophrenia. *Neuropsychopharmacology, 28*, 182–192.

Caton, C. L., Drake, R. E., Hasin, D. S., Dominquez, B., Shrout, P. E., Samet, S., Schanzer, B. (2005). Differences between early-phase primary psychotic disorders with concurrent substance use and substance-induced psychoses. *Archives of General Psychiatry, 62*, 137–145. (Published correction appears in Archives of General Psychiatry. 2005;62:493).

Chambers, J. S., & Perrone-Bizzozero, N. I. (2004). Altered myelination of the hippocampal formation in subjects with schizophrenia and bipolar disorder. *Neurochemistry Research, 29*, 2293–2302.

Chouinard, G., & Jones, B. (1980). Neuroleptic-induced supersensitivity psychosis: Clinical and pharmacologic characteristics. *The American Journal of Psychiatry, 137*, 16–20.

Chumakov, I., Blumenfeld, M., Guerassimenko, O., Cavarec, L., Palicio, M., Abderrahim, H., Bougeuelert, L., Barry, C., Tanaka, H., La Rosa, P., Puech, A., Tahri, N., Cohen-Akenine, A., Delahrosse, S., Lissarrague, S., Picord, F. P., Maurice, K., Essioux, L., Millasseau, P., Grel, P., Debaileul, V., Simon, A. M., Caterina, D., Dufaure, I., Molekzadeh, K., Belova, M., Luan, J. J., Bouillot, M., Sambucy, J. L., Primas, G., Saumier, M., Boubkiri, N., Martin-Saumier, S., Nasroune, M., Peixoto, H., Dekrye, A., Pinshot, V., Bastucci, M., Guillou, S., Chevillon, M., Sainz-Fuertes, R., Meguenni, S., Aurich-Costa, J., Chrif, D., Gimalac, A., van Duijn, C., Gauvreau, D., Ouelette, G., Fortier, I., Realson, J., Sherbatich, T., Riazanskaia, N., Rogaev, E., Raeymaekers, P., Aerssens, J., Konings, F., Luyten, W., Macciardi, F., Sham, P. C., Straub, R. E., Weinberger, D. R., Cohen, N., Dohen, D. (2002). Genetic and physiological data implicating the new human gene G72 and the gene for D-amino-acid oxidose in schizophrenia. *PNAS USA. 99*, 13675–13680.

Citrome, L., Levine, J., & Allingham, B. (2000). Changes in use of valproate and other mood stabilizers for patients with schizophrenia from 1994 to 1998. *Psychiatric Services, 51*, 634–638.

Cobb, S. (1943). *Borderlands of psychiatry*. Cambridge: Harvard University Press.

Coen, J., & Barnum, A. (2002, May 31). *Lemak gets life term for killing her 3 kids*. Chicagotribune.com.

Cohen, R. M., Semple, W. E., Gross, M., Nordahl, T. E., King, A. C., Pickar, D., Post, R. M. (1989). Evidence for common alterations in cerebral glucose metabolism in major affective disorders and schizophrenia. *Neuropsychopharmacology, 2*, 241–254.

Conrad, K. (1958). Die beginnende Schizophrenie (Stuttgart; Thieme, 1958) – from Berrios and Beer, 1994

Conwell, Y., & Thompson, C. (2008). Suicidal behaviors in elders. *Psychiatric Clinics of North America, 31*, 333–356.

Coombs, D. W., Miller, H. L., Alarcon, R., Herlihy, C., Lee, J. M., & Morrison, D. P. (1992). Presuicide attempt communications between parasuicides and consulted caregivers. *Suicide & Life-Threatening Behavior, 22*, 289–302.

Cooper, J. E., Kendell, R. E., Gurland, B. J., Sharpe. L., & Copeland, J. R. M. (1972). *Psychiatric diagnosis in New York and London* (Maudsley Monograph Series). Institute of Psychiatry London. London: Oxford University Press, *135*, 136–138.

Coryell, W., Lavori, P., Endicott, J., Keller, M., & VanEerdewegh, M. (1984). Outcome in schizoaffective, psychotic and nonpsychotic depression. Course during a six-to 24-month follow-up. *Archives of General Psychiatry, 41*, 787–791.

Coyle, J. T., Pine, D. S., Charney, D. S., Lewis, L., Nemeroff, C. B., Carlson, G. A., Joshi, P. T., Reiss, D., Todd, R. D., Hellander, M., Depression and Bipolar Support Alliance Consensus Development Panel. (2003). Depression and bipolar support alliance consensus statement on the unmet needs in diagnosis and treatment of mood disorders in children and adolescents. *Journal of American Academic Child Adolescent Psychiatry, 42*, 1494–1503.

Craddock, N. (2005). Genomewide linkage scan in schizoaffective disorder. *Archives of General Psychiatry, 62*, 1081–1088.

Craddock, N., & Owen, M. J. (2005). The beginning of the end for the Kraepelinian dichotomy. *The British Journal of Psychiatry, 184*, 384–386.

Craddock, N., & Owen, M. J. (2010a). Molecular genetics and the Kraepelinian dichotomy: One disorder, two disorders, or do we need to start thinking afresh? *Psychiatric Annals, 40*, 88–91.

Craddock, N., & Owen, M. J. (2010b). The Kraepelinian dichotomy-going, going ... but still not gone. *The British Journal of Psychiatry, 196*, 92–95.

Craddock, N., O'Donovan, M. C., & Owen, M. (2005). The genetics of schizophrenia and bipolar disorder dissecting psychosis. *Journal of Medical Genetics, 42*, 193–204.

Craddock, N., O'Donovan, M., & Owen, M. (2006). Genes for schizophrenia and bipolar disorder? Implications for psychiatric nosology. *Schizophrenia Bulletin, 32*, 9–16.

Crichton, P. (1996). First-rank symptoms or rand-and-file symptoms? *The British Journal of Psychiatry, 169*, 537–540.

Crow, T. J. (1986). The continuum of psychosis and its implication for the structure of the gene. *The British Journal of Psychiatry, 149*, 419–429.

Crow, T. J. (1990a). The continuum of psychoses and its genetic origins. The sixty-fifth Maudsley lecture. *The British Journal of Psychiatry, 156*, 788–797.

Crow, T. J. (1990b). Nature of the genetic contribution to psychotic illness: A continuum viewpoint. *Acta Psychiatrica Scandinavica, 81*, 401–408.

Crow, T. J. (2007). How and why genetic linkage has not solved the problem of psychosis: Review and hypothesis. *The American Journal of Psychiatry, 164*, 13–22.

Crow, T. J. (2010). The continuum of psychosis – 1986–2010. *Psychiatric Annals, 40*, 115–119.

Culpepper, L. (2002). Depression and chronic medical illness: Diabetes as a model. *Psychiatric Annals, 32*, 528–534.

Dalton, E. J., Cate-Carter, T. D., Mundo, E., Parikh, S. V., & Kennedy, J. L. (2003). Suicide risk in bipolar patients: The role of co-morbid substance use disorder. *Bipolar Disorder, 5*, 58–61.

Dasari, M., Friedman, L., Jesberger, J., Stuve, T. A., Findling, R. L., Swales, T. P., Schulz, S. C. (1999). A magnetic resonance imaging study of thalamic area in adolescent patients with either schizophrenia or bipolar disorder as compared to healthy controls. *Psychiatry Research, 91*, 155–162.

David, A. S. (1993). Spatial and selective attention in the cerebral hemispheres in depression, mania and schizophrenia. *Brain and Cognition, 23*, 166–180.

Davis, G. C. (2002). The Hodges psychiatry OSCE guide and emerging trends in assessment. *Academic Psychiatry, 26*, 184–186.

Demily, C., Jacquet, P., & Marie-Cardine, M. (2009). How to differentiate schizophrenia from bipolar disorder using cognitive assessment? *Encephale, 35*, 139–145.

Der, G., Gupta, S., & Murray, R. M. (1990). Is schizophrenia disappearing? *The Lancet, 335*, 513–516.

Detera-Wadleigh, S. D., Badner, J. A., Berrettini, W. H., Yoshikawa, T., Goldin, L. R., Turner, G., Rollins, D. Y., Moses, T., Sanders, A. R., Karkera, J. D., Esterling, L. F., Zeng, J., Ferraro, T. N., Guroff, J. J., Kazuba, D., Maxwell, M. E., Nurnberger, J. I., Jr., & Gershon, E. S. (1999). A high-density genome scan detects evidence for a bipolar disorder susceptibility locus on 13q32 and other potential loci on 1q32 and 18p11.2. *Proceedings of the National Academy of Sciences of the United States of America, 96*, 5604–5609.

Devinsky, O. (2008). Postictal psychosis: Common, dangerous, and treatable. *Epilepsy Currents, 8*, 31–34.

Devon, R. S., Anderson, S., Teague, P. W., Burgess, P., Kipari, T. M., Semple, C. A., Millar, J. D., Muir, W. J., Murray, V., Pelasi, A. J., Blackwood, D. H., Porteous, D. J. (2002). Identification of polymorphisms within disrupted in schizophrenia 1 and disrupted in schizophrenia 2, and an investigation of their association with schizophrenia and bipolar disorder. *Psychiatric Genetics, 11*, 71–78.

Dieperink, M. E., & Sands, J. R. (1996). Bipolar mania with psychotic features: Diagnosis and treatment. *Psychiatric Annals, 26*, 633–637.

Doran, A. R., Breier, A., & Roy, A. (1986). Differential diagnosis and diagnostic systems in schizophrenia. *Psychiatric Clinics of North America, 9*, 17–33.

Douglas, A. B. (2003). Narcolepsy: Differential diagnosis or etiology in some cases of bipolar disorder and schizophrenia? *CNS Spectrums, 8*, 120–126.

Downs, J. M., Akiskal, H. G., & Rosenthal, T. L. (1993). Presented at *the annual meeting of the American Psychiatric Association*, San Francisco. Abstract 146.

Driver, J. (2001). A selective review of selective attention research from the past century. *The British Journal of Psychiatry, 92*, 53–78.

Edwards, G. (1972). Diagnosis of schizophrenia: Anglo-American comparison. *The British Journal of Psychiatry, 120*, 385–390.

Ehrrson, H. H. (2007). The experimental induction of out-of-body experiences. *Science, 317*, 1048.

Eligon, J. (2008a, May 21). Suspect's delusions described to Judge. *The New York Times*.

Eligon, J. (2008b, October 15). Suspect in therapist death is to be institutionalized. *The New York Times*.

Evans, D. L. (2000). Bipolar disorder: Diagnostic challenges and treatment considerations. *The Journal of Clinical Psychiatry, 61*, 26–31.

Faraone, S. V., Tsuang, M. T., Gutierrez, J. M. (1987). Long-term outcome and family psychiatric illness in unipolar and bipolar disorders. *Psychopharmacological Bulletin, 23*, 465–467.

Fawcett, J. (2004). Is suicide preventable? *Psychiatric Annals, 34*, 338–339.

Fawcett, J. (2005). What do we know for sure about bipolar disorder? *The American Journal of Psychiatry, 162*, 1–2.

Fazel, S., Gulati, G., Linsell, L., Geddes, J. R., & Grann, M. (2009). Schizophrenia and violence: Systematic review and meta-analysis. *PLoS Medicine, 6*, 1–15.

Feighner, J. P., Robins, E., Guze, S. B., Woodruff, R. A., Jr., Winokur, G., & Munoz, R. (1972). Diagnostic criteria for use in psychiatric research. *Archives of General Psychiatry, 26*, 57–63.

Fink, M., & Taylor, M. A. (2006). Catatonia: Subtype or syndrome in DSM? *The American Journal of Psychiatry, 163*, 1875–1876.

First, M. B. (2006, February 16–17). Deconstructing psychosis. From the American Psychiatric Association DSM-5 Development, Fifth Diagnosis-Related Research Planning Session held under the *Conference series on the "Future of Psychiatric Diagnosis: Refining the Research Agenda"* (pp. 1–6). Arlington: APA Headquarters.

Fischer, B. A., & Carpenter, W. T. (2009). Will the Kraepelinian dichotomy survive DSM-V? *Neuropsychopharmacology, 34*, 2081–2087.

Fletcher, K. (2008, December 17). Schizophrenia drove Okie to murder, Psychiatrist says. *The Lincoln County News*.

Foderaro, L. W. (2000, May 12). Man who killed fiancée is sent to mental hospital. *The New York Times*.

Follette, W., & Cummings, N. A. (1967). Psychiatric services and medical utilization in a prepaid health plan setting. *Medical Care, 5*, 25–35.

Foussias, G., & Remington, G. (2010). Negative symptoms in schizophrenia: Avolition and Occam's razor. *Schizophrenia Bulletin, 36*, 359–369.

Fowler, R. C., McCabe, M. S., Cadoret, R. J., & Winokur, G. (1972). The validity of good prognosis schizophrenia. *Archives of General Psychiatry, 26*, 182–185.

Freudenreich, O. (2010). Differential diagnosis of psychotic symptoms: Medical "mimics". *Psychiatric Times, XXVII*, 56–61.

Freudenreich, O., Holt, D. J., Cather, C., & Goff, D. C. (2007). The evaluation and management of patients with first-episode schizophrenia: A selective, clinical review of diagnosis, treatment and prognosis. *Harvard Review of Psychiatry, 15*, 189–211.

Fried, J. P. (2002, May 26). Following up. *The New York Times*.

Funke, B., Malhotra, A. K., Finn, C. T., Plocik, A. M., Lake, S. L., Lencz, T., DeRosse, P., Kane, J. M., Kucherlapati, R. (2005). COMT genetic variation confers risk for psychotic and affective disorders: a case control study. *Behavioral and Brain Function, 1*, 19.

Gardner, A., Fahrenthold, D. A., & Fisher, M. (2011, January 13). Loughner's decent into a world of fantasy. *The Washington Post*.

Gaynes, B. N., West, S. L., Ford, C. A., Frame, P., Klein, J., & Lohr, K. N. (2004). Screening for suicide risk in adults: A summary of the evidence for the U.S. Preventive Services Task Force. *Annals of Internal Medicine, 140*, 822–835.

Gershon, S., & Yuwiler, A. (1960). Lithium ion: A specific psychopharmacological approach to the treatment of mania. *Journal of Neuropsychiatry, 1*, 229–241.

Gershon, E. S, DeLisi L. E., Hamovit, J., Nurnberger, Jr, J. I., Maxwell, M. E., Schreiber, J. (1988). A controlled family study of chronic psychoses. Schizophrenia and schizoaffective disorder. *Archives of General Psychiatry, 45,* 328–336.

Gershon, E. S., Hamovit, J., Guroff, J. J., Dibble, E., Leckman, J. F., Sceery, W., Targum, S. D., Nurnberger, J. I., Jr., Goldin, L. R., & Bunney, W. E., Jr. (1982). A family study of schizoaffective, bipolar I, bipolar II, unipolar and normal control probands. *Archives of General Psychiatry, 39,* 1157–1167.

Glahn, D. C., Bearden, C. E., Niendam, T. A., Escamilla, M. A. (2004). The feasibility of neuropsychological endophenotypes in the search of genes associated with bipolar affective disorder. *Bipolar Disorder, 6,* 171–182.

Glahn, D. C., Bearden, C. E., Barguil, M., Barrett, J., Reichenberg, A., Bowden, C. L., Soares, J. C., & Velligan, D. I. (2007). The neurocognitive signature of psychotic bipolar disorder. *Biological Psychiatry, 62,* 910–916.

Goes, F. S., Zandi, P. P., Miao, K., McMahon, F. J., Steel, J., Willour, V. L., MacKinnon, D. F., Mondimore, F. M., Schweizer, B., Nornberger, J. I., Rice, J. P., Scheftner, W., Coryell, W., Berrettini, W. H., Kelsoe, J. R., Byerley, W., Murphy, D. L., Gershon, E. S., Bipolar Disorder Phenome Group, DePalo, J. R., McInnis, M. G., & Potash, J. B. (2007). Mood-incongruent psychotic features in bipolar disorder: Familial aggregation and suggestive linkage to 2p11-q14 and 13q21-33. *The American Journal of Psychiatry, 164,* 236–247.

Goldberg, I. D., Drantz, G., & Locke, Z. (1970). Effect of a short-term outpatient psychiatric therapy befit on the utilization of medical services in a prepaid group practice medical program. *Medical Care, 8,* 419–426.

Goldman, L. S., Nielson, N. H., & Champion, H. C. (2002). Awareness, diagnosis, and treatment of depression. *Journal of General Internal Medicine, 14,* 569–580.

Goldsmith, S. K., Pellmar, T. C., Kleinman, A. M., & Bunney, W. E. (2002). *Reducing suicide: A national imperative.* Washington, DC: National Academies Press.

Gonzalez-Pinto, A., van Os, J., Perez de Heredia, J. L., Mosquera, F., Aldama, A., Lalaguna, B., Gutierrez, M., & Mico, J. A. (2003). Age-dependence of Schneiderian psychotic symptoms in bipolar patients. *Schizophrenia Research, 61,* 157–162.

Goodman, W. (1999, December 16). Television review: A new role for the family in cases of Schizophrenia. *The New York Times.*

Goodwin, F. K. (1989). The biology of recurrence: New directions for the pharmacologic bridge. *The Journal of Clinical Psychiatry, 50,* 40–44.

Goodwin, F. K., & Ghaemi, S. N. (2010). The conundrum of schizoaffective disorder: A review of the literature. *Psychiatric Annals, 40,* 168–171.

Goodwin, F. K., & Jamison, K. R. (1990). *Manic-depressive illness.* New York: Oxford University Press.

Goodwin, F. K., & Jamison, K. R. (2007). *Manic-depressive illness.* New York: Oxford University Press.

Goodwin, F. K., Fireman, B., Simon, G. E., Hunkeler, E. M., Lee, J., & Revicki, D. (2003). Suicide risk in bipolar disorder during treatment with lithium and divalproex. *The Journal of the American Medical Association, 290,* 1467–1473.

Green, E., Elvidge, G., Jacobsen, N., Glaser, B., Jones, I., O'Donovan, M. C., Kirov, G., Owen, M. J., & Craddock, N. (2005). Localization of bipolar susceptibility locus by molecular genetic analysis of the chromosome 12q23-q24 region in two pedigrees with bipolar disorder and Darier's disease. *The American Journal of Psychiatry, 162,* 35–42.

Greisinger, W. (1845). *Pathologic und Therapie der psychischen Krankheiten fur Arzte und Studierende* (1st ed.). Stuttgart: A Drabbe.

Grossman, L. S., Harrow, M., & Sands, J. R. (1986). Features associated with thought disorder in manic patients at 2-4-year follow-up. *The American Journal of Psychiatry, 143,* 306–311.

Guislain, J. (1833). *Traite Des Phrenopathies ou doctrine nouvelle des maladies mentales.* Brussels: Etablissement Encyclopedique.

Guze, S. B., & Robins, E. (1970). Suicide and primary affective disorder. *The British Journal of Psychiatry, 117,* 437–438.

Guze, S. B., Woodruff, R. A., & Clayton, P. J. (1975). The significance of psychotic affective disorders. *Archives of General Psychiatry, 32*, 1147–1150.

Hafner, H., Maurer, K., Trendier, G., an der Heiden, W., Schmidt, M., & Könnecke, R. (2005). Schizophrenia and depression: Challenging the paradigm of two separate diseases – A controlled study of schizophrenia, depression and healthy controls. *Schizophrenia Research, 77*, 11–24.

Hall, R. C. W., Popkin, M. K., DeVaul, M. K., Faillace, L. A., Stickney, S. K. (1978). Physical illness presenting as psychiatric disease. *Archives of General Psychiatry, 35*, 1315–1320.

Hamshere, M. L., Bennett, P., Williams, N., Segurado, R., Cardno, A., Norton, N., Lambert, D., Williams, H., Kirov, G., Corvin, A., Holmans, P., Jones, L., Jones, I., Gill, M., O'Donovan, M. C., Owen, M. J., & Craddock, N. (2005). Genomewide linkage scan in schizoaffective disorder. *Archives of General Psychiatry, 62*, 1081–1088.

Hanna, J., & Ferkenhoff, E. (1999, March 7). Mom charged in slayings. *Chicago Tribune*.

Harris, G. (2011, May 10, Tuesday). Antipsychotic drugs called hazardous for the elderly. *The New York Times*, p. A17.

Harrow, M., Grossman, L. S., Silverstein, M. L., & Meltzer, H. Y. (1982). Thought pathology in manic and schizophrenic patients. *Archives of General Psychiatry, 39*, 665–671.

Harrow, M., MacDonald, A. W., III, Sands, J. R., & Silverstein, M. L. (1995). Vulnerability to delusions over time in schizophrenia and affective disorders. *Schizophrenia Bulletin, 21*, 95–109.

Harrow, M., Grossman, L. S., Herbener, E. S., & Davies, E. W. (2000). Ten-year outcome: Patients with schizoaffective disorders, schizophrenia, affective disorders and mood-incongruent psychotic symptoms. *The British Journal of Psychiatry, 177*, 421–426.

Hartocollis, A. (2007, May 24). Writer is convicted in sex attack on former colleague. *The New York Times*.

Hattori, E., Liu, C., Badner, J. A., Bonner, T. I., Christian, S. L., Maheshwari, M., Detera-Wadleigh, S. D., Gibbs, R. A., Hershon, E. S. (2003). Polymorphisms at the G72/G30 gene locus, on 13q33, are associated with bipolar disorder in two independent pedigree series. *American Journal Human Genetics, 72*, 1131–1140.

Hecker, E. (1871). Die Hebephrenie. Ein Beitrag zur klinischen psychiatric. *Archiv fur Pathologische, Anatomie und Physiologie und fur Klinische Medizin, 52*, 394–429.

Hendin, H., Maltsberger, J. T., Lipschitz, A., Haas, A. P., & Kyle, J. (2001). Recognizing and responding to a suicide crisis. *Suicide & Life-Threatening Behavior, 31*, 115–128.

Henriksson, S., Boethius, G., & Isacsson, G. (2001). Suicides are seldom prescribed antidepressants: Findings from a prospective prescription database in Jamtland county, Sweden, 1985–95. *Acta Psychiatrica Scandinavica, 103*, 301–306.

Hirayasu, Y., Shenton, M. E., Salisbury, D. F., Dickey, C. C., Fischer, I. A., Mazzoni, P., Kisler, T., Akaka, H., Kwon, J. S., Anderson, J. E., Yurgelun-Todd, D., Tohen, M., McCarley, R. W. (1998). Lower left temporal lobe MRI volumes in patients with first-episode schizophrenia compared with psychotic patients with first-episode affective disorder and normal subjects. *American Journal of Psychiatry, 155*, 1384–1391.

Hirschfeld, R. M. A., Keller, M., Panico, S., Arons, B. S., Barlow, D., Davidoff, F., Endicott, J., Froom, J., Goldstein, M., Gorman, J. M., Guthrie, D., Marek, R. G., Maurer, T. A., Meyer, R., Phillips, K., Ross, J., Schwenk, T. L., Sharfstein, S. S., Thase, M. E., & Wyatt, R. J. (1997). The National Depressive and Manic-Depressive Association consensus statement on the undertreatment of depression. *The Journal of the American Medical Association, 277*, 333–340.

Hoch, P., & Rachlin, H. L. (1941). An evaluation of manic-depressive psychosis in the light of follow-up studies. *The American Journal of Psychiatry, 97*, 831–843.

Hodgkinson, C. A., Goldman, D., Jaeger, J., Persaud, S., Kane, J. M., Lipsky, R. H., & Malhotra, A. K. (2004). Disrupted in schizophrenia 1 (DISC1): Association with schizophrenia, schizoaffective disorder and bipolar disorder. *American Journal of Human Genetics, 75*, 862–872.

Honig, A., Romme, M. A. J., Ensink, B. J., Escher, S. D., Pennings, M. H., & Devries, M. W. (1998). Auditory hallucinations: A comparison between patients and non-patients. *The Journal of Nervous and Mental Disease, 186*, 646–651.

Hurwitz, N. G., & Aires, D. J. (2010). Evoked response potential endophenotypes link schizophrenia and psychotic bipolar disorder. *Psychiatric Annals, 40*, 149–153.

Hwang, M. Y., Yum, S. Y., Kwon, J. S., & Opler, L. A. (2005). Management of schizophrenia with obsessive-disorder. *Psychiatric Annals, 35*, 36–43.
ICD – World Health Organization. (2007). *The international statistical classification of diseases and related health problems* (10th rev.). Geneva: World Health Organization.
Insel, T. R. (2010). Rethinking schizophrenia. *Nature, 468*, 187–193.
Jacobs, T. J., Fogelson, S., & Charles, E. (1968). Depression ratings in hypochondria. *New York State Journal of Medicine, 25*, 3119–3122.
Jaffee, R. D. (2005). Shedding stigma of the "psycho" straight jacket. *Los Angles Times*. M1–2.
Jager, M., Bottlender, R., Strauss, A., & Moller, H. J. (2004). Fifteen-year follow-up of ICD-10 schizoaffective disorders compared with schizophrenia and affective disorders. *Acta Psychiatrica Scandinavica, 109*, 30–37.
Janicak, P. G. (guest ed.). (2011). Cases of schizophrenia. *Psychiatric Annals, 41*, 300–328.
Janzarik, W. (1969). Nosographie und Einheitspsychose. In G. Huber (Ed.), *Schizophrenie und Zyklothymie. Ergebnisse und Probleme* (pp. 22–38). Stuttgart: Thieme.
Jimenez-Jimenez, F. J., Garcia-Ruiz, P. J., & Molina, J. A. (1997). Drug-induced movement disorders. *Drug Safety, 16*, 180–204.
Johnson, G. (1970). Differential response to lithium carbonate in manic-depressive and schizoaffective disorders. *Diseases of the Nervous System, 31*, 613–615.
Johnson, K., Kovaleski, S. F., Frosch, D., & Lipton, E. (2011, January 10). Alarm grew at suspect's disturbing behavior. *The New York Times*.
Johnstone, E. C., Macmillan, J. F., & Crow, T. J. (1987). The occurrence of organic disease of possible or probable aetiological significance in a population of 268 cases of first episode schizophrenia. *Psychological Medicine, 17*, 371–379.
Jones, K. (2000, June 26). Topic: Indictment of Russell Weston Jr. (Capitol Shooter). http://projects.idc.upenn.edu.
Kahlbaum, K. (1863). *Die Gruppirung der psychischen krankheiten und die eintheilung der seelenstorungen*. Danzig: AW kafemann.
Kahlbaum, K. L. (1874). *Die Katatonie oder das spannungsirresein*. Berlin, Hirschwald.
Kalsi, G., McQuilin, A., Degn, B., Lundorf, M. D., Bass, N. J., Lawrence, J., Choudhury, K., Puri, V., Nyegaard, M., Curtis, D., Mors, O., Kruse, T., Kerwin, S., & Gurling, H. (2006). Identification of the Slynar Gene (AY070435) and related brain expressed sequences as a candidate gene for susceptibility to affective disorders through allelic and haplotypic association with bipolar disorder on chromosome 12q24. *The American Journal of Psychiatry, 163*, 1767–1776.
Kasanin, J. (1933). The acute schizoaffective psychoses. *The American Journal of Psychiatry, 13*, 97–126.
Katon, W., von Korff, M., Lin, E., Bush, T., & Ormel, J. (1992). Adequacy and duration of antidepressant in primary care. *Medical Care, 30*, 67–76.
Kendell, R. E., & Gourlay, J. (1970a). The clinical distinction between psychotic and neurotic depressions. *The British Journal of Psychiatry, 117*, 257–260.
Kendell, R. E., & Gourlay, J. (1970b). The clinical distinction between the affective psychoses and schizophrenia. *The British Journal of Psychiatry, 117*, 261–266.
Kendell, R., & Jablensky, A. (2003). Distinguishing between the validity and utility of psychiatric diagnoses. *The American Journal of Psychiatry, 160*, 4–12.
Kendler, K. S. (1991). Mood-incongruent psychotic affective illness: A historical and empirical review. *Archives of General Psychiatry, 48*, 362–369.
Kendler, K. S., McGuire, M., Gruenberg, A. M., O'Hare, A., Spellman, M., & Walsh, D. (1993). The Roscommon Family Study. IV. Affective illness, anxiety disorders and alcoholism in relatives. *Archives of General Psychiatry, 50*, 952–960.
Kendler, K. S., McGuire, M., Gruenberg, A. M., & Walsh, D. (1995). Examining the validity of DSM-III-R schizoaffective disorder and its putative subtypes in the Roscommon Family Study. *The American Journal of Psychiatry, 152*, 755–764.
Kendler, K. S., Gallagher, T. J., Ableson, J. M., & Kessler, R. C. (1996). Lifetime prevalence, demographic risk factors and diagnostic validity of non-affective psychosis as assessed in a US community sample. *Archives of General Psychiatry, 53*, 1022–1031.

Kendler, K. S., Karkowski, L. M., & Walsh, D. (1998). The structure of psychosis: Latent class analysis of probands from the Roscommon Family Study. *Archives of General Psychiatry, 55*, 492–499.

Kerr, N., Dunbar, R. I., & Bentall, R. P. (2003). Theory of mind deficits in bipolar affective disorder. *Journal of Affective Disorder, 73*, 253–259.

Kessing, L. V., & Anderson, P. K. (2004). Does the risk of developing dementia increase with the number of episodes in patients with depressive disorder and in patients with bipolar disorder? *Journal of Neurology, Neurosurgery, and Psychiatry, 75*, 1662–1666.

Kessler, R. C., Nelson, C. B., McGonagle, K. A., Liu, J., Swartz, M., & Blazer, D. G. (1996). Comorbidity of DSM-III-R major depressive disorder in the general population: Results from the U.S. National Comorbidity Survey. *British Journal of Psychiatry Supplement, 30*, 17–30.

Ketter, T., Wang, P. W., Becker, O. V., Nowakowska, C., & Yang, Y. (2004). Psychotic bipolar disorders: Dimensionally similar to or categorically different from schizophrenia? *Journal of Psychiatric Research, 38*, 47–61.

Klein, A., Williams, C., & Weil, M. (2010, March 5). 2 officers shot at Pentagon's main entrance. *The Washington Post*.

Knable, M. B., Torrey, E. F., Webster, M. J., Bartko, J. J., (2001). Multivariate analysis of prefrontal cortical data from the Stanley Foundation Neuropathology Consortium. *Brain Research Bulletin, 55*, 651–659.

Koh, P. O., Undie, A. S., Kabbani, N., Levenson, R., Goldman-Rakie, P. S., Lidow, M. S. (2003). Up-regulation of neuronal calcium sensor-1 (NCS-1) in the prefrontal cortex of schizophrenia and bipolar patients. *Proceedings of the National Academy of Sciences, 100*, 313–317.

Korn, M. L. (2004). Schizophrenia and Bipolar disorder: An evolving interface. *Medscape Psychiatry & Mental Health, 9*, 1–5.

Kraepelin, E. (1904/1913/2002). *Lectures of clinical psychiatry*. New York/Bristol: William Wood & Company/Thoemmes Press.

Kraepelin, E. (1913). *Clinical psychiatry*. New York: William Wood & Company.

Kraepelin, E. (1919/2002). *Dementia praecox and paraphrenia*. E & S Livingstone/Thoemmes Press: Edinburgh/Bristol.

Kraepelin, E. (1920/1974). Die Erscheinungsformen des Irreseins (translated by H. Marshall as: Patterns of mental disorder. In: Hirsch SR, Shepherd M. eds: Themes and Variations in European Psychiatry. Bristol, UK: Wright Publishing: 1974:7–30.). *Zeit Gesam Neurol Psychiatrie, 62*, 1–29.

Kraepelin, E. (1921/1976). *Manic depressive insanity and paranoia*. New York: Arno Press.

Kramer, M. (1961). Some problems for international research suggested by observations on differences on first-admission rates to the mental hospitals of England and Wales and of the United States. In *Proceedings of the Third World Congress of Psychiatry*. University of Toronto Press/McGill University Press, Montréal, vol. 3, pp. 153–160.

Kramer, M., Zubin, J., Cooper, J. E., et al. (1969). Cross-national study of diagnosis of the mental disorders. *The American Journal of Psychiatry, Suppl 125*, 1–46.

Kretschmeyer, E. (1919a). Die Erscheimungsformen des Irreseins. *Z Gesamte Neurol Psychiatr, 62*, 1–29.

Kretschmeyer, E. (1919b). Gedanken uber dis Fortentwicklung der psychiatrischen Systematik. Bermerkungen zu vorstehender Abhandlung. *Z Gesamte Neurol Psychiatr, 48*, 371–377.

Kruger, S., & Braunig, P. (2000). Catatonia in affective disorders: New findings and a review of the literature. *CNS Spectrums, 5*, 48–53.

Kuriansky, J. B., Deming, W. E., & Gurland, B. J. (1974). The trends in the diagnosis of schizophrenia. *The American Journal of Psychiatry, 131*, 402–408.

LaFraniere, S. (2010, November 11). Life in shadows for mentally ill in China, with violent flares. *The New York Times*.

Lake, C. R. (2008a). Hypothesis: Grandiosity and guilt cause paranoia; paranoid schizophrenia is a psychotic mood disorder; a review. *Schizophrenia Bulletin, 34*, 1151–1162.

Lake, C. R. (2008b). Disorders of thought are severe mood disorders: The selective attention defect in mania challenges the Kraepelinian dichotomy – A review. *Schizophrenia Bulletin, 34*, 109–117.

Lake, C. R. (2008c). How academic psychiatry can better prepare our students for their future patients: Part I: The failure to recognize depression and risk for suicide in primary care; problem identification, responsibility and solutions. *Behavioral Medicine, 34*, 95–100.

Lake, C. R. (2008d). How academic psychiatry can better prepare our students for their future patients: Part II: A course in ultra-brief initial diagnostic screening suitable for future primary care physicians. *Behavioral Medicine, 34*, 101–116.

Lake, C. R. (2010a). Editorial: Schizophrenia and bipolar disorder: No dichotomy: A continuum or one disease? – Part 1. *Psychiatric Annals, 40*, 72–75.

Lake, C. R. (2010b). The validity of schizophrenia vs bipolar disorder. *Psychiatric Annals, 40*, 77–87.

Lake, C. R. (2010c). Editorial: Schizophrenia and bipolar disorder: No dichotomy, a continuum, or one disease? – Part 2. *Psychiatric Annals, 40*, 129–130.

Lake, C. R. (2010d). Why the Kraepelinian dichotomy and schizophrenia have not followed the neuroses. *Psychiatric Annals, 40*, 137–142.

Lake, C. R., & Baumer, J. (2010). Academic psychiatry's responsibility for increasing the recognition of mood disorders and risk for suicide in primary care. *Current Opinion in Psychiatry, 23*, 157–166.

Lake, C. R., & Hurwitz, N. (2006a). 2 Names, 1 Disease: Does schizophrenia = psychotic bipolar disorder? *Current Psychiatry, 5*, 43–60.

Lake, C. R., & Hurwitz, N. (2006b). Schizoaffective disorders are psychotic mood disorders; there are no schizoaffective disorders. *Psychiatry Research, 143*, 255–287.

Lake, C. R., & Hurwitz, N. (2007a). The schizophrenias, the neuroses and the covered wagon. *Neuropsychiatric Disorders and Treatment, 3*, 133–143.

Lake, C. R., & Hurwitz, N. (2007b). Schizoaffective disorder merges schizophrenia and bipolar disorders as one disease – There is no schizoaffective disorder: An invited review. *Current Opinion in Psychiatry, 20*, 365–379.

Lake, C. R., Sternberg, D. E., van Kammen, D. P., Ballenger, J. C., Ziegler, M. G., Post, R. M., Kopin, I. J., & Bunney, W. E. (1980). Schizophrenia: Elevated cerebrospinal fluid norepinephrine. *Science, 207*, 331–333.

Lake, C. R., Moriarty, D. M., & Alagna, S. W. (1984). The acute psychiatric diagnostic interview. *Psychiatric Clinics of North America, 7*, 657–670.

Lapensee, M. A. (1992a). A review of schizoaffective disorder; I: Current concepts. *Canadian Journal of Psychiatry, 37*, 335–346.

Lapensee, M. A. (1992b). A review of schizoaffective disorder: II. Somatic treatment. *Canadian Journal of Psychiatry, 37*, 347–349.

Lapierre, Y. D. (1994). Schizophrenia and manic-depression: Separate illnesses or a continuum? *Canadian Journal of Psychiatry, 39*, S59–S64.

Lee, F. R. (1999, November 7). Coping; the mentally ill emerge from the shadows. *The New York Times*.

Lenggenhager, B., Tadi, T., Mdtzinger, T., & Blanke, O. (2007). Video ergo sum: Manipulating bodily self-consciousness. *Science, 317*, 1096–1099.

Leverich, G. S., Altshuler, L. L., Frye, M. A., Suppes, T., Keck, P. E., Jr., McElroy, S. L., Denicoff, K. D., Obrocea, G., Nolen, W. A., Kupka, R., Walden, J., Grunze, H., Perez, S., Luckenbaugh, D. A., & Post, R. M. (2003). Factors associated with suicide attempts in 648 patients with bipolar disorder in the Stanley Foundation Bipolar Network. *The Journal of Clinical Psychiatry, 64*, 506–515.

Lewis, N. A. (2006, April 19). Witness says Moussaoui exhibited mental illness. *The New York Times*.

Lewis, N. D. C., & Piotrowski, Z. A. (1954). Clinical diagnosis of manic-depressive psychosis. In P. H. Hoch & J. Zubin (Eds.), *Depression* (pp. 25–38). New York: Grune Stratton.

Lichtenstein, P., Yip, B. H., Bjork, C., Pawitan, Y., Cannon, T. D., Sullivan, P. F., & Hultman, C. M. (2009). Common genetic determinants of schizophrenia and bipolar disorder in Swedish families: A population-based study. *The Lancet, 373*, 234–239.

Lieberman, J. A., III. (2002). Depression: A common illness uncommonly diagnosed. *Psychiatric Annals, 32*, 522–526.

Lipkin, K. M., Dyrud, J., & Meyer, G. (1970). The many faces of mania: Therapeutic trial of lithium carbonate. *Archives of General Psychiatry, 22*, 262–267.
Longman, J. (2010, December 10). John E. du Pont, 72, dies; killed athlete. *The New York Times*.
Lonnqvist, J. K., Henriksson, M. M., Isometsa, E. T., Marttunen, M. J., Heikkinen, M. E., Aro, H. M., Kuoppasalmi, K. I. (1995). Mental disorders and suicide prevention. *Psychiatry and Clinical Neuroscience, 45*(Suppl 1), S111–S116.
Lu, M. L., Pan, J. J., Tang, H. W., Su, K. P., & Shen, W. W. (2002). Metoclopramide-induced supersensitivity psychosis. *The Annals of Pharmacotherapy, 36*, 1387–1390.
Lundquist, G. (1945). Prognosis and course in manic-depressive psychosis. *Acta Psychiatrica et Neurologica Scandinavica, 35*(Suppl), 196.
Luoma, J. B., Martin, C. E., & Pearson, J. L. (2002). Contact with mental health and primary care providers before suicide: A review of the evidence. *The American Journal of Psychiatry, 159*, 909–916.
Lyness, J. M., Kim, J., Tang, W., Tu, X., Conwell, Y., Kind, D. A., & Caine, E. D. (2007). The clinical significance of subsyndromal depression in older primary care patients. *The American Journal of Geriatric Psychiatry, 15*, 214–223.
Macgregor, S., Visscher, P. M., Knott, S. A., Thomson, P., Porteous, K. F., Millar, J. K., Devon, R. S., Blackwood, D., Muir, W. J. (2004). A genome scan and follow-up study identify a bipolar disorder susceptibility locus on chromosome 1q42. *Molecular Psychiatry, 9*, 1083–1090.
Mahendra, B. (1981). Where have all the catatonics gone. *Psychological Medicine, 11*, 669–671.
Mahgoub, N., & Serby, M. (2007). Charles Bonnet syndrome: Long-term outcome of treatment. *Psychiatric Annals, 37*, 579–580.
Maier, W. (1992). Kontinuitat und Diskontinuitat funktioneller psychosyndrome im Lichte von Familienstudien. In C. Mundt & H. Sass (Eds.), *Fur und Wider die Einheitspsychose* (pp. 99–109). New York: Georg Thieme.
Maier, W. (2006). Do schizoaffective disorders exist at all? *Acta Psychiatrica Scandinavica, 13*, 369–371.
Maier, W., Lichtermann, D., Minges, J., Hallmayer, J., Heun, R., Benkert, O., & Levinson, D. F. (1993). Continuity and discontinuity of affective disorders and schizophrenia. Results of a controlled family study. *Archives of General Psychiatry, 50*, 871–883.
Maier, W., Zobel, A., & Wagner, M. (2006). Schizophrenia and bipolar disorder: Differences and overlaps. *Current Opinion in Psychiatry, 19*, 165–170.
Maj, M., Pirozzi, R., Formicola, A. M., Bartoli, L., & Bucci, P. (2000). Reliability and validity of the DSM-IV diagnostic category of schizoaffective disorder: Preliminary data. *Journal of Affective Disorders, 57*, 95–98.
Makinen, J., Miettunen, J., Isohanni, M., & Koponen, H. (2008). Negative symptoms in schizophrenia: A review. *Nordic Journal of Psychiatry, 62*, 334–341.
Mandal, V. (2002, October 7). Families of mentally ill pay terrible toll: Psychiatric patients are killing and assaulting their families at an alarming rate. *Vancouver Sun*.
Manganis, J. (2011, January 22). *Suspect held without bail, faces mental evaluation*. http://SalemNews.com, Salem.
Mann, D. (2009, December 1). The case of Otty Sanchez. *The StandDown Texas Project*.
Mann, D. (2010, January 13). Gone baby gone. *The Texas Observer*.
Mann, J. J., Apter, A., Bertolote, J., et al. (2005). Suicide prevention strategies: A systematic review. *The Journal of the American Medical Association, 294*, 2064–2074.
Martin, M. J. (1983). A brief review of organic diseases masquerading as functional illness. *Hospital & Community Psychiatry, 34*, 328–332.
Martinez-Arán, A., Vieta, E., Reinares, M., Colom, F., Torrent, C., Sanchez-Moreno, J., Benabarre, A., Goikolea, J. M., Comes, M., & Salamero, M. (2004a). Cognitive function across manic or hypomanic, depressed and euthymic states in bipolar disorder. *The American Journal of Psychiatry, 161*, 262–270.
Martinez-Arán, A., Vieta, E., Colom, F., Torrent, C., Sanchez-Moreno, J., Reinares, M., Benabarre, S., Goikolea, J. M., Brugue, E., Daban, C., & Salamero, M. (2004b). Cognitive impairment in euthymic bipolar patients: Implication for clinical and functional outcome. *Bipolar Disorder, 6*, 224–232.

Marx, C. E., Stevens, R. D., Shampine, L. J., Uzunova, V., Trost, W. T., Butterfield, M. I., Massing, M. W., Hamer, R. M., Morrow, A. L., & Lieberman, J. A. (2006). Neuroactive steroids are altered in schizophrenia and bipolar disorder: Relevance to pathophysiology and therapeutics. *Neuwopsychopharmacology, 31*, 1249–1263.

Mason, P. S. (2004). Atypical antipsychotics in the treatment of affective symptoms: A review. *Annals of Clinical Psychiatry, 16*, 3–13.

Mays, D. (2004). Structured assessment methods may improve suicide prevention. *Psychiatric Annals, 34*, 367–372.

Mazzarini, L., & Vieta, E. (2010). Toward a valid classification of psychosis: Overcoming the schizophrenia-bipolar dichotomy. *Psychiatric Annals, 40*, 143–148.

Maziade, M., Roy, M. A., Rouillard, E., Bissonnette, L., Fournier, J. P., Roy, A., Garneau, Y., Montgrain, N., Potvin, A., Cliché, D., Dion, C., Wallot, H., Fournier, A., Nicole, L., Lavallee, J. C. (2001). A search for specific and common susceptibility loci for schizophrenia and bipolar disorder: a linkage study in 13 target chromosomes. *Molecular Psychiatry, 6*(6):684–693.

Maziade, M., Roy, M. A., Chagnon, Y. C., Cliché, D., Fournier, J. P., Montgrain, N., Dion, C., Lavalle, J. C., Garneau, Y., Gingras, N., Nicole, L., Pires, A., Ponton, A. M., Potvin, A., Wallot, H., Merette, C. (2005). Shared and specific susceptibility loci for schizophrenia and bipolar disorder: a dense genome scan in Eastern Quebec families. *Molecular Psychiatry, 10*, 486–499.

McCullum-Smith, R. E., Meador-Woodruff, J. H. (2002). Striatal excitatory amino acid transporter transcript expression in schizophrenia, bipolar disorder, and major depressive disorder. *Neuropsychopharmacology, 26*, 368–375.

McEvoy, J. P., Meyer, J. M., Goff, D. C., Nasrallah, H. A., Davis, S. M., Sullivan, L., Meltzer, H. Y., Hsiao, J., Scott Stroup, T., Lieberman, J.A. (2005). Prevalence of the metabolic syndrome in patients with schizophrenia: Baseline results from the Clinical Antipsychotic Trials of Intervention Effectiveness (CATIE) schizophrenia trial and comparison with national estimates from NHANESIII. *Schizophrenia Research, 80*, 19–32.

McGlashan, T. H., & Carpenter, W. T. (1976). Postpsychotic depression in schizophrenia. *Archives of General Psychiatry, 33*, 231–239.

McGuffin, P., Reveley, A., & Holland, A. (1982). Identical triplets: Non-identical psychosis? *The British Journal of Psychiatry, 140*, 1–6.

McGuffin, P., Rijsdijk, R., Andrew, M., Sham, P., Katz, R., & Cardno, A. (2003). The heritability of bipolar affective disorder and the genetic relationship to unipolar depression. *Archives of General Psychiatry, 60*, 497–502.

McIntosh, A. M., Harrison, L. K., Forrester, K., Lawrie, S. M., & Johnstone, E. C. (2005). Neuropsychological impairments in people with schizophrenia or bipolar disorder and their unaffected relatives. *The British Journal of Psychiatry, 186*, 378–385.

McKinley, J. C. (2010, October 20). Texas: Jordanian sentenced in bomb plot. *The New York Times*.

McQueen, M. B., Devlin, B., Faraone, S. V., Nimgaonkar, V. L., Sklar, P., Smoller, J. W., Abou Jamra, R., Albus, M., Bacanu, S. A., Baron, M., Barrett, T. B., Berrettini, W., Blacker, D., Byerley, W., Cichon, S., Coryell, W., Craddock, N., Daly, M. J., Depaulo, J. R., Edenberg, H. J., Forout, T., Gill, M., Gilliam, T. C., Hamshere, M., Jones, I., Jones, L., Juo, S. H., Kelsoe, J. R., Lambert, D., Lange, C., Lerer, B., Liu, J., Maier, W., Mackinnon, J. D., McInnis, M. G., McMahon, F. J., Murphy, D. L., Nothen, M. M., Nurnberger, Jl, Pato, C. N., Pato, M. T., Potash, J. B., Propping, P., Pulver, A. E., Rice, J. P., Rietschel, M., Scheftner, W., Schumacher, J., Segurado, R., Van Steen, K., Xie, W., Zandi, P. P., & Laird, N. M. (2005). Combined analysis from eleven linkage studies of bipolar disorder provides strong evidence of susceptibility loci on chromosomes 6q and 8q. *American Journal of Human Genetics, 77*, 582–595.

Mendlewicz, J., Fieve, R. R., Rainer, J. D., & Fleiss, J. L. (1972). Manic-depressive illness: A comparative study of patients with and without a family history. *The British Journal of Psychiatry, 120*, 523–530.

Mialet, J. P., & Pope, H. G. (1996). Impaired attention in depressive states: A non-specific deficit? *Psychological Medicine, 26*, 1009–1020.

Millar, J. K., Wilson-Annan, J. C., Anderson, S., Christie, S., Taylor, M. S., Semple, C. A. M., Devon, R. S., St Clair, D. M., Muir, W. J., Blackwood, D. H. R., Porteous, D. J. (2000).

Disruption of two novel genes by a translocation co-segregating with schizophrenia. *Human Molecular Genetics, 9,* 1415–1423.

Moller, H. J. (2003). Bipolar disorder and schizophrenia: Distinct illnesses or a continuum? *The Journal of Clinical Psychiatry, 64,* 23–27.

Moller, H. J. (2010). Is the overlap of neurobiological and psychopathological parameters large enough to give up the dichotomic classification? *Psychiatric Annals, 40,* 163–167.

Moore, R., Blackwood, N., Corcoran, R., Rowse, G., Kinderman, P., Bentall, R., & Howard, R. (2006). Misunderstanding in the intentions of others: An exploratory study of the cognitive etiology of persecutory delusions in very late-onset schizophrenia-like psychosis. *The American Journal of Geriatric Psychiatry, 14,* 410–418.

Morel, B. A. (1851). *Etudes cliniques Traite Theorique et Pratique des maladies mentales.* Paris: Vicotr Masson.

Moskvina, V., Craddock, N., Holmans, P., Nikolov, I., Pahwa, J. S., Green, E., Wellcome Trust Case Control Consortium, Owen, M. J., O'Donovan, M. C. (2009). Gene-wide analysis of genome-wide association data sets: Evidence for multiple common risk alleles for schizophrenia and bipolar disorder and for overlap in genetic risk. *Molecular Psychiatry, 14,* 252–260.

Moynihan, R., Heath, I., & Henry, D. (2002). Selling sickness: The pharmaceutical industry and disease mongering. *British Medical Journal, 324,* 886–891.

Muller, N., & Schwarz, M. J. (2008). A psychoneuroimmunological perspective in Emil Kraepelins dichotomy: Schizophrenia and major depression as inflammatory CNS disorders. *European Archives of Psychiatry and Clinical Neuroscience, 258,* 97–106.

Murphy, G. E. (1975). The physician's responsibility for suicide. II. Errors of omission. *American Journal of Internal Medicine, 82,* 305–309.

Murray, R. M., Sham, P., van Os, J., Zanelli, J., Cannon, M., & McDonald, C. (2004). A developmental model for similarities and dissimilarities between schizophrenia and bipolar disorder. *Schizophrenia Research, 71,* 405–416.

Nardi, A. E., Nascimento, I., Freire, R. C., de-Melo-Neto, V. L., Valenca, A. M., Dib, M., Soares-Filho, G. L., Veras, A. B., Mezzasalma, M. A., Lopes, F. L., de Menezes, G. B., Grivet, L. O., & Versiani, M. (2005). Demographic and clinical features of schizoaffective (Schizobipolar) disorder – A 5-year retrospective study. Support for a bipolar spectrum disorder. *Journal of Affective Disorders, 89,* 201–206.

Nasrallah, H. A. (2006). Schizophrenia is psychotic bipolar disorder? What a polarizing idea! *Current Psychiatry, 5,* 67–68.

Neumann, H. (1859). *Lehrbuch der psychiatrie.* Erlangen: Enke.

Nutting, P. A., Dickinson, L. M., Rubenstein, L. V., Keeley, R. D., Smith, J. L., & Elliott, C. E. (2005). Improving detection of suicidal ideation among depressed patients in primary care. *Annals of Family Medicine, 3,* 529–536.

Olincy, A., & Martin, L. (2005). Diminished suppression of the P50 auditory evoked potential in bipolar disorder subjects with a history of psychosis. *The American Journal of Psychiatry, 162,* 43–49.

Ollerenshaw, D. P. (1973). The classification of the functional psychoses. *The British Journal of Psychiatry, 122,* 517–530.

Oltmanns, T. F. (1978). Selective attention in schizophrenic and manic psychoses: The effect of distraction on information processing. *Journal of Abnormal Psychology, 87,* 212–225.

Ortiz, I. (2010, July 20). Psychiatrists: Rubio suffers from schizophrenia. *The Brownsville Herald.*

Osuji, I. F., & Cullum, C. M. (2005). Cognition in bipolar disorder. *Psychiatric Clinics of North America, 28,* 427–441.

Park, N., Juo, S. H., Cheng, R., Liu, J., Loth, J. E., Lilliston, B., Nee, J., Grunn, A., Kanyas, K., Lerer, B., Endicott, J., Gilliam, T. C., Baron, M. (2004). Linkage analysis of psychosis in bipolar pedigrees suggests novel putative loci for bipolar disorder and shared susceptibility with schizophrenia. *Molecular Psychiatry, 9,* 1091–1099.

Patten, J., Bozek, C., & Vogler, M. E. (2008, February 7). Teen stabs, kills therapist in Walker Street apartment. *Eagle-Tribune,* North Andover.

Pearlson, G. D., Wong, D. F., Tune, L. E., Ross, C. A., Chase. G. A., Links Jr, J. M., Dannals, R. F., Wilson, A. A., Ravert, H. T., Wagner, H. N. Jr, DePaulo, J. R. (1995). In vivo D_2 dopamine receptor density in psychotic and not nonpsychotic patients with bipolar disorder. *Archives of General Psychiatry, 52*, 471–477.

Pearlson, G. D., Barta, P. E., Powers, R. E., Menon, R. R., Richards, S. S., Aylward, E. H., Federman, E. B., Chase, G. A., Petty, R. G., Tien, A. Y., & Ziskind-Somerfeld Research Award 1996. (1997). Medial and superior temporal gyral volumes and cerebral asymmetry in schizophrenia versus bipolar disorder. *Biological Psychiatry, 41*, 1–14.

Peralta, V., & Cuesta, M. J. (1999). Diagnostic significance of Schneider's first-rank symptoms in schizophrenia. Comparative study between schizophrenia and non-schizophrenic psychotic disorders. *The British Journal of Psychiatry, 174*, 243–248.

Perea, E., Robbins, B. V., & Hutto, B. (2006). Psychosis related to ropinirole. *The American Journal of Psychiatry, 163*, 547–548.

Pierre, J. M. (2009). What do you mean, I don't have schizophrenia? *Psychiatric Times, 26*: Commentary.

Pierre, J. M., Wirshing, D. A., & Wirshing, W. C. (2003). "Iatrogenic Malingering" in VA substance abuse treatment. *Psychiatric Services, 54*, 253–254.

Pierson, A., Jouvent, R., Quintin, P., Perez-Diaz, F., Leboyer, M. (2000). Information processing deficits in relatives of manic depressive patients. *Psychological Medicine, 30*, 545–555.

Pignone, M. P., Gaynes, B. N., Rushton, J. L., Burchell, C. M., Orleans, C. T., Mulrow, C. D., & Lohr, K. N. (2002). Screening for depression in adults: A summary of the evidence for the US Preventive Services Task Force. *Annals of Internal Medicine, 136*, 765–776.

Pini, S., Cassano, G. B., Dell'Osso, L., & Amador, X. F. (2001). Insight into illness in schizophrenia, schizoaffective disorder, and mood disorders with psychotic features. *The American Journal of Psychiatry, 158*, 122–125.

Pirkis, J., & Burgess, P. (1998). Suicide and recency of health care contacts. A systematic review. *The British Journal of Psychiatry, 173*, 462–474.

Plater, F. Annales de madeicine. Praxis medica, Basel. 1625.

Politis, A., Lykouras, L., Mourtzouchou, P., & Christodoulou, G. N. (2004). Attentional disturbances in patients with unipolar psychotic depression: A selective and sustained attention study. *Comprehensive Psychiatry, 45*, 452–459.

Pope, H. G. (1983). Distinguishing bipolar disorder from schizophrenia in clinical practice: Guidelines and case reports. *Hospital & Community Psychiatry, 34*, 322–328.

Pope, H. G., & Katz, D. L. (1988). Affective and psychotic symptoms associated with anabolic steroid use. *The American Journal of Psychiatry, 145*, 487–490.

Pope, H. G., & Lipinski, J. F. (1978). Diagnosis in schizophrenia and manic-depressive illness, a reassessment of the specificity of "schizophrenic" symptoms in the light of current research. *Archives of General Psychiatry, 35*, 811–828.

Pope, H. G., & Yurgelun-Todd, D. (1990). Schizophrenic individuals with bipolar first-degree relatives: Analysis of two pedigrees. *The Journal of Clinical Psychiatry, 51*, 97–101.

Pope, H. G., Lipinski, J. F., Cowen, B. M., & Axelrod, D. T. (1980). Schizoaffective disorder: An invalid diagnosis? A comparison of schizoaffective disorder, schizophrenia, and affective disorder. *The American Journal of Psychiatry, 137*, 921–927.

Posner, M. L., & Petersen, S. E. (1990). The attention system of the human brain. *Annual Review of Neuroscience, 13*, 25–42.

Post, R. M. (1992). Transduction of psychosocial stress into the neurobiology of recurrent affective disorder. *The American Journal of Psychiatry, 149*, 999–1010.

Post, R. M. (2007). The case for polypharmacy in the treatment of bipolar disorder. *Psychiatric Times, 24*, 1–4.

Post, R. M. (2010). Overlaps between schizophrenia and bipolar disorder. *Psychiatric Annals, 41*, 106–112.

Potash, J. B., Zandi, P. P., Willour, V. L., Lan, T. H., Huo, Y., Avramopoulos, D., Shugart, Y. Y., MacKinnon, D. F., Simpson, S. G., McMahon, F. J., DePaulo, J. R., Jr, McInnis, M. G. (2003). Suggestive linkage to chromosomal regions 13q31 and 22q12 in families with psychotic bipolar disorder. *American Journal Psychiatry, 160*, 680–686.

Poyurovsky, M., Fuchs, C., & Weizman, A. (1999). Obsessive-compulsive disorder in patients with first-episode schizophrenia. *The American Journal of Psychiatry, 156*, 1998–2000.
Prestidge, B. R., & Lake, C. R. (1987). The prevalence and recognition of depression among primary care outpatients. *Journal of Family Practice, 25*, 67–72.
Prien, R. F., Caffey, E. M., Jr., & Klett, C. J. (1972). A comparison of lithium carbonate and chlorpromazine in the treatment of excited schizo-affectives. *Archives of General Psychiatry, 27*, 182–189.
Prien, R. F., Klett, C. J., & Caffey, E. M., Jr. (1973). Lithium carbonate and imipramine in prevention of affective episodes: A comparison in recurrent affective illness. *Archives of General Psychiatry, 29*, 420–425.
Prien, R. F., Kupfer, D. J., Mansky, P. A., et al. (1984). Drug therapy in the prevention of recurrences in unipolar and bipolar affective disorders: Report of the NIMH Collaborative Study Group comparing lithium carbonate, imipramine, and a lithium carbonate-imipramine combination. *Archives of General Psychiatry, 41*, 1096–1104.
Procci, W. R. (1976). Schizo-affective psychosis: Fact or fiction. *Archives of General Psychiatry, 33*, 1167–1178.
Prossin, A. R., McInnis, M. G., Anand, A., Heitzeg, M. M., & Zubieta, J. K. (2010). Tackling the Kraepelinian dichotomy: A neuroimaging review. *Psychiatric Annals, 40*, 145–162.
Quitkin, F. M., Kane, J., Rifkin, A., et al. (1981). Prophylactic lithium carbonate with and without imipramine for bipolar I patients: A double-blind study. *Archives of General Psychiatry, 38*, 902–907.
Quraishi, S., & Frangou, S. (2002). Neuropsychology of bipolar disorder: A review. *Journal of Affective Disorders, 72*, 209–226.
Raue, P. J., Brown, E. L., Meyers, B. S., & Schulberg, H. C. (2006). Does every allusion to possible suicide require the same response? *Journal of Family Practice, 55*, 605–612.
Regier, D. A., Narrow, W. E., Ray, D. S., Manderscheid, R. W., Locke, B. Z., & Goodwin, F. K. (1993). The de facto U.S. mental and addictive disorders service system: Epidemiologic catchment area prospective 1-year prevalence rates of disorders and services. *Archives of General Psychiatry, 41*, 971–978.
Rennert, H. (1965). Die Universalgenese der endogenen psychosen. Ein Beitrag zum problem "Einheitspsychose". *Fortschritte der Neurologie-Psychiatrie, 33*, 251–272.
Rennie, T. A. C. (1942). Prognosis in manic-depressive psychosis. *The American Journal of Psychiatry, 98*, 801–814.
Rice, J., Reich, T., Andreasen, N. C., Endicott, J., Van Eerdewegh, M., Fishman, R., Hirschfeld, R. M., & Klerman, G. L. (1987). Familial transmission of bipolar illness. *Archives of General Psychiatry, 44*, 441–447.
Robins, E., Murphy, G. E., Wilkinson, R. H., Jr., Gassner, S., & Kayes, J. (1959). Some clinical considerations in the prevention of suicide based on a study of 134 successful suicides. *American Journal of Public Health, 49*, 888–899.
Robinson, L. J., & Ferrier, I. N. (2006). Evolution of cognitive impairment in bipolar disorder: A systematic review of cross-sectional evidence. *Bipolar Disorder, 8*, 103–116.
Rodin, G., & Voshart, K. (1987). Depressive symptoms and functional impairment in the medically ill. *General Hospital Psychiatry, 19*, 251–258.
Roelcke, V. (1997). Biologizing social facts: An early 20th century debate on Kraepelin's concept of culture, neurasthenia, and degeneration. *Culture, Medicine and Psychiatry, 21*, 383–403.
Rohde, D. (2000, February 29). Court is told subway killer, off medication, hit a social worker. *The New York Times*.
Rosack, J. (2003). Dopamine pathway may link schizophrenia, bipolar disorder. *Psychiatric News, 38*, 21–22.
Rosack, J. (2006). Patient charged with murder of schizophrenia expert. *Psychiatric News, 41*, 1.
Rottnek, M., Riggio, S., Byne, W., Sano, M., Margolis, R. L., & Walker, R. H. (2008). Schizophrenia in a patient with spinocerebellar ataxia 2: Coincidence of two disorders or a neurodegenerative disease presenting with psychosis? *The American Journal of Psychiatry, 165*, 964–967.

Roy, P. D., Zipursky, R. B., Saint-Cyr, J. A., Bury, A., Langevin, R., Seeman, M. V. (1998). Temporal horn enlargement is present in schizophrenia and bipolar disorder. *Biological Psychiatry, 44(6)*, 418–422.

Rund, B. R., Orbeck, A. L., & Landro, N. I. (1992). Vigilance deficits in schizophrenics and affectively disturbed patients. *Acta Psychiatrica Scandinavica, 86*, 207–212.

Sadock, B. J., & Sadock, V. A. (2005). *Kaplan & Sadock's comprehensive textbook of psychiatry* (8th ed.). Philadelphia: Lippincott Williams & Wilkins.

Samuels, T., & Franey, L. (2000, February 15). Warrensburg tragedy leaves town in shock. *The Kansas City Star*.

Sands, J. R., & Harrow, M. (1994). Psychotic unipolar depression at follow-up: Factors related to psychosis in the affective disorders. *The American Journal of Psychiatry, 151*, 995–1000.

Schloesser, R. J., Huang, J., Klein, P. S., Manji, H. K. (2008). Cellular plasticity cascades in the pathophysiology and treatment of bipolar disorder. *Neuropsychopharmacology, 33*, 110–133.

Schneider, K. (1959). *Clinical psychopathology*. New York: Grune & Stratton, Inc.

Schou, M. (1967). Therapeutic and prophylactic action of lithium aga. *Activitas Nervosa Superior, 9*, 440.

Schou, M. (1968). Special review: Lithium in psychiatric therapy and prophylaxis. *Journal of Psychiatric Research, 6*, 67–95.

Schou, M. (1979). Lithium as a prophylactic agent in unipolar affective illness: Comparison with cyclic antidepressants. *Archives of General Psychiatry, 36*, 849–851.

Schretlen, D. J., Cascella, N. G., Meyer, S. M., Kingery, L. R., Testa, S. M., Munro, C. A., Pulver, A. E., Rivkin, P., Rao, V. A., Diaz-Asper, C. M., Dickerson, F. B., Yolken, R. H., & Pearlson, G. D. (2007). Neuropsychological functioning in bipolar disorder and schizophrenia. *Biological Psychiatry, 62*, 179–186.

Schulberg, H. C., Lee, P. W., Bruce, M. L., et al. (2005). Suicidal ideation and risk levels among primary-care patients with uncomplicated depression. *Annals of Family Medicine, 3*, 523–528.

Schulze, T. G., Ohlraun, S., Czerski, P., Schumacher, J., Kassem, L., Deschner, M., Gross, M., Tallius, M., Heidmann, V., Kovalenko, S., Jamra, R. A., Becker, T., Leszczynska-Rodziewicz, A., Hauser, J., & Illig, T. (2005). Genotype-phenotype studies in bipolar disorder showing association between the DAOA/G30 locus and persecutory delusions: A first step toward a molecular genetic classification of psychiatric phenotypes. *The American Journal of Psychiatry, 162*, 2101–2108.

Schumacher, J., Jamra, R. A., Freudenberg, J., Becker, T., Ohlraun, S., Otte, A. C., Tullius, M., Kovalenko, S., Bogaert, A. V., Maier, W., Rietschel, M., Propping, P., Nothen, M. M., Cichon, S. (2004). Examination fG72 and D-amino-acid oxidase as genetic risk factors for schizophrenia and bipolar affective disorder. *Molecular Psychiatry, 9*, 203–207.

Schurhoff, F., Szoke, A., Meary, A., Bellivier, F., Rouillon, F., Pauls, D., & Leboyer, M. (2003). Familial aggregation of delusional proneness in schizophrenia and bipolar pedigrees. *The American Journal of Psychiatry, 160*, 1313–1319.

Schwartz, J. E., Fennig, S., Tanenberg-Karant, M., Carlson, G., Craig, T., Galambos, N., Lavelle, J., & Bromet, E. J. (2000). Congruence of diagnoses 2 years after a first-admission diagnosis of psychosis. *Archives of General Psychiatry, 57*, 593–600.

Sereno, A. B., & Holzman, P. S. (1996). Spatial selective attention in schizophrenic, affective disorder, and normal subjects. *Schizophrenia Research, 20*, 33–50.

Sernyak, M. J., Griffin, R. A., Johnson, R. M., Pearsall, H. R., Wexler, B. E., & Woods, S. W. (1994). Neuroleptic exposure following inpatient treatment of acute mania with lithium and neuroleptic. *The American Journal of Psychiatry, 151*, 133–135.

Shahrokh, N. C., & Hales, R. E. (Eds.). (2003). *American psychiatric glossary* (8th ed.). Arlington: American Psychiatric Publishing, Inc.

Shapiro, D. R., Quitkin, F. M., & Fleiss, J. L. (1989). Response to maintenance therapy in bipolar illness: Effect of index episode. *Archives of General Psychiatry, 46*, 401–405.

Shelton, R. C., Davidson, J., Yonkers, K., Koran, L., Thase, M. E., Pearlstein, T., & Halbreich, U. (1997). The under-treatment of dysthymia. *The Journal of Clinical Psychiatry, 58*, 59–65.

Shopsin, B., Kim, S. S., & Gershon, S. (1971). A controlled study of lithium vs chlorpromazine in acute schizophrenics. *The British Journal of Psychiatry, 119*, 435–440.
Shorter, E. (2005). *A historical dictionary of psychiatry*. New York: Oxford University Press.
Simmons, J. The Raymond wood case. http://larryrobison.org/pages/raymond_wood.htm.
Simon, G. E., & VonKorff, M. (1995). Recognition, management and outcomes of depression in primary care. *Archives of Family Medicine, 4*, 99–105.
Sims, J. (1799). Pathological remarks upon various kinds of alienation of mind. Memoirs Med Soc Lond 5:372–406.
Small, J. G., Kellams, J. J., Milstem, N., et al. (1975). A placebo controlled study of lithium combined with neuroleptics in chronic schizophrenia patients. *The American Journal of Psychiatry, 132*, 1315–1317.
Smith, R. (2002). In search of "non-disease". *British Medical Journal, 324*, 883–885.
Sontag, D. (2011, June 17). A mental patient, a slain worker, troubling questions. *The New York Times*.
Specht, G. (1905). Chronische manie and paranoia. *Centralbl Nervenheilk Psychiatr, 28*, 590–597.
Sptizer, R. L., Endicott, J., & Robins, E. (1978). *Research diagnostic criteria (RDC) for a selected group of functional disorders* (3rd ed., pp. 9–11). New York: Biometrics Research New York State Psychiatric Institute.
Steiner, W., Laporta, M., & Chouinard, G. (1990). Neuroleptic-induced supersensitivity psychosis in patients with bipolar affective disorder. *Acta Psychiatrica Scandinavica, 81*, 437–440.
Stoll, A. L., Tohen, M., Baldessarini, R. J., Goodwin, D. C., Stein, S., Katz, S., Geenens, D., Swinson, R. P., Goethe, J. W., & McGlashen, T. (1993). Shifts in diagnostic frequencies of schizophrenia and major affective disorders at six North American psychiatric hospitals, 1972–1988. *The American Journal of Psychiatry, 150*, 1668–1673.
Sulzberger, A. G., & Carey, B. (2011, January 19). Getting someone to treatment can be difficult and inconclusive, experts say. *The New York Times*.
Suwalska, A., Borkowska, A., & Rybakowski, J. (2001). Cognitive deficits in the bipolar affective disorder. *Psychiatrica Poland, 35*, 657–668.
Swartz, C. M. (1995). Tardive psychopathology. *Neuropsychobiology, 32*, 115–119.
Swartz, C. M. (2001). Misdiagnosis of schizophrenia for a patient with epilepsy. *Psychiatry Services, 52*, 109–110.
Swartz, C. M. (2002a, October). Schizophrenic schizophrenia. *Psychiatric Times*, pp. 47–51.
Swartz, C. M. (2002b, November). Schizoaffective defective. *Psychiatric Times*, pp. 29–32.
Swartz, C. M. (2004, October). Antipsychotic psychosis. *Psychiatric Times*, pp. 17–20.
Swartz, C. M. (2010). Psychotic depression or schizophrenia. *Psychiatric Annals, 40*, 92–97.
Swartz, C. M., & Shorter, E. (2007). *Psychotic depression*. New York: Cambridge University Press.
Sweeney, J. A., Kmiec, J. A., & Kupfer, D. J. (2000). Neuropsychologic impairments in bipolar and unipolar mood disorders on the CANTAB neurocognitive battery. *Biological Psychiatry, 48*, 674–684.
Szasz, T. S. (1976). Schizophrenia: The sacred symbol of psychiatry. *The British Journal of Psychiatry, 129*, 308–316.
Tammeus, B. A sad testament against execution. www.kcstar.com.
Tandon, R., Keshavan, M. S., & Nasrallah, H. A. (2008). Schizophrenia, "just the facts": What we know in 2009, part 1: Overview. *Schizophrenia Research, 100*, 4–19.
Taylor, M. A. (1992). Are schizophrenia and affective disorder related? A selective review. *The American Journal of Psychiatry, 49*, 22–32.
Taylor, M. A., & Amir, N. (1994). Are schizophrenia and affective disorder related?: The problem of schizoaffective disorder and the discrimination of the psychoses by signs and symptoms. *Comprehensive Psychiatry, 35*, 420–429.
Taylor, M. A., Abrams, R. (1973). The phenomenology of mania: a new look at some old patients. *Archives of General Psychiatry, 29*, 520–522.
Taylor, M. A., Abrams, R. (1975). Manic-depressive illness and good prognosis schizophrenia. *American Journal of Psychiatry, 132*, 741–742.

Taylor, M. A., Gaztanaga, P., & Abrams, R. (1974). Manic-depressive illness and acute schizophrenia: A clinical, family history and treatment-response study. *The American Journal of Psychiatry, 131*, 678–682.

The International Schizophrenia Consortium. (2009). Common polygenic variation contributes to risk of schizophrenia and bipolar disorder. *Nature, 460*, 748–752.

Tibbo, P., Kroetsch, M., Chue, P., & Warneke, L. (2000). Obsessive-compulsive disorder in schizophrenia. *Journal of Psychiatric Research, 34*, 139–146.

Tiihonen, J., Haukka, J., Henriksson, M., Cannon, M., Kieseppa, T., Laaksonen, I., Sinivou, J., & Lonnqvist, J. (2005). Premorbid intellectual functioning in bipolar disorder and schizophrenia: Results from a cohort study of male conscripts. *The American Journal of Psychiatry, 162*, 1904–1910.

Tkachev, D. Minnack, M. L., Ryan, M. M., Wayland, M., Freeman, T., Jones, P., Starkey, M., Webster, M. J., Yolken, R. H., Bahn, S. (2003). Oligoderdrocyte dysfunction in schizophrenia and bipolar disorder. *The Lancet, 362*, 798–805.

Tohen, M., Waternaux, C. M., & Tsuang, M. T. (1990). Outcome in Mania. A 4-year prospective follow-up of 75 patients utilizing survival analysis. *Archives of General Psychiatry, 47*, 1106–1111.

Tohen, M., Tsuang, M. T., & Goodwin, D. C. (1992). Prediction of outcome in mania by mood-congruent or mood-incongruent psychotic features. *The American Journal of Psychiatry, 149*, 1580–1584.

Tohen, M., Ketter, T. A., Zarate, C. A., Suppes, T., Frye, M., Altshuler, L., Zajecka, J., Schuh, L. M., Risser, R. C., Brown, E., & Baker, R. W. (2003). Olanzapine versus divalproex sodium for the treatment of acute mania and maintenance of remission: A 47-week study. *The American Journal of Psychiatry, 160*, 1263–1271.

Tohen, M., Chengappa, K. N., Suppes, T., Baker, R. W., Zarate, C. A., Bowden, C. L., Sachs, G. S., Kupfer, D. J., Ghaemi, S. N., Feldman, P. D., Risser, R. C., Evans, A. R., Calabrese, J. R. (2004). Relapse prevention in bipolar I disorder: 18-month comparison of olanzapine plus mood stabilizer v. mood stabilizer alone. *British Journal of Psychiatry, 184*, 337–345.

Toulopoulou, T., Picchioni, M., Rijsdijk, F., Hua-Hall, M., Ettinger, U., Sham, P., & Murray, R. (2007). Substantial genetic overlap between neurocognition and schizophrenia. *Archives of General Psychiatry, 64*, 1348–1355.

Tsuang, M. T., Dempsey, G. M., & Rauscher, F. (1976). A study of "atypical schizophrenia": A comparison with schizophrenia and affective disorder by sex, age of admission, precipitant, outcome and family history. *Archives of General Psychiatry, 33*, 1157–1160.

Tsuang, M. T., Winokur, G., & Crowe, R. R. (1980). Morbidity risks of schizophrenia and affective disorders among first-degree relatives of patients with schizophrenia, mania, depression and surgical conditions. *The British Journal of Psychiatry, 137*, 497–504.

Tsuang, M. T., Stone, W. S., & Faraone, S. V. (2000). Toward reformulating the diagnosis of schizophrenia. *The American Journal of Psychiatry, 157*, 1041–1050.

Tyler, P., & Kendell, T. (2009). The spurious advance of antipsychotic drug therapy. *The Lancet, 373*, 1007.

U.S. Preventive Services Task Force. (2002). Recommendations and rationale screening for depression. *Annals of Internal Medicine, 136*, 760–764.

Ujike, H., Yamamoto, A., Tanaka, Y., Takehisa, Y., Takaki, M., Taked, T., Kodama, M., Kuroda, S. (2001). Association study of CAG repeats in the KCNN3 gene in Japanese patients with schizophrenia, schizoaffective disorder and bipolar disorder. *Psychiatry Research, 101*, 203–207.

Unknown author. (1996, February 4). A life in pieces; for du Pont heir, question was control. *The New York Times*.

Unknown author. (1996, September 22). Psychiatrists in du Pont murder case say defendant is psychotic. *The New York Times*.

Unknown author. (1997, January 28). Du Pont was insane or scheming, lawyers say. *The New York Times*.

Unknown author. (1999, October 24). Police sued in killing of mentally ill man who stabbed officer. *The New York Times*.

Unknown author. (2001, March 7). National news briefs; forced treatment backed. *The New York Times*.

Unknown author. (2001, September 15). National briefing/Rockies: Utah: More damages in gun suit. *The New York Times*.
Unknown author. (2004, March 31). *Doctor says mom who killed sons mentally ill*. Associated Press. Msnbc.com.
Unknown author. (2004, August 5). World briefing: Asia: China: School guard attacks children with knife. *The New York Times*.
Unknown author. (2004, November 23). Texan faces murder charges for cutting off baby's arm. *USA Today*.
Unknown author. (2004, November 23). *Mother confesses to severing baby's arms*. Msnbc.com.
Unknown author. (2008, December 1). *Ex-Badger Taylor charged with threatening AD, tennis star*. Associated Press, ESPN.com: College Football.
Unknown author. (2009, February 11). *Mom "euphoric" before baby died*. CBSNews.com.
Unknown author. (2009, February 11). *Andrea Yates: Where are my kids?* CBSNews.com.
Unknown author. (2009, May 1). Debra Lynn Gindorf: Quinn commutes sentence of postpartum woman who killed kids. *Huffpost Chicago*.
Unknown author. (2009, November 12). Mother competent to stand trial for allegedly decapitating baby. *Fox News*.
Urbaszewske, K. (2011, March 6). Update: Three people identified in New Orleans murder-suicide. *The Times-Picayune*.
Valles, V., van Os, J., Guillamat, R., Gutierrez, B., Campillo, M., Gento, P., & Fananas, L. (2000). Increased morbid risk for schizophrenia in families of in-patients with bipolar illness. *Schizophrenia Research, 42*, 83–90.
van Os, J., Jones, P., Lewis, G., Wadsworth, M., & Murray, R. (1997). Developmental precursors of affective illness in general population birth cohort. *Archives of General Psychiatry, 54*, 625–631.
van Os, J., Jones, P., Sham, P., Bebbington, P., & Murray, R. M. (1998). Risk factors for onset and persistence of psychosis. *Social Psychiatry and Psychiatric Epidemiology, 33*, 596–605.
van Os, J., Hanssen, M., Bijl, R. V., & Ravelli, A. (2000). Strauss (1969) revisited: A psychosis continuum in the general population? *Schizophrenia Research, 45*, 11–20.
van't Veer-Tazelaar, P. J., van Marwijk, H. W. J., van Oppen, P., van Hout, H. P. J., van der Horst, H. E., Cuijpers, P., Smit, F., & Beekman, A. T. F. (2009). Stepped-care prevention of anxiety and depression in late life. *Archives of General Psychiatry, 66*(3), 297–304.
Vedantam, S. (2002). Routine screening for depression urged. *The Washington Post, 167*, 1–2.
Velakoulis, D., Pantelis, C., McGorry, P. D., Dudgeon, P., Brewer, W., Cook, M., Desmond, P., Bridle, N., Tierney, P., Murrie, V., Singh, B., Copolov, D. (1999). Hippocampal volume in first-episode psychoses and chronic schizophrenia. *Archives of General Psychiatry, 56*, 133–140.
Vendel, C., & Williams, M. R. (2010, September 16). Sources: Nixon was target. *The Kansas City Star*.
Verdoux, H., & van Os, J. (2002). Psychotic symptoms in non-clinical populations and the continuum of psychosis. *Schizophrenia Research, 54*, 59–65.
Viguera, A. C., Baldessarini, R. J., Hegarty, J. D., van Kammen, D. P., & Tohen, M. (1997). Clinical risk following abrupt and gradual withdrawal of maintenance neuroleptic treatment. *Archives of General Psychiatry, 54*, 49–55.
Vliegen, J. (1980). *Die Einheitspsychose. Geschichte und Problem*. Stuttgart: Enke.
Vollmer-Larsen, A., Jacobsen, T. B., Hemmingsen, R., & Parnas, J. (2006). Schizoaffective disorder – The reliability of its clinical diagnostic use. *Acta Psychiatrica Scandinavica, 113*, 402–407.
Vythilingam, M., Chen, J., Bremmer, J. D., et al. (2003). Psychotic depression and mortality. *The American Journal of Psychiatry, 160*, 574–576.
Wagemaker, H., Lippmann, S., & Cade, J. R. (1985). Acutely psychotic patients: A treatment approach. *Southern Medical Journal, 78*, 833–837.
Walsh, D. (2002, March 15). *The murder conviction of Andrea Yates: A tragic case, a barbaric verdict*. World Socialist Web Site.
Ward, B. (2009, October 27). *Dr. Astrid Desrosiers talking to investigators at MGH*. Boston.com/news.

Wehr, T. A., & Goodwin, F. K. (1987). Can antidepressants cause mania and worsen the course of affective illness? *The American Journal of Psychiatry, 144*, 1403–1411.

Weinberger, D. R., Bigelow, L., Klein, S. T., & Wyatt, R. J. (1981). Drug withdrawal in chronic schizophrenia patients: In search of neuroleptic induced supersensitivity psychosis. *Journal of Clinical Psychopharmacology, 1*, 120–123.

Weiser, M., Reichenberg, A., Rabinowitz, J., et al. (2001). Association between nonpsychotic psychiatric diagnoses in adolescent males and subsequent onset of schizophrenia. *Archives of General Psychiatry, 58*, 959–964.

Weiser, M., van Os, J., & Davidson, M. (2005). Time for a shift in focus in schizophrenia: From arrow phenotypes to broad endophenotypes. *The British Journal of Psychiatry, 187*, 203–205.

Wells, K. B., Schoenbaum, M., Unutzer, J., Lagomasino, I. T., & Rubenstein, L. V. (1999). Quality of care for primary care patients with depression in managed care. *Archives of Family Medicine, 8*, 529–536.

Welner, A., Croughan, J., Fishman, R., & Robins, E. (1977a). The group of schizoaffective and related psychoses: A follow-up study. *Comprehensive Psychiatry, 18*, 413–422.

Welner, A., Welner, Z., & Leonard, M. A. (1977b). Bipolar manic-depressive disorder: A reassessment of course and outcome. *Comprehensive Psychiatry, 18*, 327–332.

Welner, A., Welner, Z., & Fishman, R. (1979). The group of schizoaffective and related psychoses: IV. A family study. *Comprehensive Psychiatry, 20*, 21–26.

Whitaker, R. (2004). The case against antipsychotic drugs: A 50-year record of doing more harm than good. *Medical Hypotheses, 62*, 5–13.

Wikipedia. (2011). *On-line encyclopedia*. Wikipedia.org.

Williams, N. M., Green, E. K., Macgregor, S., Dwyer, S., Norton, N., Williams, H., Raybould, R., Grozeva, D., Hamshere, M., Zammit, S., Jones, L., Cardno, A., Kirov, G., Jones, I., O'Donovan, M. C., Owen, M. J., & Craddock, N. (2006). Variation at the DAOA/F30 locus influences susceptibility to major mood episodes but not psychosis in schizophrenia and bipolar disorder. *Archives of General Psychiatry, 63*, 366–373.

Winokur, G. (1973). The types of affective disorders. *Journal of Nervous and Mental Disorders, 156*, 82–96.

Winokur, G. W., Clayton, P. J., & Reich, T. (1969). *Manic-depressive illness*. St. Louis: CV Mosby Co Publishers.

Woo, T. U., Walsh, J. P., Benes, F. M. (2004). Density of glutamic acid decarboxylase 67 messenger RNA-containing neurons that express the N-methyl-D-aspartate receptor subunit NR2A in the anterior cingulate cortex in schizophrenia and bipolar disorder. *Archives of General Psychiatry, 61*, 649–657.

Wu, E. Q., Birnbaum, H. G., Shi, L., Ball, D. E., Kessler, R. C., Moulis, M., & Aggarwal, J. (2005). The economic burden of schizophrenia in the United States in 2002. *The Journal of Clinical Psychiatry, 66*, 1122–1129.

Yatham, L. N. (2003). Efficacy of atypical antipsychotics in mood disorders. *Journal of Clinical Psychopharmacology, 23*, S9–S14.

Zarate, C. A., Jr., & Tohen, M. (2004). Double-blind comparison of the continued use of antipsychotic treatment versus its discontinuation in remitted manic patients. *The American Journal of Psychiatry, 161*, 169–171.

Zeller, E. (1837). Bericht uber die wirksamkeit der heilanstalt winnenthal von ihrer eroffnung den 1. Marz 1834 bis zum 28. February 1937. *Beil Med Corresp-Bl Wurtemb Arztl Ver, 7*, 321–335.

Zubieta, J. K., Huguelet, P., O'Neil, R. L., & Giordani, B. J. (2001). Cognitive function in euthymic bipolar I disorder. *Psychiatry Research, 102*, 9–20.

Zung, W., & King, R. E. (1983). Identification and treatment of masked depression in a general medical practice. *The Journal of Clinical Psychiatry, 44*, 365–368.

Zung, W. K., Magill, M., Moore, J. T., & George, D. T. (1983). Recognition and treatment of depression in a family medicine practice. *The Journal of Clinical Psychiatry, 44*, 3–6.

Index

A

Academic psychiatry, schizophrenia
    Bleuler's concept, 353
    hallucinations and delusions, 356–358
    Kraepelinian dichotomy, 353, 356
Acute dystonic reaction, 307
Addison's disease, 285
Akathisia, 304–306
Alogia, 18, 28, 224, 228
    psychotic depression, 228
    schizophrenia, 243, 264
Ambivalence, 95, 106, 121, 139
Amotivation, 299, 308, 377
Anabolic steroids, 289
Anticholinergics, 307, 338
Antipsychotic drugs, 153–155, 290–291, 297–298, 301–308
Antischizophrenia drugs
    acute dystonic reaction, 306
    adverse effects, 303–304
    akathisia, 306
    antihistamine drugs, 154
    atypical antipsychotics, 155, 308
    atypicals, 307–308
    basal ganglia enlargement, 302
    chlorpromazine, 153–155
    mania, 303
    movement disorders, 305, 306
    negative symptoms and drowsiness, 303
    Parkinsons movements, 307
    relapse rates, 302–303
    severity and frequency, 307
    tardive dyskinesia, 306
    tardive psychosis, 306
    typical *vs.* atypical, 302
Apathy, 74
Aripiprazole, 383
Asociality, 265
Atypical antipsychotics, 155, 308
Autistic thinking, 94, 95, 106
Autoimmune disorders, 282
AY070435 (Slynar), 59

B

Basal ganglia enlargement, 302
Bath salts, 289
Benzodiazepines, 383
Bipolar disorder. *See also* Mania
    definition, 24, 26–27
    diagnostic comparisons, USA *vs.* UK, 157–158
    diagnostic events and impacts, 151, 152
    diagnostic symptoms
        course and outcomes, 56, 57
        diagnostic interview, 57
        DSM diagnostic criteria, 57
        mania mean cycle length and episode number, 56, 57
        severity, 56
    diagnostic validity, 58
    DSM-I, 161
    DSM-II mental illness, 164
    DSM-IV-TR diagnostic criteria, 25
    epidemiology, 58
    genetic loci, 59
    historical perspectives, 33–37
    interrater reliabilities, 58
    lithium, 157
    mono-dizygotic twins, 58
    pharmacological consistencies, 58
    vs. schizophrenia, 378

Bipolar disorder. *See also* Mania (*cont.*)
  symptoms and course
    acute schizophrenia, 176
    affective disorder, 179
    atypical schizophrenia, 178
    classical and atypical symptoms, 176–177
    Kraepelinian dichotomy, 168
    mixed symptomatology, 175
    paranoid schizophrenia, 176
    prognosis, 175
    Schneider's first-rank symptoms, 176–177
  treatment plans
    antischizophrenia drugs, 386
    ECT, 386
    medications, 384–386
    mood-stabilizing drugs, 386
Bleuler's concept
  accessory symptoms
    catatonic conditions, 113–114
    confusional incoherence, 114
    delusions, 110–111
    depression, 112–113
    disease course, 117–118
    functional psychoses, 119
    hallucinations, 110
    manic and depressive symptoms, 119
    manic conditions, 113
    organic disease, 118
    paranoia, 114–115
    schizophrenia simplex, 115–116
    speech and writing, 111–112
  affectivity, 105
  ambivalence, 106
  autism, 106
  biography, 93–94
  disease definition, 102
  fundamental symptoms, 95, 100–101, 103
  grandiosity, 104
  hebephrenic/disorganized schizophrenia, 105–106
  manic distractibility, 103, 105
  pressure of thoughts, 112
  schizophrenias, 107–109
  schizophrenic association disturbance, 104
  schizophrenic behavior, 106
Brain's filter-prioritizer mechanism
  attention, 272
  CNS data processing, 273
  euthymia, 273
  mania, 274–276
  stimuli, 273

C
Carbamazepine, 384
Catatonic schizophrenia
  catatonic psychotic depression, 246
  delusional paranoia, 248
  DSM-IV-TR, 245–246
  DSM-5, 245
  guilt and grandiosity, 249
  validity, 247
Catechol-*O*-methyltransferase (COMT), 59
Chlorpromazine, 153–155
Chlorprothixene, 302
Chromosomal abnormalities, 282–284
Chronic traumatic head injury, 284
Clozapine, 302, 307
Corticosteroids, 282, 289

D
Delirium, 285
Delusional disorders, 24
Dementia
  APA's Psychiatric Glossary, 22
  definition, 21–22
  dementia praecox, 48–49
  organic psychoses, 48
  secondary/organic conditions, 48
  syphilis and *Treponema pallida*, 49
Dementia praecox. *See also* Kraepelinian dichotomy; Schizophrenia
  hebephrenia, 50
  melancholia, 52
  symptoms, 50
  tension insanity, 50
  waxy flexibility, 50
Dementias, 285
Demyelinating disease, 285
Disorganized schizophrenia, 248, 278–279

E
Electroconvulsive therapy (ECT), 155–156, 166
Electrolyte and fluid imbalance, 285
Endocrinopathies, 285
Epilepsy, 286
Euthymia, 273

F
Filicide, 337–348
First-line mood-stabilizing medications, 299–301
Fluphenazine, 302
Frontal lobe tumors, 288

Index

Functional psychosis
   DSM-5 and DSM-6
      catatonia, 395
      DSM specifiers, 395
      mood incongruent *vs.* congruent psychoses, 394
   hypothesized history, diagnoses, 50

G
Genetic linkage studies, 211

H
Haloperidol, 293, 302, 338
Heritability and family studies, 209–210
   genetic correlations, 208
   paranoid delusion, 208
   schizophrenia "breeds" psychotic bipolar, 211, 212
Huntington's disease, 284
Hydrocephalus, 286
Hypomania, 58

K
Kasanin's concept, 135
   biography, 123–124
   psychotic mood symptoms, 126–127
   schizoaffective disorder
      Bleuler's concept, 124–125
      diagnosis, 132
      diagnostic criteria, 132–135
      diagnostic validity, 130–131
      DSM-IV-TR diagnostic criteria for, 125
      Kraepelin's dichotomy, 124–125
      psychiatric nomenclature, 129
      PubMed literature cites of, 128–129
      schizophrenia with mood disorder, 125–126
      subtypes, 127
Kraepelinian dichotomy, 1–2, 353, 356
   biography, 63–64
   bipolar disease
      causes, 90
      prognosis, 89
   cyclothymia, 89
   dementia praecox
      ataxia of feelings, 75
      automatic obedience, 74
      bilateral castration, immunization, 84
      bodily symptoms, 75–76
      catatonia, 79–80
      catatonic excitement, 74
      circular dementia praecox, 78
      clinical forms, 76
      course and remissions, 81
      delusions, 80–81
      delusions of sin, 73
      derailments in linguistic expression, 75
      differential diagnosis, 82–83
      disturbance of sleep and appetite, 76
      emotion, 74
      exalted ideas, 73
      frequency and causes, 82
      hallucinations and delusions, 77–78
      hebephrenia, 76–77
      incoherence, 74–75
      influence on thought, 72
      issue-terminal states, 81–82
      judgment, 73
      long-term course, 83–84
      manic distractibility, 75
      manic symptoms and behavior, 74
      negativism, 74
      neologisms, 75
      paranoid dementias, 80
      paranoid schizophrenia, 85
      paraphrenia, 84–85
      periodic dementia, 79
      progressive dementia, 78
      vs. psychotic mood disorders, 71–72
      sexual ideas, 74
      sexual sensations, 72
      silly dementia, 82
      sympathetic tone, 76
      terminal dementia, 82
      train of thought and associations, 72
      volition, 74
      weakness of judgment, 82
   manic-depressive insanity, 91
      clang associations, 87
      diagnosis, 66–69
      hallucinations and delusions, 88
      inhibition of thought, 86
      insight, 88–89
      manic syndrome, 86
      periodic and circular insanity, 85–86
      pressure of activity and speech, 87
      psychotic decline, 89
      psychotic symptoms, 86
   publications of, 64
   reversal of, 90

L
Lamotragine, 301
Lexapro, 381
Lithium, 58, 380
Loxapine, 302
Lurasidone, 155
Luvox, 381

M
Major depressive disorder
  vs. bipolar disorder, 378
  chronological history
    Aretaeus of Cappadocia's view, 38
    depression, 38
    Goodwin and Jamison's view, 38
    melancholia, 38
    paranoid psychosis with mania, 38–41
    severity and chronicity identification, 41
    signs and symptom duration, 41
  definition, 24, 26
  DSM-IV-TR diagnostic criteria, 25
  misdiagnosis, negative impact, 348–351
  symptoms, 377
  treatment plans
    antidepressants, 380–381
    antischizophrenia drugs, 383–384
    aripiprazole, 383
    benzodiazepines, 383
    ECT, 381
    lithium, 380
    unipolar depression, 382
Mania
  clinical characteristics, 372–373
  disordered thought and speech, 271–272
  distractibility
    brain's filter/prioritizer, 275
    CNS data processing, 277
    mild mania, 274
    selective attention function, 274
  DSM-IV-TR, diagnostic criteria, 376–378
  schizophrenia, 275–279
Manic-depressive insanity, 91
  clang associations, 87
  diagnosis, 66–69
  hallucinations and delusions, 88
  inhibition of thought, 86
  insight, 88–89
  manic syndrome, 86
  periodic and circular insanity, 85–86
  pressure of activity and speech, 87
  psychotic decline, 89
  psychotic symptoms, 86

Mesoridazine, 302
Metabolic diseases, 287
Molecular genetic studies
  genetic linkage studies, 211
  genetic overlap, 211, 213
  genetic translocation, 213
  susceptibility genetic loci, 213
Mood disorder. *See also* Bipolar disorder
  daily mood and energy level, 374–377
  DSM-I, 161
  DSM-IV-TR specifiers for, 25
  sleep flow sheet, 374–377
  treatment plans
    bipolar disorder, 384–386
    major depressive disorder, 380–384
    mood-stabilizing drugs, 379
  types, 25
Movement disorders, 305, 306
Multiple sclerosis, 285

N
Narcolepsy, 287
Neuropsychiatric disorder, 287
Neurotransmitters, 205
Nonpsychiatric setting
  depression and suicidal risk
    Epidemiologic Catchment Area study, 389
    mania and hypomania, 392
    morbidity and mortality, 391–392
    prevalence, 390
    primary care physician, 392
  mood disorders, Academic Psychiatry, 392–393
Nutritional deficiencies, 288

O
Obsessive-compulsive disorder (OCD), 292–294

P
Pancreatic carcinoma, 288
Paranoid schizophrenia, 268
  delusional threat, 261
  mania, 249
  molecular genetic studies, 249, 250
  symptoms, 260
  take-home messages, 262
Parietal lobe tumors, 288
Parkinsons disease, 287, 305
Paxil, 381

Perphenazine, 302
Phosphofructokinase (PFK), 59
Pimozide, 302
Pristiq, 381
Prozac, 294, 381
Psychiatric disease
  diagnosis, 55–61
  diagnostic criteria, 56
  judicial sources, 395
  mood disorder (*see* Mood disorder)
  schizophrenia (*see* Schizophrenia)
Psychopharmacological studies, 206–207
  atypicals, 205
  lithium *vs.* typical antipsychotics, 204–205
  neurotransmitters, 205
  typical neuroleptics, 205
Psychosis
  Bleuler's concept, 53
  clinical characteristics, 22
  definition, 22
  diagnosis, 295–296
  functional psychosis, 23–24
  Kraepelinian dichotomy, 53
  medical and surgical causes
    autoimmune disorders, 282
    chromosomal abnormalities, 282–284
    chronic traumatic head injury, 284
    CNS HIV infection, 286
    dementias and delirium, 285
    demyelinating disease, 285
    electrolyte and fluid imbalance, 285
    endocrinopathies, 285
    epilepsy, 286
    hydrocephalus, 286
    metabolic diseases, 287
    narcolepsy, 287
    neuropsychiatric disorder, 287
    nutritional deficiencies, 288
    space-occupying lesions and structural brain abnormalities, 288
    stroke, 288
  Schneiders concept, 53
  secondary/organic causes, 23–24
  substances induced psychosis, 289–290
  tardive psychosis misdiagnosis, 290–291
Psychotherapy, 386
Psychotic depression
  misconception, 229
  negative symptoms, 229
  paranoid depression, 228
  postschizophrenic depression, 229
  prevalence, 228
  Swartz and Shorter's concept, 230

Psychotic mood disorders, 279. *See also* Mood disorder
  brain's filter-prioritizer mechanism
    attention, 272
    CNS data processing, 273
    euthymia, 273
    mania, 274–275, 277
    stimuli, 273–274
  depression, 273
  euthymia, 273
  mania, 277
  misdiagnosed as schizophrenia
    case study, 251–253
    paranoid type, 250, 254–260
  paranoid schizophrenia
    delusional threat, 261
    symptoms, 260
    take-home messages, 262
  Schneider's concept (*see* Schneider's concept)
  violence, suicide, and homicide risk
    bipolar disorder, 346
    euthymic episodes, 311
    filicide risk, 337–349
    ill murderers, 311
    killers' behaviors and symptoms, 335
    paranoid and grandiose delusions, 335
    paranoid schizophrenia, 337
    postpartum depression, 337
    psychotic murderers and their victims, 310–312
Psychotic symptoms
  psychiatrist's diagnostic plan, 378–379

Q
Quetiapine, 302, 307

R
Risperidone, 302
Ritalin, 58

S
Sarafem, 381
Schizoaffective disorder, 135
  Bleuler's concept, 124–125
  diagnosis, 132
  diagnostic criteria, 132–135
  diagnostic validity, 130–131
  DSM-IV-TR diagnostic criteria for, 125
  Kraepelin's dichotomy, 124–125
  psychiatric nomenclature, 129

Schizoaffective disorder (cont.)
  PubMed literature cites of, 128–129
  schizophrenia with mood disorder, 125–126
  subtypes, 127
Schizophrenia. *See also* Dementia praecox; Schizoaffective disorder
  academic psychiatry
    Bleuler's concept, 353
      hallucinations and delusions, 356
      Kraepelinian dichotomy, 353, 356
  antischizophrenia drugs, 365–367
  antischizophrenia medications
    antihistamine drugs, 154
    vs. atypical antipsychotics, 155
    chlorpromazine, 153–155
  Bleuler's accessory symptoms
    catatonic conditions, 113–114
    confusional incoherence, 114
    delusions, 110–120
    depression, 112–113
    disease course, 117–118
    functional psychoses, 119
    hallucinations, 110
    manic and depressive symptoms, 119
    manic conditions, 113
    organic disease, 118
    paranoia, 114–115
    schizophrenia simplex, 115–116
    speech and writing, 111–112
  Bleuler's fundamental symptoms of, 95–101
  bona fide disorder, 356
  chronicity and psychosis, 353, 354
  dementia praecox diagnoses, 353
  diagnosis, 60–61, 354
    diagnostic symptoms, 56–57
    epidemiological findings, 58
    mood symptoms, 56
    psychosis and chronicity, 55–56
  diagnostic comparisons, USA *vs.* UK, 157–158
  diagnostic events and impacts, 151
  dialectical behavior therapy, 359
  disordered thought and speech, 271–272
  DSM and ICD, 365
  DSM-I, 166
    development, 160
    manic depressive reaction, 161
    psychotic reactions, 161–162
    schizoaffective type, 161
    schizophrenic reactions, 161–163
  DSM-II
    APA, 164
    neuroses and psychoses, 164, 165
    simple type schizophrenia, 164
  DSM-IV-TR diagnostic criteria, 25
  DSM-IV-TR subtypes of, 51
  electroconvulsive therapy, 155–156, 166
  feedback loop enhancement, 355
  first-rank symptoms (*see* Schneider's concept)
  functional psychotic symptoms, 120
  Kasanin's concept (*see* Kasanin's concept)
  Kraepelinian dichotomy (*see also* Kraepelinian dichotomy)
    controversy, 30–31
    dementia praecox, 26
  mania, 275–279
  manic-depressive insanity, 353
  media emphasis, 361–363
  neuroses, 364–365
  NIMH and pharmaceutical industry, 156
  prolonged factors, 354
  psychotic depression
    misconception, 229
    negative symptoms, 229
    paranoid depression, 228
    postschizophrenic depression, 229
    prevalence, 228
    Swartz and Shorter's concept, 230
  PubMed literature cites of, 152, 153
  Schneider's concept, 166 (*see also* Schneider's concept)
  second-rank symptom, 148–149
  society's expectations, 308
  symptoms, 312–334
Schizophrenia *vs.* mood disorder, 3–11
  1990 and 2000, 189–196
  Bentall's argument, 181
  brain imaging studies, 200, 201
  brain metabolic and neurochemical studies, 198–199
  Brockington's idea, 180
  catatonic subtype
    catatonic psychotic depression, 246
    delusional paranoia, 248
    DSM-IV-TR, 242
    DSM-5, 245
    guilt and grandiosity, 249
    validity, 247
  cognitive function, selective attention, and insight studies, 220–223
  continuum concept, 181, 231–234
  disorganized subtype, 248

Index

DSM-III (1980), 182–183
DSM-III-R (1987), 184
DSM-IV (1994), 224–226
DSM-IV-TR, 225
DSM-IV-TR (2000), 225–226
DSM-5 (2013), 227–228
epidemiological studies, 202–204
    "breed true" results, 212
    cross-cultural comparison, 202–203
    single disease, 205
heritability and family studies, 208–211
    genetic correlations, 219
    paranoid delusion, 208
    schizophrenia "breeds" psychotic bipolar, 236–237
molecular genetic studies, 211–219
    genetic linkage studies, 211
    genetic overlap, 211
    genetic translocation, 213
    susceptibility genetic loci, 211–212
negative symptoms, 244, 264–266
NIMH, 180–181
paranoid subtype, 268
    mania, 249
    molecular genetic studies, 249, 250
Pope's concept, 179
positive symptoms, 244, 263, 269
psychopharmacological studies, 204–207
    atypicals, 205
    lithium vs. typical antipsychotics, 204–205
    neurotransmitters, 205
    typical neuroleptics, 205
subtypes, 241–245, 267
symptoms and course, 169–178
Szaszian idea, 179
thought pathology, 180
undifferentiated subtype, 262
Schizophrenic thought blocking, 276
Schneider's concept, 149
    biography, 137–138
    cyclothymia, 139–143
    dichotomy, 139
    first-rank symptoms
        auditory hallucinations, 143–144
        delusional perception and notion, 146
        disturbance of perception, 143
        disturbances of identity, 148
        disturbances of thinking, 145
        electrical influences, 144
        flight of ideas, 145
        lack of feelings, 147
        manic grandiosity, 147
        misidentification of delusion, 147
        mood disturbances, 147
        obsessive-compulsive disorder, 145–146
        pseudomanic schizophrenia, 145
        psychotic mania, 144
        somatic hallucinations, 144
        thought broadcasting, 145
    functional vs. organic psychoses, 139
    schizophrenia vs. mood disorders, 142
    second-rank symptom, 148–149
Selective serotonin reuptake inhibitor (SSRI), 380–381
Serotonin norepinephrine reuptake inhibitor (SNRI), 380–381
Spinocerebellar ataxia 2, 287
Stimulant drugs, 58
Stroke, 288
Supersensitivity psychosis, 282, 296

T

Tardive dyskinesia, 303, 306
Tardive psychosis, 290–291
Temporal lobe epilepsy, 286
Temporal lobe tumors, 288
Typical neuroleptics, 205

U

Undifferentiated schizophrenia, 262
Unipolar depression, treatment plans, 382
Unitary psychosis
    Cullen's concept, 45
    degeneration theory, 47
    dimensional concept, 42
    Griesinger's view, 46
    Guislain's unitarian causal theory, 46
    historical perspectives, 43–44
    Kraepelinian dichotomy, 41–42, 48
    Neumann's view, 46
    secondary/organic causes, 45
    Swartz and Shorter's concept, 45, 48

V

Valproic acid, 384
Velo-cardiofacial syndrome (VCFS), 59

Z

Ziprasidone, 302
Zoloft, 381